Handbook of Perfumes and Flavors

By

Dr. Olindo Secondini

Chemical Publishing Co., Inc.
New York, NY

ISBN 0-8206-0334-1

Printed in the United States of America

To my wife, Ann Katya

The Author

Dr. Olindo Secondini has worked in the fields of Essential Oils, Flavors, Perfumes, Cosmetics, Toiletries, and Aromatic Chemicals in the United States, Europe, Latin America, Africa, and the Middle East. He has also taught Chemistry and Chemical Engineering at several universities.

Dr. Secondini has published in various languages, particularly in Spanish with the leading newspaper "El Imparcial" of Guatemala, Central America, where he worked on research and development of natural resources.

He is a Fellow of the American Institute of Chemists.

First Foreword

By Paul B. Slawter, Jr. FAIC
Former Executive Secretary, The American Institute of Chemists
Former Editor, The Chemist

Some years ago, Dr. Olindo Secondini brought me a manuscript to consider for a publication of which I was an editor, "The Chemist," official organ of The American Institute of Chemists. Dr. Secondini was an experienced chemist in the field of essential oils, flavors, perfumes, cosmetics, toiletries, and aromatic chemicals.

I was fascinated by his story and published it in the next issue. It had a somewhat whimsical title, "Is our Sense of Scent Lost?"

The article must have made a lot of sense because we had more editorial reaction to it than to any article I had published in 60 issues over a five-year span. Dr. David W. Young, a noted American scientist, then President of the AIC, said it was the best he had ever read on this interesting subject. Several essential oil companies ordered extra copies for distribution.

Recently, Dr. Secondini brought me another manuscript, this time a formidable tome on flavors and perfumes. I must say: *This is the best* I have ever read on these interesting subjects. Dr. Secondini is to be congratulated by the likes of me and thanked by the likes of people in the business of essential oils and related materials for providing what has to be the last word on the compounding of flavors and perfumes. His entire book should be subtitled "The Gamut of Flavors and Perfumes from A to Z."

As one peruses this volume, from the history of perfumes and cosmetics to the constituents of the essential oils so important to the industry, one gets the feeling that everything, which means anything to a flavorist or a perfumer, is here for the reading.

Today, there is increased interest and awareness on the part of the general public in flavors and perfumes, which, like food and clothing, are growth industries with unlimited futures. Dr. Secondini shows how the level of production is now sufficiently large to make flavors and perfumes a most important factor in American economy and resource planning.

Its 474 pages make the publication more than a handbook for practical formulation of flavors and perfumes. It is truly a workbook of inestimable value for an industry with no place to go but upward.

Second Foreword

By Donald A. Davis
Editor, Drug & Cosmetic Industry (magazine)

There haven't been nearly enough additions to the sparse body of technical books about perfuming and flavor materials over the past two decades, though the technological advances in this area have been remarkable. In fact, it was almost as though the late Steffen Arctander had a monopoly on the subject during his long and productive lifetime. That said, it is good to have this contribution from Dr. Olindo Secondini, who has had a varied career in academia, in industry, and even in medicine.

This is far more than a simple handbook for perfumer or chemist or research worker in the field. Besides giving a comprehensive outline of each essential oil, aromatic, flavor, and fixative, it breaks down the physical and chemical character of natural materials. What is more, it provides valuable clues for the compounding or manufacture of a wide range of synthetic versions of those increasingly scarce, sometimes unbelievably expensive derivatives from rare animals or plants that grow only in remote jungles or savannahs. There is little chaff here, Dr. Secondini staying throughout with what he originally set out to do. The prediction from this quarter is that this will become a standard reference work, and remain one for years until someone equally ambitious undertakes to do another 30 or 40 years hence. One interesting addition not usually seen in such a book is a small section suggesting new kinds of perfumes, some oriented toward fragrances far different than are encountered in any now on the market. Such targets of opportunity seem worthy of attention by some innovative compounder—and reflect well on the author's imagination.

Third Foreword

By David W. Young, Sc.D., P.E.
Vice President, Young & Kather Associates, Inc.
Member of Board of Directors, ACC&CE

This book is based on a fresh approach to the analysis and interpretation of odor evaluation tests. Utilizing his years of experience, observation, and personal judgment, the author presents new insights and attitudes regarding the nature and method of odor evaluation testing. Dr. Secondini published a similar article in "The Chemist," the official publication of the AIC.

This book is strictly practical while at the same time provides indispensable technical and scientific details. The book presents important information for all. The chemist will require this work as well as the student of chemistry. It is a fresh theme in the area of industrial chemistry.

I strongly recommend this book to anyone involved in the application of odors for commercial use.

Fourth Foreword

By Annette Green, Executive Director, The Fragrance Foundation

In the last twenty-five years, the universe of olfaction has expanded beyond anyone's imagination and the pleasures of fragrance, in particular, have captured the minds and hearts of people in every culture, every environment, every social level.

As we enter an even more highly developed technological decade, it becomes increasingly clear that many of the challenges we will all face will call on a completely new mindset in interpreting sensory needs and providing a vast range of experiences which will be resolved through sensory experiences.

It has never been more imperative to provide scientists, students, perfumers, and scholars with the most effective and authoritative tools. They must not only provide the broadest possible perspectives of the extremely complex field of fragrance creation (historically, culturally, scientifically), but also create an environment for higher consciousness and creativity.

I believe Dr. Secondini has accomplished this monumental feat in his extraordinary work which is represented in this volume. I salute him and thank him for his masterful contribution to the world of fragrance and the sensory lives of societies of the future.

Preface

In line with the human necessities, flavors and perfumes, like the food and clothing industries, are omnipresent and fast growing.

The correlated literature, however, although necessary for bringing up-to-date information for research and development, is comparatively slow and rather scarce. Even educational institutions are still not interested in giving courses in this important field of daily consumption comprehending biological, botanical, and chemical sciences.

This book provides a general orientation to the subject and information on the compounding of basic flavors for food and floral perfumes for personal use, for cosmetics, soaps, disinfectants, deodorants, and antipollutants. All are concisely described in the 995 formulas of perfumes and flavors and the related material reported in this book.

Regardless of scientific and technical education, or experience in this field, this book can contribute to the necessary knowledge for the compounding of any flavor or perfume. However, since the perception of taste and odor is intrinsically individual, a creative technique is indispensable for improving and expanding on this very fascinating industrial activity.

The author, who has many years of practical experience in this field, gratefully acknowledges and thanks the authors of the very valuable books listed in the bibliography, which have amply helped in the compilation of this book.

Olindo Secondini

Explanatory Notes

1. CLASSIFICATION OF FORMULAS

The formulas, as reported in this book, are classified in four categories:

1. ***Essences:*** Compounds made with natural products, such as Essential Oils, Balsams, Resinoids
2. ***Extracts:*** Made from barks, roots, leaves, seeds, buds, fruits, flowers, in their natural state.
3. ***Imitation:*** A mixture of essences, extracts, and esters in prevalence.
4. ***Synthetics:*** A duplication of the natural product, made generally with a combination of esters. Esters are fragrant compounds formed by the reaction between an acid and an alcohol. For example, ethyl acetate is made by heating acetic acid and ethyl alcohol in the presence of sulfuric acid and distilling. The synthetic formula, when there is more than one of the same species, has a progressive number.

2. COMPOSITION

All the formulas are of a general orientative nature. It remains exclusively to the compounder to improve each one, either reducing, increasing, or modifying the components in each formula, in accordance with his taste and olfactory stimulus. Good flavors, or perfumes, are not derived from the best formulas. The success, in compounding the ingredients (which must be excellent in taste and odor) depends on the sense of taste and scent of the compounder.

3. TURBIDITY

The ingredients must be blended thoroughly and totally clear in an absolute pure and odorless solvent such as ethyl alcohol 95% from grain, propylene glycol, neutral glycerin, distilled water, and other solvents. Many of the formulas will probably give turbidity in their compounding. This can be eliminated, or at least reduced, by increasing the amount of solvent, or by repeated filtration.

4. UNSPECIFIED UNITS FOR WEIGHTS, VOLUMES, OR PERCENTAGES

The unit measures in the manufacture of synthetic aromatic basic material, or formulas for flavors and perfumes, could either be in kilograms, if the material is solid, or liters, if the material is liquid.

The amount of *1000*, for instance, with unspecified unit, could be either 1000 kilograms or 1000 grams (1 kilogram); or 1000 liters or 1000 milliliters (1 liter).

As standard practice in the use of all components no units are specified. The same chosen unit must be applied to all items in the required material or formulas.

Example:

1.	Distilled Water	1000
2.	Ethyl Alcohol	1000
3.	Sugar	500

In this case, because the units are unspecified, all components are measured by weight, which will be either in kilograms or grams. The formula must therefore be understood as:

1.	Distilled Water	1000 grams
2.	Ethyl Alcohol	1000 grams
3.	Sugar	500 grams

The unspecified units facilitate any system of measure, particularly those of foreign countries. Therefore, the unspecified amount could be: kilograms, grams, liters, milliliters, ounces, etc.

In this book all unspecified amounts must be understood as *parts by weight.*

5. USES OF THE FORMULAS FOR ESSENCES

The amount of any formulas, to be basically employed in making essences, is in the proportion of 2 or 3 parts (2 or 3 grams × 1 kilogram (1000 grams) of solvent).

6. CONCRETE, ABSOLUTE, RESINOID

Concrete—a waxy solid obtained from roses by extraction without solvents, or after removing the solvent; the essential oil. Absolute—free from admixture with other substances, e.g., absolute alcohol which is dehydrated as ethyl alcohol 99% pure. Resinoid—any thermosetting synthetic natural, vegetable-derived resin. The best known are rosin and balsam from coniferous trees. Their use is in varnishes and adhesives.

7. TINCTURES

Tincture—an alcoholic or aqueous-alcoholic solution of vegetable material.

All tinctures are made by maceration, stirring every day for one hour, until total dissolution is obtained in flavor and odor (approximately one week) and filtering at the end until completely clear.

8. UNSPECIFIED NATURAL PRODUCTS (OIL OR CONCRETE)

When a natural product, such as carnation, gardenia, etc. is not specified, either as an oil or concrete, it refers to its imitation or synthetic formula reported in the book.

9. COLORS

In coloring flavors or perfumes, only certified colors or the natural, legally exempted from certification colors must be used. The color must be added before filtration, which is necessary even if the product appears clear.

10. TEMPERATURE

The temperature is in Centigrade (°C), with the exception of flash point TCC (Tagliabue Closed Cup) given in Fahrenheit (°F). Specific gravity is given at 25/25°C. Refractive index and optical rotation are at 20°C. Different temperatures are specified in parenthesis.

11. SOLUBILITY

Number refers to the amount of alcohol, or other solvent, needed to dissolve the material. Example 2/70% means two volumes of alcohol at 70%; 3/80% means three volumes of alcohol at 80%; 2–8/70% means that the volume of alcohol may be from two to eight volumes at 70%.

12. FORM OF THE MATERIAL

If it is not liquid, a specification is given either as a powder, crystals, etc.

13. HABITAT

When the habitat is not specified, worldwide existence is assumed.

14. SOLUTION

When not specified, the solvent for solutions is ethyl alcohol 95%.

15. NATURAL PRODUCTS

For natural products, when particular parts, e.g., oil, concrete, bark, flowers, leaves, resinoid, roots, tops are not specified, they must be used in their total natural state.

16. CAS NUMBERS

Whereever possible, the American Chemical Society's Chemical Abstract Service (CAS) registry numbers have been included to facilitate accurate identification of a given chemical substance.

17. ABBREVIATIONS

C .... degrees Centigrade
cc .... cubic centimeter
CC .... closed cup
cl .... centiliter
cml .... centimilliliter
EDTA .... ethylene diamine tetraacetate
F .... degrees Fahrenheit
FDA .... Food and Drug Administration
g .... gram
gal .... gallon
h .... hour
kg .... kilogram
l .... liter
max .... maximum
min .... minimum, minutes
ml .... milliliter
OC .... open cup
sol'n. .... solution
TCC .... Tagliabue Closed Cup
> .... greater than

NOTICE

Table of Contents

Chapter I:

ODORS

Introduction

"The Rose distills a healing balm
The beating pulse of pain to calm"
—Alexander Farkas

From early Spring to late Fall, scent is all around us, particularly in the Southern states, where plants are more extensively flowering and where Spring starts earlier and Fall lasts longer. The color of all these flowers, in their beautiful multivariety, is overwhelming. But very few people will probably pay any attention to their odors.

Paradoxically, even though odors—currently called perfumes—are extensively used by almost everyone, either applying them directly to the body, or indirectly through the use of soaps, creams, powders, detergents, etc., the human sense of smell has degenerated during the last centuries, and is in danger of being lost.

The impact of pollution has already had a deleterious effect, beginning during the Industrial Revolution when people started to desert farms and countryside in order to find work in the growing factories and continuing through this century with the evolution of mechanical transportation. Our cities are now filthy with smoke of factories and exhaust from cars. Parks and countrysides smell of pesticides and chemical fertilizers. Highways offend our sight and nose with the bodies of innocent animals killed by our crushing transportation.

The first men who populated our planet certainly had a better sense of smell, as wild animals still have. Early man had to use primarily smell and taste in order to investigate what kind of food he could use for his nourishment. Forced to select organic materials which could be poisonous, putrefied, and so forth, the nose was the master guide with the sense of taste as supervisor.

Until the beginning of this century, flowers and herbs were still collected for their scent and aroma, and preserved in order to be used during the nonflowering seasons. Cities had herbal shops for this purpose, and druggists and pharmacists stored them in their laboratories. Since the beginning of civilization men of science and lovers of nature have attempted to distinguish and classify odors. A fundamental classification of odors is reported throughout history.

EARLY HISTORY OF PERFUMES

Early in the history of humanity it appears that men burned various kinds of woods for warmth and light during the nights and cold winter seasons. Thus, they accidentally discovered the pleasant smell of the smoke that drifted through the air over the flames from some of the naturally perfumed woods. The French name "parfum" comes from the Latin preposition "per" meaning *through* and the substantive "fumus" meaning *smoke.*

Primitive men also accidentally discovered that putting resinous wood in water made it oily and odorous. Rubbing the body with the resinous material produced a feeling of pleasure by improving their body odor and protecting their skin. The development of perfumes, therefore, can be traced as far back as the beginning of the history of humanity.

Perfumes have been found in the Egyptian pharaohs' tombs. The Ebers' papyrus, which refers to the beginning of recorded history in the Nile Valley, contains formulas in which botanicals, minerals, and animal products were employed. They are still utilized today in the manufacture of perfumes.

Ancient Greeks and Romans learned from the Egyptians. For many centuries perfumes remained an exclusive oriental art. During the period of the Crusades in the early decades of the thirteenth century, perfumes were brought from Palestine to Europe. Trade in spices followed.

In the 1500's perfumes became popular through those made by a certain René, a perfumer from Florence, Italy. René travelled to France with Catherine de Medicis when she went to marry Prince Henry, who later became Henry II of France.

HISTORY OF THE WATER COLOGNE

The perfume which rapidly became the most popular was "Eau de Cologne." The name derives from the fact that the product was initially made in the city of Cologne (Köln), Germany, on the Rhine river, in the early 1700's.

It was first prepared in the town of Cologne by Jean Marie Farina. He was born in Italy in the town of Saint Marie Major, and went to Cologne to trade perfumes. He first prepared this very famous composition in 1709. It is known, however, that the "Eau de Cologne" was first marketed by Paul de Feminis in Milan, Italy, and it was afterwards made in Cologne from 1690. The formula was then passed to his nephew Jan Antoine Farine, who started manufacturing it in Paris in 1806.

The popularity of "Eau de Cologne" since the early 18th century is due to its fresh and clean smell. Many manufacturers in Cologne and elsewhere have continued its trade worldwide. It has perpetuated as a standard type of a lightly refreshing scent. It is a water-alcohol solution of a concentrated citrus essence prevalently extracted from lemon, bergamot, orange flowers, and blended with some lavender and orris roots, with traces of benzoin as a fixative. The finest "Eau de Cologne" is produced by distilling pure ethyl alcohol with the previously mentioned ingredients. Some neroli is further added. The distillate is then left to mature for at least one year.

THE PERFUME INDUSTRY

Alexander Farkas, in the introduction to his book *Perfume Through the Ages,* says:

> "The perfume industry is perhaps the most romantic of all industries."

It is indeed true that the perfume industry, even from the chemical point of view, is the most fascinating.

The art of blending natural essences and synthetic odorants to obtain a stable, odoriferous alcohol solution embraces all kinds of organic chemicals, and more extensively than in any other branch of the chemical industry. The psychological influence of a perfume determines its appeal for the customer, and thus its success. Today, all kinds of papers are perfumed to improve their salability. Perfumed merchandise is preferred, and outsells its odorless counterpart by a large margin.

The products of the perfume industry are classified as:

1. Gaseous: Aerosols
2. Liquids: Lotions, Perfumes
3. Pastes: Creams, Toothpastes
4. Solids: Soaps, Powders

THE COSMETICS INDUSTRY

Cosmetics are preparations applied to the surface of the body for the purpose of enhancing its appearance. Cosmetic products aid the whole human body—face, hair, teeth, hands, feet—with the triple purpose of preserving, restoring, or simulating beauty. In a larger sense, cosmetics are products of perfumery. Perfumes of natural origin, such as essential oils, and of synthetic production are usually employed in cosmetics. Cosmetics are liquids, solids, creams, pastes, and powders.

Cosmetics can be generally classified as:

1. Cutaneous cosmetics: Lipsticks, creams, soaps, toilet water
2. Capillary cosmetics: Brilliantines, shampoos, depilatories
3. Dental cosmetics: Toothpastes, liquids, powders

In accordance with their specific properties and intended application, cosmetics may be classified in various categories:

1. Creams
2. Lotions
3. Eye makeup and other eye preparations
4. Lipsticks and other lip preparations
5. Nail preparations
6. Face and body makeup
7. Perfumes and scented preparations
8. Bath preparations
9. Skin cleanser and other skin preparations

10. Shampoo and hair rinses
11. Hair preparations
12. Depilatories
13. Shaving preparations
14. Deodorants and antiperspirants
15. Suntan preparations
16. Miscellaneous: rubbing alcohols, mouthwashes, toothpastes, tooth powders, denture cleaners, face and body powders.

Historical Classification of Odors

CLASSIFICATION OF ARISTOTLE (384–322 B.C.)

The Greek philosopher Aristotle, the greatest influential thinker of Western culture, was the first to classify odors.

He classified odors in six groups in accordance with the sensations:

1. Sweet odors
2. Acid odors
3. Severe odors
4. Fatty odors
5. Sour odors
6. Fetid odors

CLASSIFICATION OF LINNAEOUS (1707–1778)

Linnaeous, the celebrated Swedish botanist, based his odor classification on seven groups:

1. Aromatic odors: Clove, laurel
2. Fragrant odors: Jasmine, lily
3. Ambrosiac odors: Moss, amber
4. Alliaceous odors: Garlic, asafoetida
5. Fetid odors: Valerian
6. Repulsive odors: Solanaceous
67. Distusting odors: Hellebore

Many others have attempted to classify odors, but very few have achieved a passable classification.

CLASSIFICATION OF FOURCROY (1755–1809)

Antoine Francois Fourcroy, a French chemist and politician, founded the French Museum of Natural Sciences, and with Antoine Laurent Lavoisier and C.I. Bertholett, the

Annals of Chemistry in 1783.

Fourcroy divided the odors by:

1. Extractive odors
2. Volatile odors
3. Aromatic odors
4. Acidous odors
5. Hydrosulfurous odors

CLASSIFICATION OF PIESSE (1820–1882)

George William Septimus Piesse, a chemist-perfumer of London, attempted to match the odors with the musical notes:

do, re, mi, fa, sol, la, si or
C, D, E, F, G, A, B

by matching heavy odors with heavy notes, sweet odors with light notes, and so on for the intermediates.

CLASSIFICATION OF RIMMEL (1820–1887)

Eugene Rimmel, in his fascinating *Book of Perfumes* (1865), which went through many editions, described the use of perfumes from ancient times among Egyptians, Jews, Asiatics, Greeks, Romans, Far East, and developing countries.

Rimmel grouped all odors according to the maxim: odors more or less close to each other. The terms "isotonic odors" from the Greek word "isotonos" meaning *same tone* and "iso-osmatic," more appropriately meaning *same odor* from the Greek word "osme" *(odor)* may be applied here.

1. Rose : Geranium
2. Jasmine : Ylang ylang
3. Orange : Acacia
4. Tuberose : Narcissus, lily
5. Violet : Iris
6. Vanilla : Styrax, Peru balsam, heliotrope
7. Cinnamon : Cassia
8. Sandal : Vetiver
9. Lemon : Bergamot
10. Lavender : Spike
11. Mint : Basil, thyme
12. Anise : Coriander
13. Bitter almond : Laurel
14. Musk : Civet
15. Fruit : Apple, pineapple
16. Clove : Pink carnation

TREBLE OR G CLEF

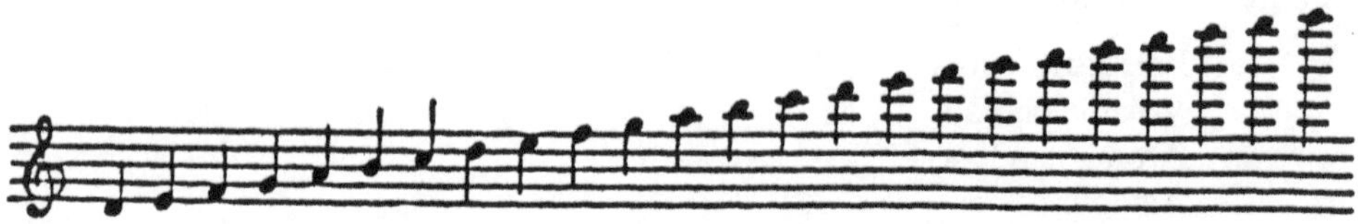

D Violet
E Acacia
F Tuberose
G Orange flower
A Vernal grass (new hay)
B Southernwood
C Camphor
D Almond
E Portugal
F Jonquil
G Syringa
A Tonquin bean
B Mint
C Jasmine
D Bergamot
E Cedrac
F Ambergris
G Magnolia
A Lavender
B Peppermint
C Pineapple
D Citronella
E Verbena
F Civet

BASS OR F CLEF

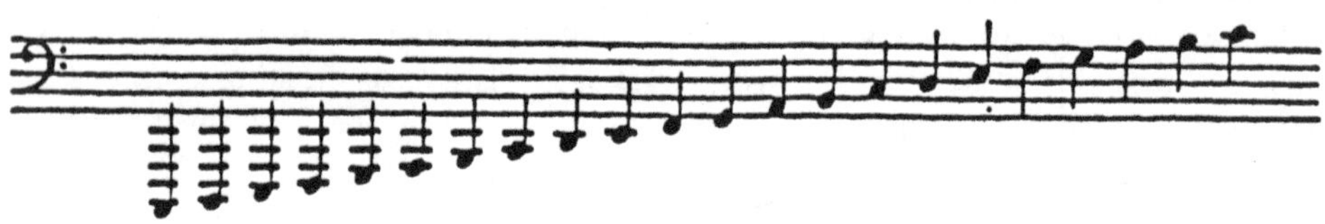

C Patchouli
D Vanilla
E Wallflower
F Benzoin
G Plumeria alba (frangipani plant)
A Storax
B Clove
C Santal
D Clematis
E Calamus
F Castor
G Pergalaria
A Balsam of Peru
B Stocks and pinks
C Geranium
D Heliotrope
E Orris
F Musk
G Sweet pea
A Tolu
B Cinnamon
C Rose

The "Odorphone" of Piesse from the book The *Science and Art of Perfumery* by Edward Sagarin, McGraw-Hill Books, 1945.

17. Camphor : Rosemary
18. Amber : Ambergris

An arrangement of isotonic or iso-osmatic odors:

1. Folial-nutty
2. Verdure
3. Oakmoss-lichen
4. Fern
5. Earthy
6. Fungal
7. Rooty
8. Woody
9. Smoky
10. Leather
11. Animal
12. Resinous
13. Spicy-nutty
14. Balsamic
15. Herbaceous
16. Amber
17. Honey
18. Aldehydic
19. Citrus
20. Fruity
21. Oenanthic

CLASSIFICATION OF ZWAARDEMAKER (1857–1930)

Hendrick Zwaardemaker, a German rhinolaryngologist, was the maker of the first olfactometer. In his book *Die Physiologie des Geruchs* (1895) (The Physiology of Perfumes), Zwaardemaker classified odors according to their major content:

1. Amyl acetate
2. Nitrobenzene
3. Terpineol
4. Ethyl sulfate
5. Guaiacol
6. Valerianic acid
7. Pyridine
8. Skatol

He further classified the odors in nine groups:

1. Ethereal: a) Fruits; b) Beeswax; c) Ethers
2. Aromatic: a) Camphor; b) Cloves; c) Lavender; d) Lemon; e) Bitter almond

3. Balsamic or fragrant: a) Flowers; b) Violet; c) Vanilla and Coumarin
4. Ambrosial: a) Amber; b) Musk
5. Alliaceous: a) Sulfureted hydrogen; b) Arsine; c) Chlorine
6. Empyreumatic*: a) Roast coffee; b) Benzene
7. Caprylic: a) Cheese; b) Rancid fat
8. Repulsive: a) Deadly nightshade; b) Bedbug
9. Nauseating or fetid: a) Carrion; b) Faeces

CLASSIFICATION OF HENNING (1885-?)

Hans Henning, a German chemist, in his 1916 book *Der Geruch* ("The Odors"), made a more realistic classification of the odors:

1. Flowery: Heliotrope, coumarin, geranium
2. Fruity: Orange oil, bergamot oil, citronellal
3. Resinous or balsamic: Turpentine, eucalyptus oil, Canada balsam
4. Burnt: Pyridine, tar
5. Putrefaction/Foul: Sulfureted hydrogen, carbon disulfide
6. Spicy: Cloves, fennel, anise

Henning pictured his classification as an olfactory prism where all odors appear longitudinally and diametrically, approximating: Flowery—Fruity; Spicy—Resinous; Burnt—Foul.

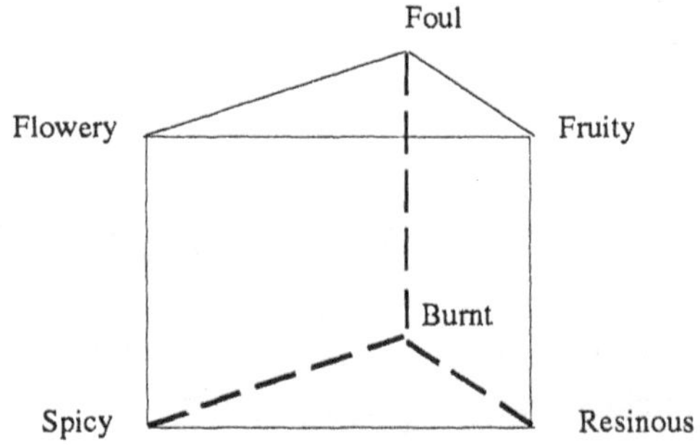

Henning's Olfactory Prism

The fundamental classes are joined by intermediate odors, converging into each other. According to Henning, each of the six odor types occupy a corner of the prism, and all odors, fundamentals and intermediates, irradiate on the surface of the prism.

* Empyreumatic, from the Greek word "Empyreuma." A peculiar odor of animal or vegetable matter when charred in a closed vessel, it is technically formed by dry distillation. In technological perfumery, it refers to the odor and taste of slightly burnt animal or vegetable substances. It is related to crude products of destructive distillation such as juniper tar, birch tar, rectified cod oil, tobacco, leather, dried hay, fern, mushroom, caramel, malt, coffee, and the characteristic odor of fried potatoes or grilled steak.

CLASSIFICATION OF CROKER AND HENDERSON

E.C. Croker and L. Henderson in 1935 classified the odors in four large groups, assigning to each group a common odor's number, from zero to eight, indicating intensity, with the rose as zero.

1. Fragrant—floral, 6
2. Acid, 4
3. Burnt—hot, 2
4. Caprylic—fat (putrid, disagreeable), 3

CLASSIFICATION OF CERBELAUD (1871–?)

René Cerbelaud, a French chemical engineer, classified all odors in 45 groups. The grouping was based on botanical families of similar odor, specifying the intrinsic constituents of each group.

CLASSIFICATION OF GATTEFOSSÉ (1881–?)

René Maurice Gattefossé, a French chemical engineer, reduced the 45 groups of Cerbelaud to 15 botanical family odor groups. The 15 botanical families were grouped according to odor and constituents' similarity. Gattefossé's classification appears to be the most precise and practical:

Gattefossé's Floral Families of Odors

Number	Family	Variety	Common Odor Due to Similar Constituents
1.	Jasmines	Jasmine, lilac, lily of the valley, cyclamen, ylang ylang, amaryllis	Benzyl acetate and other esters, hydroxycitronellol, linalool, terpineol
2.	Orange	Neroli, orange flower, petitgrain, acacia, sweet pea	Nerol, methyl anthranilate, farnesol
3.	Narcissus	Narcissus, tuberose, hyacinth, jonquil, glycine, gardenia, honeysuckle, magnolia, genista (broom)	Paracresyl esters, phenyl acetic esters

Number	Family	Variety	Common Odor Due to Similar Constituents
4.	Rose	Rose, geranium, palmarosa	Phenyl ethyl alcohol, geraniol, citronellol, rhodinol, diphenyl oxide
5.	Violet	Violet, iris (orris), mignonette, reseda	Irone, ionone, methyl ionone, methyl heptyne carbonate
6.	Mimosa	Mimosa, cassia	Paramethylacetophenone
7.	Citrus	Bergamot, verbena, melissa (balm mint)	Citral, citronellol, limonene, linalool
8.	Aurantiae	Orange, tangerine, lemon	Methyl anthranilate, aldehyde C-10
9.	Lavender	Lavender, hyssop, laurel	Linalyl acetate and other esters, terpenyl acetate
10.	Mint	Mint, spearmint	Pulegone, menthol, menthone
11.	Spice	Cinnamon, clove, bay, tarragon, thyme, oregano	Cinnamic aldehyde, eugenol, thymol
12.	Woods	Pine, juniper, rosemary, vetiver, patchouli	Borneol and acetates, camphor
13.	Vanilla	Vanilla, heliotrope	Vanillin, heliotropine
14.	Anise	Anise, fennel, Chinese anise	Anethole
15.	Amber	Clary sage, labdanum	Musk ambrette, musk ketone, ambergris

CLASSIFICATION OF BILLOT

Marcel Billot, a French chemical engineer, classified the odors in eight series:

1. Floral
2. Balsamic
3. Frutal
4. Empyreumatic
5. Comestible
6. Woody
7. Rural
8. Repulsive

CLASSIFICATION OF AMOORE

Amoore, in 1952, suggested that there are seven primary classes of odors:

1. Ethereal
2. Camphoraceous
3. Musky
4. Floral
5. Minty
6. Pungent
7. Putrid

CLASSIFICATION OF REDGROVE

Herbert Stanley Redgrove, an English chemist and writer, classified the odors in classes and types, giving examples of odors of the same class:

Class	Types	Odor of the Same Class
Violet	Violet	Cassie*, orris root, mignonette
Spice	Cinnamon	Cassia**, nutmeg, mace, pimento
Clove	Clove	Carnation, clove
Citrine	Lemon	Bergamot, orange, limette
Aniseed	Aniseed	Badiene, caraway, dill, coriander, fennel
Mint	Peppermint	Spearmint, balm, rue, sage
Fruit	Pear	Apple, pineapple, quince

* Cassie (*Acacia farnesiana*)
** Cassia (*Cinnamommum cassia*, of China)

Subjective Classification of the Odors

The classification of odors, from the author's viewpoint, should be done subjectively, that is, to consider basically the human sensations:

APERITIF ODORS

They give to the human organism the perception of substances adaptable to his nourishment, and they stimulate the appetite:

1. Fresh fruit odors: lower fatty acid ethers
2. Odors developed by the roasting of meats and fats: upper fatty acid ethers
3. Odors developed by the roasting of carbohydrates: furans

BALSAMIC ODORS

They give to the human organism the perception of good fresh air, or of substances that ordinarily stimulate breathing:

1. Fresh floral odors: countryside in bloom, terpenes, alcohols, ethers, aromatic derivatives
2. Resin odors: woods, forests, aromatic derivatives
3. Odor of fresh air early in the morning; odor of pure, light air; odor of ozone, which we perceive in the morning, especially after getting out of the bedroom; odor of air after storms
4. Odor of algae: volatile compounds of algae in decomposition

BODY ODORS

They are peculiar to the human body:

1. Women's odor: bouquet formed by the perspiration glands in which the odors of butyric and valerianic ethers are prevalent.
2. Hair odors: predominately sulfur.
3. Animal odors: civet, musk, amber.

DISGUSTING ODORS

They are emitted by substances introduced into the human organism and which are chemically and bacterially dangerous, or by compounds which accompany such substances:

1. Odor of albuminous substances, odor of substances in putrefaction (e.g., fecal substances which are generally formed by nitrogen, nitrosulfates, amino sulfates, or phosphates).
2. Fatty acids in putrefaction.
3. Fungi odors

IRRITATING ODORS

These odors derive from substances which have a very violent and destructive action on the mucosae, thus endangering the organism:

1. Hygroscopic substances: acids, bases, anhydrides.
2. Oxidant substances: halogens, nitrogenous and sulfurous compounds.

General Classification of Odorous Substances

Notwithstanding all the previously enunciated classifications of the odors by very competent experts, no perfect classification has yet been devised. It is extremely difficult to achieve perfection in the classification of naturally occurring substances.

Müller carried out an investigation of 1266 different types of blooming flowers with the following results:

14	closely resembled heliotrope
63	were fairly similar to heliotrope
64	had honey-like odors
18	had jasmine odors
19	had balsamic odors
211	had cabbage-like odors
138	had spicy odors
32	had narcotic odors
12	had orange flower odors
695	were nonodorous

Müller also examined the odors of 738 different types of leaves and noted that in 350 cases the odor was of β-hexylene aldehyde which has a typical "green" or "fresh" odor.

Müller concluded that:

1. Not all flowers have a pleasant odor
2. Many flowers are nonodorous
3. Many have cabbage-like odors
4. Only the minority of the flowers have pleasant odors.

Odorous substances are, therefore, simply classified by origin of extraction:

1. Vegetal origin: essential oils from all parts of a plant.
2. Animal origin: derived from organs, animal parts, or animal products: castoreum, civet, musk, ambergris.
3. Artificial origin: constituents of essential oils synthetically produced by chemical reactions.

THE ODOR THEORY

The volatile portion of a substance perceptible by the sense of smell is called "odor" from the Latin word "odor."

Substances have osmophoric elements which combine with the osmoreceptors of the nasal membranes giving the sensation of odor. The perception of odor is limited by the quantity of nasal receptors in each individual. Therefore, odors can be perceived by some as pleasantly suave (eusomophores*) and by others as obnoxious or bad (cacosmophores*) depending on the number of osmoreceptors in their noses.

The odor theory states that:

1. Substances that emit smells are called *osmyls.*
2. Organs that receive smells are called *osphrenes.*
3. Osphrenes transmit the smells sent by the osmyls to the brain.

These principles embrace various fields of science—chemistry, physics, biology, and anatomy—and comprise altogether the science of smell, more appropriately called "osmics' science," from the Greek word "osme" ("smell").

John H. Kenneth, M.A. of Edinburgh, Scotland, published in 1922 a list of 1500 references all related to the sense of smell under the title *Osmics, The Science of Smell.*

ODOR DETERMINATION

The persistance of an odor can be determined by placing a definite quantity of essential oil or perfume on a filter paper and exposing it to the air. The test compared the odor at timed intervals.

Among the most persistent essential oils, in decreasing order, are:

1. Patchouli
2. Sandalwood
3. Cinnamon
4. Cassia
5. Citronella
6. Oregano
7. Thyme
8. Neroli

ODOR CONCENTRATION

The concentration, intensity, or strength of an odor is determined in terms of the minimum perceptible amount. The unity of intensity, called "olfactometer," refers to the minimum perceptible concentration in grams per milliliters of air:

---

* From the Greek: Caco = bad; eu = good; phoresis = carrying.

ODORS

Odor	mg/liter of air
Musk	0.0004
Iodoform	0.018
Diamyl sulfide	0.001
Propyl mercaptan	0.006
Butyric acid	0.009
Amyl isovalerate	0.012
Valeric acid	0.029
Peppermint oil	0.03
Methyl salicylate	0.1
Acetic ether	0.68
Chloroform	3.3

AROMATHERAPY

R.M. Gattefossé, in his book *Aromatherapie, Les Huiles Essentielles, Hormones Vegetales*, considers the use of the essential oils for their benefic therapeutic effects in the following areas of medicine:

1. Respiratory system
2. Nervous system
3. Skin
4. Hair
5. Veneral diseases
6. Obstetrics and gynecology
7. Hemorrhoids
8. Cancer
9. Various ulcers
10. Hydrotherapy, particularly for rheumatism
11. Tooth therapy
12. Veterinary medicine

Marguerite Maurey, in her book *The Secret of Life and Youth*, considers the use of essential oils in the following branches of medicine:

1. Surgery: tissue regeneration, application in preoperational cases, action on the underlying tissue, cicatrization, burns
2. Radiology: old burns from x-rays, preservation of the skin and tissue in the course of x-ray treatment, protection against ultraviolet and infrared radiation, the skin and its sensitivity
3. Dermatology: eczema, acne
4. Gynecology: local treatment, uterine erosion
5. General medicine: muscular refection, ganglia in children, hematoma, bone

tumors, encapsulated tumors, aromatherapy in homeopathic treatment

6. Psychiatry: analysis, relaxation, ageing of emotions
7. Hydrotherapy and spa treatment: thermal cures, steam baths, underwater massages
8. Physiotherapy: massage, absorption of essential oils after exposure to ultraviolet radiation, mobilization, sprains
9. Sports medicine
10. Cosmetics

ANTISEPTIC VALUE OF THE ESSENTIAL OILS

Essential oils can be employed as antiseptics, particularly for microorganisms such as *Staphylococcus pyogenes aureus, Streptococcus pyogenes, Penicillium glaucum,* and *Aspergillus albus.*

Examples of the antiseptic value of certain essential oils follows:

Highest 100%:	Clove, wintergreen, sassafras, sandalwood, mint, thyme, cinnamon, camphor
Good 70%:	Eucalyptus, sage, lavender, violet
Fair 50%:	Juniper, rose, bergamot, patchouli, vanilla, verbena
Low 10%:	Neroli, geranium, vetiver, jasmine, opopanax, origanum, lemongrass

Chapter II:
NATURAL ESSENCES

Introduction

ESSENTIAL OILS

Essential oils, or volatile oils, are odoriferous liquids obtained from vegetal sources. They volatilize without decomposition. They are the source of terpenes. Terpenes are volatile and low in strength and odor. They decompose on exposure to light, moisture, and air, causing the oil to spoil.

Terpeneless essential oils (from which the terpenes have been removed by fractional distillation) have more solubility, concentration, and fragrance.

Essential oils are very numerous and they are found in all parts of a plant.

DERIVATION

1. ***Flowering Plants, Shrubs and Trees:***
   Carnation, cassie, cananga, hyacith, jasmine, jonquil, mimosa, narcissus, orange flower, reseda, rose, tuberose, violet, ylang ylang.
2. ***Leaves:***
   Bay cinnamon, cedar, patchouli, bitter orange, wintergreen, eucalyptus.
3. ***Woods:***
   Amyris, cade, cedar, birch, bois de rose, camphor, guaiac, laurel, linaloe, santal, sassafrass.
4. ***Barks:***
   Birch, cascarilla, cassia, cedar, cinnamon, cypress.
5. ***Fresh Fruits' Peels:***
   Bergamot, citron, grapefruit, lemon, limes, mandarin, orange, tangerine.
6. ***Grass:***
   Citronella, gingergrass, lemongrass, palmarosa.
7. ***Seeds:***
   Ambrette, angelica, cardamom, carrot, croton, cumin, dill, mustard, parsley, bitter almond.
8. ***Dried Leaves:***
   Cherry laurel, eucalyptus, niaouli, patchouli

9. ***Dried Fruits:***
   Coriander, anise, juniper, nutmeg.
10. ***Dried Buds and Berries:***
   Clove, cubeb, juniper, pimenta.
11. ***Balsams:***
   Copaiba, labdanum, Peru, Tolu, Gilead.
12. ***Gums:***
   Elemi, galbanum, mastic, myrrh, olibanum, opoponax, styrax.
13. ***Roots and Rhizomes:***
   Angelic, calamus, costus, ginger, orris, valerian, vetiver
14. ***Herbs' Flowers:***
   Basil, chamomile, dill, estragon, fennel, geranium, lavandin, lavender and spike lavender, lovage, marjoram, origanum, parsley, pennyroyal, peppermint, rosemary, sage (Clary, Dalmation), spearmint, tansy, thyme, verbena, wormseed, wormwood.

CHARACTERISTICS

Essential oils differ widely from one another both in property and composition. The essential oil extracted from one organ of a plant differs from those of other organs of the same plant. The essential oil of the roots of a cinnamon plant, for instance, is different in composition from that of the bark and that of the leaves. The essential oil of the orange flower is different from that of the peels of the orange fruit.

The essential oil of the same organ of a plant of the same species is also different because of differences in soils where the plant is located, its physiological conditions, and even the atmospheric conditions and seasons in which the collection is made for the ulterior extraction of the essential oil.

Some essential oils are colorless, while others are green or dark brown. Generally, they are lighter than water, with a few, such as the cinnamon oil, being heavier.

Chemically, essential oils are hydrocarbons. They are different from the fixed oils, such as linseed oil or coconut oil, or from fatty oils, such as cotton oil or olive oil. The difference lies in the fact that essential oils are volatile, nongreasy, and consequently not saponifiable. An exception is the essential oil of wintergreen, which is a single compound of methyl salicylate. All other essential oils are mixtures of many constituents. Mostly essential oils have fluid constituents. There are some exceptions in which solid compounds, called *stearoptenes*, are present in solution, and these can be separated by chilling the oil ("Otto" Rose oil is an example.).

METHOD OF EXTRACTION OF THE ESSENTIAL OILS

Essential oils are industrially extracted by the following processes:

1. Distillation with water.
2. Steam distillation.
3. Vacuum distillation.
4. Squeezing the peels of the fruits by hand or mechanically over a sponge. This

process is mostly applied to citrus products.
5. Solvent extraction.
6. Maceration of the flowers and leaves in neutral fat and further dissolving it in a solvent.
7. Cold enfleurage, employed for the very delicate type of oil which is easily destroyed even by moderate heat.
8. By mixing the flowers with a neutral fat until it becomes strongly saturated with the odor, and then dissolving it with a solvent.
9. Enfleurage at moderate temperature between 50–70 C.

ANALYSIS OF THE ESSENTIAL OILS

The analysis is intended to ascertain if the organoleptic characteristics of the essential oil in examen correspond to the standards as specified in the official Pharmacopeia and National Formulary, or any other official standards as specified by the manufacturing associations.

The analysis combines qualitative and quantitative chemistry: physical for the organoleptic standards, instrumental for spectrometry and chromatography, computerized automatic control, etc.

Specifically the analysis includes:

1. Specific gravity
2. Optical index
3. Refractive index
4. Boiling point
5. Solidifying point or freezing point
6. Solubility
7. Saponification number
8. Acetylation
9. Aldehyde and ketones determination
10. Esters and alcohols determination
11. Phenols determination
12. Iodine determination
13. Acids determination
14. Melting point
15. Absorption
16. Flax point
17. Polymerization
18. Viscosimetry
19. Colorimetry
20. Spectrophotometry
21. Chromatography
22. Microscopy
23. Computerized automatic control
24. Search for adulteration through fractional distillation

An accurate and complete analysis would give assurance in the use of the material in medicine, pharmacy, food, flavors, perfumes, and cosmetics.

Because essential oils are very expensive, particularly those with low yields in extraction, adulteration is very common, even when official standards are maintained. Therefore, in the analysis of essential oils, deep expertise, specific knowledge of the essential oil, and, above all, a good sense of smell are necessary. In some cases, the application of fractional distillation may be very useful in obtaining an accurate separation of all components in analysis.

Constituents of the Essential Oils

Chemically the essential oils are mixtures of various substances which may be divided into two classes: nonoxygenated and oxygenated.

1. The *nonoxygenated* are hydrocarbons of the class commonly known as *terpenes*, and are of little importance as perfume material.
2. The *oxygenated* bodies, probably formed by the oxidation of the hydrocarbons, are:
    a. *Alcohols*, formed by the first step in oxidation
    b. *Aldehydes* and *ketones*, formed by the further oxidation of the alcohols
    c. *Acids*, formed from the aldehydes by a further addition of oxygen
    d. *Esters*, derived from the combination of alcohols and acids
    e. *Ethers*, derived from alcohols by the elimination of water

1. Hydrocarbon Constituents of Essential Oils

HYDROCARBONS	ESSENTIAL OILS
1. Pinene	Turpentine
2. Camphene	Ginger, spike, citronella, valerian
3. Fenchene	Turpentine
4. Limonene	Orange peels, lemon, bergamot, fir, camphor
5. Silvestrene	Turpentine
6. Phellandrene	Fennel, elemi, eucalyptus
7. Terpinene	Cardamom
8. Terpinolene	Cardamom
9. Cadinene	Cade
10. Caryophyllen	Clove
11. Cumene	Cumin, cyminum thyme
12. Styrene	Styrax

2. *Alcohol—Acid—Ester Constituents of Essential Oils*

	ALCOHOLS	ACIDS		ESSENTIAL OILS
1.	Methyl			Clove
		Salicylic		Wintergreen
		Benzoic		Niobe
2.	Ethyl	Formic		Rum
		Acetic		White wine, vinegar, cognac
		Butyric		Pineapple
		Isovaleric		Apple
		Pelargonic		Cognac
3.	Isobutyl			Fusel
		Isobutyric		Chamomile
		Angelic		Chamomile
4.	Isoamyl	Acetic		Pear
		Isovaleric		Apple
		Caprylic }	Oenanthic	Cognac
		Caprinic }	Ether	
5.	Rhodinol			Rose, geranium, citronella,
	Geraniol			lemongrass
		Acetic		Neroli (orange flower)
6.	Linalol			Linaloes, bergamot, lavender, neroli, jasmine
		Acetic		Bergamot, neroli
7.	Citronellol			Rose, citronella
8.	Furfurol			Coffee
9.	Borneol			Camphor, rosemary
		Acetic		Pine
		Isovaleric		Valerian
10.	Terpineol			Cajeput, cardamom
11.	Menthol			Peppermint
12.	Eucalyptol (Cineol)			Wormseed, eucalyptus
13.	Peruviol			Balsam Peru
14.	Benzyl			Jasmine
		Acetic		Jasmine
		Benzoic		Balsam Peru
15.	Cinnamic	Cinnamic		Styrax

3. *Aldehyde Constituents of Essential Oils*

	ALDEHYDES	ESSENTIAL OILS
1.	Citral	Lemon, lemongrass
2.	Citronellal	Citronella, lemon, eucalyptus
3.	Furfural	Clove
4.	Benzaldehyde	Bitter almond, laurel
5.	Phenylacetaldehyde	Neroli (orange flower), hyacinth
6.	Cinnamic	Cassia, cinnamon
7.	Cuminic	Caraway
8.	Salicylic	Spiraea, *Crepis foetida*
9.	Anisic	Hawthorn
10.	Vanillin	Vanilla, benzoin, balsam Peru, beet sugar
11.	Heliotropin	Spiraea

4. *Acid and Acid Anhydride Constituents of Essential Oils*

	ACIDS AND ACID ANHYDRIDES	ESSENTIAL OILS
1.	Angelic	Chamomile
2.	Tiglic	Chamomile, croton
3.	Benzoic	Balsam Peru, benzoin, balsam Tolu
4.	Cinnamic	Balsam Peru, balsam Tolu, benzoin, styrax
5.	Coumarin	Tonka beans, woodruff (*Asperula odorata*)

5. *Ketone Constituents of Essential Oils*

	KETONES	ESSENTIAL OILS
1.	Methylamyl	Clove
2.	Methylnonyl	Rue
3.	Methylheptenone	Linaloes, lemongrass
4.	Pseudo-ionone	Linaloes, lemongrass
5.	Carvone	Caraway
6.	Camphor	Camphor
7.	Fenchone	Fennel, thuja
8.	Thujone (Tanacetone)	Thuja, tansy, absinthe
9.	Pulegone	Pennyroyal
10.	Menthone	Peppermint
11.	Irone	Orris root
12.	Ionone	Orris root

6. *Phenol and Phenol Ester Constituents of Essential Oils*

	PHENOLS AND PHENOL ESTERS	ESSENTIAL OILS
1.	*p*-Cresol methyl ether	Ylang-ylang
2.	Guaiacol	Beech tar, birch tar
3.	Creosol	Birch tar
4.	Anethol	Anise, fennel
5.	Chavicol	Betel
6.	Estragol	Estragon
7.	Eugenol	Clove
8.	Thymol	Thyme
9.	Safrol	Sassafrass, camphor

7. *Nitrogenous Compound Constituents of Essential Oils*

	NITROGENOUS COMPOUNDS	ESSENTIAL OILS
1.	Trimethylamine	Chenopodium
2.	Prussic acid	Bitter almond, laurel
3.	Allyl mustard oil	Mustard, horseradish, *Alliaria officinalis*
4.	Pyrrol	Unripe orange
5.	Indole	Jasmine
6.	Benzyl cyanide	Cress (*Lepdium sativum, Tropaeolum majus*)
7.	Mandelic nitrile	Almond
8.	Tonquinol	Baur's musk
9.	Anthranilic methyl ester	Jasmine, orange flower

ESSENTIAL OILS' DESCRIPTION FORMAT

NAME

CLASSIFICATION: Botanical or zoological: Family, Genus, Species, Variety
SOURCE: Habitat, part of plant or body
CHEMICAL CONSTITUENTS:
CHARACTERISTICS: Form, color, odor, taste
PHYSICAL PROPERTIES: Specific gravity, refractive index, optical rotation, other
SOLUBILITY: Water, alcohol, ether, chloroform, other solvent
USES: Flavors, perfumes pharmaceuticals, medicine, other
WARNINGS AND CAUTION:

Essential Oils Directory

ALMOND, BITTER

BOTANICAL: *Family: Rosaceae; Genus: Prunus; Species: Amygdalus, Communis; Variety: Amara*

SOURCE: *Habitat:* Italy, Spain, Southern France; *Part of Plant:* Meal; Seeds; Kernels of Almond, Apricot, Cherries, Plums, Peaches

CHEMICAL CONSTITUENTS: Benzaldehyde 95%, Hydrocyanic acid, Phenoxy acetonitrile

CHARACTERISTICS: *Color:* Colorless to yellow. It changes on exposure to air; *Odor:* Benzaldehyde; *Taste:* Bitter

PHYSICAL PROPERTIES: *Specific gravity:* 1.038–1.060; *Refractive index:* 1.5428–1.5439; *Optical rotation:* Inactive; *Boiling point:* 179 C

SOLUBILITY: Slightly sol. in water; sol. in ether, chloroform, oils; sol. in alcohol (2/70%).

USES: *Flavors:* Liqueurs, soft drinks; *Perfumes: Cosmetics*

WARNINGS AND CAUTION: Use only if it is totally free of hydrocyanic acid

AMBERGRIS (TINCTURE)

ZOOLOGICAL: *Family: Physeteridae; Genus: Physeter; Species: Macrocephalus*

SOURCES: *Habitat:* Afloat in the oceans and in the sea shores; *Part of the Body:* Excretion from sperm whale's intestinal tract

CHEMICAL CONSTITUENTS: Cholesterol 80%, benzoic acid, 5 β-cholestan-3 α-ol, fatty oil, ambrein, liquid paraffin

CHARACTERISTICS: *Color:* Greyish-black, waxy opaque; *Odor:* Woody, reminiscent of seaweeds

PHYSICAL CONSTANTS: *Specific gravity:* 0.80–0.92; *Melting point:* 60 C

SOLUBILITY: Insoluble in water; sol. in ether, chloroform, volatile oils, hot alcohol

USES: As tincture and essence for fixing odors (fixative)

AMBRETTE, SEED

BOTANICAL: *Family: Malvaceae; Genus: Mallow; Species: Hibiscus; Variety: Abelmoschus* or *moschatus*

SOURCES: *Habitat:* Java, Indonesia, India, Central and South America; *Part of the Plant:* Seeds

CHEMICAL CONSTITUENTS: Farnesol, δ-7-hexadeceno-lactone, ambrettolid

CHARACTERISTICS: *Form:* Powder; *Color:* White to yellow; *Odor:* Heavy musk; *Taste:* Cognac

PHYSICAL CONSTANTS: *Specific gravity:* 0.908–0.918; *Refractive index:* 1.4742–1.4764; *Optical rotation:* +1 to +1.34; *Congealing point:* 83.4 C

SOLUBILITY: Insoluble in water; sol. in oils, benzyl benzoate, diethyl phthalate, dimethyl phthalate, methyl carbinol; sparingly sol. in alcohol, ether, chloroform

USES: Fixative

ANGELICA, ROOT

BOTANICAL: *Family: Umbelliferae; Genus: Archangelica; Species: Officinalis*
SOURCES: *Habitat:* Mainly in Europe; *Part of the Plant:* Roots
CHEMICAL CONSTITUENTS: Phellandrene, exaltolide, δ-7-hexadecenolactone
CHARACTERISTICS: *Color:* Yellow; *Odor:* Musky, strong, aromatic, agreeable; *Taste:* Spicy
PHYSICAL CONSTANTS: *Specific gravity:* 0.857–0.915 (15 C); *Refractive index:* 1.476–1.480; *Optical rotation:* +16 to +32
SOLUBILITY: Sol. in alcohol (6/90%)
USES: *Flavors:* Liqueurs; *Medicine:* Medicine

ANGELICA, SEED

BOTANICAL: *Family: Umbelliferae; Genus: Archangelica; Species: Officinalis*
SOURCES: *Habitat:* Europe, mainly in Saxony; *Part of the Plant:* Seeds
CHEMICAL CONSTITUENTS: Phellandrene, exaltolide, δ-7-hexadecenolactone, valeric acid, farnesol
CHARACTERISTICS: *Color:* Yellow. It darkens on aging; *Odor:* Spicy, finer than the oil from the roots; *Taste:* Spicy
PHYSICAL CONSTANTS: *Specific gravity:* 0.851–0.890 (15 C); *Refractive index:* 1.476–1.488; *Optical rotation:* +13 to +15 (15 C)
SOLUBILITY: Sol. in alcohol (5–9/90%)
USES: *Flavors:* Liqueurs; *Medicine:* Medicine

ANGOSTURA

BOTANICAL: *Family: Rutaceae; Genus: Galipea; Species: Officinalis; Variety: Cusparia trifoliata, febrifuga*
SOURCES: *Habitat:* Venezuela, Brazil; *Part of the Plant:* Bark
CHEMICAL CONSTITUENTS: Cadinene, angosturin, quinoline, cusparine, galipine, galipoidine, galipoline
CHARACTERISTICS: *Color:* Yellow; *Odor:* Musty, unpleasant; *Taste:* Bitter, pungent, tonic, stimulant
PHYSICAL CONSTANTS: *Specific gravity:* 0.928–0.960 (15 C); *Refractive index:* 1.5060–1.5085; *Optical rotation:* –7.30 to –50
SOLUBILITY: Soluble in alcohol
USES: *Flavors:* Liqueurs bitter type; *Medicine:* Antipyretic, febrifugo

ANISE, SEED

BOTANICAL: *Family: Umbelliferae; Genus: Pimpinella; Species: Anisum or anisatum*
SOURCES: *Habitat:* Western Asia, India, Egypt, Southern Europe; *Part of the Plant:* Dried seeds
CHEMICAL CONSTITUENTS: Anethole 90%, estragole, acetaldehyde, safrole, methylchavicol, anisaldehyde, anisole, ethyl anisate
CHARACTERISTICS: *Form:* Thick; solidifies to a crystalline mass at 15 C; *Color:* Colorless; *Odor:* Characteristic anise; *Taste:* Sweet
PHYSICAL CONSTANTS: *Specific gravity:* 0.978–0.988; *Refractive index:* 1.5530–1.5600; *Optical rotation:* –2 to +2; *Boiling point:* 210 C

SOLUBILITY: Slightly soluble in water; sol. in ether, chloroform; sol. in alcohol (3/90%)
USES: *Flavors:* Liqueurs, candies, cookies; *Perfumes:* Perfumes, dentifrices; *Other:* Source of anethole

ANISE, STAR
BOTANICAL: *Family: Magnoliaceae; Genus: Ilicium; Species: Verum*
SOURCES: *Habitat:* China, U.S.S.R., Spain; *Part of the Plant:* Seeds from the tree
CHEMICAL CONSTITUENTS: Anethole 90%, estragole, acetaldehyde, safrole, eugenol, methylchavicol, anisaldehyde
CHARACTERISTICS: *Form:* Thick; it solidifies to a crystalline mass at 15 C; *Color:* Colorless; *Odor:* Characteristic anise; *Taste:* Sweet
PHYSICAL CONSTANTS: *Specific gravity:* 1.006; *Refractive index:* 1.553–1.556; *Optical rotation:* –8; *Melting point:* 14–18 C; *Solidification point:* –10 to –15 C; *Boiling point:* 210 C
SOLUBILITY: Soluble in alcohol
USES: *Perfumes:* Perfumes; *Medicine:* As a carminative and expectorant; *Other:* Source of anethole

ARTEMISIA
BOTANICAL: *Family: Compositae; Genus: Artemisia; Species: Vulgaris; Variety: Alba*
SOURCES: *Habitat:* Morocco, Algeria, Yugoslavia, France; *Part of the Plant:* Dried herb
CHEMICAL CONSTITUENTS: Thujone
CHARACTERISTICS: *Color:* Colorless; it turns yellow on exposure; *Odor:* Spicy, herbaceous; *Taste:* Bitter
PHYSICAL CONSTANTS: *Specific gravity:* 0.925–0.955 (15 C); *Refractive index:* 1.460–1.474
SOLUBILITY: Slightly soluble in water; soluble in ether; sol. in alcohol (2/80%)
USES: *Perfumes:* Perfumes

ASARUM
SYNONYMS: Canada "snake root"
BOTANICAL: *Family: Aristolochiaceae; Genus: Asarum; Species: Canadense*
SOURCES: *Habitat:* Canada, North Carolina, Kansas; *Part of the Plant:* Rhizomes, leaves
CHEMICAL CONSTITUENTS: Pinene, methyl eugenol, borneol, linalool, geraniol, terpineol
CHARACTERISTICS: *Color:* Yellowish to brown; *Odor:* Aromatic; *Taste:* Burning, unpleasant
PHYSICAL CONSTANTS: *Specific gravity:* 0.947–0.998 (15 C); *Refractive index:* 1.4843–1.5015; *Optical rotation:* Inactive –11.20
SOLUBILITY: Insoluble in water; sol. in alcohol (2/70%)
USES: *Perfumes:* Perfumery

ASAFOETIDA (RESINOID)

BOTANICAL: *Family: Umbelliferae; Genus: Ferula; Species: Narthex*
SOURCES: *Habitat:* Afghanistan; *Part of the Plant:* Rhizomes, roots
CHEMICAL CONSTITUENTS: Pinene, diallyl sulfide, perulic acid, asaresinotannol, vanillin, sulfur: 8.9–31.4%
CHARACTERISTICS: *Color:* Colorless to yellow; *Odor:* Onion, garlic; *Taste:* Bitter, acrid
PHYSICAL CONSTANTS: *Specific gravity:* 0.915–0.993 (15 C); *Refractive index:* 1.492–1.5259; *Optical rotation:* +10.58 to 17.3
SOLUBILITY: Soluble in alcohol, ether, chloroform, benzene
USES: *Flavors:* Flavors for foods, Worcestershire sauce; *Medicine:* Carminative, antispasmodic, expectorant

BALM

SYNONYMS: Melissa
BOTANICAL: *Family: Labiatae; Genus: Melissa; Species: Officinalis; Variety: Calamintha*
SOURCES: *Part of the Plant:* Leaves and tops
CHEMICAL CONSTITUENTS: Citral
CHARACTERISTICS: *Color:* Yellow to yellowish-green; *Odor:* Lemon; *Taste:* Lemon
PHYSICAL CONSTANTS: *Specific gravity:* 0.890–0.925; *Refractive index:* 1.4738–1.4820; *Optical rotation:* +2 to –8; *Congealing point:* +12 C
SOLUBILITY: Insoluble in water; soluble in alcohol
USES: *Flavors:* Food flavoring; *Medicine:* Carminative, febrifuge

BASIL, SWEET

BOTANICAL: *Family: Labiatae; Genus: Ocimum; Species: Basilicum*
SOURCES: *Habitat:* Europe, Reunion; *Part of the Plant:* Leaves
CHEMICAL CONSTITUENTS: Estragole, linalool, cineol, camphor, methylchavicol, pinene, eugenol
CHARACTERISTICS: *Color:* Yellowish to green; *Odor:* Camphoraceous
PHYSICAL CONSTANTS: *Specific gravity:* 0.904–0.930 (15 C); *Refractive index:* 1.480–1.484; *Optical rotation:* –6 to –22
SOLUBILITY: Insoluble in water; sol. in in alcohol 2/80%, ether, chloroform
USES: *Flavors:* Flavoring food and liqueurs; *Perfumes:* Perfumery, mignonette type; *Medicine:* Medicine

BAY

SYNONYMS: Sweet bay
BOTANICAL: *Family: Myrtaceae; Genus: Pimenta or myrica; Species: Acris*
SOURCES: *Habitat:* West Indies, Central and South America; *Part of the Plant:* Leaves
CHEMICAL CONSTITUENTS: Eugenol 40–45%, chavicol, methyl eugenol, methyl chavicol, citral, *l*-phellandrene, pinene, myrcene, phenols 50–65%
CHARACTERISTICS: *Color:* Yellow to brownish; it darkens on exposure; *Odor:* Clove-like; *Taste:* Sharp, spicy

PHYSICAL CONSTANTS: *Specific gravity:* 0.962–0.990; *Refractive index:* 1.500–1.520; *Optical rotation:* 0–3 (25 C)
SOLUBILITY: Insoluble in water; soluble in alcohol, carbon disulfide, glacial acetic acid
USES: F*lavors:* Flavors; *Perfumes:* Perfumes, preparation of bay rum; *Pharmaceuticals:* Pharmaceuticals aromatic aid

BEESWAX (ABSOLUTE)
ZOOLOGICAL (Bees): *Family: Apoidea; Genus: Apis; Species: Mellifera*
SOURCES: Honey bees' wax comb, melting in hot water and cooling in molds
CHEMICAL CONSTITUENTS: Cerolein, cerotic acid, myricyl alcohol, melissic acid, and various alkanes
CHARACTERISTICS: *Color:* Yellowish to brownish; *Odor:* Honey-like with herbaceous reminiscence; *Taste:* Sweet, slightly balsamic
PHYSICAL CONSTANTS: *Specific gravity:* 0.950–0.960; *Melting point:* 62–65 C
SOLUBILITY: Insoluble in water; soluble in ether, chloroform, carbon disulfide, oils, hot alcohol
USES: *Flavors:* Food additive; *Perfumes:* Floral fine fragrance; *Pharmaceuticals:* Pharmaceutic acid; *Medicine:* Ointments; *Other:* Cosmetics

BENZOIN, SIAM (RESINOID)
BOTANICAL: *Family: Styracaceae; Genus: Benzoin; Species: Siam*
SOURCES: *Habitat:* Asia; *Part of the Plant:* Bark's resin of Liquidambar orientalis tree
CHEMICAL CONSTITUENTS: Benzoic acid, cinnamic acid, vanillin
CHARACTERISTICS: *Form:* Almond-shaped tears; *Color:* Pale reddish brown; *Odor:* Chocolate-vanilla; *Taste:* Slightly acrid
SOLUBILITY: Insoluble in water; Soluble in carbon disulfide, hot alcohol
USES: *Flavors:* Flavoring; *Perfumes:* Perfumery; *Medicine:* Medicine

BENZOIN, SUMATRA (RESINOID)
BOTANICAL: *Family: Styracaceae; Genus: Benzoin; Species: Sumatra*
SOURCES: *Habitat:* Asia; *Part of the Plant:* Bark's resin of Liquidambar orientalis tree
CHEMICAL CONSTITUENTS: Benzoic acid, cinnamic acid, vanillin
CHARACTERISTICS: *Form:* Almond-shaped tears; *Color:* Pale reddish brown; *Odor:* Chocolate-vanilla; *Taste:* Slightly acrid
SOLUBILITY: Insoluble in water; Soluble in carbon disulfide, hot alcohol
USES: *Perfumes:* As a fixative; *Medicine:* Medicine; *Other:* Cosmetics

BERGAMOT
BOTANICAL: *Family: Rutaceae; Genus: Citrus; Species: Aurantium; Variety: Bergamia*
SOURCES: *Habitat:* Sicily, Calabria; *Part of the Plant:* Peels
CHEMICAL CONSTITUENTS: Limonene, linalyl acetate 40%, linalool, bisabolene, pinene

CHARACTERISTICS: *Color:* Yellowish-green; *Odor:* Citrus; *Taste:* Sharp, bitter
PHYSICAL CONSTANTS: *Specific gravity:* 0.875–0.880; *Refractive index:* 1.4650–1.4675; *Optical rotation:* +8 to +24
SOLUBILITY: Insoluble in water; soluble in alcohol 2/80%
USES: *Flavors:* Flavors; *Perfumes:* Perfumery; *Other:* Deodorant, odor masking

BIRCH, TAR
BOTANICAL: *Family: Betulaceae; Genus: Betula; Species: Alba*
SOURCES: *Habitat:* Europe; *Part of the Plant:* Wood, bark
CHEMICAL CONSTITUENTS: Phenols, guaiacol, cresol, creosol, xylenol, pyrocatechol, betulin
CHARACTERISTICS: *Color:* Yellowish-brown; *Odor:* Woody, tarry, smokey, leather; *Taste:* Poisonous
PHYSICAL CONSTANTS: *Specific gravity:* 0.886–0.950; *Refractive index:* 1.5350–1.5380; *Boiling point:* 218–222 C
SOLUBILITY: Soluble in ether, chloroform, glacial acetic acid, amyl alcohol, benzene, carbon disulfide, turpentine
USES: *Perfumes:* Small quantities; *Medicine:* External use; *Other:* Disinfectant—preserving leather and wood
WARNING AND CAUTION: Poisonous

BORONIA (ABSOLUTE)
BOTANICAL: *Family: Rutaceae; Genus: Boronia; Species: Megastigma*
SOURCES: *Habitat:* Western Australia; *Part of the Plant:* Flowers
CHEMICAL CONSTITUENTS: beta-Ionone; alpha-ionone (little)
CHARACTERISTICS: *Color:* Dark green; *Odor:* Spicy, herbaceous, fruity, woody; *Taste:* Sweet
SOLUBILITY: Soluble in alcohol, ether, chloroform
USES: *Flavors:* Raspberry, strawberry, plum, peach, black currant; *Perfumes:* Chypre, fougere, violet, mimosa, honeysuckle, sweet pea; *Other:* Blend with clary sage, bergamot, costus, sandalwood, helichrysum, amylcinnamic aldehyde, linalool, salicylates, etc.

BROOM (ABSOLUTE)
BOTANICAL: *Family: Leguminosae; Genus: Spartium; Species: Genista*
SOURCES: *Habitat:* Mediterranean area; *Part of the Plant:* Flowers' blossom
CHARACTERISTICS: *Odor:* Hay-like; *Taste:* Sweet
PHYSICAL CONSTANTS: *Specific gravity:* 0.9335 (15 C); *Refractive index:* 1.4712; *Optical rotation:* –9 to –10
USES: *Perfumes:* Perfumes

BRUYERE (ABSOLUTE)
SYNONYMS: Brier, tree; heath, white heath; heather shrub
BOTANICAL: *Family: Ericaceae; Genus: Erica; Species: Arborea*
SOURCES: *Habitat:* Southern Europe; *Part of the Plant:* Roots
CHARACTERISTICS: *Odor:* Spicy, herbaceous, mild balsamic

USES: *Perfumes:* Chypre-type perfumes; *Other:* Pipes are made from the roots for smoking tobacco

BUCHU, LEAF

BOTANICAL: *Family: Rutaceae; Genus: Barosma; Species: Betulina, crenulata, seratifolia*

SOURCES: *Habitat:* South Africa; *Part of the Plant:* Fresh leaves

CHEMICAL CONSTITUENTS: Diosphenol (barosma champhor), diosmin, *l*-menthone, hesperidin, mucilage, resin

CHARACTERISTICS: *Odor:* Minty, champhor-like, strong, black currant reminiscent

PHYSICAL CONSTANTS: *Specific gravity:* 0.935–0.970; *Refractive index:* 1.4740–1.4870; *Optical rotation:* –15 to –25

USES: *Perfumes:* Perfumes in a small amount due to its intensity; *Medicine:* Antiseptic (urinary)

CABREUVA

BOTANICAL: *Family: Leguminosae; Genus: Myrocarpus; Species: Frondosus or fastigiatus*

SOURCES: *Habitat:* Southern Brazil, Paraguay, northern Argentina; *Part of the Plant:* Wood and sawdust

CHARACTERISTICS: *Odor:* Woody

PHYSICAL CONSTANTS: *Specific gravity:* 0.893; *Refractive index:* 1.4845; *Optical rotation:* +8 to 0

SOLUBILITY: Sol. in alcohol (6/70%)

USES: *Perfumes:* Perfumes of woody fragrance

CADE

SYNONYMS: Juniper wood; tar oil

BOTANICAL: *Family: Cupressaceae or Pinaceae or Coniferae; Genus: Juniperus; Species: Oxycedrus; Variety: Communis*

SOURCES: *Habitat:* Mainly in Europe; *Part of the Plant:* Wood

CHEMICAL CONSTITUENTS: 1-β-Caryophyllene, *l*-cadinene, cedrene, carvone, cresol, cadinol

CHARACTERISTICS: *Color:* Dark brown; *Odor:* Smoky, leathery, tarry; *Taste:* Burning

PHYSICAL CONSTANTS: *Specific gravity:* 0.952–0.961; *Refractive index:* 1.5110–1.5200; *Optical rotation:* +4.17 to +4.40

SOLUBILITY: Slightly soluble in water; soluble in ether, chloroform, glacial acetic acid; soluble in alcohol (0.5/90% to 5/95%)

USES: *Perfumes:* Perfumery, in small amount for leather, fougere, pine, basic compositions; soaps; *Pharmaceuticals:* Pharmaceuticals

WARNING AND CAUTION: Not for preserving catgut or silk

CAJEPUT

SYNONYMS: Cajuput

BOTANICAL: *Family: Myrtaceae; Genus: Melaleuca; Species: Leucadendron*

SOURCES: *Habitat:* Indonesia, Australia, Malaysia; *Part of the Plant:* Fresh leaves and twigs
CHEMICAL CONSTITUENTS: Eucalyptol (cineol) 50–60%, *l*-pinene, terpineol; valeric, butyric, benzoic aldehydes
CHARACTERISTICS: *Color:* Bluish-green (crude); colorless or yellowish (rectified); *Odor:* Camphor; *Taste:* Bitter, aromatic, burning
PHYSICAL CONSTANTS: *Specific gravity:* 0.912–0.925 (15 C); *Refractive index:* 1.4660–1.4710; *Optical rotation:* 0 to –4
SOLUBILITY: Slightly soluble in water; soluble in alcohol (1/80%), ether, chloroform, carbon disulfide, benzyl benzoate, fixed oils, diethyl phthalate; slightly soluble in mineral oils; insoluble in glycerin
USES: *Perfumes:* Perfumery; *Medicine:* Medicine

CALAMUS
SYNONYMS: Sweet flag
BOTANICAL: *Family: Araceae or Aroidae; Genus: Acorus; Species: Calamus*
SOURCES: *Habitat:* Korea, India, U.S.S.R.; *Part of the Plant:* Rhizomes
CHEMICAL CONSTITUENTS: Asarone (2,4,5-trimethoxy-1-propenylbenzene), eugenol, acetic acid, heptyl acid (esters)
CHARACTERISTICS: *Form:* Viscid; *Color:* Yellow to brownish; *Odor:* Aromatic; *Taste:* Bitter
PHYSICAL CONSTANTS: *Specific gravity:* 0.959–0.970 (15 C); *Refractive index:* 1.507–1.515; *Optical rotation:* +9 to +31
SOLUBILITY: Slightly soluble in water; soluble in alcohol
USES: *Flavors:* Liqueurs; *Perfumes:* Perfumery; *Medicine:* Medicine

CALENDULA (CONCRETE, ABSOLUTE)
BOTANICAL: *Family: Compositae; Genus: Calendula; Species: Officinalis*
SOURCES: *Habitat:* Europe, North America; *Part of the Plant:* Flowers
CHARACTERISTICS: *Odor:* Intense herbaceous
USES: Perfumes: Due to its scarcity is rarely employed in composition of perfumes

CAMPHOR
BOTANICAL: *Family: Lauraceae; Genus: Cinnamomum; Species: Camphora*
SOURCES: *Habitat:* Java, Sumatra, China, Japan, Formosa, Brazil; *Part of the Plant:* Wood
CHEMICAL CONSTITUENTS: *d*-Pinene, camphor, phellandrene, eucalyptol, eugenol, acetaldehyde, terpineol, cineol, cadinene
CHARACTERISTICS: *Color:* Colorless; *Odor:* Camphor; *Taste:* Bitter; in large amount is poisonous
PHYSICAL CONSTANTS: *Specific gravity:* 0.875–0.900; *Refractive index:* 1.465–1.470; *Optical rotation:* +9 to +24; *Melting point:* 175 C
SOLUBILITY: Insoluble in water; soluble in alcohol, ether, chloroform, oils
USES: Perfu*mes:* Mouth washes; *Medicine:* In solution as mild antiseptic, ointments; *Other:* Cheap soaps, shoe polish, deodorant for minerals and lubricating oils, detergents, solvent for paints

WARNING AND CAUTION: Large doses of camphor are poisonous, causing delirium and confusion

CANANGA

BOTANICAL: *Family: Anonaceae; Genus: Cananga or Uvaria; Species: Odorata*
SOURCES: *Habitat:* Madagascar, Java, Philippines, Comoro Islands; *Part of the Plant:* Flowers
CHEMICAL CONSTITUENTS: Linalyl benzoate, linalyl acetate, linalool, geraniol, nerol, farnesol, cadinene, eugenol
CHARACTERISTICS: *Odor:* Warm, floral, jasmine-like
PHYSICAL CONSTANTS: *Specific gravity:* 0.930–0.956; *Refractive index:* 1.495–1.505; *Optical rotation:* –25 to –19
USES: *Perfumes:* Perfumery

CARAWAY

BOTANICAL: *Family: Umbelliferae; Genus: Carum; Species: Carvi*
SOURCES: *Habitat:* Europe, mainly in Yugoslavia and Poland; *Part of the Plant:* Dried seeds
CHEMICAL CONSTITUENTS: *l*-Carvone 53–63%, *d*-limonene, carveol
CHARACTERISTICS: *Color:* Colorless or yellowish, darker and thicker on aging; *Odor:* Spicy, characteristic; *Taste:* Spicy
PHYSICAL CONSTANTS: *Specific gravity:* 0.900–0.910; *Refractive index:* 1.4840–1.4880; *Optical rotation:* +70 to +80; *Boiling point:* 175–230 C
SOLUBILITY: Slightly soluble in water; soluble in alcohol
USES: *Flavors:* Cookies, candies, liqueurs; *Perfumes:* Soaps; *Medicine:* As a carminative

CARDAMOM

BOTANICAL: *Family: Zingiberaceae; Genus: Elettaria; Species: Cardamomum* (Annomum, East Indies), *Rublatum, Bengala; Variety: Maton*
SOURCES: *Habitat:* Malabar, Ceylon, India, Tanzania, Guatemala; *Part of the Plant:* Seeds
CHEMICAL CONSTITUENTS: Terpinene, dipentene, limonene, eucalyptol, borneol, cineol, sabinene; *d*-α terpineol, *l*-terpinene-ol formate and acetate
CHARACTERISTICS: *Color:* Colorless or yellowish; *Odor:* Aromatic; *Taste:* Pleasant
PHYSICAL CONSTANTS: *Specific gravity:* 0.917–0.947; *Refractive index:* 1.4630–1.4660; *Optical rotation:* +22 to +44 (25 C)
SOLUBILITY: Insoluble in water; soluble in alcohol (4/70%)
USES: *Flavors:* Curry sauces, baked goods, liqueurs; *Pharmaceuticals:* Pharmaceutical syrups

CARROT

BOTANICAL: *Family: Umbelliferae; Genus: Daucus; Species: Carota*
SOURCES: *Habitat:* Oil produced only in France, Hungary, Yugoslavia, U.S.S.R.; *Part of the Plant:* Seeds

CHEMICAL CONSTITUENTS: Carotene, pinene, limonene; palmitic, butyric, isobutyric acids
CHARACTERISTICS: *Color:* Light yellow; *Odor:* Spicy; *Taste:* Spicy
PHYSICAL CONSTANTS: *Specific gravity:* 0.870–0.944; *Refractive index:* 1.482–1.491; *Optical rotation:* –8 to –37
SOLUBILITY: Soluble in alcohol
USES: *Flavors:* Liqueurs; *Perfumes:* Little amount

CASCARILLA
BOTANICAL: *Family: Euphorbiaceae; Genus: Croton; Species: Eluteria; Variety: Bennet*
SOURCES: *Habitat:* West Indies; *Part of the Plant:* Dried bark
CHEMICAL CONSTITUENTS: Cascarillic acid
CHARACTERISTICS: *Color:* Light yellow to brown-greenish; *Odor:* Spicy; *Taste:* Spicy
PHYSICAL CONSTANTS: *Specific gravity:* 0.890–0.925; *Refractive index:* 1.4885–1.4895; *Optical rotation:* +2 to +5
SOLUBILITY: Insoluble in water; soluble in alcohol, ether, fixed oils, mineral oils
USES: *Flavors:* Food, tobacco; *Medicine:* Medicine

CASSIA
SYNONYMS: Chinese cinnamon
BOTANICAL: *Family: Lauraceae; Genus: Cinnamomum; Species: Cassia*
SOURCES: *Habitat:* China, southeast Asia; *Part of the Plant:* Leaves, twigs, stalks
CHEMICAL CONSTITUENTS: Cinnamic aldehyde, cinnamic alcohol, phenyl propyl cinnamate, coumarin, benzaldehyde, salicylic aldehyde
CHARACTERISTICS: *Odor:* Intense spicy, characteristic of cinnamon; *Taste:* Spicy
PHYSICAL CONSTANTS: *Specific gravity:* 1.055–1.070; *Refractive index:* 1.602–1.606; *Optical rotation:* –1 to +6
SOLUBILITY: Soluble in alcohol (1–2/80%)
USES: *Flavors:* Flavors; *Perfumes:* Perfumes

CASSIE (CONCRETE, ABSOLUTE)
BOTANICAL: *Family: Leguminosae; Genus: Acacia; Species: Farnesiana*
SOURCES: *Habitat:* Mediterranean area, West Indies; *Part of the Plant:* Flowers
CHARACTERISTICS: *Odor:* Spicy-floral
PHYSICAL CONSTANTS: *Specific gravity:* 1.055–1.070; *Refractive index:* 1.5120–1.5140; *Optical rotation:* –1 to +6
USES: *Perfumes:* Fine perfumes, such as jasmine and rose

CASTOREUM
ZOOLOGICAL: *Family: Beaver; Genus: Castor; Species: Fiber*
SOURCES: *Habitat:* Canada, U.S.S.R.; *Part of the Body:* Pods of the secretion of the perineal glands of the beaver
CHARACTERISTICS: *Color:* Orange-brown, creamy; *Odor:* Strong leather-like; it becomes pleasant on dilution; *Taste:* Bitter

USES: *Perfumes:* As a tincture in fougere, chypre, and oriental-type perfumes

CEDARLEAF

SYNONYMS: Thuja
BOTANICAL: *Family: Pinaceae; Genus: Thuja; Species: Occidentalis*
SOURCES: *Habitat:* North America, Canada; *Part of the Plant:* Leaves
CHEMICAL CONSTITUENTS: α-Pinene, δ-thujone 60%, α-fenchone
CHARACTERISTICS: *Color:* Colorless, yellowish, or greenish; *Odor:* Lavender-like; *Taste:* Bitter, camphoraceous, toxic
PHYSICAL CONSTANTS: *Specific gravity:* 0.915–0.935 (15 C); *Refractive index:* 1.4560–1.4590; *Optical rotation:* –5 to +1.4 (25 C)
SOLUBILITY: Insoluble in water; soluble in alcohol (4/70%), ether, chloroform, carbon disulfide, fixed oils, mineral oils
USES: *Flavors:* Flavors; *Perfumes:* Perfumes; *Medicine:* Medicine; *Other:* Substitute for lavender oil
WARNING AND CAUTION: Toxic—ingestion of large amounts causes convulsion, death

CEDARWOOD

BOTANICAL: *Family: Pinaceae or Cupressaceae; Genus: Juniperus; Species: Virginiana*
SOURCES: *Habitat:* U.S.A.; *Part of the Plant:* Wood
CHEMICAL CONSTITUENTS: Cedrene, cedrol, cedrenol, cedryl acetate
CHARACTERISTICS: *Form:* Viscid; *Color:* Colorless, yellowish, or greenish; *Odor:* Persistent, agreeable; *Taste:* Acrid
PHYSICAL CONSTANTS: *Specific gravity:* 0.940–0.960 (15 C); *Refractive index:* 1.495–1.510; *Optical rotation:* –27 to –45
SOLUBILITY: Insoluble in water; soluble in alcohol (10–20/90%), ether, fixed oils
USES: *Perfumes:* Soaps; *Medicine:* Sanitary supplies; *Other:* Insect repellent, microscopy, lens clearing agent

CELERY

BOTANICAL: *Family: Umbelliferae; Genus: Apium; Species: Graveolens; Variety: Green or white*
SOURCES: *Habitat:* Central and eastern Europe, India, California; *Part of the Plant:* Seeds
CHEMICAL CONSTITUENTS: *d*-Limonene, phenols, sedanolide (tetrahydrobutyl phthalide), sedanolic acid
CHARACTERISTICS: *Color:* Colorless or greenish-yellow; *Odor:* Characteristic; *Taste:* Sweet spicy
PHYSICAL CONSTANTS: *Specific gravity:* 0.9236 (15 C); *Refractive index:* 1.478–1.486; *Optical rotation:* +60 to +82
SOLUBILITY: Slightly soluble in water; soluble in alcohol, ether, chloroform
USES: *Flavors:* Soft drinks; *Medicine:* Medicine

CHAMOMILE, GERMAN

BOTANICAL: *Family: Compositae; Genus: Matricaria; Species: Chamomile; Variety: Blue chamomile, German chamomile*
SOURCES: *Habitat:* Germany, Hungary, Egypt, U.S.S.R.; *Part of the Plant:* Flowers
CHEMICAL CONSTITUENTS: Amyl, butyl, butyric, angelic, tiglic acids and esters; anthemol, anthemene, azulene
CHARACTERISTICS: *Form:* Viscid butter-like; *Color:* Deep blue; it turns green or brown on exposure; *Odor:* Characteristic, herbaceous; *Taste:* Bitter, aromatic
PHYSICAL CONSTANTS: *Specific gravity:* 0.922–0.956; *Refractive index:* 1.364; *Optical rotation:* Slightly dextro
SOLUBILITY: Insoluble in water; soluble in alcohol (6/90%), fixed oils
USES: *Flavors:* Flavors; *Medicine:* Medicine

CHAMOMILE, ROMAN

BOTANICAL: *Family: Compositae; Genus: Anthemis; Species: Nobilis; Variety: Romana*
SOURCES: *Habitat:* England, Bulgaria, Yugoslavia, Hungary, France, Italy; *Part of the Plant:* Dried flowers
CHEMICAL CONSTITUENTS: Amyl, butyl, butyric, angelic, tiglic acids and esters; anthemol, anthemene, azulene
CHARACTERISTICS: *Color:* Light blue or greenish, turning brownish on exposure; *Odor:* Herbaceous, aromatic; *Taste:* Bitter, tea-like
PHYSICAL CONSTANTS: *Specific gravity:* 0.905–0.915; *Refractive index:* 1.442–1.448; *Optical rotation:* –2.30 to +3; *Boiling point:* 190 C
SOLUBILITY: Insoluble in water; soluble in alcohol (6–10/70% or 1/90%), fixed oils, mineral oils
USES: *Flavors:* Flavors; *Perfumes:* Perfumes; *Medicine:* Medicine

CHAMPACA (CONCRETE, ABSOLUTE)

BOTANICAL: *Family: Magnoliaceae; Genus: Michelia; Species: Champaca*
SOURCES: *Habitat:* Philippines, Indonesia; *Part of the Plant:* Flowers
CHEMICAL CONSTITUENTS: Benzoic acid and esters, benzaldehyde, benzyl alcohol, isoeugenol
CHARACTERISTICS: *Color:* Light yellow or reddish-yellow to brownish; *Odor:* Floral-herbaceous, magnolia-like
PHYSICAL CONSTANTS: *Specific gravity:* 0.906–0.935; *Refractive index:* 1.4640–1.4688; *Optical rotation:* –12 to –52
SOLUBILITY: Slightly soluble in water, alcohol; soluble in ether, chloroform
USES: *Perfumes:* Perfumery

CHENOPODIUM

BOTANICAL: *Family: Chenopodiaceae; Genus: Chenopodium; Species: Ambrosioides; Variety: Anthelminticum*
SOURCES: *Part of the Plant:* Fresh seeds and leaves
CHEMICAL CONSTITUENTS: Ascaridole 60–70%, *p*-cymene, α-terpinene, *l*-limonene, methadiene

CHARACTERISTICS: *Color:* Colorless or yellowish; *Odor:* Disagreeable, penetrating; *Taste:* Pungent, bitter, burning
PHYSICAL CONSTANTS: *Specific gravity:* 0.950–0.980; *Refractive index:* 1.4723–1.4790; *Optical rotation:* –4 to –8
SOLUBILITY: Insoluble in water; sol. in alcohol (8/70%); partially soluble in glacial acetic acid
USES: *Medicine:* Anthelmintic

CINNAMON, BARK
BOTANICAL: *Family: Lauraceae; Genus: Cinnamomum; Species: Ceylanicum; Variety: Breyne*
SOURCES: *Habitat:* Sri Lanka, Madagascar, southern India, Comoro Islands, Seychelles; *Part of the Plant:* Bark
CHEMICAL CONSTITUENTS: Cinnamic aldehyde 70%, eugenol 18%, phellandrene, benzaldehyde, linalool, camphor
CHARACTERISTICS: *Color:* Light yellow turning reddish on aging; *Odor:* Spicy; *Taste:* Spicy
PHYSICAL CONSTANTS: *Specific gravity:* 1.014–1.040; *Refractive index:* 1.569–1.584
SOLUBILITY: Insoluble in water; soluble in alcohol (1–2/80%), all oils
USES: *Flavors:* Flavors; *Perfumes:* Perfumes; *Medicine:* As a carminative

CINNAMON, LEAF
BOTANICAL: *Family: Lauraceae; Genus: Cinnamomum; Species: Ceylanicum; Variety: Breyne*
SOURCES: *Habitat:* Sri Lanka, southern India, Madagascar, Seychelles and Comoro Islands; *Part of the Plant:* Leaves and twigs
CHEMICAL CONSTITUENTS: Cinnamic alcohol, safrole, linalool, cinnamic aldehyde 6%, cinnamyl acetate 6%, eugenol 70–90%, benzyl benzoate, cinnamyl formate, α-methyl cinnamic aldehyde
CHARACTERISTICS: *Color:* Yellowish or brownish, turning darker and thicker on exposure; *Odor:* Cinnamon; *Taste:* Pungent
PHYSICAL CONSTANTS: *Specific gravity:* 1.045–1.063; *Refractive index:* 1.525–1.540; *Optical rotation:* 1.30–2
SOLUBILITY: Slightly soluble in water; sol. in alcohol (equal volumes), glacial acetic acid, oils
USES: *Flavors:* Foods; *Perfumes:* Perfumes; *Medicine:* As a carminative

CISTUS (RESINOID)
SYNONYMS: Labdanum
BOTANICAL: *Family: Cistaceae; Genus: Cistus; Species: Ladaniferus*
SOURCES: *Habitat:* Mediterranean area: Spain, Portugal, southern France; *Part of the Plant:* Gum from leaves and twigs of the shrubs
CHARACTERISTICS: *Odor:* Ambra-like, warm spicy, balsamic
PHYSICAL CONSTANTS: *Specific gravity:* 0.947–0.980; *Refractive index:* 1.4919–1.5048; *Optical rotation:* +2.20 to +6.32
USES: *Perfumes:* Perfumes

CITRONELLA

BOTANICAL: *Family: Graminaceae; Genus: Cymbopogon or Andropogon; Species: Nardus*

SOURCES: *Habitat:* China, Taiwan, Indonesia, Ceylon, Java, Brazil, Colombia, Guatemala; *Part of the Plant:* Grass

CHEMICAL CONSTITUENTS: Ceylon: Geraniol 60%, citronellal 15%, camphene 10–15%, dipentene, linalool, borneol; Java: Geraniol 25–45%, citronellal 25–50%

CHARACTERISTICS: *Color:* Colorless to pale yellow turning reddish on aging; *Odor:* Lemon-like; *Taste:* Bitter, pungent

PHYSICAL CONSTANTS: Ceylon: *Specific gravity:* 0.897–0.912; *Refractive index:* 1.479–1.485; *Optical rotation:* –6 to –14; Java: *Specific gravity:* 0.885–0.900; *Refractive index:* 1.468–1.472; *Optical rotation:* –2 to –5

SOLUBILITY: Slightly soluble in water; soluble in alcohol (10/80%)

USES: *Perfumes:* For soaps; *Medicine:* Medicine; *Other:* Insect repellent, disinfectants, denatured alcohol; source of citronellal, geraniol

CIVET (ABSOLUTE)

ZOOLOGICAL: *Family: Viverridae; Genus: Civettictis; Species: civetta*

SOURCES: *Habitat:* Ethiopia; *Part of the Body:* Glandular secretion from a pouch near the sexual organ of the civet cat

CHARACTERISTICS: *Color:* Yellowish; *Odor:* Powerful musky

PHYSICAL CONSTANTS: *Specific gravity:* 0.9135; *Refractive index:* 1.4666–1.4678; *Optical rotation:* ± 0.4

USES: *Perfumes:* Perfumes

CLARY SAGE (ABSOLUTE)

BOTANICAL: *Family: Labiatae; Genus: Salvia; Species: Sclarea*

SOURCES: *Habitat:* France, Spain, U.S.S.R.; *Part of the Plant:* Flowering tops

CHEMICAL CONSTITUENTS: Linalyl acetate, linalool, nerolidol, santalene

CHARACTERISTICS: *Color:* Yellowish or greenish-yellow; *Odor:* Spicy, hay-like, citrus reminiscent; *Taste:* Camphoraceous

PHYSICAL CONSTANTS: *Specific gravity:* 0.900–0.910; *Refractive index:* 1.4613–1.4700; *Optical rotation:* –11.22 to –32.38

SOLUBILITY: Soluble in alcohol (1/80%)

USES: *Perfumes:* Fougere, chypre, colognes

CLOVE BUD

BOTANICAL: *Family: Myrtaceae; Genus: Eugenia; Species: Caryophyllata (Caryophyllus aromaticus)*

SOURCES: *Habitat:* Indonesia, Sri Lanka, Madagascar, Tanzania, Zanzibar; *Part of the Plant:* Dried buds

CHEMICAL CONSTITUENTS: Eugenol 82–87%, acetyl eugenol 10%, cayophyllene, furfural, vanillin, methyl amyl ketone

CHARACTERISTICS: *Color:* Colorless to pale yellow, turning darker and thicker on exposure or aging; *Odor:* Characteristic of clove; *Taste:* Pungent spicy

PHYSICAL CONSTANTS: *Specific gravity:* 1.038–1.060; *Refractive index:* 1.530–

1.535; *Optical rotation:* –1 to –10
SOLUBILITY: Insoluble in water; soluble in alcohol (2/70%), ether, glacial acetic acid
USES: *Flavors:* Flavors; *Perfumes:* Tooth powders, dentifrices, soaps; *Medicine:* Microscopy; *Other:* Source of vanillin (via isoeugenol)

CLOVE LEAF
BOTANICAL: *Family: Myrtaceae; Genus: Eugenia; Species: Caryophyllata*
SOURCES: *Habitat:* Indonesia, Tanzania, Madagascar, Sri Lanka; *Part of the Plant:* Leaves
CHEMICAL CONSTITUENTS: Eugenol, acetyl eugenol, caryophyllene, furfural (all in smaller amounts than the buds)
CHARACTERISTICS: *Color:* Colorless to pale yellow; *Odor:* Clove characteristic; *Taste:* Pungent spicy
PHYSICAL CONSTANTS: *Specific gravity:* 1.036–1.044; *Refractive index:* 1.5312–1.5339; *Optical rotation:* –0.40 to +1.36
SOLUBILITY: Soluble in alcohol (1/70%)
USES: *Perfumes:* As a spicy-herbaceous perfume

COPAIBA BALSAM
BOTANICAL: *Family: Leguminosae; Genus: Copaifera; Species: Officinalis*
SOURCES: *Habitat:* Brazil, Venezuela, Colombia, Amazon Valley, Orinoco Banks; *Part of the Plant:* Balsam from oleoresin
CHEMICAL CONSTITUENTS: Caryophyllene, illuric, metacopaivic acid (Maracaibo balsam), copaivic and oxycopaivic acids (Peru balsam)
CHARACTERISTICS: *Color:* Colorless to yellowish or bluish; *Odor:* Pepper-like; *Taste:* Bitter
PHYSICAL CONSTANTS: *Specific gravity:* 0.88–0.91 (15 C); *Refractive index:* 1.494–1.500; *Optical rotation:* –7 to –33; *Boiling point:* 250–275 C
SOLUBILITY: Insoluble in water; soluble in alcohol (5–6/95%), ether, chloroform, carbon disulfide, oils
USES: *Flavors:* Flavors; *Perfumes:* Perfumes, fixative; *Medicine:* Medicine

CORIANDER
BOTANICAL: *Family: Umbelliferae; Genus: Coriandrum; Species: Sativum*
SOURCES: *Habitat:* Southeastern Europe, France, Italy, Morocco, Tunisia, U.S.S.R., India; *Part of the Plant:* Dried fruits
CHEMICAL CONSTITUENTS: *d*-Linalool and acetate, pinene
CHARACTERISTICS: *Color:* Colorless or pale; *Odor:* Spicy, aromatic; *Taste:* Spicy
PHYSICAL CONSTANTS: *Specific gravity:* 0.863–0.875; *Refractive index:* 1.4620–1.4720; *Optical rotation:* +8 to +13
SOLUBILITY: Soluble in alcohol (3/70%), ether, chloroform, glacial acetic acid
USES: *Flavors:* Flavors, food, alcoholic beverages; *Medicine:* As a carminative

COSTUS
BOTANICAL: *Family: Compositae; Genus: Saussurea; Species: Lappa*
SOURCES: *Habitat:* China, India, Himalaya; *Part of the Plant:* Roots

CHEMICAL CONSTITUENTS: Phellandrene, camphene, costus acid, costus lactone, ionone
CHARACTERISTICS: *Odor:* Woody, slightly animalic
PHYSICAL CONSTANTS: *Specific gravity:* 1.000–1.045; *Refractive index:* 1.5159–1.5280; *Optical rotation:* +12 to +14.14
SOLUBILITY: Soluble in alcohol (0.5/90%)
USES: *Perfumes:* Scarcely employed in perfumery

CRAVO
BOTANICAL: *Family: Rutaceae; Genus: Citrus; Species: Aurantium; Variety: Reticulata*
SOURCES: *Habitat:* Brazil; *Part of the Plant:* Ripe fruits' peels
CHARACTERISTICS: *Odor:* Fresh fruity orange-mandarin-like
USES: *Perfumes:* Cologne-type

CUBEB
BOTANICAL: *Family: Piperaceae; Genus: Piper; species: Cubeba; Variety: Singapore*
SOURCES: *Habitat:* Singapore; *Part of the Plant:* Unripe fruits
CHEMICAL CONSTITUENTS: *d-l*-Limonene, pinene, cadinene, camphor, dipentene
CHARACTERISTICS: *Color:* Colorless, pale greenish, or yellowish; *Odor:* Pepper; *Taste:* Warm camphoraceous
PHYSICAL CONSTANTS: *Specific gravity:* 0.905–0.925; *Refractive index:* 1.480–1.502; *Optical rotation:* –20 to –40
SOLUBILITY: Insoluble in water; soluble in alcohol (10 volumes), ether, chloroform
USES: *Flavors:* Flavors; *Medicine:* Urinary antiseptic

CUMIN
BOTANICAL: *Family: Umbelliferae; Genus: Cuminum; Species: Cyminum*
SOURCES: *Habitat:* Mediterranean area, India; *Part of the Plant:* Fruits
CHEMICAL CONSTITUENTS: Cuminaldehyde 30–40%, *p*-cymene, β-pinene, dipentene, cumene
CHARACTERISTICS: *Color:* Colorless to yellow; *Odor:* Strong spicy-green with anise reminiscence; *Taste:* Sharp, spicy
PHYSICAL CONSTANTS: *Specific gravity:* 0.900–0.935; *Refractive index:* 1.495–1.509; *Optical rotation:* +4 to +8
SOLUBILITY: Insoluble in water; soluble in alcohol (10/80%)
USES: *Flavors:* Food flavoring; *Perfumes:* Perfumery

CURCUMA
SYNONYMS: Turmeric
BOTANICAL: *Family: Scitaminaceae; Genus: Curcuma; Species: Longa; Variety: Aromatica*
SOURCES: *Habitat:* Southern Asia, India, Korea; *Part of the Plant:* Dried rhizomes
CHARACTERISTICS: *Odor:* Spicy, fresh fruity
PHYSICAL CONSTANTS: *Specific gravity:* 0.930–0.969 (15 C); *Refractive index:* 1.5030; *Optical rotation:* –25 to +8.6

USES: *Perfumes:* Scarcely used; *Other:* Condiment, coloring from the rhizomes (curcumin)

CYPRESS

BOTANICAL: *Family: Pinaceae or Coniferae; Genus: Cupressus; Species: Sempervirens*

SOURCES: *Habitat:* Mediterranean area, mainly in Algeria and southern France; *Part of the Plant:* Leaves and twigs, fresh shoots

CHEMICAL CONSTITUENTS: Furfural, δ-pinene, δ-camphene, cymene, δ-terpineol, *l*-cadinene, sylvestrene, camphor

CHARACTERISTICS: *Color:* Yellowish; *Odor:* Pine-like; *Taste:* Camphoraceous

PHYSICAL CONSTANTS: *Specific gravity:* 0.88–0.89; *Refractive index:* 1.474–1.480; *Optical rotation:* +4 to +18; *Boiling point:* 160–250 C

SOLUBILITY: Slightly soluble in water; soluble in alcohol (2–6/90%), chloroform

USES: *Perfumes:* Perfumes; *Medicine:* Medicine

DAVANA

BOTANICAL: *Family: Compositae; Genus: Artemisia; Species: Pallens*

SOURCES: *Habitat:* Southern India; *Part of the Plant:* Herb

CHARACTERISTICS: *Odor:* Herbaceous, tea-like, with whiskey reminiscence

PHYSICAL CONSTANTS: *Specific gravity:* 0.961–0.990 (15 C); *Refractive index:* 1.4874–1.5003; *Optical rotation:* –25 to –48

SOLUBILITY: Soluble in alcohol (10/70%)

USES: *Perfumes:* Scarcely employed

DILL

BOTANICAL: *Family: Umbelliferae; Genus: Anethum or Peucedanum; Species: Graveolens*

SOURCES: *Habitat:* U.S.A. and Balkans; *Part of the Plant:* Crushed dried fruits and seeds

CHEMICAL CONSTITUENTS: Carvone 50%, *d*-limonene, phellandrene, terpenes

CHARACTERISTICS: *Color:* Colorless or pale yellow; *Odor:* Spicy, reminiscent of mint; *Taste:* Sweet spicy

PHYSICAL CONSTANTS: *Specific gravity:* 0.900–0.915; *Refractive index:* 1.481–1.492; *Optical rotation:* +70 to +80

SOLUBILITY: Insoluble in water; soluble in alcohol (1/90%)

USES: *Flavors:* Flavoring; *Perfumes:* Perfumery; *Medicine:* As a carminative

DWARF PINE

BOTANICAL: *Family: Pinaceae; Genus: Pinus; Species: Pumilio; Variety: Montana, mugho*

SOURCES: *Habitat:* European Alps; *Part of the Plant:* Fresh leaves

CHEMICAL CONSTITUENTS: *l*-Pinene, *l*-phellandrene, sylvestrene, dipentene, cadinene, bornyl acetate 5–7%

CHARACTERISTICS: *Color:* Colorless or pale yellow; *Odor:* Pine-like, pleasant, aromatic; *Taste:* Bitter pungent

PHYSICAL CONSTANTS: *Specific gravity:* 0.853–0.869; *Refractive index:* 1.4750–1.4800; *Optical rotation:* –5 to –12 (25 C)
SOLUBILITY: Insoluble in water; soluble in ether, chloroform
USES: *Flavors:* Flavors; *Perfumes:* Perfumery; *Medicine:* Medicine

ELEMI (RESINOID)
BOTANICAL: *Family: Burseraceae or Terebinthaceae; Genus: Canarium or Villosum; Species: Luzonicum or commune*
SOURCES: *Habitat:* Philippines; *Part of the Plant:* Gum of Manila elemi tree
CHEMICAL CONSTITUENTS: Phellandrene, *d*-limonene
CHARACTERISTICS: *Color:* Colorless or pale yellow; *Odor:* Fresh lemon-like; *Taste:* Spicy, peppery green
PHYSICAL CONSTANTS: *Specific gravity:* 0.870–0.910; *Refractive index:* 1.479–1.489; *Optical rotation:* +35 to +55
SOLUBILITY: Soluble in alcohol, ether, chloroform, carbon disulfide
USES: *Flavors:* Flavors; *Perfumes:* Perfumes as freshener; *Medicine:* Medicine

ESTRAGON
SYNONYMS: Tarragon
BOTANICAL: *Family: Compositae; Genus: Artemisia; Species: Dracunculus*
SOURCES: *Habitat:* Italy, Yugoslavia, France, Spain; *Part of the Plant:* Whole plant
CHEMICAL CONSTITUENTS: Estragole, ocimene, phellandrene
CHARACTERISTICS: *Odor:* Anise-like, herbaceous; *Taste:* Celery-like
PHYSICAL CONSTANTS: *Specific gravity:* 0.920–0.940; *Refractive index:* 1.5028–1.5138; *Optical rotation:* +2 to +9
USES: *Perfumes:* Fresh spicy base

EUCALYPTUS CITRIODORA
BOTANICAL: *Family: Myrtaceae; Genus: Eucalyptus; Species: Citriodora*
SOURCES: *Habitat:* Australia, Europe, northern Africa, southern U.S.A., Brazil, South Africa, China, India; *Part of the Plant:* Leaves and twigs
CHEMICAL CONSTITUENTS: Limonene, dipentene, citronellal, geraniol, pinene, cineol, isopulegol, guaiacol
CHARACTERISTICS: *Odor:* Rose-like with citronella reminiscence
PHYSICAL CONSTANTS: *Specific gravity:* 0.862–0.874; *Refractive index:* 1.450–1.459; *Optical rotation:* –1 to +8.5
SOLUBILITY: Soluble in alcohol (1.5–4.2/70%)
USES: *Perfumes:* Household products; *Other:* Source of citronellal

EUCALYPTUS DIVES
BOTANICAL: *Family: Myrtaceae; Genus: Eucalyptus; Species: Dives*
SOURCES: *Habitat:* Australia; *Part of the Plant:* Leaves and twigs
CHEMICAL CONSTITUENTS: Piperitone, phellandrene
CHARACTERISTICS: *Odor:* Mint-like, with fresh grass reminiscence
PHYSICAL CONSTANTS: *Specific gravity:* 0.8630–0.8772; *Refractive index:* 1.4784–1.4812; *Optical rotation:* 43–78

SOLUBILITY: Soluble in alcohol (1.3–10/70%)
USES: *Flavors:* Flavors; *Other:* Source of piperitone

EUCALYPTUS GLOBULUS
BOTANICAL: *Family: Myrtaceae; Genus: Eucalyptus; Species: Globulus*
SOURCES: *Habitat:* Australia, Spain, Portugal; *Part of the Plant:* Fresh leaves and twigs
CHEMICAL CONSTITUENTS: Cineol (eucalpytol) 70–90%, α-pinene, phellandrene, terpineol, citronellal, geranyl acetate, eudesmol, eudesmyl acetate, piperitone, isovaleric aldehyde
CHARACTERISTICS: *Color:* Colorless or pale yellow; *Odor:* Camphoraceous; *Taste:* Spicy, pungent, cooling
PHYSICAL CONSTANTS: *Specific gravity:* 0.905–0.925; *Refractive index:* 1.4580–1.4700; *Optical rotation:* –5 to +5; *Melting point:* –15.4 C
SOLUBILITY: Insoluble in water; soluble in alcohol (5/70%), oils, fats
USES: *Flavors:* Flavors; *Perfumes:* Perfumery, soaps; *Medicine:* Expectorant; dressing for wounds

EUCALYPTUS STAIGERIANA
BOTANICAL: *Family: Myrtaceae; Genus: Eucalyptus; Species: Staigeriana*
SOURCES: *Habitat:* Australia, Brazil; *Part of the Plant:* Leaves
CHEMICAL CONSTITUENTS: Citral, *l*-limonene, geraniol, geranyl acetate, sesquiterpenes
CHARACTERISTICS: *Odor:* Lemon fresh; *Taste:* Herbaceous
PHYSICAL CONSTANTS: *Specific gravity:* 0.871–0.883 (15 C); *Refractive index:* 1.4793–1.4814; *Optical rotation:* –26.4 to +37.5
SOLUBILITY: Soluble in alcohol (1–8/80%)
USES: *Perfumes:* Citrus-type; *Other:* Source of citral

FENNEL BITTER (WILD)
BOTANICAL: *Family: Umbelliferae; Genus: Foeniculum (Anethum foeniculum); Species: Vulgare; Variety: Amara*
SOURCES: *Habitat:* Mediterranean area; *Part of the Plant:* Seeds
CHEMICAL CONSTITUENTS: Anethole 60%, fenchene 20%, pinene, limonene, dipentene, phellandrene, camphene
CHARACTERISTICS: *Color:* Colorless or pale yellow; *Odor:* Aromatic, camphor-like; *Taste:* Bitter, changing to sweetish and spicy
PHYSICAL CONSTANTS: *Specific gravity:* 0.953–0.973 (15 C); *Refractive index:* 1.528–1.538; *Optical rotation:* +12 to +24; *Congealing point:* 3 C
SOLUBILITY: Insoluble in water; soluble in alcohol (1/90% or 5/80%), ether, chloroform
USES: *Flavors:* Liqueurs; *Perfumes:* Perfumes; *Medicine:* As a carminative; to cover unpleasant taste of medicines; *Other:* Source of anethole

FENNEL SWEET
BOTANICAL: *Family: Umbelliferae; Genus: Foeniculum (Anethum foeniculum); Species: Vulgare; Variety: Dulce*

SOURCES: *Habitat:* Mediterranean area; *Part of the Plant:* Seeds
CHEMICAL CONSTITUENTS: Anethole 60%, fenchene 20%, pinene, limonene, dipentene, phellandrene, camphene
CHARACTERISTICS: *Odor:* Characteristic anise-like; *Taste:* Sweet
PHYSICAL CONSTANTS: *Specific gravity:* 0.976–0.980; *Refractive index:* 1.5250–1.5370; *Optical rotation:* +5 to +16.30; *Congealing point:* 10–14.5 C
SOLUBILITY: Insoluble in water; soluble in alcohol (1/90% or 5/80%), ether, chloroform
USES: *Flavors:* Liqueurs; *Perfumes:* Herbaceous type; *Other:* Source of anethole

FENUGREEK (RESINOID)
BOTANICAL: *Family: Leguminosae; Genus: Trigonella; Species: Foenumgraecum*
SOURCES: *Habitat:* Southeastern Europe, Middle East, northern Africa, India; *Part of the Plant:* Seeds
CHEMICAL CONSTITUENTS: Trigonellin (alkaloid), sapogenin dioscenin (steroid)
CHARACTERISTICS: *Odor:* Woody; *Taste:* Walnut-like
USES: *Flavors:* Flavoring, in small amount in various types of culinary spices (no curry); *Medicine:* Emollient and flavoring agent in medicine; *Other:* Maple syrup imitation

FIR NEEDLE
BOTANICAL: *Family: Pinaceae; Genus: Abies; Species: Alba; Variety: Balsamea, pectinata, picea*
SOURCES: *Habitat:* Canada; *Part of the Plant:* Needles and twigs
CHEMICAL CONSTITUENTS: *l*-Pinene, *l*-limonene, *l*-bornyl acetate
CHARACTERISTICS: *Color:* Colorless to yellowish; *Odor:* Balsamic; *Taste:* Camphoraceous
PHYSICAL CONSTANTS: *Specific gravity:* 0.860–0.875 (15 C); *Refractive index:* 1.4730–1.4760; *Optical rotation:* –20 to +24
SOLUBILITY: Insoluble in water; soluble in alcohol (5/90%), ether, fixed oils
USES: *Flavors:* Flavors; *Perfumes:* Perfumes; *Medicine:* Expectorant

FIR NEEDLE, SIBERIAN
BOTANICAL: *Family: Pinaceae; Genus: Abies; Species: Siberica*
SOURCES: *Habitat:* Siberia; *Part of the Plant:* Fresh leaves and twigs
CHEMICAL CONSTITUENTS: Bornyl acetate, pinene, camphene, dipentene, phellandrene
CHARACTERISTICS: *Color:* Colorless to yellowish; *Odor:* Camphoraceous; *Taste:* Pungent
PHYSICAL CONSTANTS: *Specific gravity:* 0.905–0.925 (15 C); *Refractive index:* 1.466–1.476; *Optical rotation:* –32 to +45
SOLUBILITY: Insoluble in water; soluble in alcohol (equal volumes 90%), fixed oils
USES: *Flavors:* Flavors; *Perfumes:* Perfumes; *Medicine:* Expectorant

FLEABANE

SYNONYMS: Erigeron
BOTANICAL: *Family: Compositae; Genus: Coryza, Erigeron, Leptilon; Species: Canadensis*
SOURCES: *Habitat:* Canada; *Part of the Plant:* Flowering herbs
CHEMICAL CONSTITUENTS: *d*-Limonene, terpineol, aldehydes
CHARACTERISTICS: *Color:* Yellowish, turning darker and thicker on exposure and aging; *Odor:* Aromatic persistent; *Taste:* Slightly pungent
PHYSICAL CONSTANTS: *Specific gravity:* 0.845–0.865; *Optical rotation:* +45 to +83; *Boiling point:* 175–180 C
SOLUBILITY: Soluble in alcohol (equal volumes), ether, chloroform
USES: *Flavors:* Flavoring

FLOUVE

BOTANICAL: *Family: Graminaceae; Genus: Anthoxanthum; Species: Odoratum; Variety: Sweet vernal grass*
SOURCES: *Habitat:* Southern France; *Part of the Plant:* Dried grass
CHARACTERISTICS: *Odor:* Herbaceous hay-like, reminiscent of mimosa
USES: *Perfumes:* Fougere, chypre, oriental types

GALBANUM (RESINOID)

BOTANICAL: *Family: Umbelliferae; Genus: Rubricaulis or Peucedarum; Species: Galbaniflora, galbaniflorum, or galbaniflua; Variety: Ferula*
SOURCES: *Habitat:* Iran; *Part of the Plant:* Gum by solvent extraction
CHEMICAL CONSTITUENTS: Pinene, cadinene, dipentene, cadinol
CHARACTERISTICS: *Odor:* Woody, pine needle-like, balsamic; *Taste:* Spicy, bitter, acrid
PHYSICAL CONSTANTS: *Specific gravity:* 0.890–0.955; *Refractive index:* 1.4820–1.506; *Optical rotation:* –10 to +20
USES: *Perfumes:* Herbaceous and pine type

GARDENIA

BOTANICAL: *Family: Rubiaceae; Genus: Gardenia; Species: Grandiflora; Variety: Jasminoides*
SOURCES: *Part of the Plant:* Flowers
CHEMICAL CONSTITUENTS: Benzyl acetate, linalool, methyl anthranilate, linalyl acetate, terpineol, methyl phenyl carbinyl acetate
USES: *Perfumes:* Perfumery; *Other:* Due to the very little yield (about 1 kg from 500 kg of flowers) the extraction of essential oil, concrete, or absolute, is very limited.

GARLIC

BOTANICAL: *Family: Liliaceae; Genus: Allium; Species: Sativum*
SOURCES: *Part of the Plant:* Bulb and the entire plant
CHEMICAL CONSTITUENTS: Diethyl disulfide, allyl propyl disulfide, allyl sulfide, diallyl disulfide, diallyl trisulfide, diallyl polysulfide
CHARACTERISTICS: *Form:* Liquid; *Color:* Pale or yellowish; *Odor:* Strong, sulfur-

like, penetrating; *Taste:* Strong, sulfur-like
PHYSICAL CONSTANTS: *Specific gravity:* 1.055–1.098 (15 C); *Refractive index:* 1.5578–1.5745; *Optical rotation:* inactive ± 0
SOLUBILITY: Soluble in alcohol, ether, carbon disulfide
USES: *Medicine:* Anthelmintic, rubefacient, bactericide

GERANIUM
BOTANICAL: *Family: Geraniaceae; Genus: Pelargonium; Species: Odoratissimum, roseum, graveolens, capitatum*
SOURCES: *Habitat:* Morocco, Egypt, U.S.S.R., France, China, Reunion, Madagascar, Algeria; *Part of the Plant:* Leaves and stalks harvested when the plant is in blossom
CHEMICAL CONSTITUENTS: Geraniol, linalool, citronellol, rhodinol
CHARACTERISTICS: *Color:* Colorless, greenish, or brownish; *Odor:* Rose-like
PHYSICAL CONSTANTS: *Specific gravity:* 0.894–0.905 (15 C); *Refractive index:* 1.465–1.470; *Optical rotation:* –7 to –11
SOLUBILITY: Slightly soluble in water; soluble in alcohol (3/10%), ether, chloroform
USES: *Flavors:* Flavors; *Perfumes:* Perfumery; *Other:* Source of geraniol and rhodinol

GINGER
BOTANICAL: *Family: Zingiberaceae; Genus: Zingiber; Species: Officinalis (Amonum zingiber)*
SOURCES: *Habitat:* India, China, western Africa, West Indies; *Part of the Plant:* Dried rhizomes
CHEMICAL CONSTITUENTS: *l*-Zingiberene, zingerone, *d*-camphene, cineol, borneol, citral, phellandrene, aldehyde C-12 MNA
CHARACTERISTICS: *Form:* Viscid; *Color:* Yellowish; *Odor:* Aromatic; *Taste:* Burning
PHYSICAL CONSTANTS: *Specific gravity:* 0.875–0.885 (15 C); *Refractive index:* 1.4880–1.4950; *Optical rotation:* –25 to –45
SOLUBILITY: Insoluble in water; slightly soluble in alcohol; soluble in ether, carbon disulfide, benzyl benzoate, diethyl phthalate, mineral oils
USES: *Flavors:* Liqueurs, soft drinks, flavors; *Other:* Mouthwashes

GINGERGRASS
BOTANICAL: *Family: Graminaceae; Genus: Cymbopogon; Species: Martini; Variety: Sofia*
SOURCES: *Habitat:* India; *Part of the Plant:* Fresh grass
CHEMICAL CONSTITUENTS: *d*-Limonene, dipentene, *d*-α-phellandrene, *d-l*-carvone, geraniol
CHARACTERISTICS: *Odor:* Herbaceous-rosy, reminiscent of bread when dry
PHYSICAL CONSTANTS: *Specific gravity:* 0.900–0.953 (15 C); *Refractive index:* 1.4780–1.4930; *Optical rotation:* +54 to 30
SOLUBILITY: Soluble in alcohol (2–3/70% or 0.5–1.5/80%)
USES: *Perfumes:* Little amount employed in perfumery

GRAPEFRUIT

SYNONYMS: Shaddock
BOTANICAL: *Family: Rutaceae; Genus: Citrus; Species: Decumana*
SOURCES: *Habitat:* Israel, U.S.A.; *Part of the Plant:* Peels' fruits
CHEMICAL CONSTITUENTS: α-Pinene, *d*-limonene, linalool, citral, geraniol
CHARACTERISTICS: *Odor:* Citrus; *Taste:* Fresh, bitter
PHYSICAL CONSTANTS: *Specific gravity:* 0.855–0.860; *Refractive index:* 1.4750–1.4785; *Optical rotation:* +91.45 to +94.36
SOLUBILITY: 90% insoluble in alcohol
USES: *Flavors:* Nonalcoholic beverages; *Perfumes:* Colognes

GUAIACWOOD

BOTANICAL: *Family: Zygophyllaceae; Genus: Bulnesia; Species: Sarmienti*
SOURCES: *Habitat:* Paraguay, Argentina; *Part of the Plant:* Branches, wood, sawdust
CHEMICAL CONSTITUENTS: Guaiol, bulnesol (sesquiterpenes)
CHARACTERISTICS: *Odor:* Balsamic; *Taste:* Sweet, tea-like
PHYSICAL CONSTANTS: *Specific gravity:* 0.965–0.970; *Refractive index:* 1.5030–1.5040; *Optical rotation:* –6 to –7
SOLUBILITY: Insoluble in water; soluble in alcohol, ether, chloroform
USES: *Perfumes:* Household products

GURJUN (BALSAM)

BOTANICAL: *Family: Diperocarpaceae; Genus: Dipterocarpus; Species: Turbinatus or tuberculatus*
SOURCES: *Habitat:* Southeastern Asia, mainly in India; *Part of the Plant:* Balsam from the trunk of the tree
CHARACTERISTICS: *Form:* Viscous; *Color:* Yellow; *Odor:* Woody, reminiscent of patchouli
PHYSICAL CONSTANTS: *Specific gravity:* 0.95–0.97; *Refractive index:* 1.510–1.516
SOLUBILITY: Solubility in alcohol (not completely 90%, 7–10/95%)
USES: *Perfumes:* As a fixative

HELICHRYSUM (CONCRETE, ABSOLUTE)

BOTANICAL: *Family: Compositae; Genus: Helichrysum; Species: Angustifolium*
SOURCES: *Habitat:* Italy and all Mediterranean area; *Part of the Plant:* Herb
CHEMICAL CONSTITUENTS: Neryl acetate, *d*-α-pinene, nerol
CHARACTERISTICS: *Odor:* Honey-like, with a chamomile and tea reminiscence
PHYSICAL CONSTANTS: *Specific gravity:* 0.901–0.911 (15 C); *Refractive index:* 1.4735–1.4759; *Optical rotation:* –2.20 to +0.10
SOLUBILITY: Soluble in alcohol (0.5/90%)
USES: *Perfumes:* Herbaceous type; *Other:* Isolation of nerol

HOP

BOTANICAL: *Family: Moraceae or Cannabinaceae; Genus: Humulus; Species: Lupulus; Variety: Americanus*

SOURCES: *Habitat:* Germany, eastern Europe, America; *Part of the Plant:* Ripe and fresh flower tops
CHEMICAL CONSTITUENTS: Humulene 65–70% (α-caryophyllene), geraniol
CHARACTERISTICS: *Color:* Yellowish to brownish; *Odor:* Strong penetrating; *Taste:* Pungent
PHYSICAL CONSTANTS: *Specific gravity:* 0.855–0.880 (15 C); *Refractive index:* 1.4775–1.490; *Optical rotation:* –2 to +2
SOLUBILITY: Insoluble in water; slightly soluble in alcohol; soluble in ether
USES: *Flavors:* Aromatizing beer and tobacco; flavoring agent

HYACINTH (ABSOLUTE)
BOTANICAL: *Family: Lilyaceae; Genus: Hyacinthus; Species: Orientalis*
SOURCES: *Habitat:* Extensively cultivated in Holland; *Part of the Plant:* Flowers' blossom
CHEMICAL CONSTITUENTS: Benzyl acetate, benzyl benzoate, benzyl alcohol, cinnamyl acetate and alcohol, vanillin, phenyl ethyl alcohol, benzoic acid, eugenol, dimethyl anthranilate, hydroquinone
CHARACTERISTICS: *Odor:* Powerful, characteristic, reminiscent of styrax, sweet
PHYSICAL CONSTANTS: *Specific gravity:* 1.0423; *Refractive index:* 1.4981; *Optical rotation:* 0 to +12
USES: *Perfumes:* Green, floral type

HYSSOP
BOTANICAL: *Family: Labiatae; Genus: Hyssopus; Species: Officinalis*
SOURCES: *Habitat:* Mediterranean area; *Part of the Plant:* Herb flowers and stocks
CHEMICAL CONSTITUENTS: Pinene 50%, sesquiterpenes
CHARACTERISTICS: *Color:* Colorless or greenish-yellow; *Odor:* Sharp, camphor-like
PHYSICAL CONSTANTS: *Specific gravity:* 0.925–0.940 (15 C); *Refractive index:* 1.48315–1.48441; *Optical rotation:* –17 to +23; *Boiling point:* 200 C
SOLUBILITY: Insoluble in water; soluble in alcohol (2–4/80%), ether, chloroform
USES: *Flavors:* Liqueurs, flavors; *Medicine:* Medicine

JASMINE (ABSOLUTE)
BOTANICAL: *Family: Oleaceae; Genus: Jasminum; Species: Officinalis; Variety: Grandiflorum (Spanish)*
SOURCES: *Habitat:* East Indies, Mediterranean area; *Part of the Plant:* Flowers extraction through solvent
CHEMICAL CONSTITUENTS: Jasmone, indole, methyl anthranilate, benzyl acetate, linalyl acetate, linalool
CHARACTERISTICS: *Color:* Colorless to yellowish; *Odor:* Characteristic jasmine, honey floral-like
PHYSICAL CONSTANTS: *Specific gravity:* 0.92290–0.9550 (15 C); *Refractive index:* 1.4822–1.4935; *Optical rotation:* +2.23 to +4.95; *Congealing point:* 47–51 C; *Melting point:* 49–52 C
SOLUBILITY: Soluble in alcohol

USES: *Flavors:* Flavors; *Perfumes:* Perfumery

JUNIPER BERRY

BOTANICAL: *Family: Pinaceae, Coniferae, or Cupressaceae; Genus: Juniperus; Species: Communis*

SOURCES: *Habitat:* Europe, mainly Italy, Yugoslavia, Hungary, Czechoslovakia; *Part of the Plant:* Dried berries

CHEMICAL CONSTITUENTS: Pinene, cadinene, camphene, terpineol, camphor

CHARACTERISTICS: *Color:* Colorless to greenish-yellow; it becomes darker and thicker on exposure; *Odor:* Turpentine-like; *Taste:* Bitter, burning

PHYSICAL CONSTANTS: *Specific gravity:* 0.854–0.879; *Refractive index:* 1.478–1.4840; *Optical rotation:* –1 to 0

SOLUBILITY: Insoluble in water; soluble in alcohol (5–10/90%), chloroform, fixed oils, mineral oils, carbon disulfide, benzene, amyl alcohol

USES: *Flavors:* Liqueurs, flavoring; *Perfumes:* Perfumery; *Medicine:* Diuretic; *Other:* Preserving catgut ligature

LAUREL

BOTANICAL: *Family: Lauraceae; Genus: Laurus; Species: Nobilis*

SOURCES: *Habitat:* Mediterranean area; *Part of the Plant:* Fresh green leaves and twigs

CHEMICAL CONSTITUENTS: Eugenol, methyl ether, pinene, myrcene, cineol

CHARACTERISTICS: *Color:* Bright yellow; *Odor:* Aromatic; *Taste:* Bitter

PHYSICAL CONSTANTS: *Specific gravity:* 0.924–0.932; *Refractive index:* 1.4650–1.4700; *Optical rotation:* –18 to +15

SOLUBILITY: Slightly soluble in water; soluble in alcohol (2/70%), ether, chloroform, benzene

USES: *Flavors:* Flavors; *Perfumes:* Perfumes; *Medicine:* Medicine

LAVANDIN

BOTANICAL: *Family: Labiatae; Genus: Lavandula; Species: Officinalis; Variety: Latifolia*

SOURCES: *Habitat:* France, Spain; *Part of the Plant:* Dried flowers and stalks of the shrubs

CHEMICAL CONSTITUENTS: Borneol, cineol, linalool, pinene, camphene

CHARACTERISTICS: *Odor:* Characteristic with a camphoraceous reminiscence

PHYSICAL CONSTANTS: *Specific gravity:* 0.900–0.922; *Refractive index:* 1.404–1.468; *Optical rotation:* –5.45 to +16.44

SOLUBILITY: Soluble in alcohol (1.5–3/70%)

USES: *Perfumes:* Inexpensive perfumes

LAVENDER

BOTANICAL: *Family: Labiatae; Genus: Lavandula; Species: Vera; Variety: Officinalis*

SOURCES: *Habitat:* Mediterranean area, Yugoslavia, U.S.S.R., Australia, mainly France, Spain, Italy; *Part of the Plant:* Fresh flowering tops and stalks

CHEMICAL CONSTITUENTS: Cineol, linalyl acetate 30–40%, linalool, geraniol, pinene, limonene, borneol, coumarin
CHARACTERISTICS: *Color:* Colorless, yellowish, or greenish-yellow; *Odor:* Warm camphoraceous, floral-herbaceous; *Taste:* Bitter, strongly aromatic burning
PHYSICAL CONSTANTS: *Specific gravity:* 0.875–0.888; *Refractive index:* 1.459–1.470; *Optical rotation:* –3 to –10
SOLUBILITY: Insoluble in water; soluble in alcohol (4/70%)
USES: *Perfumes:* Perfumes

LEMON

BOTANICAL: *Family: Rutaceae; Genus: Citrus; Species: Limonum; Variety: Medica*
SOURCES: *Habitat:* Mediterranean area, Brazil, Argentina, west Africa, U.S.A.; *Part of the Plant:* Peels of fresh fruits by expression
CHEMICAL CONSTITUENTS: Limonene 90%, terpinene, phellandrene, citral 2.2–3.8%, citronellal, geranyl acetate, *d-l*-pinene, geraniol; octyl, nonyl, decyl aldehydes; sesquiterpenes
CHARACTERISTICS: *Color:* Pale to deep yellow or greenish-yellow; *Odor:* Citrus; *Taste:* Pungent, bitter
PHYSICAL CONSTANTS: *Specific gravity:* 0.849–0.855; *Refractive index:* 1.474-1.467; *Optical rotation:* +57 to +65.6
SOLUBILITY: Slightly soluble in water; soluble in alcohol (3 volumes), carbon disulfide, glacial acetic acid
USES: *Flavors:* Flavors, soft drinks, liqueurs, pastry, food; *Perfumes:* Perfumes, especially colognes; *Other:* Polishes

LEMONGRASS

SYNONYMS: Verbena
BOTANICAL: *Family: Graminaceae; Genus: Cymbopogon; Species: Citratus; Variety: Flexuous*
SOURCES: *Habitat:* India, China, Brazil, Guatemala, West Indies; *Part of the Plant:* Fresh or partially dried grass
CHEMICAL CONSTITUENTS: Citral 75–85%, methyl heptenone, citronellal, geraniol, limonene, dipentene
CHARACTERISTICS: *Color:* Reddish-yellow or brownish-red; *Odor:* Strong, citrus-like; *Taste:* Bitter, pungent
PHYSICAL CONSTANTS: *Specific gravity:* 0.895–0.908; *Refractive index:* 1.483–1.489; *Optical rotation:* –3 to +1
SOLUBILITY: Insoluble in water; soluble in alcohol (3/70%), ether, chloroform, fixed oils; slightly soluble in glycerol
USES: *Flavors:* Flavors; *Perfumes:* Perfumery; *Pharmaceuticals:* Synthesis of Vitamin A; *Other:* Source of citral and ionones

LIME

BOTANICAL: *Family: Rutaceae; Genus: Citrus; Species: Aurantifolia; Variety: Swingle*
SOURCES: *Habitat:* Italy, West Indies, Mexico, Brazil; *Part of the Plant:* Crushed

fruits, or by expression of the peels from ripe fruits

CHEMICAL CONSTITUENTS: Citral 0.5–2.5% by distillation, 2.6–6.6% by expression; limonene, terpineol

CHARACTERISTICS: *Color:* Colorless to greenish-yellow; *Odor:* Fresh citrus, intense; *Taste:* Bitter, pungent

PHYSICAL CONSTANTS: Distillation: *Specific gravity:* 0.855–0.863; *Refractive index:* 1.4477–1.4745; *Optical rotation:* +34 to +47; Expression: *Specific gravity:* 0.880–0.884 (15 C); *Refractive index:* 1.482–1.486; *Optical rotation:* +32 to +38

SOLUBILITY: Insoluble in water; soluble in alcohol (4–10/90%), fixed oils, mineral oils

USES: *Flavors:* Flavors; *Perfumes:* Perfumery, soaps, cosmetics

LINALOE WOOD

SYNONYMS: Boi de rose

BOTANICAL: *Family: Burseraceae; Genus: Bursera; Species: Delpechiana*

SOURCES: *Habitat:* Mexico; *Part of the Plant:* Fruits and woods

CHEMICAL CONSTITUENTS: Linalool, geraniol, methyl heptenone, terpineol

CHARACTERISTICS: *Color:* Colorless to yellowish; *Odor:* Floral rose-citrus, soft, sweet; *Taste:* Rose-citrus

PHYSICAL CONSTANTS: *Specific gravity:* 0.876–0.883; *Refractive index:* 1.460–1.463; *Optical rotation:* –5 to –13

SOLUBILITY: Insoluble in water; soluble in alcohol, fixed oils, propylene glycol

USES: *Flavors:* Flavors; *Perfumes:* Perfumery, soaps

LITSEA CUBEBA

BOTANICAL: *Family: Lauraceae; Genus: Litsea; Species: Cubeba*

SOURCES: *Habitat:* China, southeast Asia; *Part of the Plant:* Ripe fruit

CHEMICAL CONSTITUENTS: Citral

CHARACTERISTICS: *Odor:* Lemon-like, floral

USES: *Perfumes:* Citrus type; *Other:* Source of citral

LOVAGE

BOTANICAL: *Family: Umbelliferae; Genus: Levisticum; Species: Officinalis*

SOURCES: *Habitat:* Europe; *Part of the Plant:* All fresh plant and roots

CHEMICAL CONSTITUENTS: *d*-α–Terpineol, eugenol, carvacrol, coumarin, sesquiterpenes, acetic acid, isovaleric acid, benzoic acid, myristic acid, butyric acid

CHARACTERISTICS: *Odor:* Powerful, sweet-spicy reminiscent of celery and angelica, with a mossy tone

PHYSICAL CONSTANTS: *Specific gravity:* 1.034–1.057; *Refractive index:* 1.5502–1.5591; *Optical rotation:* +0.40 to +1.20

SOLUBILITY: Soluble in alcohol (1–2/80%)

USES: *Perfumes:* Herbal and spicy

MACE

SYNONYMS: Nutmeg

BOTANICAL: *Family: Myristaceae; Genus: Myristica; Species: Fragrans*

SOURCES: *Habitat:* Indonesia, Sri Lanka, West Indies; *Part of the Plant:* Dried seeds and peels
CHEMICAL CONSTITUENTS: Pinene, dipentene, camphene, cymene, linalool, geraniol, terpineol, borneol, safrol, eugenol, isoeugenol, myristicina
CHARACTERISTICS: *Odor:* Characteristic spicy
PHYSICAL CONSTANTS: *Specific gravity:* 0.865–0.932; *Refractive index:* 1.4780–1.4895; *Optical rotation:* +9 to +30
SOLUBILITY: Soluble in alcohol (3/90%), fixed oils
USES: *Flavors:* Flavors; *Perfumes:* Perfumery, spicy colognes

MANDARIN
BOTANICAL: *Family: Rutaceae; Genus: Citrus; Species: Nobilis; Variety: Madurensis or reticulata*
SOURCES: *Habitat:* Italy, Spain, Brazil, Argentina; *Part of the Plant:* Fresh peels by mechanical pressure
CHEMICAL CONSTITUENTS: Methyl anthranilate, limonene, geraniol, citral, citronellol, aldehyde C_9–C_{10}
CHARACTERISTICS: *Odor:* Fresh citrus, with a refreshing tone
PHYSICAL CONSTANTS: *Specific gravity:* 0.854–0.859; *Refractive index:* 1.475–1.478; *Optical rotation:* +65 to +75
SOLUBILITY: Soluble in alcohol (1.5/95%)
USES: *Flavors:* Liqueurs; *Perfumes:* Cologne type

MARJORAM
BOTANICAL: *Family: Labiatae; Genus: Origanum; Species: Marjorana*
SOURCES: *Habitat:* Germany, France, Spain, Tunisia, Hungary, Egypt; *Part of the Plant:* Fresh and dried leaves and flowering tops
CHEMICAL CONSTITUENTS: Terpenes 40%, terpinene, *d*-terpineol
CHARACTERISTICS: *Color:* Colorless, yellow, or greenish-yellow; *Odor:* Strong penetrating, camphoraceous
PHYSICAL CONSTANTS: *Specific gravity:* 0.888–0.912 (20 C); *Refractive index:* 1.4630–1.4660; *Optical rotation:* +13 to +18; Spanish type: *Specific gravity:* 0.907–0.915; *Refractive index:* 1.4630–1.4660; *Optical rotation:* +5 to +10
SOLUBILITY: Insoluble in water; soluble in alcohol (2/80%), ether, chloroform
USES: *Flavors:* Flavors; *Perfumes:* Perfumery, soaps; *Medicine:* Medicine; *Other:* Microscopy

MATE (ABSOLUTE)
BOTANICAL: *Family: Aquifoliaceae; Genus: Ilex; Species: Paraguariensis*
SOURCES: *Habitat:* Paraguay, Argentina, southern Brazil; *Part of the Plant:* Flowers, leaf stems
CHEMICAL CONSTITUENTS: Caffeine, purines, tannin, chlorogenic acid and derivatives
CHARACTERISTICS: *Odor:* Herbaceous, hay, tea-like
USES: *Perfumes:* Fantasy compositions

MENTHA CITRATA

BOTANICAL: *Family: Labiatae; Genus: Mentha; Species: Citrata; Variety: Viridis or acquatica*
SOURCES: *Habitat:* Western U.S.; *Part of the Plant:* Whole plant
CHEMICAL CONSTITUENTS: Linalool, linalyl acetate
CHARACTERISTICS: *Odor:* Refreshing, bergamot-rosewood-like
PHYSICAL CONSTANTS: *Specific gravity:* 0.916–0.924 (15 C); *Refractive index:* 1.4582–1.4598; *Optical rotation:* –7 to –8
SOLUBILITY: Soluble in alcohol (1.5–2/70%, 5/60%)
USES: *Perfumes:* Fresh type

MIGNONETTE (ABSOLUTE)

SYNONYMS: Reseda
BOTANICAL: *Family: Resedaceae; Genus: Reseda; Species: Odorata*
SOURCES: *Habitat:* North America, Europe; *Part of the Plant:* Flowers and top leaves by petroleum ether extraction
CHEMICAL CONSTITUENTS: Aldehyde C-8, C-10, eugenol, caprylic acid
CHARACTERISTICS: *Form:* Viscous liquid or paste; *Color:* Dark orange or olive-brown; *Odor:* Intense, herbaceous-green
PHYSICAL CONSTANTS: *Specific gravity:* 0.966–0.972 (15 C); *Refractive index:* 1.4886–1.4944; *Optical rotation:* +27.42 t +37.16
USES: *Perfumes:* Perfumery

MIMOSA (CONCRETE, ABSOLUTE)

BOTANICAL: *Family: Leguminosae; Genus: Mimosa; Species: Decurrens; Variety: Farnesiana or dealbata*
SOURCES: *Habitat:* Northern Italy, southern France; *Part of the Plant:* Flowers and twigs
CHEMICAL CONSTITUENTS: Palmitic aldehyde, oenanthic acid, anisic acid, acetic acid, palmitic acid, phenols
CHARACTERISTICS: *Odor:* Powerful, persistent green floral
PHYSICAL CONSTANTS: *Specific gravity:* 1.04–1.05; *Refractive index:* 1.513; *Optical rotation:* +15.40 to +22.40; *Melting point:* 52.5 C
USES: *Perfumes:* Fine floral type

MONARD

SYNONYMS: Horsemint
BOTANICAL: *Family: Labiatae; Genus: Monarda; Species: Punctata*
SOURCES: *Habitat:* North America; *Part of the Plant:* Whole plant
CHEMICAL CONSTITUENTS: *d*-Limonene, carvacrol, linalool, thymol 60%, cymene
CHARACTERISTICS: *Color:* Yellowish to brownish; *Odor:* Mint-like; *Taste:* Thyme-like
PHYSICAL CONSTANTS: *Specific gravity:* 0.930–0.940 (15 C); *Refractive index:* 1.467; *Optical rotation:* Slightly dextro
SOLUBILITY: Slightly soluble in water; soluble in alcohol, ether
USES: *Other:* Source of thymol

MUSK (TINCTURE)

ZOOLOGICAL: *Family: Cervidae; Genus: Moschus; Species: Moschiferus*

SOURCES: *Habitat:* Nepal, China, Tibet mountains; *Part of the Body:* Glandular secretion from an internal pouch between the legs of the male musk deer

CHARACTERISTICS: *Odor:* Penetrating woody

SOLUBILITY: Soluble in water

USES: *Perfumes:* As a fixative in expensive fantasy type

MUSTARD

SYNONYMS: Sinapsis oil

BOTANICAL: *Family: Cruciferae; Genus: Brassica, Lobularia, or Sweet alysum; Species: Alba* (white), *nigra* (black), *juncea* (green), *lobularia* (maritima)

SOURCES: *Part of the Plant:* Seeds from *Brassica alba* and *nigra*

CHEMICAL CONSTITUENTS: Allyl isothiocarbimida, carbon disulfide, allyl thiocyanate, myrosin (enzyme), sinigrin (glucoside)

CHARACTERISTICS: *Color:* Yellowish, brown-yellow, greenish-brown; *Odor:* Pungent; *Taste:* Acrid

PHYSICAL CONSTANTS: *Specific gravity:* 0.914–0.916 (15 C); *Refractive index:* 1.4655–1.4670 (40 C); *Optical rotation:* ± 0; *Solidification point:* –8 to –16 C

SOLUBILITY: Slightly soluble in alcohol; soluble in ether, chloroform

USES: *Flavors:* Manufacture of oleomargarine, salad oils condiment; *Perfumes:* Soap; *Medicine:* Counterirritant and stimulant; *Other:* The black mustard seeds are employed in commercial mustard products

MYRRH (RESINOID)

BOTANICAL: *Family: Burseraceae; Genus: Commiphora; Species: Myrrha*

SOURCES: *Habitat:* Somalia, Ethiopia, north Africa; *Part of the Plant:* Gum resin

CHEMICAL CONSTITUENTS: Cuminic aldehyde, bisabolene, pinene, *d-l*-limonene, eugenol, *n*-cresol, myrrhin, myrrholic acid-gum 57–61%

CHARACTERISTICS: *Form:* Tears; *Color:* Brown; *Odor:* Balsamic, spicy, camphoraceous; *Taste:* Bitter

PHYSICAL CONSTANTS: *Specific gravity:* 0.988–1.045; *Refractive index:* 1.5180–1.5280; *Optical rotation:* –90 to –30; *Boiling point:* 220–235 C

SOLUBILITY: Insoluble in water; soluble in alcohol (8–10/90%); partially soluble in ether

USES: *Flavors:* Dentifrices; *Perfumes:* Perfumery; *Pharmaceuticals:* Protective pharmaceuticals; *Medicine:* Carminative; *Other:* Dentistry for carious teeth

WARNING AND CAUTION: Low toxicity

MYRTLE

BOTANICAL: *Family: Myrtaceae; Genus: Myrtus; Species: Communis*

SOURCES: *Habitat:* Mediterranean area; *Part of the Plant:* Blossoms, leaves, twigs

CHEMICAL CONSTITUENTS: Cineol, borneol, cuminic aldehyde, eugenol, eucalyptol, dipentene, camphor, metracresol, pinene

CHARACTERISTICS: *Form:* Viscid; *Color:* Yellowish to greenish; *Odor:* Fragrant, strong, camphoraceous

PHYSICAL CONSTANTS: *Specific gravity:* 0.900–0.915; *Refractive index:* 1.519–1.5275; *Optical rotation:* +10 to +30; *Boiling point:* 220–235 C
SOLUBILITY: Insoluble in water; soluble in alcohol (80%), ether, chloroform, fixed oils
USES: *Flavors:* Flavors; *Perfumes:* As a fixative; *Medicine:* Medicine

NARCISSUS (CONCRETE, ABSOLUTE)
BOTANICAL: *Family: Amaryllidaceae; Genus: Narcissus; Species: Poeticus*
SOURCES: *Habitat:* France, Morocco, Egypt; *Part of the Plant:* Flowers
CHEMICAL CONSTITUENTS: Eugenol, benzyl alcohol, cinnamyl alcohol, benzaldehyde, benzoic acid
CHARACTERISTICS: *Odor:* Characteristic, hay-like
PHYSICAL CONSTANTS: *Specific gravity:* 0.9714; *Refractive index:* 1.5050; *Optical rotation:* –5.48
USES: *Perfumes:* Floral type

NEPETA
SYNONYMS: Catnip
BOTANICAL: *Family: Labiatae; Genus: Nepeta; Species: Cataria*
SOURCES: *Habitat:* North America, Europe; *Part of the Plant:* Spikes
CHEMICAL CONSTITUENTS: Menthol, caprylic acid, valeric acid, carvacrol, pulegone, thymol, caryophyllene, neptalactone
CHARACTERISTICS: *Odor:* Strong-scented mint
PHYSICAL CONSTANTS: *Specific gravity:* 0.986–1.83; *Refractive index:* 1.4872–1.4913; *Optical rotation:* +1.20 to +13.20
SOLUBILITY: Soluble in alcohol (0.5–1/80%)
USES: *Medicine:* Diaphoretic and expectorant

NEROLI
BOTANICAL: *Family: Rutaceae; Genus: Citrus; Species: Aurantium; Variety: Bigaradia*
SOURCES: *Habitat:* Morocco, Algeria, Egypt, southern France; *Part of the Plant:* Unopened flowers
CHEMICAL CONSTITUENTS: Pinene, dipentene, geraniol, nerol, geranyl acetate, neryl acetate, indole, farnesol, alcohol C_{10}, ethyl benzoate
CHARACTERISTICS: *Odor:* Characteristic
PHYSICAL CONSTANTS: *Specific gravity:* 0.870–0.881; *Refractive index:* 1.467–1.474; *Optical rotation:* +1.37 to +12
SOLUBILITY: Soluble in alcohol (1–2.5/80%)
USES: *Perfumes:* Colognes

NIAOULI
BOTANICAL: *Family: Myrtaceae; Genus: Melaleuca; Species: Viridiflora*
SOURCES: *Part of the Plant:* Leaves
CHEMICAL CONSTITUENTS: Cineol 65%, terpineol 30%, limonene, *d*-pinene
CHARACTERISTICS: *Color:* Slightly yellow; *Odor:* Aromatic mint; *Taste:* Pungent,

refreshing peppermint-like
PHYSICAL CONSTANTS: *Specific gravity:* 0.908–0.932 (15 C); *Refractive index:* 1.465–1.472; *Optical rotation:* –3.34 to +0.42
SOLUBILITY: Insoluble in water; soluble in alcohol (1/80%), ether, benzene
USES: *Medicine:* Anthelmintic

NUTMEG
BOTANICAL: *Family: Myristaceae; Genus: Myristica; Species: Fragrans; Variety: Officinalis*
SOURCES: *Habitat:* Indonesia, Sri Lanka, East Indies, West Indies; *Part of the Plant:* Dried kernels and seeds
CHEMICAL CONSTITUENTS: *d*-Camphene 8%, *d*-pentene, *d*-borneol, *l*-terpineol, geraniol 6%, safrol, myristicin 4%, trimyristin, *d*-pinene 8%, camphene 60–68%, elemicin
CHARACTERISTICS: *Form:* Soft solid; *Color:* Colorless or orange-red to reddish-brown; *Odor:* Nutmeg characteristic; *Taste:* Warm, spicy
PHYSICAL CONSTANTS: West Indian (expressed): *Specific gravity:* 0.990–0.995; *Refractive index:* 1.470–1.488; *Optical rotation:* +8 to +30; *Melting point:* 45–51 C; East Indian (distilled): *Specific gravity:* 0.859–0.924; *Refractive index:* 1.469–1.476; *Optical rotation:* +25 to +45; *Melting point:* 45–51 C
SOLUBILITY: Insoluble in water; soluble in alcohol (1–3/90%), carbon disulfide, glacial acetic acid
USES: *Flavors:* Flavors; *Perfumes:* Perfumery; *Medicine:* Medicine as a carminative or rubefacient
WARNING AND CAUTION: Ingestion of large amount produces narcosis, delirium, death

OAKMOSS (RESINOID, ABSOLUTE)
BOTANICAL: *Family: Usneaceae; Genus: Evernia; Species: Prunastri*
SOURCES: *Habitat:* Central and southern Europe, mainly in Yugoslavia, France, and Morocco; *Part of the Plant:* Moss growing on oak tree
CHEMICAL CONSTITUENTS: Cineol, geraniol, citronellol, vanillin, methyl nonyl ketone, palmitic acid
CHARACTERISTICS: *Odor:* Woody, leather, and slightly phenolic
PHYSICAL CONSTANTS: *Melting point:* 48–50 C
USES: *Perfumes:* As a fixative

OLIBANUM (RESINOID)
SYNONYMS: Frankincense
BOTANICAL: *Family: Burseraceae or Terebintaceae; Genus: Boswellia or Bhaudayana; Species: Carterii; Variety: Serrata*
SOURCES: *Habitat:* Somalia, Ethiopia, Saudi Arabia; *Part of the Plant:* Oleoresin formed on the bark of the tree
CHEMICAL CONSTITUENTS: Pinene, camphene, phellandrene, dipentene, *d*-limonene (East Africa)
CHARACTERISTICS: *Color:* Colorless or yellowish; *Odor:* Balsamic, lemon-like; *Taste:* Lemon-like

PHYSICAL CONSTANTS: *Specific gravity:* 0.869–0.889; *Refractive index:* 1.4685–1.4820; *Optical rotation:* –15 to +35
SOLUBILITY: Insoluble in water; soluble in alcohol (4–6/90%), ether, chloroform, carbon disulfide
USES: *Flavors:* Flavors; *Perfumes:* Perfumes; *Medicine:* Medicine

ONION
BOTANICAL: *Family: Liliaceae; Genus: Allium; Species: Cepa*
SOURCES: *Part of the Plant:* Crushed seed
CHEMICAL CONSTITUENTS: Allyl propyl disulfide, s-(1-propenyl) cysteine sulfoxide, 1-propenyl sulfeneic acid (lacrimatory)
CHARACTERISTICS: *Color:* Pale yellow; *Odor:* Very strong and characteristic; *Taste:* Sweetish
PHYSICAL CONSTANTS: *Specific gravity:* 1.047–1.098 (15 C); *Refractive index:* 1.5373–1.5588; *Optical rotation:* +1.3 to +3.53; *Solidification point:* –15 C
SOLUBILITY: Soluble in ether, chloroform, carbon disulfide
USES: *Flavors:* Flavors, culinary

OPOPANAX (RESINOID)
BOTANICAL: *Family: Burseraceae; Genus: Commiphora; Species: Erythraea; Variety: Glabrescens*
SOURCES: *Habitat:* Somalia and Ethiopia; *Part of the Plant:* Oleoresin from the bark of the tree
CHEMICAL CONSTITUENTS: Bisabolene
CHARACTERISTICS: *Color:* Pale yellow or olive yellowish to dark greenish; *Odor:* Sweet balsamic; *Taste:* Spicy, warm, reminiscent of wine
PHYSICAL CONSTANTS: *Specific gravity:* 0.8835–0.9170; *Refractive index:* 1.49039–1.49535; *Optical rotation:* –12.11 to +19.28
SOLUBILITY: Soluble in alcohol (1–10/90%)
USES: *Flavors:* Liqueurs; *Perfumes:* As a fixative for oriental type

ORANGE BITTER
BOTANICAL: *Family: Rutaceae; Genus: Citrus; Species: Aurantium or bigaradia; Variety: Amara*
SOURCES: *Habitat:* Sicily, Calabria, France, Spain, Morocco, Egypt; *Part of the Plant:* Fresh peels of bitter orange fruits expressed by hands or machine
CHEMICAL CONSTITUENTS: *d*-Limonene 90%, citral, aldehyde C-10, methyl anthranilate, linalool, terpineol
CHARACTERISTICS: *Color:* Pale to yellow; *Odor:* Citrus; *Taste:* Bitter
PHYSICAL CONSTANTS: *Specific gravity:* 0.842–0.848; *Refractive index:* 1.4725–1.4755; *Optical rotation:* +88 to +98
SOLUBILITY: Slightly soluble in water; soluble in alcohol (4 volumes), glacial acetic acid
USES: *Flavors:* Flavoring; *Perfumes:* Perfumery; *Medicine:* Medicine

ORANGE FLOWERS (CONCRETE, ABSOLUTE)

BOTANICAL: *Family: Rutaceae; Genus: Citrus; Species: Aurantium or bigaradia; Variety: Amara*

SOURCES: *Habitat:* Mediterranean area, mainly Italy, France, Spain, Algeria, Morocco; *Part of the Plant:* Fresh orange flowers

CHEMICAL CONSTITUENTS: Limonene, *l*-linalool, geraniol, linalyl acetate 7–18%, methyl anthranilate, nerol, neroli camphor

CHARACTERISTICS: *Color:* Yellowish, fluorescent, becoming brown on exposure; *Odor:* Intense, very pleasant; *Taste:* Bitter, aromatic

PHYSICAL CONSTANTS: *Specific gravity:* 0.863–0.880; *Refractive index:* 1.475; *Optical rotation:* +1.5 to +9.8

SOLUBILITY: Slightly soluble in water; soluble in alcohol ($1\frac{1}{2}$–2/80%) with a violet fluorescence

USES: *Flavors:* Flavors; *Perfumes:* Perfumery

ORANGE SWEET

BOTANICAL: *Family: Rutaceae; Genus: Citrus; Species: Aurantium; Variety: Dulcis*

SOURCES: *Habitat:* Mediterranean area, Brazil, South Africa, U.S.; *Part of the Plant:* Fresh peels of ripe fruits of sweet orange

CHEMICAL CONSTITUENTS: *d*-Limonene 90%, citral, aldehyde C-10, methyl anthranilate, linalool, terpineol

CHARACTERISTICS: *Color:* Yellow to deep orange; *Odor:* Characteristic orange; *Taste:* Sweet

PHYSICAL CONSTANTS: *Specific gravity:* 0.842–0.846; *Refractive index:* 1.4723–1.4737; *Optical rotation:* +94 to +99

SOLUBILITY: Insoluble in water; soluble in alcohol (8/90%), carbon disulfide, glacial acetic acid (1 volume)

USES: *Flavors:* Flavors; *Perfumes:* Perfumery; *Medicine:* Expectorant

OREGANO

BOTANICAL: *Family: Labiatae; Genus: Origanum; Species: Vulgare; Variety: Capitatus*

SOURCES: *Habitat:* Middle East, Spain, France, Balkans; *Part of the Plant:* Flowering herb and tops

CHEMICAL CONSTITUENTS: Carvacrol, terpenes, cymene, linalool

CHARACTERISTICS: *Color:* Light yellow, becoming darker on aging; *Odor:* Spicy; *Taste:* Bitter, strong, spicy

PHYSICAL CONSTANTS: *Specific gravity:* 0.870–0.910 (15 C); *Refractive index:* 1.5020–1.5080; *Optical rotation:* –2 to +3

SOLUBILITY: Slightly soluble in water; soluble in alcohol (2/70%), fixed oils, mineral oils

USES: *Flavors:* Flavoring foods; *Perfumes:* Perfumery

WARNING AND CAUTION: May be toxic by ingestion

ORRIS

BOTANICAL: *Family: Iridaceae; Genus: Orris; Species: Pallida; Variety: Florentina or germanica*

SOURCES: *Habitat:* Italy, Germany; *Part of the Plant:* Rhizomes

CHEMICAL CONSTITUENTS: Myristic acid 85%, methyl myristate, oleic anhydride, iridin, ionone, methyl esters

CHARACTERISTICS: *Form:* Semisolid; *Color:* Yellowish; *Odor:* Violet; *Taste:* Fatty

PHYSICAL CONSTANTS: *Specific gravity:* 0.930–0.940; *Refractive index:* 1.495–1.4960; *Optical rotation:* +14 to +30; *Melting point:* 38–50 C

SOLUBILITY: Soluble in alcohol, ether, chloroform

USES: *Flavors:* Flavors; *Perfumes:* Perfumes; *Other:* Tooth powders

WARNING AND CAUTION: Strong allergen

OSMANTHUS (CONCRETE, ABSOLUTE)

BOTANICAL: *Family: Oleaceae; Genus: Osmanthus; Species: Fragrans*

SOURCES: *Habitat:* Japan, China, India; *Part of the Plant:* Flowers

CHARACTERISTICS: *Odor:* Plum and raisin-like

USES: *Perfumes:* Fantasy perfumes

PALMAROSA

BOTANICAL: *Family: Graminaceae; Genus: Cymbopogon; Species: Martini; Variety; Motia*

SOURCES: *Habitat:* India, Brazil, Central America; *Part of the Plant:* Leaves, fresh or dried, harvested before flowering

CHEMICAL CONSTITUENTS: Geraniol, dipentene, farnesol, methyl heptenone, ethyl acetate, capryl acetate

CHARACTERISTICS: *Color:* Colorless or yellowish; *Odor:* Rose-like; *Taste:* Rose-like, herbaceous

PHYSICAL CONSTANTS: *Specific gravity:* 0.885–0.897 (15 C); *Refractive index:* 1.4730–1.4775; *Optical rotation:* –2 to +3

SOLUBILITY: Insoluble in water; soluble in alcohol (2/70%), benzyl benzoate, fixed oils, propylene glycol, mineral oils

USES: *Flavors:* Flavors; *Perfumes:* Perfumery; *Other:* Source of geraniol

PARSLEY

BOTANICAL: *Family: Umbelliferae; Genus: Petroselinum; Species: Hortense, sativum, or carum*

SOURCES: *Habitat:* Middle East, France, Balkans, and almost worldwide; *Part of the Plant:* Dried seeds or herb

CHEMICAL CONSTITUENTS: Apiol, terpenes, *l*-pinene, α-pinene, palmitic acid, myristicin

CHARACTERISTICS: *Form:* Viscid; *Color:* Colorless or greenish-yellow; *Odor:* Strong, characteristic; *Taste:* Mild green

PHYSICAL CONSTANTS: Seeds: *Specific gravity:* 1.040–1.100 (15 C); *Refractive index:* 1.510–1.519; *Optical rotation:* –5 to –11; Herb: *Specific gravity:* 1.043–1.110;

Refractive index: 1.512–1.528; *Optical rotation:* –4 to –10
SOLUBILITY: Slightly soluble in water; soluble in alcohol (4–8/80%), ether
USES: *Flavors:* Flavoring for meat, sauces, pickles; seasoning; spice combinations; *Perfumes:* Herbal type; *Medicine:* Medicine

PARSNIP

BOTANICAL: *Family: Umbelliferae; Genus: Pastinaca; Species: Sativa*
SOURCES: *Habitat:* Eastern Europe, southeast Asia, Central America; *Part of the Plant:* Fruits, flowers, roots
CHEMICAL CONSTITUENTS: Octyl butyrate, octyl propionate, propionic acid, heptylic acid, caproic acid (hexyl)
CHARACTERISTICS: *Odor:* Aromatic, spicy, herbaceous
PHYSICAL CONSTANTS: *Specific gravity:* 0.8970 (15 C); *Refractive index:* 1.43007; *Optical rotation:* +0.6
SOLUBILITY: Soluble in alcohol (1–2/80%)
USES: *Perfumes:* Spicy, herbal type, rarely employed

PATCHOULI

BOTANICAL: *Family: Labiatae; Genus: Pogostemon; Species: Cablin*
SOURCES: *Habitat:* East Indies, Indonesia, Philippines, China, Madagascar; *Part of the Plant:* Dried leaves
CHEMICAL CONSTITUENTS: Patchouli alcohol, patchoulene, azulene, eugenol, sesquiterpenes, cinnamic aldehyde, cadinene
CHARACTERISTICS: *Color:* Yellowish or greenish to dark brown; *Odor:* Intense, persistent, fragrant, improving on aging; *Taste:* Camphoraceous
PHYSICAL CONSTANTS: *Specific gravity:* 0.975–0.987 (15 C); *Refractive index:* 1.5099–1.5111; *Optical rotation:* –67 to –43
SOLUBILITY: Insoluble in water; soluble in alcohol (10/90%), ether, chloroform, benzyl benzoate, fixed oils, mineral oils
USES: *Flavors:* Flavors; *Perfumes:* Oriental type; fixative; soaps; cosmetics; *Other:* Scent of Indian fabrics and shawls, in incense

PENNYROYAL

BOTANICAL: *Family: Labiatae; Genus: Mentha* (European), *Hedeoma* (American); *Species: Pulegium* (European), *Pulegioides* (American)
SOURCES: *Habitat: Mentha pulegium:* Japan, Spain, Morocco, Tunisia; *Part of the Plant:* From the flowering leaves and tops of *Mentha pulegium* or *Hedeoma pulegioides*
CHEMICAL CONSTITUENTS: Pulegon 85%; ketones, acetic, formic, isoheptoic acids; limonene; dipentene; menthol; menthone
CHARACTERISTICS: *Color:* Pale yellow or greenish, bluish fluorescent; *Odor:* Aromatic mint-like; *Taste:* Pungent mint-like
PHYSICAL CONSTANTS: European: *Specific gravity:* 0.890–0.900 (15 C); *Refractive index:* 1.4750–1.4960; *Optical rotation:* +14 to +28; American: *Specific gravity:* 0.920–0.935; *Refractive index:* 1.4830–1.4875; *Optical rotation:* +18 to +22

SOLUBILITY: Slightly soluble in water; soluble in alcohol (3/70%), ether, chloroform, fixed oils

USES: *Flavors:* Flavoring; *Perfumes:* Perfumery; *Other:* Insectifuge; source of pulegone and derivatives

PEPPER, BLACK

BOTANICAL: *Family: Piperaceae; Genus: Piper; Species: Nigrum*

SOURCES: *Habitat:* India, Indonesia, southeast Asia, Brazil; *Part of the Plant:* Unripe berries

CHEMICAL CONSTITUENTS: Piperine, *d-l*-limonene, *l*-phellandrene, caryophyllene

CHARACTERISTICS: *Color:* Colorless or yellowish, greenish; *Odor:* Pepper characteristic; *Taste:* Spicy

PHYSICAL CONSTANTS: *Specific gravity:* 0.890–0.900 (15 C); *Refractive index:* 1.4935–1.4977; *Optical rotation:* –3 to +5

SOLUBILITY: Soluble in water, alcohol (15/90%), fixed oils, mineral oils, propylene glycol

USES: *Flavors:* Flavoring foods

PEPPERMINT, ARVENSIS

BOTANICAL: *Family: Labiatae; Genus: Mentha; Species: Arvensis*

SOURCES: *Habitat:* Japan, China, Korea, Taiwan, Brazil, Paraguay; *Part of the Plant:* Dried herb

CHEMICAL CONSTITUENTS: 2,4-Dimethyl acetophenone, 2-*p*-tolyl propionaldehyde, menthol 50%, menthyl acetate, menthyl isovalerate, menthone, pinene (inactive), *l*-limonene, cadinene, phellandrene, acetaldehyde, isovaleric aldehyde, amyl alcohol, dimethyl sulfide

CHARACTERISTICS: *Form:* Liquid, thicker on aging and exposure; *Color:* Colorless or pale yellow, darker on aging and exposure; *Odor:* Strong, penetrating mint; *Taste:* Pungent with coolness sensation

PHYSICAL CONSTANTS: *Specific gravity:* 0.896–0.908; *Refractive index:* 1.460–1.471; *Optical rotation:* –18 to –32

SOLUBILITY: Slightly soluble in water; soluble in alcohol (4/90%), ether, chloroform

USES: *Flavors:* Liqueurs, candies, tobacco; *Perfumes:* Perfumes, soaps; *Medicine:* As a carminative; *Other:* Source of menthol; in mouthwashes, dentifrices

PEPPERMINT, PIPERITA

BOTANICAL: *Family: Labiatae; Genus: Mentha; Species: Piperita*

SOURCES: *Habitat:* Italy, Spain, France, Balkans, U.S.A; *Part of the Plant:* Partially dried, harvested about the flowering period

CHEMICAL CONSTITUENTS: Menthol, carvone, cineol, thymol, pinene, limonene, acetic acid, isovalerianic acid

CHARACTERISTICS: *Odor:* Powerful, balsamic, persistent specific mint

PHYSICAL CONSTANTS: *Specific gravity:* 0.900–0.927; *Refractive index:* 1.460–1.471; *Optical rotation:* –35 to –5

SOLUBILITY: Soluble in alcohol (3–4/70%)

USES: *Flavors:* Foods, beverages, liqueurs

PERILLA

BOTANICAL: *Family: Labiatae; Genus: Perilla; Species: Frutescens; Variety: Ocimoides*

SOURCES: *Habitat:* Japan, China, India; *Part of the Plant:* Leaves and flowers

CHEMICAL CONSTITUENTS: Perillic aldehyde, linoleic and linoleic acids

CHARACTERISTICS: *Form:* Liquid; *Color:* Light yellow; *Odor:* Mint; *Taste:* Mint

PHYSICAL CONSTANTS: *Specific gravity:* 0.923–0.938 (15 C); *Refractive index:* 1.4971–1.5048; *Optical rotation:* –73.10 to +96.32

SOLUBILITY: Soluble in alcohol (0.5/90%)

USES: *Perfumes:* Scarcely used

PERU BALSAM

BOTANICAL: *Family: Leguminosae; Genus: Myroxylon; Species: Peruifera or Pereira* (San Salvador)

SOURCES: *Habitat:* Central America; *Part of the Plant:* Oleoresin

CHEMICAL CONSTITUENTS: Benzyl benzoate, benzyl cinnamate, cinnamein, cinnamic acid and esters, benzoic acid and esters, styracine, vanillin, perins

CHARACTERISTICS: *Form:* Viscid; *Color:* Dark; *Odor:* Hyacinth-like; *Taste:* Warm bitter, persistent

PHYSICAL CONSTANTS: *Specific gravity:* 1.095–1.110; *Refractive index:* 1.5670–1.5790; *Optical rotation:* –1 to +2; *Melting point:* 38–60 C

SOLUBILITY: Insoluble in water; soluble in alcohol, ether, chloroform, glacial acetic acid; partially soluble in petroleum ether and fixed oils

USES: *Flavors:* Chocolate flavor; *Perfumes:* Perfumery; *Medicine:* Skin ulcer therapy; *Other:* Deodorants

PETITGRAIN

BOTANICAL: *Family: Rutaceae; Genus: Citrus; Species: Aurantium; Variety: Amara*

SOURCES: *Habitat:* Italy, Algeria, Morocco, Egypt, France, Brazil, Paraguay; *Part of the Plant:* Leaves, twigs, and unripe fruits of bitter orange tree

CHEMICAL CONSTITUENTS: Linalyl acetate 40–80%, geraniol, geranyl acetate, limonene, mircene, linalool, methyl anthranilate

CHARACTERISTICS: *Color:* Yellowish; *Odor:* Neroli-like; *Taste:* Bitter

PHYSICAL CONSTANTS: *Specific gravity:* 0.887–0.900 (15 C); *Refractive index:* 1.4580–1.4640; *Optical rotation:* –4 to +1

SOLUBILITY: Slightly soluble in water; soluble in alcohol (2/80%)

USES: *Flavors:* Flavors; *Perfumes:* Eau de cologne, soaps, synthetic neroli, creams

PIMENTO

SYNONYMS: Allspice

BOTANICAL: *Family: Myrtaceae; Genus: Pimenta; Species: Officinalis; Variety: Dioica*

SOURCES: *Habitat:* West Indies, Central America, India, Reunion; *Part of the Plant:* Dried, crushed unripe berries, and from the leaves

CHEMICAL CONSTITUENTS: Eugenol 65–75%, phellandrene, caryophyllene,

cineol, eugenol methyl ether, palmitic acid, sesquiterpenes
CHARACTERISTICS: *Color:* Colorless to brownish or reddish; it becomes darker on aging and on exposure; *Odor:* Nutmeg, peppermint, cinnamon, clove-like (allspice); *Taste:* Pungent
PHYSICAL CONSTANTS: *Specific gravity:* 1.018–1.048; *Refractive index:* 1.5270–1.5400; *Optical rotation:* 0 to –4
SOLUBILITY: Soluble in alcohol (2/70%)
USES: *Flavors:* Flavors; *Medicine:* Medicine

PINE
BOTANICAL: *Family: Coniferae; Genus: Pinus; Species: Palustris, ponderosa,* and other
SOURCES: *Habitat:* U.S.A, France, Finland, U.S.S.R., Portugal; *Part of the Plant:* Wood chips
CHEMICAL CONSTITUENTS: Bornyl acetate, cadinene, pinene, sylvestrene, dipentene, phellandrene
CHARACTERISTICS: *Color:* White or yellowish; *Odor:* Fresh, camphoraceous
PHYSICAL CONSTANTS: *Specific gravity:* 0.905–0.925; *Refractive index:* 1.470–1.472; *Optical rotation:* –43 to +37
SOLUBILITY: Soluble in alcohol (0.5–1/90%)
USES: *Perfumes:* Soaps, detergents, low-cost perfumes

PINE NEEDLE
BOTANICAL: *Family: Pinaceae; Genus: Pinus; Species: Sylvestris*
SOURCES: *Habitat:* Europe, U.S.S.R.; *Part of the Plant:* Needles and twigs
CHEMICAL CONSTITUENTS: Dipentene, pinene, sylvestrene, cadinene, bornyl acetate 3.0–3.5%
CHARACTERISTICS: *Color:* Yellowish; *Odor:* Fresh, pungent, characteristic; *Taste:* Bitter
PHYSICAL CONSTANTS: *Specific gravity:* 0.884–0.886 (15 C); *Refractive index:* 1.4730–1.4785; *Optical rotation:* +7.3 to +10
SOLUBILITY: Insoluble in water; soluble in alcohol (10/90%), fixed oils
USES: *Perfumes:* Perfumery

ROSE (CONCRETE, ABSOLUTE)
BOTANICAL: *Family: Rosaceae; Genus: Rosa; Species: Gallica, damascena, centifolia, alba*
SOURCES: *Habitat:* Europe, Middle East, southern France, Algeria, Morocco, Egypt, Italy, Bulgaria, Turkey; *Part of the Plant:* Petals
CHEMICAL CONSTITUENTS: Geraniol 70–75%, citronellol, terpenes, phenyl ethyl alcohol, verol, eugenol, linalool, aldehyde C-9, farnesol
CHARACTERISTICS: *Form:* Viscous semisolid at room temperature; *Color:* Colorless or pale yellow, pale green, pale red; *Odor:* Fragrant, rose characteristic; *Taste:* Mild sweet
PHYSICAL CONSTANTS: *Specific gravity:* 0.848–0.861 (30 C); *Refractive index:* 1.457–1.463 (30 C); *Optical rotation:* –1 to –4 (25 C); *Congealing point:* 18–22 C

SOLUBILITY: Slightly soluble in water; sparingly soluble in alcohol; soluble in chloroform, fatty oils
USES: *Perfumes:* Perfumery, toilet preparations; *Pharmaceuticals:* Lozenges; *Medicine:* Ointments

ROSEMARY
BOTANICAL: *Family: Labiatae; Genus: Rosmarinus; Species: Officinalis*
SOURCES: *Habitat:* France, Spain, Tunisia, Italy, Yugoslavia; *Part of the Plant:* Fresh flowering tops and leaves
CHEMICAL CONSTITUENTS: Borneol 10%, bornyl acetate 2.5%, camphor, eucalpytol, pinene, camphene
CHARACTERISTICS: *Color:* Colorless or pale yellow; *Odor:* Camphoraceous, pungent; *Taste:* Warm, aromatic, camphoraceous
PHYSICAL CONSTANTS: *Specific gravity:* 0.894–0.912; *Refractive index:* 1.464–1.476; *Optical rotation:* –5 to +10 (25 C)
SOLUBILITY: Insoluble in water; soluble in alcohol (10/80%), glacial acetic acid
USES: *Flavors:* Foods; *Perfumes:* Low-cost soaps; *Medicine:* Liniments, carminative, rubefacient; *Other:* Hair lotions washer

ROSEWOOD
BOTANICAL: *Family: Lauraceae; Genus: Aniba; Species: Rosaeodora*
SOURCES: *Habitat:* Central America, Brazil, Mexico; *Part of the Plant:* Chipped wood
CHEMICAL CONSTITUENTS: Alcohols, linalool
CHARACTERISTICS: *Odor:* Slightly rose-like, with a sweet tone
PHYSICAL CONSTANTS: *Specific gravity:* 0.868–0.889; *Refractive index:* 1.4620–1.4685; *Optical rotation:* –4 to –5
SOLUBILITY: Soluble in alcohol (6/60% or 2/70%), fixed oils, propylene glycol, benzyl benzoate; slightly soluble in glycerin
USES: *Perfumes:* Colognes and fantasy type

RUE
BOTANICAL: *Family: Rutaceae; Genus: Ruta; Species: Graveolens*
SOURCES: *Part of the Plant:* Fresh flowers
CHEMICAL CONSTITUENTS: Methyl nonyl ketone 90%, methyl anthranilate, methyl heptyl ketone, alismone
CHARACTERISTICS: *Color:* Pale yellow to amber with fluorescence; *Odor:* Unpleasant, but on dilution it becomes pleasant; *Taste:* Sharp
PHYSICAL CONSTANTS: *Specific gravity:* 0.832–0.842 (15 C); *Refractive index:* 1.4300–1.4400; *Optical rotation:* +8 to +10
SOLUBILITY: Insoluble in water; soluble in alcohol (3/70%)
USES: *Perfumes:* Perfumery; *Other:* Isolation of methyl nonyl ketone
WARNING AND CAUTION: Contact produces erythema, vesication; ingestion causes epigastric pain, nausea, vomiting, convulsion, death

SAFFRON
SYNONYMS: Crocus
BOTANICAL: *Family: Iridaceae; Genus: Crocus; Species: Sativus*

SOURCES: *Habitat:* Western Asia, southern Europe; *Part of the Plant:* Dried stigma
CHEMICAL CONSTITUENTS: Picrocrocin, safranal, glucoside crocetin
CHARACTERISTICS: *Color:* Orange-brown; *Odor:* Strong, aromatic characteristic; *Taste:* Bitter, aromatic
USES: *Flavors:* Flavors; coloring for foods; *Medicine:* Carminative, emmenagogue

SAGE

BOTANICAL: *Family: Labiatae; Genus: Salvia; Species: Officinalis* (Dalmatian); *Lavandulaefolia* (Spanish); *Variety: Dalmatian* (Dalmatian), *Spanish* (Spanish)
SOURCES: *Habitat:* Southeastern Europe, especially in Dalmatia and Spain; *Part of the Plant:* Dried leaves
CHEMICAL CONSTITUENTS: Pinene, cineol, linalool, thujone, aldehyde C_{12} MNA, dimethyl benzyl carbinyl acetal, borneol, linalyl acetate, salvene
CHARACTERISTICS: *Color:* Yellowish or greenish-yellow; *Odor:* Spicy, herbaceous, camphoraceous; *Taste:* Camphoraceous
PHYSICAL CONSTANTS: Dalmatian: *Specific gravity:* 0.903–0.925; *Refractive index:* 1.4570–1.4690; *Optical rotation:* +2 to +29; Spanish: *Specific gravity:* 0.900–0.925; *Refractive index:* 1.4575–1.4690; *Optical rotation:* +2 to +25
SOLUBILITY: Insoluble in water; soluble in alcohol (10/70%), mineral oils
USES: *Flavors:* Food flavoring; *Perfumes:* Herbaceous type; as a fixative; *Medicine:* Medicine

SANDALWOOD

BOTANICAL: *Family: Santalaceae; Genus: Santalum* (East Indies), *Amyris* (West Indies); *Species: Album* (East Indies), *Balsamifera* (West Indies); *Variety: East Indies, West Indies*
SOURCES: *Habitat: Santalum album:* Indonesia, southeast Asia, Mysore Province; *Amyris balsamifera:* Indonesia, West Indies; *Part of the Plant:* Wood
CHEMICAL CONSTITUENTS: Santalene, santalone, cadinene, diacetyl, santalol, santalyl acetate, β–caryophyllene, *d*-cadinene, cadinol
CHARACTERISTICS: *Form:* Viscid; *Color:* Pale yellow; *Odor:* Characteristic resinous, faint aromatic, persistent; *Taste:* Harsh, resinous, woody
PHYSICAL CONSTANTS: East Indies: *Specific gravity:* 0.965–0.980; *Refractive index:* 1.500–1.510; *Optical rotation:* –15 to –20 (25 C); West Indies: *Specific gravity:* 0.943–0.968; *Refractive index:* 1.508–1.513; *Optical rotation:* +10 to +46 (25 C)
SOLUBILITY: Slightly soluble in water; soluble in alcohol (5/70% or 1–3/80%); insoluble in glycerin
USES: *Flavors:* Flavors; *Perfumes:* Perfumery, woody type; *Medicine:* Diuretic and antiseptic

SARSAPARILLA

BOTANICAL: *Family: Liliaceae; Genus: Smilax; Species: Aristolochiaefolia; Variety: Medica*
SOURCES: *Habitat:* Brazil, Honduras, Guatemala, Mexico, Jamaica, southern U.S.; *Part of the Plant:* Dried roots

CHEMICAL CONSTITUENTS: Glucosides: sarsaponin, smilacin (parillin), paroparic acid, resin
USES: *Flavors:* Soft drinks, root beer; *Pharmaceuticals:* Flavoring agent; *Medicine:* Medicaments

SASSAFRAS
BOTANICAL: *Family: Lauraceae; Genus: Sassafras; Species: Officinalis; Variety: Albidum, variifolium*
SOURCES: *Habitat:* North America; *Part of the Plant:* Barks of the roots
CHEMICAL CONSTITUENTS: Safrole 80%, pinene, eugenol, phellandrene, *d*-camphora, sesquiterpenes, dihydrosafrole, isosafrole
CHARACTERISTICS: *Color:* Yellow to reddish-yellow; *Odor:* Characteristic aromatic; *Taste:* Warm aromatic
PHYSICAL CONSTANTS: *Specific gravity:* 1.065–1.077; *Refractive index:* 1.5250–1.5350; *Optical rotation:* +2 to +4
SOLUBILITY: Slightly soluble in water; soluble in alcohol (2/90%), ether, chloroform, glacial acetic acid, carbon disulfide
USES: *Perfumes:* Perfumes, soaps; *Medicine:* Carminative; anti-infective; pediculicide; *Other:* Masking disagreeable odors
WARNING AND CAUTION: Not for use in food and beverages—toxic by ingestion (FDA)

SAVIN
BOTANICAL: *Family: Pinaceae; Genus: Juniperus; Species: Sabina*
SOURCES: *Habitat:* Europe, northern Asia, North America; *Part of the Plant:* Fresh tops
CHEMICAL CONSTITUENTS: Sabinol, sabinyl acetate, cadinene, pinene, decylic nono terpene, podophyllotoxin, sabinene
PHYSICAL CONSTANTS: *Specific gravity:* 0.903–0.923 (15 C); *Refractive index:* 1.470–1.478; *Optical rotation:* +40 to +60
SOLUBILITY: Slightly soluble in water; soluble in alcohol, ether, chloroform
USES: *Medicine:* Emmenagogue, anthelmintic, antirheumatic

SAVORY
BOTANICAL: *Family: Labiatae; Genus: Satureja; Species: Hortensis*
SOURCES: *Habitat:* France, Yugoslavia, U.S.A; *Part of the Plant:* Twigs and leaves
CHARACTERISTICS: *Color:* Light yellow to dark brown; *Odor:* Aromatic, thyme, oregano-like; *Taste:* Oregano-like
PHYSICAL CONSTANTS: *Specific gravity:* 0.875–0.954; *Refractive index:* 1.4860–1.5050; *Optical rotation:* –5 to +4
SOLUBILITY: Soluble in alcohol (2/80%), fixed oils, mineral oils; insoluble in glycerin
USES: *Flavors:* Flavors

SILVER FIR NEEDLE
BOTANICAL: *Family: Pinaceae; Genus: Abies; Species: Alba*

SOURCES: *Habitat:* Central Europe; *Part of the Plant:* Needles and twigs
CHEMICAL CONSTITUENTS: Santene, *l*-α-pinene, β-pinene, *l*-camphene, α-phellandrene, dipentene, *l*-bornyl acetate, terpinyl acetate, bisabolene
CHARACTERISTICS: *Odor:* Balsamic, characteristic of pine needles
PHYSICAL CONSTANTS: *Specific gravity:* 0.905–0.925; *Refractive index:* 1.469–1.473; *Optical rotation:* –37 to +43
SOLUBILITY: Soluble in alcohol (10–14/80%)
USES: *Perfumes:* Detergents, disinfectants, deodorants

SPEARMINT

BOTANICAL: *Family: Labiatae; Genus: Mentha; Species: Spicata*
SOURCES: *Habitat:* China, Japan, Brazil, U.S.; *Part of the Plant:* Flowering tops
CHEMICAL CONSTITUENTS: *l*-Carvone 50–65%, *l*-limonene, pinene, linalool, carvyl acetate, *l*-carvyl propionate, dihydrocarvyl acetate
CHARACTERISTICS: *Color:* Colorless, yellow, or greenish-yellow; *Odor:* Spearmint characteristic; *Taste:* Spearmint
PHYSICAL CONSTANTS: *Specific gravity:* 0.917–0.934; *Refractive index:* 1.4820–1.4900; *Optical rotation:* –48 to +59
SOLUBILITY: Slightly soluble in water; soluble in alcohol (equal volumes 80% alcohol), ether, chloroform
USES: *Flavors:* Flavors; *Medicine:* Medicine

SPIKE LAVENDER

BOTANICAL: *Family: Labiatae; Genus: Lavandula; Species: Spica; Variety: Latifolia*
SOURCES: *Habitat:* Mediterranean area, mainly in Spain, Morocco, southern France, Yugoslavia; *Part of the Plant:* Flowering tops
CHEMICAL CONSTITUENTS: Eucalyptol 35%, camphor, linalool, borneol, terpineol, *d*-camphene, sesquiterpenes, linalyl acetate 3%
CHARACTERISTICS: *Color:* Colorless or pale yellow; *Odor:* Lavender, eucalyptol, camphoraceous; *Taste:* Warm, bitter, camphoraceous
PHYSICAL CONSTANTS: *Specific gravity:* 0.900–0.920 (15 C); *Refractive index:* 1.4462–1.469; *Optical rotation:* –4 to +6
SOLUBILITY: Insoluble in water; soluble in alcohol (3/70%), fixed oils, propylene glycol; slightly soluble in glycerin and mineral oils
USES: *Flavors:* Flavors; *Perfumes:* Soaps, bath preparations, lavender-type perfumes; *Other:* Odor-masking sprays; disinfectants; denaturant for alcohol

SPRUCE

SYNONYMS: Hemlock
BOTANICAL: *Family: Pinaceae; Genus: Picea; Species: Alba, nigra*; *Tsuga canadensis* is Canada hemlock
SOURCES: *Habitat:* Canada; *Part of the Plant:* Needles and branches
CHEMICAL CONSTITUENTS: Bornyl acetate, cadinene, pinene
CHARACTERISTICS: *Color:* Colorless to light yellow; *Odor:* Agreeable, characteristic
PHYSICAL CONSTANTS: *Specific gravity:* 0.907–0.920 (15 C); *Refractive index:*

1.4675–1.4700; *Optical rotation:* –18 to –25
SOLUBILITY: Soluble in alcohol (1/90%); slightly soluble in propylene glycol
USES: *Perfumes:* Soaps, cosmetics; *Medicine:* Liniments
WARNING AND CAUTION: Low toxicity

STORAX (RESINOID)
SYNONYMS: Styrax, Styrol
BOTANICAL: *Family: Hamamelidaceae; Genus: Liquidambar; Species: Orientalis; Variety: Styraciflua*
SOURCES: *Habitat:* Middle East, Iran, Honduras, Guatemala; *Part of the Plant:* Inner bark and gum
CHEMICAL CONSTITUENTS: Phenyl ethylene, styrene, cinnamic acid and esters, phenyl propyl cinnamate, ethyl cinnamate, benzyl cinnamate 5–15%, α–β–storesin and its cinnamic esters 33–50%, styracin 5–10%, vanillin (traces)
CHARACTERISTICS: *Form:* Thick semiliquid; *Color:* Gray; *Odor:* Aromatic; *Taste:* Sweet aromatic
PHYSICAL CONSTANTS: *Specific gravity:* 0.890–0.900; *Refractive index:* 1.539–1.565; *Optical rotation:* –35 to –0.30; *Boiling point:* 150–300 C
SOLUBILITY: Insoluble in water; soluble in warm alcohol (1/70%); soluble in ether, acetone, carbon disulfide
USES: *Flavors:* Flavors; *Perfumes:* Perfumery; *Pharmaceuticals:* Fumigating powders and tablets; *Medicine:* Expectorant; *Other:* Microscopy

TAGETES
BOTANICAL: *Family: Compositae; Genus: Tagetes; Species: Glandulifera or patula*
SOURCES: *Habitat:* Italy, Spain, South Africa; *Part of the Plant:* Flowers
CHEMICAL CONSTITUENTS: Tagetone, *d*-limonene, 2,6-dimethyl-7-octene-4-one
CHARACTERISTICS: *Odor:* Intense aromatic, fruits reminiscent
PHYSICAL CONSTANTS: *Specific gravity:* 0.922; *Refractive index:* 1.5112; *Optical rotation:* +1.30
SOLUBILITY: Soluble in alcohol (1/90%)
USES: *Perfumes:* Cosmetics and fine fragrance compositions

TAMARIND
BOTANICAL: *Family: Leguminosae; Genus: Tamarindus; Species: Indica*
SOURCES: *Habitat:* East Indies, India, Africa, West Indies; *Part of the Plant:* Pulp of the fruits
CHEMICAL CONSTITUENTS: Tartaric acid 10%, citric and malic acids 25–40%, invert sugar, pectin
CHARACTERISTICS: *Odor:* Agreeable, characteristic
SOLUBILITY: Soluble in water, alcohol, ether, chloroform
USES: *Flavors:* Soft drinks, liqueurs; *Medicine:* Mild laxative; *Other:* Seed kernels powder as sizing agent

TANSY
BOTANICAL: *Family: Compositae; Genus: Tanacetum; Species: Vulgare and huronense*

SOURCES: *Habitat:* Europe, North America; *Part of the Plant:* Leaves and tops
CHEMICAL CONSTITUENTS: Thujone, borneol, camphor
CHARACTERISTICS: *Form:* Liquid; *Color:* Yellow which becomes brown on exposure; *Odor:* Camphoraceous strong; *Taste:* Poisonous
PHYSICAL CONSTANTS: *Specific gravity:* 0.925–0.950; *Refractive index:* 1.4588; *Optical rotation:* +30 to +44
SOLUBILITY: Insoluble in water; soluble in alcohol, ether, chloroform, carbon disulfide
USES: *Medicine:* Medicine
WARNING AND CAUTION: Highly toxic by ingestion

THYME
BOTANICAL: *Family: Labiatae; Genus: Thymus; Species: Vulgaris; Variety: Gracilis*
SOURCES: *Habitat:* France, Spain, Algeria, Yugoslavia; *Part of the Plant:* Flowering herb
CHEMICAL CONSTITUENTS: Borneol, thymol, carvacrol, bornyl acetate, pinene, linalool
CHARACTERISTICS: *Color:* Colorless to reddish-brown; *Odor:* Pleasant oregano-like; *Taste:* Sharp
PHYSICAL CONSTANTS: *Specific gravity:* 0.910–0.935; *Refractive index:* 1.4950–1.5050; *Optical rotation:* –8 to +5
SOLUBILITY: Slightly soluble in water; soluble in alcohol (2/80%)
USES: *Flavors:* Flavors; *Perfumes:* Perfumery, cosmetics, toilet soaps; *Medicine:* Medicine

TOBACCO (ABSOLUTE)
BOTANICAL: *Family: Solanaceae; Genus: Nicotiniana; Species: Tabacum*
SOURCES: *Habitat:* America (native), worldwide; *Part of the Plant:* Leaves
CHEMICAL CONSTITUENTS: Nicotine, nornicotine, nicotianine, nicotelline, and other alkaloids; an albumin, myosmine; tannin, ammonia, glutamine; traces of zinc, iodine, copper, manganese, carbohydrates (lignin, pentosans, starch, glucose)
CHARACTERISTICS: *Odor:* Warm, aromatic, characteristic of tobacco
USES: *Flavors:* Flavoring tobacco; *Perfumes:* Masculine-type perfumes

TOLU BALSAM (RESINOID)
BOTANICAL: *Family: Leguminosae; Genus: Myroxylon; Species: Balsamum; Variety: Genuinum* (New Granada, Venezuela); also *Toluifera balsamum*
SOURCES: *Habitat:* Central and South America; *Part of the Plant:* Oleoresin exudation
CHEMICAL CONSTITUENTS: Benzyl benzoate, benzyl cinnamate, farnesol, cinnamic acid, benzoic acid, benzyl esters, cinnamein
CHARACTERISTICS: *Form:* Semifluid or semisolid resinous mass; *Color:* Yellowish-brown; *Odor:* Hyacinth-like; *Taste:* Aromatic
PHYSICAL CONSTANTS: *Specific gravity:* 0.945–1.090; *Refractive index:* 1.544–1.560; *Optical rotation:* –2 to +1
SOLUBILITY: Insoluble in water; soluble in alcohol, ether, chloroform, benzene,

glacial acetic acid; partially soluble in carbon disulfide, sodium hydroxide
USES: *Flavors:* Chewing gums; *Perfumes:* Perfumery; *Medicine:* Expectorant ingredient

TONKA BEANS (ABSOLUTE)
BOTANICAL: *Family: Leguminosae; Genus: Dipteryx; Species: Odorata; Variety: Oppositifolia*
SOURCES: *Habitat:* Africa, South America, especially in Brazil, tropical America, Guiana, and Venezuela; *Part of the Plant:* Beans
CHARACTERISTICS: *Color:* Black-brownish; *Odor:* Warm, coumarin-vanilla-like; *Taste:* Bitterish
USES: *Flavors:* Flavoring; *Perfumes:* Toilet powders; perfumes of fantasy type; *Medicine:* Medicine; *Other:* Natural coumarin production

TREEMOSS (RESINOID, ABSOLUTE)
BOTANICAL: *Family: Lichens; Genus: Evernia or Urnea; Species: Furfuracea or barbata*
SOURCES: *Habitat:* Central and southern Europe, France, Morocco, Yugoslavia; *Part of the Plant:* From the bark of spruce and fir trees growing in the humid forests
CHEMICAL CONSTITUENTS: Phenols
CHARACTERISTICS: *Odor:* Phenolic, tar-like
USES: *Perfumes:* Fixative in many compositions, particularly of fougere and chypres types

TUBEROSE (CONCRETE, ABSOLUTE)
BOTANICAL: *Family: Amaryllidaceae; Genus: Polianthes; Species: Tuberosa*
SOURCES: *Habitat:* Central America, France, Morocco, Egypt, India, Comoro Islands; *Part of the Plant:* Flowers by enfleurage
CHEMICAL CONSTITUENTS: Methyl anthranilate, methyl benzoate, benzyl alcohol
CHARACTERISTICS: *Color:* Colorless to very light; *Odor:* Heavy, honey-like, floral, jasmine
PHYSICAL CONSTANTS: *Specific gravity:* 1.007–1.035 (15 C); *Refractive index:* 1.5136–1.5352; *Optical rotation:* –3.21 to –2.30
SOLUBILITY: Soluble in alcohol
USES: *Flavors:* Flavors; *Perfumes:* Extensively in floral fragrances

TURPENTINE (RECTIFIED)
BOTANICAL: *Family: Pinaceae; Genus: Pinus; Species: Palustris; heterphylla; echinata*
SOURCES: *Part of the Plant:* Oleoresin
CHEMICAL CONSTITUENTS: Pinene, sylvestrene, dipentene
CHARACTERISTICS: *Color:* Colorless; *Odor:* Camphoraceous, characteristic, penetrating; *Taste:* Bitter, becoming stronger on aging and exposure
PHYSICAL CONSTANTS: *Specific gravity:* 0.860–0.875 (15 C); *Refractive index:* 1.463–1.483; *Flash point:* 90–115 F
SOLUBILITY: Insoluble in water; soluble in alcohol (5 volumes), ether, chloroform,

carbon disulfide, oils
USES: *Other:* Source of terpineol
WARNING AND CAUTION: Highly toxic by ingestion; moderately toxic by inhalation and skin absorption

VALERIAN

BOTANICAL: *Family: Valerianaceae; Genus: Valeriana; Species: Officinalis; Variety: Angustifolia, Japanese*
SOURCES: *Habitat:* Poland, Hungary, France, Belgium, Japan, China, U.S.S.R., Madagascar, Haiti, Tahiti; *Part of the Plant:* Dried rhizomes and roots
CHEMICAL CONSTITUENTS: Borneol, bornyl acetate, camphene, pinene, isovalerianic esters; valeric, formic, malic, acetic acids; valerianin, chatinine, alkaloids; tannin, resin; *l*-limonene
CHARACTERISTICS: *Color:* Yellowish or brownish; *Odor:* Penetrating characteristic; *Taste:* Pungent
PHYSICAL CONSTANTS: *Specific gravity:* 0.930–0.960; *Refractive index:* 1.470–1.486; *Optical rotation:* –14 to –8
SOLUBILITY: Slightly soluble in water; soluble in alcohol (1.5/90%), ether, chloroform
USES: *Flavors:* Flavors; *Perfumes:* Tobacco perfume, soaps; *Pharmaceuticals:* Pharmaceuticals; *Medicine:* Sedative; *Other:* Industrial odorant

VANILLA (RESINOID)

BOTANICAL: *Family: Orchidaceae; Genus: Vanilla; Species: Planifolia*
SOURCES: *Habitat:* Central America, Mexico, Indonesia, Madagascar, West Indies; *Part of the Plant:* Pods
CHEMICAL CONSTITUENTS: Anisic alcohol, anisic aldehyde, anisic acid, coniferin, resin, sugar, vanillin
CHARACTERISTICS: *Odor:* Warm, balsamic, intense, sweet characteristic
USES: *Flavors:* Flavoring foods; *Perfumes:* Fine perfumes; *Other:* Source of vanillin

VASSOURA

BOTANICAL: *Family: Compositae; Genus: Baccharis; Species: Dracunculifolia*
SOURCES: *Habitat:* Brazil; *Part of the Plant:* Green leaves
CHARACTERISTICS: *Odor:* Spicy, woody
USES: *Flavors:* As spice component

VERBENA

BOTANICAL: *Family: Verbenaceae; Genus: Lippia; Species: Citriodora, triphylla*
SOURCES: *Habitat:* South America, southern France, Algeria, Morocco; *Part of the Plant:* Leaves
CHEMICAL CONSTITUENTS: Citral 20–38%, *d*-verbenone, verbenalin, linalool 3.5–11%, geraniol, limonene, sesquiterpenes, methyl heptenone
CHARACTERISTICS: *Color:* Reddish; *Odor:* Lemongrass-like
PHYSICAL CONSTANTS: *Specific gravity:* 0.895–0.920; *Refractive index:* 1.482–1.488; *Optical rotation:* –10 to +18; *Boiling point:* 200 C
SOLUBILITY: Soluble in alcohol (1–5/90%)

USES: *Perfumes:* Perfumes; *Medicine:* Tonic and diaphoretic; *Other:* Not a commercial essential oil due to its scarcity and high cost

VETIVER

BOTANICAL: *Family: Graminaceae; Genus: Vetiveria; Species: Zizanoides*
SOURCES: *Habitat:* Indonesia, Reunion, Haiti, Brazil, China, Angola
CHEMICAL CONSTITUENTS: Vetiverol, vetivenyl vetivenate, vetivene, khusol, kusinol (Indian type); vetivenic, palmitic, benzoic acids; vetiver acetate, vetacetal
CHARACTERISTICS: *Form:* Viscous; *Color:* Brown to reddish; *Odor:* Harsh aromatic, violet-like; *Taste:* Woody
PHYSICAL CONSTANTS: *Specific gravity:* 0.990–1.040 (15 C); *Refractive index:* 1.5200–1.5280; *Optical rotation:* +15 to +45
SOLUBILITY: Insoluble in water, glycerin, propylene glycol; soluble in alcohol (3/80%), benzyl benzoate, mineral oils (slightly turbid), diethyl phthalate
USES: *Perfumes:* Perfumes mostly of the chypre type; soaps

VIOLET (CONCRETE, ABSOLUTE)

BOTANICAL: *Family: Violaceae; Genus: Viola* (blue violet)*; Species: Odorata, papilionaceae; Variety: Pansy* (violet tricolor)
SOURCES: *Habitat:* Italy, southern France, and almost worldwide; *Part of the Plant:* Leaves
CHARACTERISTICS: *Odor:* Intense, herbaceous, peppery, iris-like
PHYSICAL CONSTANTS: *Specific gravity:* 0.920 (17C); *Optical rotation:* +104 (15 C)
USES: *Perfumes:* Special violet-type perfumes

WALLFLOWER

BOTANICAL: *Family: Cruciferae; Genus: Cheiranthus, Erysimum; Species: Cheiri*
SOURCES: *Part of the Plant:* Flowers
CHEMICAL CONSTITUENTS: Nerol, geraniol, indole, methyl anthranilate
CHARACTERISTICS: *Odor:* Fragrant
PHYSICAL CONSTANTS: *Specific gravity:* 1.001; *Refractive index:* 1.4920
USES: *Perfumes:* Perfumery

WINTERGREEN

BOTANICAL: *Family: Ericaceae; Genus: Gaultheria; Species: Procumbens; Variety: Fragrantissima* (Indian)
SOURCES: *Part of the Plant:* Leaves
CHEMICAL CONSTITUENTS: Methyl salicylate 90%, arbutin, ericolin, urson
CHARACTERISTICS: *Color:* Colorless, yellowish, or reddish; *Odor:* Methyl salicylate; *Taste:* Astringent
PHYSICAL CONSTANTS: *Specific gravity:* 1.180–1.185; *Refractive index:* 1.535–1.538; *Optical rotation:* Inactive; *Boiling point:* 220–224 C; *Melting point:* –8.6 C
SOLUBILITY: Slightly soluble in water; soluble in alcohol (7/70%), ether, glacial acetic acid
USES: *Flavors:* Flavors, dentifrices; *Perfumes:* Perfumes; *Medicine:* Antipyretic; antiseptic; antirheumatic liniments; *Other:* Insecticides

WARNING AND CAUTION: Highly toxic by ingestion; it's use is restricted by FDA

WORMSEED

BOTANICAL: *Family: Compositae; Genus: Artemisia; Species: Maritima; Variety: Panniflora, stechmanniana, pauciflora*
SOURCES: *Habitat:* Europe; *Part of the Plant:* Flowers
CHEMICAL CONSTITUENTS: Eucalyptol (cineol)
CHARACTERISTICS: *Color:* Pale yellow to yellowish-green; *Odor:* Unpleasant; *Taste:* Bitter
PHYSICAL CONSTANTS: *Specific gravity:* 0.915–0.940; *Refractive index:* 1.46201
SOLUBILITY: Insoluble in water; soluble in alcohol, ether
USES: *Medicine:* Anthelmintic

WORMWOOD

BOTANICAL: *Family: Compositae; Genus: Artemisia; Species: Absinthum*
SOURCES: *Habitat:* Europe; *Part of the Plant:* Fresh or dry leaves and tops
CHEMICAL CONSTITUENTS: Thujyl alcohol, thujyl acetate, thujone, phellandrene, cadinene
CHARACTERISTICS: *Color:* Brownish to dark green; *Odor:* Unpleasant; *Taste:* Bitter
PHYSICAL CONSTANTS: *Specific gravity:* 0.925-0.955 (15 C); *Refractive index:* 1.4660–1.4770
SOLUBILITY: Slightly soluble in water; soluble in alcohol (2/80%), ether, benzyl benzoate, diethyl phthalate, fixed oils (with opalescence)
USES: *Medicine:* Anthelmintic; antimalaric
WARNING AND CAUTION: Highly toxic by ingestion; small amount may be fatal. In vermouth, it is only in traces, since it can cause stupor, convulsion, death

WOODRUFF

SYNONYMS: Petit muguet
BOTANICAL: *Family: Rubiaceae; Genus: Asperula; Species: Odorata*
SOURCES: *Habitat:* Europe, Siberia, northern Africa, Australia; *Part of the Plant:* Dried leaves
CHEMICAL CONSTITUENTS: Coumarin, tannin, asperuloside, fatty oil
CHARACTERISTICS: *Odor:* Muguet-like; *Taste:* Bitter, astringent
USES: *Flavors:* Flavoring May wine with the dried leaves in sachets; *Perfumes:* Fragrant compositions

YLANG YLANG

SYNONYMS: Flower of flowers
BOTANICAL: *Family: Anonaceae; Genus: Cananga; Species: Odorata; Variety: Genuina*
SOURCES: *Habitat:* Indonesia, Philippines, Comoro Islands; *Part of the Plant:* Fresh flowers
CHEMICAL CONSTITUENTS: Benzyl benzoate, benzyl alcohol, sesquiterpenes, linalool, geraniol, pinene, cadinene, acetic acid, benzoic acid, cresol methyl ether, phenol

CHARACTERISTICS: *Color:* Yellowish; *Odor:* Jasmine-like, very fragrant
PHYSICAL CONSTANTS: Manila: *Specific gravity:* 0.911-0.958 (30 C); *Refractive index:* 1.4747–1.4940; *Optical rotation:* –27 to –49; Reunion-Bourbon: *Specific gravity:* 0.932–0.962 (15 C); *Refractive index:* 1.491–1.500; *Optical rotation:* –34 to –64
SOLUBILITY: Soluble in benzyl benzoate, fixed oils, diethyl phthalate
USES: *Flavors:* Flavors; *Perfumes:* Perfumery of very delicate type
NOTE: The first fraction of distillation is called ylang ylang oil. Subsequent fractions are called cananga oil.

Chapter III:

SYNTHETIC ESSENCES

Introduction

The synthetic odorants are artificially prepared substances. The odors are similar to those of flowers, fruits, or other natural aromatic material, such as the essential oils. Many are the artificial reproduction of the constitutents of the essential oils such as:

Linalyl acetate, constituent of bergamot and lavender;
Benzaldehyde, constituent of bitter almond;
Methyl salicylate, constituent of wintergreen;
Vanillin, constituent of vanilla;
Coumarin, constituent of Tonka beans;
Heliotropin, constituent of heliotrope.

There are, however, many synthetic products with a strong, fruity, floral odor which are not found in nature. The artificial essences are prepared by blending various aromatic substances with similar odor to those of the natural flowers or fruits.

The preparations are made by mixing artificial products (sometimes natural products are included) with ethyl alcohol as a solvent, in minimal amounts until the compound becomes completely clear. These essences are considerably more concentrated and stronger in odor intensity than the perfumes, extracts, bouquets, colognes, etc.

The separation from the essential oils by fractional distillation is expensive and yields minimal quantities. Therefore, synthetic products, mostly derived from benzene, through synthesis with natural constituent fragrance of the essential oils, are frequently used in the manufacture of many perfume and flavor components. The compounds that have been isolated from the essential oils include the hydrocarbon series known as terpenes, and in addition, many nitro-sulfo-halogenated compounds.

Materials Employed as Odorants

From the chemical standpoint there are two groups of materials employed as odorants:

I. *Aliphatic* (fat like) from Greek word "aliphe" fat.
Compounds related to methane (CH_4)

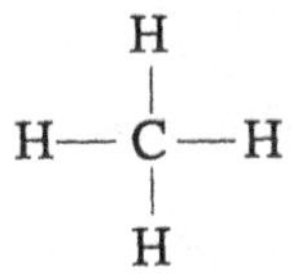

The name of this group is derived from the similarity of the vegetal and animal fats present.

II. *Aromatic*.
Compounds related to benzene (C_6H_6).

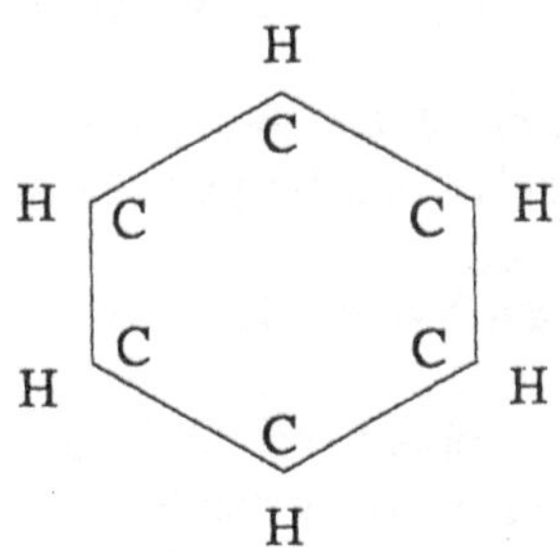

This group has been so named because almost all of its products are characterized by fragrant odors (aromatic).

Both groups are divided into: *hydrocarbons, esters, acetates, acids, alcohols, aldehydes, ethers, ketones, lactones, phenols, nitro compounds, halogenated compounds, sulfurous compounds.*

Hydrocarbons. Of the aliphatic hydrocarbon series few essential oils are found in nature, e.g., paraffins, terpenes, and sesquiterpenes. Of the aromatic hydrocarbon series more abundant in the essential oils are terpenes and sesquiterpenes with others in lesser amounts.

Esters. Esters are the most characteristic fruit odoring liquid employed in the preparation of flavors and some perfumes.

The term "ester" refers to a product of condensation by heating an alcohol and an acid, usually in the presence of a small amount of sulfuric acid, with the elimination of water, followed by purification by distillation, after the addition of alkali and charcoal. The combination generally includes a variety of alcohols and acids for each preparation.

Acetates. Specific esters, generically termed "acetates," are also employed because of their fruity or flowery odor. The term "acetate" refers to the combination with acetic acid.

Acids. Acids are ordinarily found in essential oils esterified with alcohols. In the free state, very small amounts are found due to the decomposition of the esters. Exceptions are the free acids found in larger quantity in orris oil as myristic acid, and in Mexican valerian oil as valerianic acid.

The product of the condensation reaction producing esters is classified with a binomial combination reflecting the two materials employed in the preparation of the ester. For example, the combination of methyl alcohol and formic acid yields methyl formate. Products of formic acid would be ethyl formate, propyl formate, or amyl formate, etc., according to the alcohol employed.

Alcohols. Alcohols are found in essential oils, either in the free state or in combination with various acids as esters. Alcohols, with a characteristic peculiar odor, are extensively employed in perfume compounding.

Aldehydes. Many aldehydes are extensively employed both in flavor and perfume manufacturing. The word "aldehyde" derives from alcohol deprived of hydrogen. Aldehydes are formed from alcohols by dehydrogenation or oxidation.

Ethers. Ethers are derived from alcohols by concentration with the elimination of water.

Ketones. Ketones are liquids, or solids of low melting point, with a pleasant odor. They are derived from organic acids and alcohol by gently heating in the presence of a metallic catalyst.

Lactones. Lactones are products of condensation of an oxacid with elimination of water.

Phenols. Phenols are products of oxidation of hydrocarbons by means of alkali.

Nitro compounds. Nitro compounds are combinations of ketones and lactones with the odor of natural musk (animal or plant type), through nitro-oxidation.

Halogenated compounds. These are combinations containing halogens (bromine, chlorine, fluorine, iodine). They produce a pleasant odor.

Sulfurous compounds. Compounds in which the odor of sulfur is prominent.

Of these organic chemicals, those employed most often in compounding of flavors and perfumes are further described.

Chemical Components of Flavors and Perfumes

Note: Specific gravity at 25/25 C
Refractive index at 20 C
Flash point: TCC (Tag closed cup)

ACETALDEHYDE
SYNONYMS: Ethanal; acetic aldehyde; ethyl aldehyde
CHEMICAL FORMULA: C_2H_4O
CAS NUMBER: 75-07-0
CLASSIFICATION: Aldehyde
OCCURRENCE: Synthetic
CHARACTERISTICS: *Form:* Liquid; *Color:* Colorless; *Odor:* Pungent aromatic
PHYSICAL CONSTANTS: *Specific gravity:* 0.788; *Refractive index;* 1.3316; *Boiling point:* 21 C
SOLUBILITY: Miscible with water, alcohol
USES: Perfumes, flavors
WARNINGS AND CAUTION:Toxic in large doses

ACETATE C-8
SYNONYMS: Octyl acetate
CHEMICAL FORMULA: $C_{10}H_{20}O_2$
CLASSIFICATION: Acetate
OCCURRENCE: Green tea
CHARACTERISTICS: *Form:* Liquid; *Color:* Colorless; *Odor:* Floral, fatty jasmine, orange
PHYSICAL CONSTANTS: *Specific gravity:* 0.865, 0.868; *Refractive index;* 1.4180, 1.4210; *Flash point:* 185 F
SOLUBILITY: Soluble in alcohol (4 parts/70%)
USES: Jasmine, rose, cassie, chypre, fougere, neroli type perfumes

ACETATE C-9
SYNONYMS: Nonyl acetate
CHEMICAL FORMULA: $C_{11}H_{22}O_2$
CLASSIFICATION: Acetate
OCCURRENCE: Synthetic
CHARACTERISTICS: *Form:* Liquid; *Color:* Colorless; *Odor:* Fruity-floral
PHYSICAL CONSTANTS: *Specific gravity:* 0.864, 0.868; *Refractive index;* 1.4220, 1.4260; *Flash point:* 212 F
SOLUBILITY: Soluble in alcohol (6 parts/70% or 1 part/80%)
USES: Lavender, rose, gardenia, orange flower type perfumes

ACETATE C-10
SYNONYMS: Decyl acetate
CHEMICAL FORMULA: $C_{12}H_{24}O_2$

CLASSIFICATION: Acetate
OCCURRENCE: Synthetic
CHARACTERISTICS: *Form:* Liquid; *Color:* Colorless; *Odor:* Floral, orange-rose
PHYSICAL CONSTANTS: *Specific gravity:* 0.862, 0.866; *Refractive index;* 1.4250, 1.4300; *Flash point:* 212 F
SOLUBILITY: Soluble in alcohol (4 parts/80%)
USES: Rose, geranium, jasmine, muguet, orange flower type perfumes

ACETATE C-11
SYNONYMS: Undecenyl acetate; 10-undecen-1-yl acetate
CHEMICAL FORMULA: $C_{13}H_{24}O_2$
CLASSIFICATION: Acetate
OCCURRENCE: Synthetic
CHARACTERISTICS: *Form:* Liquid; *Color:* Colorless; *Odor:* Floral, fatty
PHYSICAL CONSTANTS: *Specific gravity:* 0.876, 0.880; *Refractive index;* 1.4380, 1.4420; *Flash point:* 212 F
SOLUBILITY: Soluble in alcohol (2 parts/80%)
USES: Eau de cologne-type perfumes

ACETATE C-12
SYNONYMS: Dodecyl acetate; lauryl acetate
CHEMICAL FORMULA: $C_{14}H_{28}O_2$
OCCURRENCE: Synthetic
CLASSIFICATION: Acetate
CHARACTERISTICS: *Form:* Liquid; *Color:* Colorless; *Odor:* Citrus-rose
PHYSICAL CONSTANTS: *Specific gravity:* 0.860, 0.865; *Refractive index;* 1.4320, 1.4360; *Flash point:* 212 F
SOLUBILITY: Soluble in alcohol (4 parts/80%)
USES: Rose, gardenia, carnation, and other floral type perfumes

ACETATE PA
CLASSIFICATION: Acetate
OCCURRENCE: Synthetic
CHARACTERISTICS: *Form:* Liquid; *Color:* Colorless; *Odor:* Fruity, pineapple
PHYSICAL CONSTANTS: *Specific gravity:* 1.100–1.105; *Refractive index:* 1.5130–1.5180; *Flash point:* > 212 F
SOLUBILITY: Clearly soluble in alcohol (2 parts/80%)
USES: Cologne and oriental heavy scents

ACETIC GLACIAL (PURE)
CHEMICAL FORMULA: $C_2H_4O_2$
CAS NUMBER: 64-19-7
CLASSIFICATION: Acid
OCCURRENCE: Synthetic
CHARACTERISTICS: *Form:* Liquid; *Color:* Colorless; *Odor:* Very pungent
PHYSICAL CONSTANTS: *Specific gravity:* 1.051; *Refractive index;* 1.3718; *Optical*

rotation: 1049 D; *Flash point:* 110 F
SOLUBILITY: Soluble in water, alcohol, ether, glycerin, carbon tetrachloride
USES: Manufacture of acetates, solvents, preserving food

ACETOPHENONE
CHEMICAL FORMULA: C_8H_8O
CAS NUMBER: 98-86-2
CLASSIFICATION: Ketone
OCCURRENCE: Labdanum, green tea, orris, castoreum
CHARACTERISTICS: *Form:* Semisolid; *Color:* Colorless; *Odor:* Mimosa, hawthorn
PHYSICAL CONSTANTS: *Specific gravity:* 1.025–1.028; *Refractive index;* 1.5330–1.5350; *Congealing point:* 19 C; *Flash point:* 177 F
SOLUBILITY: Soluble in alcohol (5 parts/50%)
USES: Hawthorn, new mown hay, syringa, lilac, fougere-type perfumes; soaps

ALCOHOL C-7
SYNONYMS: 1-Heptanol; heptyl alcohol
CHEMICAL FORMULA: $C_7H_{16}O$
CLASSIFICATION: Alcohol
OCCURRENCE: Leaves of *Litsea zeylanic*
CHARACTERISTICS: *Form:* Liquid; *Color:* Colorless; *Odor:* Citrus, strong fatty
PHYSICAL CONSTANTS: *Specific gravity:* 0.820–0.824; *Refractive index;* 1.4230–1.4270; *Flash point:* 170 F
SOLUBILITY: Soluble in alcohol (2 parts/60% or 1 part/70%)
USES: Oriental, spicy, citrus, carnation, and jasmine-type perfumes

ALCOHOL C-8
SYNONYMS: 1-Octanol; *n*-octyl alcohol; *n*-caprylic alcohol
CHEMICAL FORMULA: $C_8H_{18}O$
CLASSIFICATION: Alcohol
OCCURRENCE: Sweet orange, grapefruit, green tea, *Heracleum villosum,* and esterified in various oils
CHARACTERISTICS: *Form:* Liquid; *Color:* Colorless; *Odor:* Citrus, strong fatty
PHYSICAL CONSTANTS: *Specific gravity:* 0.822–0.828; *Refractive index;* 1.4280–1.4310; *Flash point:* 184 F
SOLUBILITY: Soluble in alcohol (6 parts/50% or 3 parts/60%)
USES: Colognes, rose, jasmine-type perfumes

ALCOHOL C-9
SYNONYMS: 1-Nonanol; nonyl alcohol; pelargonic alcohol
CHEMICAL FORMULA: $C_9H_{20}O$
CLASSIFICATION: Alcohol
OCCURRENCE: Sweet orange, oakmoss
CHARACTERISTICS: *Form:* Liquid; *Color:* Colorless; *Odor:* Citrus, rosy
PHYSICAL CONSTANTS: *Specific gravity:* 0.824–0.830; *Refractive index;* 1.4310–1.4350; *Flash point:* 210 F

SOLUBILITY: Soluble in alcohol (3 parts/60%)
USES: Colognes, neroli, rose, reseda, orange, gardenia, tuberose, jasmine-type perfumes

ALCOHOL C-10
SYNONYMS: Decyl alcohol; *n*-decyl alcohol; 1-decanol; capric alcohol
CHEMICAL FORMULA: $C_{10}H_{22}O$
CLASSIFICATION: Alcohol
OCCURRENCE: Sweet orange, almond tree flowers, ambrette seed oils
CHARACTERISTICS: *Form:* Liquid; *Color:* Colorless; *Odor:* Orange flower
PHYSICAL CONSTANTS: *Specific gravity:* 0.826–0.832; *Refractive index;* 1.4350–1.4390; *Flash point:* 220 F
SOLUBILITY: Soluble in alcohol (4 parts/60%)
USES: Citrus, violet, orange flower, jonquil, orris, lilac, jasmine, rose-type perfumes

ALCOHOL C-11 (UNDECYLENIC)
SYNONYMS: *n*-Undecylenic alcohol; 10-undecen-1-ol
CHEMICAL FORMULA: $C_{11}H_{22}O$
CLASSIFICATION: Alcohol
OCCURRENCE: Leaves of *Litsea odorifera*
CHARACTERISTICS: *Form:* Liquid; *Odor:* Flowery, herbaceous, slightly fruity, somewhat citrus odor
PHYSICAL CONSTANTS: *Specific gravity:* 0.842–0.846; *Refractive index:* 1.4490–1.4540; *Melting point:* –3 C min.; *Flash point:* > 212 F
SOLUBILITY: Soluble in alcohol (2 parts/70%)
USES: Tuberose, gardenia, jasmine, lilac, green notes in small quantities

ALCOHOL C-11 (UNDECYLIC)
SYNONYMS: Undecyl alcohol; 1-undecanol
CHEMICAL FORMULA: $C_{11}H_{24}O$
CLASSIFICATION: Alcohol
OCCURRENCE: Synthetic
CHARACTERISTICS: *Form:* Liquid; *Color:* Colorless; *Odor:* Citrus
PHYSICAL CONSTANTS: *Specific gravity:* 0.828–0.834; *Refractive index;* 1.4370–1.4430; *Flash point:* 212 F
SOLUBILITY: Soluble in alcohol (4 parts/60%)
USES: Acacia, cassie, tuberose, floral types

ALCOHOL C-12
SYNONYMS: Dodecyl alcohol; 1-dodecanol; lauryl alcohol
CHEMICAL FORMULA: $C_{12}H_{26}O$
CLASSIFICATION: Alcohol
OCCURRENCE: Lime oil, *Furcrae gigantea* flowers
CHARACTERISTICS: *Form:* Liquid; *Color:* Colorless; *Odor:* Tuberose, violet, fatty
PHYSICAL CONSTANTS: *Specific gravity:* 0.830–0.836; *Refractive index;* 1.4400–1.4440; *Flash point:* 212 F

SOLUBILITY: Soluble in alcohol (2 parts/70%)
USES: Tuberose, reseda, muguet, narcissus, violet, rose-type perfumes

ALCOHOL C-16
SYNONYMS: Cetyl alcohol
CHEMICAL FORMULA: $C_{16}H_{34}O$
CLASSIFICATION: Alcohol
OCCURRENCE: Whale oil, spermaceti, and natural waxes
CHARACTERISTICS: *Form:* Wax; *Color:* White; *Odor:* Odorless
PHYSICAL CONSTANTS: *Specific gravity:* 0.8176 (49.5 C); *Refractive index;* 1.4283; *Melting point:* 47 C; *Congealing point:* 46 C; *Boiling point:* 344 C
SOLUBILITY: Soluble in alcohol (1 part/90%)
USES: Cosmetics, shaving creams

ALDEHYDE C-7
SYNONYMS: Heptanol; *n*-heptaldehyde; oenanthaldehyde; oenanthol
CHEMICAL FORMULA: $C_7H_{14}O$
CLASSIFICATION: Aldehyde
OCCURRENCE: Hyacinth oils (traces), ylang ylang
CHARACTERISTICS: *Form:* Liquid; *Color:* Colorless or yellowish; *Odor:* Harsh, pungent, acidic-fruity
PHYSICAL CONSTANTS: *Specific gravity:* 0.814–0.819; *Refractive index;* 1.4120–1.4200; *Flash point:* 95 F
SOLUBILITY: Soluble in alcohol (2 parts/70%)
USES: Traces in perfume, orange flower, fixative

ALDEHYDE C-8
SYNONYMS: Octanal; caprylic aldehyde; caprylaldehyde
CHEMICAL FORMULA: $C_8H_{16}O$
CLASSIFICATION: Aldehyde
OCCURRENCE: Citrus, rose, lavender, lemongrass, *Pinus jeffrey*
CHARACTERISTICS: *Form:* Liquid; *Color:* Colorless; *Odor:* Sharp citrus, rosaceous-fruity, jasmine-waxy
PHYSICAL CONSTANTS: *Specific gravity:* 0.818–0.825; *Refractive index;* 1.4180–1.4220; *Flash point:* 131 F
SOLUBILITY: Soluble in alcohol (2 parts/70%)
USES: Citrus, jasmine, neroli, rose-type perfumes; fixative

ALDEHYDE C-9
SYNONYMS: Nonanal; pelargonaldehyde; *n*-nonyl aldehyde
CHEMICAL FORMULA: $C_9H_{18}O$
CLASSIFICATION: Aldehyde
OCCURRENCE: Citrus, rose, orris, ginger, *Pinus sabinian*
CHARACTERISTICS: *Form:* Liquid; *Color:* Colorless; *Odor:* Sharp-fatty lily, rose, orris, orange, verbena
PHYSICAL CONSTANTS: *Specific gravity:* 0.820–0.828; *Refractive index;* 1.4220–

1.4260; *Flash point:* 161 F
SOLUBILITY: Soluble in alcohol (3 parts/70%)
USES: Citrus, rose, orris, heliotrope, jasmine, tuberose-type perfumes; fixative

ALDEHYDE C-10

SYNONYMS: Decanal; capric aldehyde; capraldehyde; *n*-decyl aldehyde
CHEMICAL FORMULA: $C_{10}H_{20}O$
CLASSIFICATION: Aldehyde
OCCURRENCE: Citrus, lavender, juniperus, coriander, cassie, orris, lemongrass, savin, acacia, *Pinus* various species
CHARACTERISTICS: *Form:* Liquid; *Color:* Colorless; *Odor:* Fatty, orange, lemon, rose, waxy
PHYSICAL CONSTANTS: *Specific gravity:* 0.822–0.830; *Refractive index;* 1.4270–1.4300; *Flash point:* 183 F
SOLUBILITY: Soluble in alcohol (1 part/80%)
USES: Citrus, lavender, cassie, jasmine, violet, clary sage, rose, neroli, cyclamen, lilac

ALDEHYDE C-11 (UNDECYLENIC)

SYNONYMS: Undecylenaldehyde; undecenal; hendecenal; 10-undecenal
CHEMICAL FORMULA: $C_{11}H_{20}O$
CLASSIFICATION: Aldehyde
OCCURRENCE: Synthetic
CHARACTERISTICS: *Form:* Liquid; *Color:* Colorless or yellowish; *Odor:* Rosy, violet, tuberose, orris, slightly green-fruity
PHYSICAL CONSTANTS: *Specific gravity:* 0.841–0.848; *Refractive index;* 1.4410–1.4460; *Flash point:* 197 F
SOLUBILITY: Soluble in alcohol (2 parts/80%)
USES: Floral perfumes, tuberose, woody compositions; fixative for patchouli, sandalwood, orris, oakmoss, clary sage compositions

ALDEHYDE C-11 (UNDECYLIC)

SYNONYMS: Undecylic aldehyde; undecanal; hendecanal
CHEMICAL FORMULA: $C_{11}H_{22}O$
CLASSIFICATION: Aldehyde
OCCURRENCE: Synthetic
CHARACTERISTICS: *Form:* Liquid; *Color:* Colorless or yellowish; *Odor:* Citrus, woody, fatty
PHYSICAL CONSTANTS: *Specific gravity:* 0.825–0.832; *Refractive index;* 1.4310–1.4350; *Flash point:* 180 F
SOLUBILITY: Soluble in alcohol (5 parts/70%)
USES: Floral and fantasy perfumes

ALDEHYDE C-12 (LAURIC)

SYNONYMS: Lauric aldehyde; dodecanal; lauraldehyde; *n*-dodecyl aldehyde
CHEMICAL FORMULA: $C_{12}H_{24}O$
CLASSIFICATION: Aldehyde

OCCURRENCE: Citrus, rue, *Pinus* various species
CHARACTERISTICS: *Form:* Liquid; *Color:* Colorless; *Odor:* Woody, green, herbaceous, fatty, tuberose flowers, violet on dilution
PHYSICAL CONSTANTS: *Specific gravity:* 0.826–0.834; *Refractive index;* 1.4330–1.4380; *Flash point:* 212 F
SOLUBILITY: Soluble in alcohol (2 parts/80% or 1 part/90%)
USES: Lilac, jasmine, tuberose, muguet, violet, reseda, cassie, chypre, new mown hay, fern, pine; traces in petitgrain; fixative

ALDEHYDE C-12 (MNA)
SYNONYMS: Methyl *n*-nonyl acetaldehyde; 2-methylendecanal; 2-methylundecanal
CHEMICAL FORMULA: $C_{12}H_{24}O$
CLASSIFICATION: Aldehyde
OCCURRENCE: Synthetic
CHARACTERISTICS: *Form:* Liquid; *Color:* Colorless or yellowish; *Odor:* Ginger, sage, orange, amber, moss, tuberose
PHYSICAL CONSTANTS: *Specific gravity:* 0.822–0.830; *Refractive index;* 1.4310–1.4360; *Flash point:* 157 F
SOLUBILITY: Soluble in alcohol (4 parts/80%)
USES: Chypre-like fine perfumes, tuberose, orchid, honeysuckle, sweet pea; fixative

ALDEHYDE C-14 (MYRISTIC)
SYNONYMS: *n*-Tetradecyl aldehyde; myristaldehyde
CHEMICAL FORMULA: $C_{14}H_{28}O$
CLASSIFICATION: Aldehyde
OCCURRENCE: *Pinus sabinian*, *Ocotea usambarensis*, camphora tree, formosa oils
CHARACTERISTICS: *Form:* Liquid; *Color:* Colorless or yellowish; *Odor:* Orris, strong fatty
PHYSICAL CONSTANTS: *Specific gravity:* 0.825–0.835; *Refractive index;* 1.4380–1.4450; *Flash point:* 212 F
SOLUBILITY: Soluble in alcohol (1 part/80%)
USES: Orris, cassie, violet-type perfumes

ALDEHYDE C-14 (PURE)
SYNONYMS: Peach aldehyde; γ-undecalactone; 4-hydroxyundecanoic acid lactone
CHEMICAL FORMULA: $C_{11}H_{20}O$
CLASSIFICATION: Aldehyde
OCCURRENCE: Synthetic
CHARACTERISTICS: *Form:* Liquid; *Color:* Yellowish; *Odor:* Peach-like
PHYSICAL CONSTANTS: *Specific gravity:* 0.940–0.944; *Refractive index;* 1.4500–1.4540; *Flash point:* 212 F
SOLUBILITY: Soluble in alcohol (5 parts/60%), benzyl alcohol, benzyl benzoate, and other organic solvents
USES: Fruity flavors, jasmine, lilac, chypre compositions

ALDEHYDE C-16 (PURE)

SYNONYMS: Ethyl α, β-epoxy-β methylhydocinnamate; ethyl methyl phenyl glycidate; strawberry aldehyde
CHEMICAL FORMULA: $C_{12}H_{14}O_2$
CLASSIFICATION: Aldehyde
OCCURRENCE: Synthetic
CHARACTERISTICS: *Form:* Liquid; *Color:* Yellowish; *Odor:* Strong strawberry
PHYSICAL CONSTANTS: *Specific gravity:* 1.0887–1.0920; *Refractive index;* 1.5040–1.5090; *Flash point:* 212 F
SOLUBILITY: Soluble in alcohol (4 parts/70%)
USES: Flavors; rose centifolia, hyacinth, acacia, cyclamen, strawberry, jasmine, lilac, orange flower-type perfumes

ALDEHYDE C-18

SYNONYMS: γ-Nonalactone; coconut aldehyde; nonanolide-1-4; prunolide
CHEMICAL FORMULA: $C_9H_{16}O_2$
CLASSIFICATION: Aldehyde
OCCURRENCE: Synthetic
CHARACTERISTICS: *Form:* Liquid; *Color:* Yellowish; *Odor:* Coconut
PHYSICAL CONSTANTS: *Specific gravity:* 0.958–0.965; *Refractive index;* 1.4460–1.4500; *Flash point:* 212 F
USES: Gardenia, tuberose, oriental, heavy floral type perfumes

ALDEHYDE C-19

SYNONYMS: Benzyl isobutyrate
CLASSIFICATION: Aldehyde
OCCURRENCE: Synthetic
CHARACTERISTICS: *Odor:* Fruity, floral; pineapple
USES: Woody and spicy floral perfumes

ALDEHYDE C-20

SYNONYMS: Ethyl-*p*-methyl β-phenyl glycidate; raspberry aldehyde
CLASSIFICATION: Aldehyde
OCCURRENCE: Synthetic
CHARACTERISTICS: *Odor:* Raspberry
USES: Chypres and ionone compositions

ALLYL SULFIDE

SYNONYMS: Thioallyl ether; "oil garlic;" diallyl sulfide; 3,3′-thiobis (1-propene)
CHEMICAL FORMULA: $C_6H_{10}S$
CLASSIFICATION: Sulfurous compound
OCCURRENCE: Garlic (natural)
CHARACTERISTICS: *Form:* Liquid; *Color:* Yellow; *Odor:* Garlic
PHYSICAL CONSTANTS: *Specific gravity:* 0.888 (27/4 C); *Refractive index;* 1.4877 (27 C); *Boiling point:* 139 C
SOLUBILITY: Slightly soluble in water; miscible with alcohol, ether, chloroform,

carbon tetrachloride
USES: Culinary food; medicine
WARNINGS AND CAUTION: Artificial oil of garlic is toxic by ingestion; it is strongly irritating to the eyes and skin

AMBRETTOLIDE
CHEMICAL FORMULA: $C_{16}H_{28}O_2$
CLASSIFICATION: Lactone
OCCURRENCE: Ambrette seed
CHARACTERISTICS: *Form:* Liquid; *Color:* Colorless; *Odor:* Floral, ambrette seed
PHYSICAL CONSTANTS: *Specific gravity:* 0.954–0.957; *Refractive index;* 1.4800–1.4810
SOLUBILITY: Soluble in alcohol (9 parts/80% or 1 part/90%)
USES: Fixative

AMYL BENZOATE
SYNONYMS: Isopentyl benzoate; isoamyl benzoate
CHEMICAL FORMULA: $C_{12}H_{16}O_2$
CAS NUMBER: 94-46-2
CLASSIFICATION: Benzoate
OCCURRENCE: Synthetic
CHARACTERISTICS: *Form:* Liquid; *Color:* Colorless; *Odor:* Fruity, balsamic; slightly pungent
PHSYICAL CONSTANTS: *Specific gravity:* 0.986–0.990; *Refractive index:* 1.4920–1.4950; *Flash point:* > 212 F
SOLUBILITY: Clearly soluble in alcohol (3 parts/80%)
USES: Clover, orchis, tobacco, oriental compositions; fixative

AMYL BUTYRATE
CHEMICAL FORMULA: $C_9H_{18}O_2$
CAS NUMBER: 106-27-4
CLASSIFICATION: Ester
OCCURRENCE: Oil of cocoa and oil of eucalpytus
CHARACTERISTICS: *Form:* Liquid; *Color:* Colorless; *Odor:* Apricot-like
PHYSICAL CONSTANTS: *Specific gravity:* 0.861–0.864; *Refractive index;* 1.4090–1.4130; *Flash point:* 148 F
SOLUBILITY: Soluble in alcohol (5 parts/70%)
USES: Flavors; hawthorn, new mown hay, fougère scents

AMYL CINNAMIC ALDEHYDE
SYNONYMS: Buxine; α-pentylcinnamaldehyde; α-amylcinnamaldehyde; α-*n*-amyl-β-phenylacrolein; jasmine aldehyde
CHEMICAL FORMULA: $C_{14}H_{18}O$
CLASSIFICATION: Aldehyde
OCCURRENCE: Synthetic
CHARACTERISTICS: *Form:* Liquid; *Color:* Clear yellow; *Odor:* Floral, jasmine,

lily
PHYSICAL CONSTANTS: *Specific gravity:* 0.963–0.968; *Refractive index:* 1.5540–1.5590; *Flash point:* 221 F
SOLUBILITY: Clearly soluble in alcohol (6 parts/80%)
USES: Jasmine and many other floral compositions

AMYL PHENYL ACETATE
SYNONYMS: Isopentyl phenylacetate; isoamyl phenylacetate
CHEMICAL FORMULA: $C_{13}H_{18}O_2$
CLASSIFICATION: Phenyl acetate
OCCURRENCE: Synthetic
CHARACTERISTICS: *Form:* Liquid; *Color:* Colorless; *Odor:* Sweet, honey
PHYSICAL CONSTANTS: *Specific gravity:* 0.975–0.977; *Refractive index:* 1.4850–1.4870; *Flash point:* > 212 F
SOLUBILITY: Clearly soluble in alcohol (3 parts/80%)
USES: Sweet pea, lily of the valley, tobacco; flavors

AMYL PROPIONATE
SYNONYMS: Isopentyl propionate; isoamyl propionate
CHEMICAL FORMULA: $C_8H_{16}O_2$
CLASSIFICATION: Propionate
OCCURRENCE: Synthetic
CHARACTERISTICS: *Form:* Liquid; *Color:* Colorless; *Odor:* Fruity, apricot, pineapple
PHYSICAL CONSTANTS: *Specific gravity:* 0.865–0.869; *Refractive index:* 1.4060–1.4090; *Flash point:* 116 F
SOLUBILITY: Clearly soluble in alcohol (3 parts/70%)
USES: Modifier for top notes in perfumes and flavors

ANETHOLE
SYNONYMS: Isoestragole; anise camphor; *p*-methoxypropenyl benzene
CHEMICAL FORMULA: $C_{10}H_{12}O$
CLASSIFICATION: Ether
OCCURRENCE: Anise seed, star anise, fennel leaves
CHARACTERISTICS: *Form:* Liquid at room temperature; *Color:* Colorless; *Odor:* Anise
PHYSICAL CONSTANTS: *Specific gravity:* 0.984–0.987; *Refractive index;* 1.5570–1.5610; *Optical rotation:* ± 0.15; *Flash point:* 212 F
SOLUBILITY: Soluble in alcohol (2 parts/90%)
USES: Liquors, liqueurs, perfumes, soaps

ANGELIC ACID
CHEMICAL FORMULA: $C_5H_8O_2$
CLASSIFICATION: Acid
OCCURRENCE: Roots of *Archangelica* or *Anthemis nobilis*
CHARACTERISTICS: *Form:* Crystals; *Color:* Colorless; *Odor:* Spicy

PHYSICAL CONSTANTS: *Specific gravity:* 0.9539 (76.4 C); *Refractive index;* 1.4434 (47 C); *Melting point:* 45 C; *Boiling point:* 185 C
SOLUBILITY: Soluble in alcohol, ether, hot water
USES: Flavoring medicine

ANISIC ACID
CHEMICAL FORMULA: $C_8H_8O_3$
CLASSIFICATION: Acid
OCCURRENCE: Oxidation of anethole
CHARACTERISTICS: *Form:* Crystals, powder, or needles; *Color:* White; *Odor:* Anise
PHYSICAL CONSTANTS: *Specific gravity:* 1.385; *Melting point:* 184 C; *Boiling point:* 275–280 C
SOLUBILITY: Soluble in alcohol, ether
USES: Antirheumatic, repellent, antiseptic

ANISIC ALCOHOL
SYNONYMS: Anisyl alcohol; anise alcohol; *p*-methoxybenzyl alcohol
CHEMICAL FORMULA: $C_8H_{10}O_2$
CLASSIFICATION: Alcohol
OCCURRENCE: Vanilla pods
CHARACTERISTICS: *Form:* Liquid; *Color:* Colorless; *Odor:* Rosy, lilac-vanilla; suggesting hawthorn
PHYSICAL CONSTANTS: *Specific gravity:* 1.111–1.114; *Refractive index:* 1.541–1.545; *Boiling point:* 255–265 C; *Congealing point:* 24 C
SOLUBILITY: Soluble in alcohol (1 volume/50%)
USES: Jasmine, lilac, muguet, sweet pea, gardenia; flavors; pharmaceutical intermediate
WARNINGS AND CAUTION: Flammable, moderate risk

ANISIC ALDEHYDE
SYNONYMS: Aubepine; *p*-anisaldehyde; *p*-methoxybenzaldehyde
CHEMICAL FORMULA: $C_8H_8O_2$
CLASSIFICATION: Aldehyde
OCCURRENCE: Fennel, anise seed, star anise, mimosa, acacia, *Magnolia salicifolia* leaves, vanilla beans, *Agastache rugosa*
CHARACTERISTICS: *Form:* Liquid; *Color:* Colorless or yellowish; *Odor:* Strong hawthorn
PHYSICAL CONSTANTS: *Specific gravity:* 1.119–1.123; *Refractive index;* 1.5710–1.5740; *Flash point:* 248 F
SOLUBILITY: Soluble in alcohol (2 parts/60%)
USES: Floral, new mown hay, fougere, clover, heliotrope, hawthorn-type perfumes

ANISOLE
SYNONYMS: Methyl phenyl ether; methoxybenzene
CHEMICAL FORMULA: C_7H_8O
CAS NUMBER: 100-66-3
CLASSIFICATION: Ether

OCCURRENCE: Synthetic
CHARACTERISTICS: *Form:* Liquid; *Color:* Colorless; *Odor:* Sharp anise phenolic
PHYSICAL CONSTANTS: *Specific gravity:* 0.990–0.993; *Refractive index;* 1.5150–1.5180; *Flash point:* 123 F
SOLUBILITY: Soluble in alcohol (6 parts/70%)
USES: Lilac, spicy perfumes, soaps

ANISYL ACETATE
SYNONYMS: *p*-Methoxybenzyl acetate
CHEMICAL FORMULA: $C_{10}H_{12}O_3$
CLASSIFICATION: Acetate
OCCURRENCE: Synthetic
CHARACTERISTICS: *Form:* Liquid; *Color:* Colorless; *Odor:* Lilac-hawthorn
PHYSICAL CONSTANTS: *Specific gravity:* 1.104–1.107; *Refractive index:* 1.5110–1.5160; *Flash point:* > 212 C
SOLUBILITY: Clearly soluble in alcohol (6 parts/60%)
USES: Lilac, honeysuckle, acacia, violet, gardenia, floral bouquet

ANISYL FORMATE
SYNONYMS: *p*-Methoxybenzyl formate
CHEMICAL FORMULA: $C_9H_{10}O_3$
CLASSIFICATION: Formate
OCCURRENCE: Synthetic
CHARACTERISTICS: *Form:* Liquid; *Color:* Colorless; *Odor:* Floral, sweet, hawthorn, syringa
PHYSICAL CONSTANTS: *Specific gravity:* 1.138–1.142; *Refractive index:* 1.5220–1.5240; *Flash point:* 212 F
SOLUBILITY: Clearly soluble in alcohol (3 parts/70%)
USES: Lilac, tuberose, gardenia, ylang ylang, heliotrope, jasmine compositions; flavors: berry, currant, vanilla, licorice

ANTHRANILIC ACID
CHEMICAL FORMULA: $C_7H_7NO_2$
CAS NUMBER: 118-92-3
CLASSIFICATION: Acid
OCCURRENCE: Synthetic
CHARACTERISTICS: *Form:* Crystals or powder; *Color:* White or yellowish; *Odor:* Slightly orange
PHYSICAL CONSTANTS: *Melting point:* 144–146 C
SOLUBILITY: Soluble in hot water, alcohol, ether
USES: Perfumes, pharmaceuticals

BENZALDEHYDE
CHEMICAL FORMULA: C_7H_6O
CAS NUMBER: 100-52-7
CLASSIFICATION: Aldehyde

OCCURRENCE: Bitter almonds, peach, cherries, plum seeds and kernels
CHARACTERISTICS: *Form:* Liquid; *Color:* Colorless; *Odor:* Bitter almond
PHYSICAL CONSTANTS: *Specific gravity:* 1.041–1.046; *Refractive index;* 1.5440–1.5465; *Flash point:* 148 F
SOLUBILITY: Soluble in alcohol (3 parts/60%)
USES: Traces in various types of perfume

BENZOIC ACID
CHEMICAL FORMULA: $C_7H_6O_2$
CAS NUMBER: 65-85-0
CLASSIFICATION: Acid
OCCURRENCE: It occurs naturally in benzoic resin
CHARACTERISTICS: *Form:* Scales, needles, crystals; *Color:* White; *Odor:* Benzaldehyde
PHYSICAL CONSTANTS: *Specific gravity:* 1.2659; *Melting point;* 121 C; *Boiling point:* 249.2 C
SOLUBILITY: Soluble in alcohol, ether, chloroform, benzene
USES: Perfumes, tobacco curing, preservative for food, benzoates

BENZYL ACETATE
SYNONYMS: Phenylmethyl acetate; acetic acid phenyl methyl ester
CHEMICAL FORMULA: $C_9H_{10}O_2$
CLASSIFICATION: Acetate
OCCURRENCE: Jasmine, ylang ylang, hyacinth, gardenia, neroli, tuberose
CHARACTERISTICS: *Form:* Liquid; *Color:* Colorless; *Odor:* Jasmine
PHYSICAL CONSTANTS: *Specific gravity:* 1.052–1.054; *Refractive index:* 1.5010–1.5030; *Flash point:* 216 F
SOLUBILITY: Clearly soluble in alcohol (6 parts/60%)
USES: Jasmine, rosy, muguet compositions; widely used in a variety of soap and cosmetic perfumes

BENZYL BENZOATE
CHEMICAL FORMULA: $C_{14}H_{12}O_2$
CAS NUMBER: 120-51-4
CLASSIFICATION: Benzoate
OCCURRENCE: Tolu and Peru balsam, jasmine, ylang ylang, tuberose, hyacinth, jonquil, carnation, cinnamon leaves and oil
CHARACTERISTICS: *Form:* Liquid; *Color:* Colorless; *Odor:* Faintly balsamic
PHYSICAL CONSTANTS: *Specific gravity:* 1.116–1.120; *Refractive index:* 1.5680–1.5700; *Flash point:* 298 F
SOLUBILITY: Clearly soluble in alcohol (2 parts/90%)
USES: Solvent for synthetic musks, vanillin, heliotropin; fixative for floral compositions

BENZYL CINNAMATE
SYNONYMS: Cinnamein; 3-phenyl-2-propenoic acid phenyl methyl ester
CHEMICAL FORMULA: $C_{16}H_{14}O_2$

CLASSIFICATION: Cinnamate
OCCURRENCE: Peru and Tolu balsam, storax
CHARACTERISTICS: *Form:* Crystals or fused solid; *Color:* Melt; *Odor:* Sweet balsamic
PHYSICAL CONSTANTS: *Boiling point:* 244 C; *Flash point:* > 212 F; *Congealing point:* 33 C max.
SOLUBILITY: 1 g is soluble in 5 ml of 95% alcohol; insoluble in water
USES: Oriental types; flavors; fixative

BENZYL FORMATE
CLASSIFICATION: Formate
OCCURRENCE: Synthetic
CHARACTERISTICS: *Form:* Liquid; *Color:* Colorless; *Odor:* Powerful, fruity, spicy, jasmine
PHYSICAL CONSTANTS: *Specific gravity:* 1.083–1.092; *Refractive index:* 1.5100–1.5140; *Flash point:* 180 F
USES: Extensively used in perfume compounding and flavors

BENZYL PHENYL ACETATE
SYNONYMS: Benzyl α-toluate
CHEMICAL FORMULA: $C_{15}H_{14}O_2$
CLASSIFICATION: Phenyl acetate
OCCURRENCE: Synthetic
CHARACTERISTICS: *Form:* Liquid; *Color:* Colorless; *Odor:* Sweet, floral, honey
PHYSICAL CONSTANTS: *Specific gravity:* 1.095–1.099; *Refractive index:* 1.5530–1.5580; *Flash point:* > 212 F
SOLUBILITY: Clearly soluble in alcohol (3 parts/90%)
USES: Floral compositions for soaps and cosmetics

BENZYL PROPIONATE
CHEMICAL FORMULA: $C_{10}H_{12}O_2$
CLASSIFICATION: Propionate
OCCURRENCE: Synthetic
CHARACTERISTICS: *Form:* Liquid; *Color:* Colorless; *Odor:* Jasmine, floral, sweet
PHYSICAL CONSTANTS: *Specific gravity:* 1.028–1.032; *Refractive index:* 1.4950–1.4990; *Flash point:* 213 F
SOLUBILITY: Clearly soluble in alcohol (4 parts/70%)
USES: Jasmine, rose, and many floral types especially for soaps; also in fruit flavors

BENZYL SALICYLATE
SYNONYMS: Benzyl *o*-hydroxybenzoate
CHEMICAL FORMULA: $C_{14}H_{12}O_3$
CLASSIFICATION: Salicylate
OCCURRENCE: Ylang ylang oil, carnation
CHARACTERISTICS: *Form:* Liquid, solidyfing at cool room temperature; *Color:* Colorless; *Odor:* Sweet, faintly balsamic, woody, floral

PHYSICAL CONSTANTS: *Specific gravity:* 1.176–1.180; *Refractive index:* 1.580–1.581; *Flash point:* > 212 F; *Boiling point:* 208 C (26 mm)
SOLUBILITY: Clearly soluble in alcohol (4 parts/95%)
USES: As a solvent for synthetic musks; fixative and diluent in many floral compositions, e.g., lilac, carnation, lily, jasmine

BENZYL VALERIANATE
SYNONYMS: Benzylvaleriniac ether; benzyl valerate
CHEMICAL FORMULA: $C_{12}H_{16}O_2$
CLASSIFICATION: Valerate (valerianate)
OCCURRENCE: Synthetic
CHARACTERISTICS: *Form:* Liquid; *Color:* Colorless; *Odor:* Fruity, musky, rosaceous
PHYSICAL CONSTANTS: *Specific gravity:* 0.985–0.988; *Refractive index:* 1.4860–1.4890; *Flash point:* > 212 F
SOLUBILITY: Clearly soluble in alcohol (2 parts/80% or 1 part/90%)
USES: In small quantities in florals, particularly rose types; also in oriental-type perfumes

BORNYL ACETATE
CHEMICAL FORMULA: $C_{12}H_{20}O_2$
CLASSIFICATION: Acetate
OCCURRENCE: Synthetic
CHARACTERISTICS: *Form:* Liquid; *Color:* Colorless; *Odor:* Fruity, musk, rosaceous
PHYSICAL CONSTANTS: *Specific gravity:* 0.981–0.984; *Refractive index:* 1.462–1.465; *Flash point:* 185 F
SOLUBILITY: Soluble in alcohol (3 volumes/70%); miscible with 95% alcohol
USES: Oriental-type perfumes; perfumery, flavoring; nitrocellulose solvent
WARNINGS AND CAUTION: Moderately toxic by ingestion; flammable

BROMO STYROL
CHEMICAL FORMULA: C_8H_7Br
CLASSIFICATION: Halogenated compound
OCCURRENCE: Synthetic
CHARACTERISTICS: *Form:* Liquid; *Color:* Clear, yellow, or brownish; *Odor:* Hyacinth-like
PHYSICAL CONSTANTS: *Specific gravity:* 1.402–1.422; *Refractive index;* 1.6020–1.6080; *Congealing point:* –2 C; *Flash point:* 212 F
SOLUBILITY: Soluble in alcohol (5 parts/90%)
USES: Lilac, hyacinth-type perfumes
WARNINGS AND CAUTION: Causes irritation

BUTYL BENZOATE
CHEMICAL FORMULA: $C_{11}H_{14}O_2$
CLASSIFICATION: Ester

OCCURRENCE: Benzoic acid and butyl alcohol
CHARACTERISTICS: *Form:* Liquid; *Color:* Colorless; *Odor:* Pleasant
PHYSICAL CONSTANTS: *Specific gravity:* 1.00 (20 C); *Melting point:* –22 C; *Boiling point:* 247.3 C; *Flash point:* 225 F
SOLUBILITY: Alcohol, ether
USES: Flavors, perfumes

BUTYRIC ACID
CHEMICAL FORMULA: $C_4H_8O_2$
CAS NUMBER: 107-92-6
CLASSIFICATION: Acid
OCCURRENCE: Fermentation of molasses, starch
CHARACTERISTICS: *Form:* Oily clear liquid; *Odor:* Rancid, unpleasant
PHYSICAL CONSTANTS: *Specific gravity:* 0.964; *Refractive index;* 1.399; *Melting point:* –4.7 to –7.9 C; *Boiling point:* 163 C; *Flash point:* 170 F
SOLUBILITY: Soluble in water, alcohol, ether
USES: Flavoring candies, syrups, liqueurs; synthesis of butyrate esters

BUTYRIC ALDEHYDE
SYNONYMS: Butanal; butaldehyde; *n*-butanal; *n*-butyl aldehyde
CHEMICAL FORMULA: C_4H_8O
CAS NUMBER: 123-72-8
CLASSIFICATION: Aldehyde
OCCURRENCE: Synthetic
CHARACTERISTICS: *Form:* Liquid; *Color:* Colorless; *Odor:* Pungent
PHYSICAL CONSTANTS: *Specific gravity:* 0.8048 (20 C); *Refractive index;* 1.379; *Congealing point:* –99 C; *Boiling point:* 75.7 C; *Flash point:* 20 F
SOLUBILITY: Soluble in alcohol, ether; slightly soluble in water
USES: Solvents, colored soaps

CADINENE
CHEMICAL FORMULA: $C_{15}H_{24}$
CLASSIFACTION: Sesquiterpene hydrocarbon
OCCURRENCE: Juniperus berries, cedar leaf, cubebe, cade oils
CHARACTERISTICS: *Form:* Liquid; *Color:* Colorless; *Odor:* Slightly pleasant
PHYSICAL CONSTANTS: *Specific gravity:* 0.9819 (20 C); *Refractive index;* 1.5079; *Optical rotation:* –251; *Boiling point:* 274.5 C
SOLUBILITY: Alcohol, ether, chloroform
USES: Perfumery
WARNINGS AND CAUTION: Low toxicity by ingestion

CAPRIC ACID
CHEMICAL FORMULA: $C_{10}H_{20}O_2$
CAS NUMBER: 334-48-5
CLASSIFICATION: Acid
OCCURRENCE: Coconut oil

CHARACTERISTICS: *Form:* Crystals; *Color:* White; *Odor:* Unpleasant
PHYSICAL CONSTANTS: *Specific gravity:* 0.8858 (40 C); *Refractive index;* 1.4288 (40 C); *Melting point:* 31.5 C; *Boiling point:* 268–270 C
SOLUBILITY: Soluble in alcohol, ether, chloroform, benzene, carbon disulfide
USES: Perfumes, flavor

CAPROIC ACID
SYNONYMS: Hexanoic acid; hexoic acid
CHEMICAL FORMULA: $C_6H_{12}O_2$
CAS NUMBER: 142-62-1
CLASSIFICATION: Acid
OCCURRENCE: Fermentation of butyric and other natural fatty acids
CHARACTERISTICS: *Form:* Liquid; *Color:* Colorless or yellowish; *Odor:* Unpleasant
PHYSICAL CONSTANTS: *Specific gravity:* 0.9276 (20/4 C); *Refractive index:* 1.4168 (20 C); *Flash point:* 215 F; *Boiling point:* 205 C
SOLUBILITY: Soluble in alcohol, ether; slightly soluble in water
USES: Flavors, pharmaceuticals; manufacture of rubber chemicals, varnish driers, resins, and pharmaceuticals
WARNINGS AND CAUTION: Strong irritant

CAPRYLIC ACID
SYNONYMS: Octanoic acid
CHEMICAL FORMULA: $C_8H_{16}O_2$
CLASSIFICATION: Acid
OCCURRENCE: Saponification and further distillation of coconut oil
CHARACTERISTICS: *Form:* Liquid; *Color:* Colorless; *Odor:* Rancid, disagreeable
PHYSICAL CONSTANTS: *Specific gravity:* 0.910 (20/4 C); *Refractive index:* 1.4280 (20 C); *Flash point:* 270 F; *Melting point:* 16 C; *Boiling point:* 237 C
SOLUBILITY: Soluble in alcohol, ether, chloroform, carbon disulfide, acetic acid; slightly soluble in water
USES: Perfumes, pharmaceuticals, flavors, antiseptics, and fungicides

CARVACROL
CHEMICAL FORMULA: $C_{10}H_{14}O$
CAS NUMBER: 499-75-2
CLASSIFICATION: Phenol
OCCURRENCE: Camphor, origanum, caraway, savory
CHARACTERISTICS: *Form:* Liquid; *Color:* Colorless or yellowish; *Odor:* Spicy, thyme-like
PHYSICAL CONSTANTS: *Specific gravity:* 0.974–0.979; *Refractive index;* 1.5210–1.5260; *Flash point:* 212 F
SOLUBILITY: Soluble in alcohol (4 parts/60%)
USES: Perfumery; antiseptic, vermifuge, fungicide

CARYOPHYLLENE
CHEMICAL FORMULA: $C_{15}H_{24}$

CLASSIFACTION: Sesquiterpene hydrocarbon
OCCURRENCE: Various essential oils, mainly clove oil
CHARACTERISTICS: *Form:* Liquid; *Color:* Colorless; *Odor:* Clove-turpentine
PHYSICAL CONSTANTS: *Specific gravity:* 0.897–0.910; *Refractive index;* 1.4980–1.5040; *Flash point:* 207 F; *Boiling point:* 129–130 C
SOLUBILITY: Benzene, chloroform, alcohol (4 parts/95%)
USES: Flavors, perfumes

CEDRENE
CHEMICAL FORMULA: $C_{15}H_{24}$
CLASSIFACTION: Sesquiterpene hydrocarbon
OCCURRENCE: Red cedar oil
CHARACTERISTICS: *Form:* Crystalline; *Color:* Colorless; *Odor:* Camphor
PHYSICAL CONSTANTS: *Specific gravity:* 0.984 (15 C); *Boiling point:* 237 C
SOLUBILITY: Alcohol
USES: Perfumery, odorant for disinfectants

CEDRYL ACETATE
CHEMICAL FORMULA: $C_{17}H_{28}O_2$
CLASSIFICATION: Acetate
OCCURRENCE: Synthetic
CHARACTERISTICS: *Form:* White crystal; *Color:* Slightly yellow to brownish yellow when liquefied; *Odor:* Light cedar-vetiver
PHYSICAL CONSTANTS: *Specific gravity:* 0.967–0.985; *Refractive index:* 1.4990–1.5060; *Optical rotation:* –10 to –20
SOLUBILITY: 1 g is clearly soluble in 6 ml of 90% alcohol
USES: Woody and heavy oriental perfumes, tobacco, leather

CINNAMIC ACID
CHEMICAL FORMULA: $C_9H_8O_2$
CAS NUMBER: 621-82-9
CLASSIFICATION: Acid
OCCURRENCE: Styrax; Peru, Tolu balsams; cinnamon and cocoa leaves
CHARACTERISTICS: *Form:* Crystalline scales; *Color:* White; *Odor:* Cinnamon
PHYSICAL CONSTANTS: *Specific gravity:* 1.2475; *Freezing point:* 133 C; *Boiling point:* 300 C
SOLUBILITY: Soluble in benzene, ether, acetone, acetic acid, carbon disulfide, oils
USES: Perfumes, medicine

CINNAMIC ALDEHYDE
CHEMICAL FORMULA: C_9H_8O
CAS NUMBER: 104-55-2
CLASSIFICATION: Aldehyde
OCCURRENCE: Cassia, cinnamon barks, roots, and leaves; patchouli, myrrh, hyacinth, narcissus
CHARACTERISTICS: *Form:* Liquid; *Color:* Yellow; *Odor:* Cinnamon

PHYSICAL CONSTANTS: *Specific gravity:* 1.047–1.051; *Refractive index;* 1.6200–1.6230; *Flash point:* 268 F
SOLUBILITY: Soluble in alcohol (6 parts/60% or 2 parts/70%)
USES: Spicy perfumes, flavors

CINNAMYL ACETATE
SYNONYMS: 3-Phenyl-2-propen-1-yl acetate
CHEMICAL FORMULA: $C_{11}H_{12}O_2$
CLASSIFICATION: Acetate
OCCURRENCE: Cassia oil
CHARACTERISTICS: *Form:* Liquid; *Color:* Slightly yellow; *Odor:* Warm balsamic-floral
PHYSICAL CONSTANTS: *Specific gravity:* 1.047–1.051; *Refractive index:* 1.5400–1.5430; *Flash point:* > 212 F
SOLUBILITY: Clearly soluble in alcohol (5 parts/70%)
USES: Hyacinth, rose, woody, spicy, and floral oriental compositions, basically as a fixative

CINNAMYL BENZOATE
CLASSIFICATION: Benzoate
OCCURRENCE: Synthetic
CHARACTERISTICS: *Odor:* Spicy, balsamic
USES: Oriental, woody-floral types

CINNAMYL CINNAMATE
SYNONYMS: Styracin; cinnamic acid cinnamyl ester; cinnyl cinnamate
CHEMICAL FORMULA: $C_{18}H_{16}O_2$
CAS NUMBER: 122-69-0
CLASSIFICATION: Cinnamate
OCCURRENCE: Peru and styrax
CHARACTERISTICS: *Form:* Crystal; *Odor:* Cinnamon, sweet
SOLUBILITY: Soluble in alcohol, ether, benzene; insoluble in water
USES: Fixative and flavors; perfumery; flavoring

CINNAMYL FORMATE
SYNONYMS: 3-Phenyl-2-propen-1-yl formate
CHEMICAL FORMULA: $C_{10}H_{10}O_2$
CLASSIFICATION: Formate
OCCURRENCE: Synthetic
CHARACTERISTICS: *Form:* Liquid; *Color:* Colorless to slightly yellow; *Odor:* Cinnamon, balsamic
PHYSICAL CONSTANTS: *Specific gravity:* 1.074–1.079; *Refractive index:* 1.5500–1.5560; *Flash point:* 212 F
SOLUBILITY: Clearly soluble in alcohol (10 parts/70% or 2 parts/80%)
USES: Sandal, patchouli, vetiver, and heavy oriental perfumes

CITRAL

SYNONYMS: Geranial; neral
CHEMICAL FORMULA: $C_{10}H_{16}O$
CAS NUMBER: 5392-40-5
CLASSIFICATION: Aldehyde
OCCURRENCE: Lemongrass, verbena, geranium, ginger, lavender, pepper, bay, melissa
CHARACTERISTICS: *Form:* Liquid; *Color:* Yellowish; *Odor:* Strong citrus lemon
PHYSICAL CONSTANTS: *Specific gravity:* 0.885–0.890; *Refractive index;* 1.4860–1.4900; *Flash point:* 208 F
SOLUBILITY: Soluble in alcohol (10 parts/60%, 2 parts/70%, 1 part/95%), benzyl benzoate, diethyl phthalate, glycerin, propylene glycol, mineral oils, fixed oils
USES: Citrus, cologne-type perfumes; source of ionones

CITRIC ACID

CHEMICAL FORMULA: $C_6H_8O_7$
CLASSIFICATION: Acid
OCCURRENCE: Fermentation of citrus juice or molasses, of carbohydrates
CHARACTERISTICS: *Form and Color:* Colorless crystals or white granular powder; *Odor:* Odorless
PHYSICAL CONSTANTS: *Specific gravity:* 1.542; *Melting point:* 153 C
SOLUBILITY: Soluble in water, alcohol, ether
USES: Beverages, flavors, syrups, elixirs

CITRONELLAL

CHEMICAL FORMULA: $C_{10}H_{18}O$
CAS NUMBER: 8000-29-1
CLASSIFICATION: Aldehyde
OCCURRENCE: Citronella, eucalyptus, citriodora, *Pinus jeffrey*
CHARACTERISTICS: *Form:* Liquid; *Color:* Colorless or yellowish; *Odor:* Strong lemon-citronella, rosy
PHYSICAL CONSTANTS: *Specific gravity:* 0.848–0.856; *Refractive index;* 1.4460–1.4520; *Optical rotation:* +5 to +11; *Flash point:* 178 F
SOLUBILITY: Soluble in alcohol (5 parts/70%), miscible in alcohol (95%)
USES: Perfumes

CITRONELLYL ACETATE

SYNONYMS: 3,7-Dimethyl-6-octen-1-yl acetate
CHEMICAL FORMULA: $C_{12}H_{22}O_2$
CAS NUMBER: 150-84-5
CLASSIFICATION: Acetate
OCCURRENCE: Citronella oil, geranium oil
CHARACTERISTICS: *Form:* Liquid; *Color:* Colorless; *Odor:* Fresh fruity, rosy
PHYSICAL CONSTANTS: *Specific gravity:* 0.883–0.888; *Refractive index:* 1.4400–1.4470; *Optical rotation:* –1 to +4; *Flash point:* > 212 F
SOLUBILITY: Clearly soluble in alcohol (9 parts/70% or 2 parts/80%)

USES: Rose, muguet, lavender, carnation, chypre, geranium; flavors

CITRONELLYL BUTYRATE

SYNONYMS: 3,7-Dimethyl-6-octen-1-yl butyrate
CHEMICAL FORMULA: $C_{14}H_{26}O_2$
CLASSIFICATION: Butyrate
OCCURRENCE: Citronella (Ceylon)
CHARACTERISTICS: *Form:* Liquid; *Color:* Colorless; *Odor:* Fruity, rosy
PHYSICAL CONSTANTS: *Specific gravity:* 0.873–0.883; *Refractive index:* 1.4440–1.4480; *Flash point:* 212 F
SOLUBILITY: Clearly soluble in alcohol (3 parts/80%)
USES: Rose, muguet, geranium; flavors

CITRONELLYL FORMATE

SYNONYMS: 3,7-Dimethyl-6-octen-1-yl formate
CHEMICAL FORMULA: $C_{13}H_{20}O_2$
CAS NUMBER: 105-85-1
CLASSIFICATION: Formate
OCCURRENCE: Geranium oil
CHARACTERISTICS: *Form:* Liquid; *Color:* Colorless; *Odor:* Rose, citrus
PHYSICAL CONSTANTS: *Specific gravity:* 0.887–0.900; *Refractive index:* 1.4430–1.4480; *Flash point:* 198 F
SOLUBILITY: Clearly soluble in alcohol (3 parts/80%)
USES: Eau de cologne, rose, muguet, lavender, hyacinth, and citrus-type perfumes

CITRONELLYL PROPIONATE

SYNONYMS: 3,7-Dimethyl-6-octenyl propionate
CHEMICAL FORMULA: $C_{13}H_{24}O_2$
CLASSIFICATION: Propionate
OCCURRENCE: Synthetic
CHARACTERISTICS: *Form:* Liquid; *Color:* Colorless; *Odor:* Fruity, rosy
PHYSICAL CONSTANTS: *Specific gravity:* 0.877–0.883; *Refractive index:* 1.4430–1.4490; *Flash point:* > 212 F
SOLUBILITY: Clearly soluble in alcohol (4 parts/80%)
USES: In oriental, muguet, and rose perfumes

CITRONELLYL VALERIANATE

CLASSIFICATION: Valerate (valerianate)
OCCURRENCE: Synthetic
CHARACTERISTICS: *Odor:* Rosy
USES: Tobacco perfumes

COUMARIN

SYNONYMS: Cumarin; benzopyrone; tonka bean camphor; coumarinic anhydride
CHEMICAL FORMULA: $C_9H_6O_2$
CAS NUMBER: 91-64-5

CLASSIFICATION: Lactone
OCCURRENCE: Tonka beans, Peru balsam, cassia, lavender, lovage, orchid, vernal grass, sundry ferns, melilot
CHARACTERISTICS: *Form:* Crystals; *Color:* White; *Odor:* New mown hay
PHYSICAL CONSTANTS: *Melting point:* 68 C
SOLUBILITY: Soluble 1 g/15 ml 95% alcohol
USES: Chypre, fougere, lavender, new mown hay-type perfumes

COUMARIN ACID
CHEMICAL FORMULA: $C_9H_8O_3$
CLASSIFICATION: Acid
CHARACTERISTICS: *Form:and Color:* Colorless needles or prisms or white needles
PHYSICAL CONSTANTS: *Melting point:* 191–208 C
SOLUBILITY: Soluble in hot water
USES: Perfumery

***p*-CRESYL ACETATE**
SYNONYMS: *p*-Tolyl acetate
CHEMICAL FORMULA: $C_9H_{10}O_2$
CLASSIFICATION: Acetate
OCCURRENCE: Ylang ylang, cananga, wallflower
CHARACTERISTICS: *Form:* Liquid; *Color:* Colorless; *Odor:* Narcissus, strong pungent; it becomes more floral on dilution
PHYSICAL CONSTANTS: *Specific gravity:* 1.044–1.049; *Refractive index:* 1.4990–1.5020; *Flash point:* 186 F
SOLUBILITY: Clearly soluble in alcohol (2 parts/70%)
USES: Narcissus, hyacinth, lily, and other floral compositions

***p*-CRESYL PHENYL ACETATE**
SYNONYMS: *p*-Tolyl phenyl acetate
CHEMICAL FORMULA: $C_{15}H_{14}O_2$
CLASSIFICATION: Phenyl acetate
OCCURRENCE: Synthetic
CHARACTERISTICS: *Form:* Crystals; *Color:* White; *Odor:* Light narcissus
PHYSICAL CONSTANTS: *Congealing point:* 73.7 C min.
SOLUBILITY: 1 g is clearly soluble in 45 ml of 95% alcohol
USES: Lily, narcissus, hyacinth, jasmine, floral soaps

CUMINIC ALDEHYDE
CHEMICAL FORMULA: $C_{10}H_{12}O$
CAS NUMBER: 122-03-2
CLASSIFICATION: Aldehyde
OCCURRENCE: Cumin, eucalyptus, cinnamon oils
CHARACTERISTICS: *Form:* Liquid; *Color:* Colorless or yellowish; *Odor:* Strong, characteristic
PHYSICAL CONSTANTS: *Specific gravity:* 0.976–0.980; *Refractive index;* 1.5290–

1.5340; *Flash point:* 212 F
SOLUBILITY: Soluble in alcohol (4 parts/70%)
USES: Cassie, mimosa, hawthorn, lily, violet-type perfumes

CYMOL
SYNONYMS: Cymene; isopropyltoluene; methylisopropylbenzene; methyl (1-methyethyl) benzene
CHEMICAL FORMULA: $C_{10}H_{14}$
CAS NUMBER: *m-* 535-77-3; *o-* 527-84-4; *p-* 99-87-6; mixed 25155-15-1
CLASSIFACTION: Aromatic hydrocarbon
OCCURRENCE: Eucalyptus, cumin, thyme oils
CHARACTERISTICS: *Form:* Liquid; *Color:* Colorless transparent; *Odor:* Aromatic
PHYSICAL CONSTANTS: *Specific gravity:* 0.8551, 0.8740; *Refractive index:* 1.489; *Boiling point:* 177 C; melting point –182 C; *Flash point:* 117 F
SOLUBILITY: Alcohol, ether. chloroform
USES: Solvent

DIMETHYL BENZYL CARBINYL ACETATE
SYNONYMS: α,α-Dimethylphenethyl acetate; 1,1-dimethyl-2-phenyl acetate
CHEMICAL FORMULA: $C_{12}H_{16}O_2$
CLASSIFICATION: Acetate
OCCURRENCE: Synthetic
CHARACTERISTICS: *Form:* Fused solid melting at warm temperature; *Color:* Colorless; *Odor:* Sage-floral, woody
PHYSICAL CONSTANTS: *Specific gravity:* 0.995–0.999 (supercooled); *Refractive index:* 1.4900–1.4940 (supercooled); *Flash point:* > 212 F; *Congealing point:* 29.5 C min.
SOLUBILITY: Clearly soluble in alcohol (4 parts/70%)
USES: Muguet, geranium, hyacinth, rose, and other greenish floral-type perfumes

DIMETHYL OCTANOL
SYNONYMS: Pelargol; dihydrocitronellol; 3,7-dimethyl-1-octanol; tetrahydrogeraniol
CHEMICAL FORMULA: $C_{10}H_{22}O$
CLASSIFICATION: Acetate
OCCURRENCE: Synthetic
CHARACTERISTICS: *Form:* Liquid; *Color:* Colorless; *Odor:* Rosy, sweet
PHYSICAL CONSTANTS: *Specific gravity:* 0.828–0.840; *Refractive index:* 1.4350–1.4400; *Flash point:* 192 F
USES: Rose or lavender

DIMETHYL PHENYL CARBINYL ACETATE
CLASSIFICATION: Acetate
OCCURRENCE: Synthetic
CHARACTERISTICS: *Odor:* Rosaceous-green
USES: Rose

DIPHENYL OXIDE

SYNONYMS: Phenyl ether; diphenyl ether; phenoxybenzene; phenyl ether
CHEMICAL FORMULA: $C_{12}H_{10}O$
CAS NUMBER: 101-84-8
CLASSIFICATION: Ether
OCCURRENCE: Synthetic
CHARACTERISTICS: *Form:* Solid (melting at room temperature); *Color:* Colorless; *Odor:* Geranium leaf, strong
PHYSICAL CONSTANTS: *Specific gravity:* 1.072–1.074; *Congealing point:* 26.5 C; *Flash point:* 239 F
SOLUBILITY: Soluble in alcohol (5 parts/90%)
USES: Perfumes, soaps, rose and foin coupé types

EPOXY LINALYL ACETATE

SYNONYMS: Linalool oxide acetate
CLASSIFICATION: Acetate
OCCURRENCE: Synthetic
CHARACTERISTICS: *Odor:* Fresh floral, slightly woody
USES: Lavender-type perfumes

ETHYL ACETOACETATE

SYNONYMS: Diacetic ester; aceto acetic ester; 3-oxobutanoic acid ethyl ester
CHEMICAL FORMULA: $C_6H_{10}O_3$
CLASSIFICATION: Acetate
OCCURRENCE: Synthetic
CHARACTERISTICS: *Form:* Liquid; *Color:* Colorless; *Odor:* Fresh, sweet, fruity
PHYSICAL CONSTANTS: *Specific gravity:* 1.0250 (20/4 C); *Boiling point:* 180–181 C
SOLUBILITY: Soluble in alcohol, water
USES: Flavors
WARNINGS AND CAUTION: Moderately toxic by ingestion and inhalation; irritant to skin and eyes

ETHYL ALCOHOL

SYNONYMS: Ethanol; grain alcohol
CHEMICAL FORMULA: C_2H_6O
CAS NUMBER: 64-17-5
CLASSIFICATION: Alcohol
OCCURRENCE: Spirit of wine, grain
CHARACTERISTICS: *Form:* Liquid; *Color:* Colorless; *Odor:* Vinous
PHYSICAL CONSTANTS: *Specific gravity:* 0.816 (15.56 C); *Refractive index;* 1.3651 (15 C); *Congealing point:* –114 C; *Boiling point:* 78.3 C; *Flash point:* 55 F
SOLUBILITY: Miscible with water, ether, chloroform, acetone
USES: Colognes, liquors, liqueurs, beverages, cosmetics, antiseptics, medicine, solvent

ETHYL ANISATE

SYNONYMS: Ethyl *p*-methoxybenzoate
CHEMICAL FORMULA: $C_{10}H_{12}O_3$
CLASSIFICATION: Anisate
OCCURRENCE: Synthetic
CHARACTERISTICS: *Form:* Liquid; *Color:* Colorless to slightly yellow; *Odor:* Fruity, anise, tarragon
PHYSICAL CONSTANTS: *Specific gravity:* 1.101–1.104; *Refractive index:* 1.5220–1.5260; *Flash point:* > 212 F
SOLUBILITY: Clearly soluble in alcohol (7 parts/60% or 2 parts/70%)
USES: Lilac, carnation, ylang ylang, muguet, jasmine, fern, lily of the valley, chypres

ETHYL ANTHRANILATE

SYNONYMS: Ethyl *o*-aminobenzoate
CHEMICAL FORMULA: $C_9H_{11}NO_2$
CAS NUMBER: 87-25-2
CLASSIFICATION: Anthranilate
OCCURRENCE: Synthetic
CHARACTERISTICS: *Form:* Liquid; *Color:* Slightly yellow to brownish; *Odor:* Sweet flowery, grape, faintly wintergreen
PHYSICAL CONSTANTS: *Specific gravity:* 1.115–1.120; *Refractive index:* 1.5630–1.5660; *Flash point:* 210 F
SOLUBILITY: Clearly soluble in alcohol (7 parts/60% or 2 parts/70%)
USES: Orange flower, acacia, jasmine; flavors

ETHYL BENZOATE

CHEMICAL FORMULA: $C_9H_{10}O_2$
CAS NUMBER: 93-89-0
CLASSIFICATION: Ester
OCCURRENCE: Benzoic acid and ethyl alcohol in presence of sulfuric acid
CHARACTERISTICS: *Form:* Liquid; *Color:* Colorless; *Odor:* Aromatic
PHYSICAL CONSTANTS: *Specific gravity:* 1.043–1.046; *Refractive index;* 1.503–1.506; *Melting point:* –34 C; *Boiling point:* 211 C, 213 C; *Flash point:* 190 F
SOLUBILITY: Soluble in alcohol (3 parts/70%), ether, chloroform
USES: Flavors, perfumes, essence de niobe, peau d'espagne, artificial fruit essences, extensively in ylang ylang and in perfumes for soap

ETHYL CAPROATE

SYNONYMS: Ethyl hexoate; ethyl hexanoate; hexanoic acid ethyl ester
CHEMICAL FORMULA: $C_8H_{16}O_2$
CAS NUMBER: 123-66-0
CLASSIFICATION: Caproate
OCCURRENCE: Synthetic
CHARACTERISTICS: *Form:* Liquid; *Color:* Colorless to yellowish; *Odor:* Fruity, herbaceous pleasant
PHYSICAL CONSTANTS: *Specific gravity:* 0.873; *Boiling point:* 167 C
SOLUBILITY: Soluble in alcohol and ether; insoluble in water and glycerin

USES: Organic synthesis; artificial fruit essences
WARNINGS AND CAUTION: Low toxicity; combustible

ETHYL CINNAMATE

SYNONYMS: Ethyl phenylacrylate; 3-phenyl-2 propenoic acid ethyl ester
CHEMICAL FORMULA: $C_{11}H_{12}O_2$
CLASSIFICATION: Cinnamate
OCCURRENCE: Storax oil and *Kaempferia galanga*
CHARACTERISTICS: *Form:* Liquid; *Color:* Colorless; *Odor:* Sweet balsamic, honey
PHYSICAL CONSTANTS: *Specific gravity:* 1.045–1.048; *Refractive index:* 1.5590–1.5610; *Flash point:* > 212 F
SOLUBILITY: Clearly soluble in alcohol (5 parts/70%)
USES: Heavy oriental bouquet; floral, e.g., narcissus; soaps; toilet water; powder perfumes; fixative; flavors

ETHYL FORMATE

CHEMICAL FORMULA: $C_3H_6O_2$
CAS NUMBER: 109-94-4
CLASSIFICATION: Formate
OCCURRENCE: Geranium oil
CHARACTERISTICS: *Form:* Liquid; *Color:* White; *Odor:* Aroamtic pleasant, light leaf, rose, and tea rose
PHYSICAL CONSTANTS: *Specific gravity:* 0.9236 (20/20 C); *Refractive index:* 1.35975 (20 C); *Flash point:* –4 F (closed cup); *Boiling point:* 54.3 C; *Melting point:* –80.5 C
SOLUBILITY: Miscible with benzene, ether, alcohol; slightly in water
USES: Rose, orange flower, lavender, colognes; use in food restricted to 0.0015%
WARNINGS AND CAUTION: Highly flammable; dangerous fire and explosion hazard; narcotic irritating to skin and eyes

ETHYL HEXYL CARBINYL ACETATE

SYNONYMS: 3-Nonanyl acetate
CLASSIFICATION: Acetate
OCCURRENCE: Synthetic
CHARACTERISTICS: *Odor:* Fruity, floral, waxy
USES: Rose, carnation, lavender, fougere, chypre, orange flower, and other perfumes

ETHYL LINALYL ACETATE

CLASSIFICATION: Acetate
OCCURRENCE: Synthetic
CHARACTERISTICS: *Odor:* Floral, faintly fruity
USES: Numerous applications in perfumery

ETHYL PHENYL ACETATE

SYNONYMS: Ethyl α-toluate; benzeneacetic acid ethyl ester

CHEMICAL FORMULA: $C_{10}H_{12}O_2$
CAS NUMBER: 101-97-3
CLASSIFICATION: Phenyl acetate
OCCURRENCE: Synthetic
CHARACTERISTICS: *Form:* Liquid; *Color:* Colorless; *Odor:* Sweet honey, rose
PHYSICAL CONSTANTS: *Specific gravity:* 1.027–1.032; *Refractive index:* 1.4960–1.4980; *Flash point:* 212 F
USES: Sweet pea, rose, orange blossom, floral types

ETHYL SALICYLATE
SYNONYMS: Ethyl *o*-hydroxybenzoate; salicylic ether; sal ethyl
CHEMICAL FORMULA: $C_9H_{10}O_2$
CAS NUMBER: 118-61-6
CLASSIFICATION: Salicylate
OCCURRENCE: Synthetic
CHARACTERISTICS: *Form:* Liquid; *Color:* Colorless; *Odor:* Mild wintergreen
PHYSICAL CONSTANTS: *Specific gravity:* 1.126–1.129; *Refractive index:* 1.5210–1.5230; *Flash point:* > 212 F
SOLUBILITY: Clearly soluble in alcohol (4 parts/80%)
USES: Acacia, cassie, ylang ylang, oakmoss

EUGENOL
SYNONYMS: 4-Allyl-2-methoxyphenol; eugenic acid; 4-allylguaiacacol
CHEMICAL FORMULA: $C_{10}H_{12}O_2$
CAS NUMBER: 97-53-0
CLASSIFICATION: Phenol
OCCURRENCE: Clove, cinnamon leaf, pimento, ylang ylang, patchouli, rose, violet, orange flower, acacia
CHARACTERISTICS: *Form:* Liquid; *Color:* Yellowish; *Odor:* Spicy, characteristic
PHYSICAL CONSTANTS: *Specific gravity:* 1.064–1.068; *Refractive index;* 1.5400–1.5420; *Optical rotation:* –1.30; *Flash point:* 230 F
SOLUBILITY: Soluble in alcohol (2 parts/60%)
USES: Carnation, oriental, spicy-type perfumes

EUGENOL ACETATE
SYNONYMS: 4-Allyl-2-methoxyphenyl acetate; eugenyl acetate; acetyl eugenol; aceteugenol
CHEMICAL FORMULA: $C_{12}H_{14}O_3$
CLASSIFICATION: Acetate
OCCURRENCE: Clove bud oil
CHARACTERISTICS: *Form:* Liquid or fused solid; *Color:* Slightly yellow; *Odor:* Carnation, spicy mild clove
PHYSICAL CONSTANTS: *Specific gravity:* 1.077–1.082 (supercooled); *Congealing point:* 25 C min.
SOLUBILITY: Clearly soluble in alcohol (5 parts/70%)
USES: Fixative for carnation-type perfumes and as enhancer of green-herbaceous types

FENCHENE

CHEMICAL FORMULA: $C_{10}H_{16}$
CLASSIFACTION: Terpene hydrocarbon
OCCURRENCE: Various essential oils
CHARACTERISTICS: *Form:* Liquid; *Color:* Colorless; *Odor:* Aromatic
PHYSICAL CONSTANTS: *Specific gravity:* 0.854, 0.866; *Boiling point:* 146 C, 152 C
SOLUBILITY: Alcohol
USES: Perfumes

FORMIC ACID

CHEMICAL FORMULA: CH_2O_2
CAS NUMBER: 64-18-6
CLASSIFICATION: Acid
OCCURRENCE: Synthetic
CHARACTERISTICS: *Form:* Liquid; *Color:* Colorless; *Odor:* Pungent
PHYSICAL CONSTANTS: *Specific gravity:* 1.2201; *Refractive index:* 1.3719; *Melting point:* 8.3 C; *Boiling point:* 100.8 C; *Flash point:* 156 F
SOLUBILITY: Soluble in water, alcohol, ether
USES: Food preservative; formates and esters

FUMARIC ACID

SYNONYMS: Boletic acid; lichenic acid; allomaleic acid; *trans*-butenedioic acid
CHEMICAL FORMULA: $C_4H_4O_4$
CAS NUMBER: 110-17-8
CLASSIFICATION: Acid
OCCURRENCE: Synthetic; occurs in many plants
CHARACTERISTICS: *Form:* Crystals; *Color:* Colorless
PHYSICAL CONSTANTS: *Specific gravity:* 1.635; *Melting point:* 287 C; *Sublimation point:* 290 C
SOLUBILITY: Slightly soluble in water; insoluble in chloroform and benzene
USES: Substitute for citric and tartaric acids; food and oil drier

GERANIOL

CHEMICAL FORMULA: $C_{10}H_{18}O$
CLASSIFICATION: Alcohol
OCCURRENCE: Palmarosa rose, geranium, citronella, verbena, lemongrass, linaloe, petitgrain
CHARACTERISTICS: *Form:* Liquid; *Color:* Colorless; *Odor:* Rose-like
PHYSICAL CONSTANTS: *Specific gravity:* 0.870–0.880; *Refractive index;* 1.4710–1.4760; *Optical rotation:* ±2; *Flash point:* 217 F
SOLUBILITY: Soluble in alcohol (2 parts/70%)
USES: Floral, especially rose, cosmetics, soaps

GERANYL ACETATE

SYNONYMS: *trans*-3,7-Dimethyl-2,6-octadienyl acetate; geraniol acetate
CHEMICAL FORMULA: $C_{12}H_{20}O_2$

CAS NUMBER: 105-87-3
CLASSIFICATION: Acetate
OCCURRENCE: Lemon, petitgrain, lavender, lemongrass, and others
CHARACTERISTICS: *Form:* Liquid; *Color:* Colorless to slightly yellow; *Odor:* Rosy, woody, fruity, lavender
PHYSICAL CONSTANTS: *Specific gravity:* 0.900–0.910; *Refractive index:* 1.4570–1.4620; *Optical rotation:* ± 1; *Flash point:* 228 F
SOLUBILITY: Clearly soluble in alcohol (2 parts/80%)
USES: Extensively used in perfume compositions

GERANYL BUTYRATE
SYNONYMS: *trans*-3,7-Dimethyl-2,6-octadienyl butyrate; geraniol butyrate
CHEMICAL FORMULA: $C_{14}H_{24}O_2$
CLASSIFICATION: Butyrate
OCCURRENCE: *Darwinia grandiflora*
CHARACTERISTICS: *Form:* Liquid; *Color:* Colorless to slightly yellow; *Odor:* Apricot, fruity, rosy
PHYSICAL CONSTANTS: *Specific gravity:* 0.891–0.896; *Refractive index:* 1.4560–1.4620; *Optical rotation:* ± 1; *Flash point:* 200 F
SOLUBILITY: Clearly soluble in alcohol (7 parts/80% or 1 part/90%)
USES: Rose, peonia, cassie, lavender; apple, peach, apricot flavors

GERANYL CAPROATE
CLASSIFICATION: Caproate
OCCURRENCE: Synthetic
CHARACTERISTICS: *Odor:* Rose, geranium, fruity
USES: Oriental compositions

GERANYL PHENYL ACETATE
SYNONYMS: *trans*-3,7-Dimethyl-2,6-octadienyl phenyl acetate
CHEMICAL FORMULA: $C_{18}H_{24}O_2$
CLASSIFICATION: Phenyl acetate
OCCURRENCE: Synthetic
CHARACTERISTICS: *Form:* Liquid; *Color:* Yellow; *Odor:* Honey, rose, geranium, peach
PHYSICAL CONSTANTS: *Specific gravity:* 0.971–0.978; *Refractive index:* 1.5070–1.5110; *Optical rotation:* ± 1; *Flash point:* 210 F
SOLUBILITY: Clearly soluble in alcohol (4 parts/90%)
USES: Rose, floral perfumes; flavors

GERANYL PROPIONATE
SYNONYMS: *trans*-3,7-Dimethyl-2,6-octadienyl propionate; geraniol propionate
CHEMICAL FORMULA: $C_{13}H_{22}O_2$
CLASSIFICATION: Propionate
OCCURRENCE: Synthetic
CHARACTERISTICS: *Form:* Liquid; *Color:* Colorless to slightly yellow; *Odor:* Fruity, rose, fresh

PHYSICAL CONSTANTS: *Specific gravity:* 0.896–0.909; *Refractive index:* 1.4570–1.4620; *Optical rotation:* ±1; *Flash point:* 210 F
SOLUBILITY: Clearly soluble in alcohol (3 parts/80%)
USES: Gardenia, lavender, rose, and other floral types; flavors

HELIOTROPIN
SYNONYMS: Piperonal; 3,4-methylenedioxybenzaldehyde; piperonyl aldehyde; protocatechuic aldehyde methylene ether
CHEMICAL FORMULA: $C_8H_6O_3$
CLASSIFICATION: Aldehyde
OCCURRENCE: Vanilla tahitiana, sassafras, violet, and others
CHARACTERISTICS: *Form:* Crystalline; *Color:* White; turns red-brown on exposure to light; *Odor:* Heliotrope, floral
PHYSICAL CONSTANTS: *Boiling point:* 263 C; *Melting point:* 35.5–37 C; *Congealing point:* 30–35 C
SOLUBILITY: Soluble in alcohol (4 parts/95%); insoluble in water and glycerol
USES: Lilac, sweet pea, heliotrope, lily of the valley, honeysuckle, and other fine perfumes; flavoring; medicine
WARNINGS AND CAUTION: Combustible; low toxicity

HEPTANE
CHEMICAL FORMULA: C_7H_{16}
CLASSIFICATION: Aliphatic hydrocarbon
OCCURRENCE: Needles *Pinus sabiana*
CHARACTERISTICS: *Form:* Liquid; *Color:* Colorless; *Odor:* Camphor
PHYSICAL CONSTANTS: *Specific gravity:* 0.68368 (20 C); *Refractive index:* 1.38764; *Boiling point:* 98 C
SOLUBILITY: Soluble in alcohol, chloroform, ether; insoluble in water
USES: Solvent, anesthetic
WARNINGS AND CAUTION: Flammable; dangerous fire risk; moderately toxic by inhalation

HEPTANOIC ACID
SYNONYMS: Oenanthic acid; enanthic acid; oenanthylic acid; *n*-heptoic acid
CHEMICAL FORMULA: $C_7H_{14}O_2$
CAS NUMBER: 111-14-8
CLASSIFICATION: Acid
OCCURRENCE: Synthetic
CHARACTERISTICS: *Form:* Liquid; *Color:* Clear; *Odor:* Unpleasant
PHYSICAL CONSTANTS: *Specific gravity:* 0.9181 (20/4 C); *Refractive index:* 1.4229; *Melting point:* –7.0 C; *Boiling point:* 221.9 C
SOLUBILITY: Soluble in alcohol, ether; insoluble in water
USES: Organic synthesis

INDOLE
CHEMICAL FORMULA: C_8H_7N
CAS NUMBER: 120-72-9

CLASSIFICATION: Nitro compound
OCCURRENCE: Citrus, jasmine, neroli, jonquil, wallflower
CHARACTERISTICS: *Form:* Crystalline; *Color:* White or brownish; *Odor:* Sharp jasmine-like on dilution
PHYSICAL CONSTANTS: *Congealing point:* 48–51 C
SOLUBILITY: Soluble 1 g/3 ml 70% alcohol
USES: Floral, jasmine, lilac, honeysuckle-type perfumes

IONONE
CHEMICAL FORMULA: $C_{13}H_{20}O$
CAS NUMBER: 8013-90-9
CLASSIFICATION: Ketone
OCCURRENCE: Boronia, violet, costus root
CHARACTERISTICS: *Form:* Liquid; *Color:* Yellowish; *Odor:* Violet
PHYSICAL CONSTANTS: *Specific gravity:* 0.927–0.933; *Refractive index;* 1.4970–1.5010; *Flash point:* 212 F
SOLUBILITY: Soluble in alcohol (3 parts/70%)
USES: Violet-type perfumes; soaps

ISOAMYL ACETATE
CHEMICAL FORMULA: $C_7H_{14}O_2$
CAS NUMBER: 123-92-2
CLASSIFICATION: Acetate
OCCURRENCE: Synthetic
CHARACTERISTICS: *Form:* Liquid; *Color:* Colorless; *Odor:* Pear, banana
PHYSICAL CONSTANTS: *Specific gravity:* 0.876 (15/4 C); *Refractive index:* 1.400 (21 C); *Flash point:* 80 F; *Boiling point:* 142 C
SOLUBILITY: Slightly soluble in water; miscible with alcohol and ether
USES: Flavoring; perfumes; solvents
WARNINGS AND CAUTION: Flammable; dangerous fire risk; moderately toxic and irritating

ISOAMYL SALICYLATE
SYNONYMS: Amyl salicylate
CHEMICAL FORMULA: $C_{12}H_{16}O_3$
CAS NUMBER: 87-20-7
CLASSIFICATION: Salicylate
OCCURRENCE: Synthetic
CHARACTERISTICS: *Form:* Liquid; *Color:* White, sometimes with faint yellow tinge; *Odor:* Herbaceous, woody, orchid
PHYSICAL CONSTANTS: *Specific gravity:* 1.053–1.059 (15 C); *Refractive index*1.5050–1.5080 (n 20/D): *Optical rotation:* 0 to + 2.30; *Boiling point:* 280 C
SOLUBILITY: Soluble in alcohol, ether; insoluble in water and glycerol
USES: Soap perfumes, orchid, fern, new mown hay, hyacinth, cyclamen, camellia, carnation, wallflower, chrysanthemum, mimosa, chypre; spicy, woody, oriental compositions

WARNINGS AND CAUTION: Combustible; low toxicity

ISOBUTYL ACETATE

CHEMICAL FORMULA: $C_6H_{12}O_2$
CAS NUMBER: 110-19-0
CLASSIFICATION: Acetate
OCCURRENCE: Synthetic
CHARACTERISTICS: *Form:* Liquid; *Color:* Colorless; *Odor:* Fruity
PHYSICAL CONSTANTS: *Specific gravity:* 0.8685 (15 C); *Refractive index:* 1.392; *Flash point:* 88 F; *Boiling point:* 116–117 C; *Melting point:* –99 C
SOLUBILITY: Soluble in alcohols, ether, and hydrocarbons; immiscible with water
USES: Strawberry, raspberry, and other fruit flavors; solvent for nitrocellulose
WARNINGS AND CAUTION: Flammable; dangerous fire risk

ISOBUTYL BENZOATE

CHEMICAL FORMULA: $C_{11}H_{14}O_2$
CLASSIFICATION: Benzoate
OCCURRENCE: Synthetic
CHARACTERISTICS: *Form:* Liquid; *Color:* Colorless; *Odor:* Rosy, geranium green eglantine
PHYSICAL CONSTANTS: *Specific gravity:* 0.994–0.997; *Refractive index:* 1.4930–1.4960; *Flash point:* 205 F
SOLUBILITY: Clearly soluble in alcohol (2 parts/80%)
USES: Sweet pea, carnation, rose, orange blossom, amber, incense; flavors

ISOBUTYL CINNAMATE

SYNONYMS: Labdanol
CHEMICAL FORMULA: $C_{13}H_{16}O_2$
CAS NUMBER: 122-67-8
CLASSIFICATION: Cinnamate
OCCURRENCE: Synthetic
CHARACTERISTICS: *Form:* Liquid; *Color:* Colorless; *Odor:* Fruity, balsamic
PHYSICAL CONSTANTS: *Specific gravity:* 1.001–1.004; *Refractive index:* 1.5390–1.5410; *Flash point:* > 212 F
SOLUBILITY: Clearly soluble in alcohol (3 parts/80%)
USES: Oriental-woody such as vetiver, coumarin, vanilla, patchouli, oakmoss, heliotropin, treflé, orchid; flavors: chocolate, cherry, plum, and others

ISOBUTYL PHENYL ACETATE

SYNONYMS: Eglantine; isobutyl α-toluate
CHEMICAL FORMULA: $C_{12}H_{16}O_2$
CLASSIFICATION: Phenyl acetate
OCCURRENCE: Synthetic
CHARACTERISTICS: *Form:* Liquid; *Color:* Colorless; *Odor:* Honey, musky, rose, eglantine
PHYSICAL CONSTANTS: *Specific gravity:* 0.984–0.986; *Refractive index:* 1.4860–

1.4875; *Flash point:* > 212 F
SOLUBILITY: Clearly soluble in alcohol (8 parts/70% or 2 parts/80%)
USES: Rose, orchid, sweet pea, tuberose

ISOBUTYL QUINOLINE
SYNONYMS: 2-Isobutylquinoline; α-isobutylquinoline
CHEMICAL FORMULA: $C_{13}H_{15}N$
CLASSIFICATION: Nitro compound
OCCURRENCE: Synthetic
CHARACTERISTICS: *Form:* Liquid; *Color:* Yellowish or brownish; *Odor:* Woody
PHYSICAL CONSTANTS: *Specific gravity:* 0.989–0.993 (α-isobutyl quinoline), 0.991–0.996 (isobutyl quinoline); *Refractive index;* 1.5730–1.5760 (α-isobutyl quinoline), 1.5730–1.5780 (isobutyl quinoline); *Flash point:* 212 F
SOLUBILITY: Clearly soluble in alcohol (3 parts/70%)
USES: Wood-like, patchouli, vetiver component

ISOBUTYL SALICYLATE
SYNONYMS: Isobutyl *o*-hydroxybenzoate
CHEMICAL FORMULA: $C_{11}H_{14}O_3$
CAS NUMBER: 87-19-4
CLASSIFICATION: Salicylate
OCCURRENCE: Synthetic
CHARACTERISTICS: *Form:* Liquid; *Color:* Colorless; *Odor:* Clover, orchid, herbaceous
PHYSICAL CONSTANTS: *Specific gravity:* 1.061–1.065; *Refractive index:* 1.5070–1.5100; *Flash point:* > 212 F
SOLUBILITY: Clearly soluble in alcohol (9 parts/80% or 2 parts/90%)
USES: Blends well with clary sage, lavender, orchid, carnation, and wood oil; musk ambrette, coumarin, resins, and balsams

ISOPROPYL ANTHRANILATE
CLASSIFICATION: Anthranilate
OCCURRENCE: Synthetic
CHARACTERISTICS: *Odor:* Neroli, hawthorn, honey
USES: Mandarin, jasmine

LACTIC ACID
CHEMICAL FORMULA: $C_3H_6O_3$
CAS NUMBER: 50-21-5
CLASSIFICATION: Acid
OCCURRENCE: Fermentation of starch, molasses, or potatoes; synthetically from sulfite pulp liquor
CHARACTERISTICS: *Form:* Syrup; *Color:* Colorless or yellowish; *Odor:* Acidic
PHYSICAL CONSTANTS: *Specific gravity:* 1.2; *Melting point:* 18 C; *Boiling point:* 122 C
SOLUBILITY: Soluble in water, alcohol, ether, acetone, glycerin

USES: Flavors; preservative acidulant in beverages

LAURIC ACID

CHEMICAL FORMULA: $C_{12}H_{24}O_2$
CAS NUMBER: 143-07-7
CLASSIFICATION: Acid
OCCURRENCE: From coconut, laurel oils
CHARACTERISTICS: *Form and Color:* Colorless needles or white powder; *Odor:* Bay oil-like
PHYSICAL CONSTANTS: *Specific gravity:* 0.833; *Refractive index:* 1.4323 (45 C); *Melting point:* 44 C; *Boiling point:* 225 C
SOLUBILITY: Soluble in alcohol, ether, benzene
USES: Soaps, cosmetics, detergents, insecticides

LINALOOL

CHEMICAL FORMULA: $C_{10}H_{18}O$
CAS NUMBER: 78-70-6
CLASSIFICATION: Alcohol
OCCURRENCE: Rosewood, lavender, citrus, jasmine, geranium
CHARACTERISTICS: *Form:* Liquid; *Color:* Colorless; *Odor:* Floral
PHYSICAL CONSTANTS: *Specific gravity:* 0.859–0.867; *Refractive index;* 1.4610–1.4640; *Optical rotation:* –12 to –18; *Flash point:* 175 F
SOLUBILITY: Soluble in alcohol (2 parts/70%)
USES: Lilac, muguet, lavender, citrus, sweet pea-type perfumes

LINALYL ACETATE

SYNONYMS: 3,7-Dimethyl-1,6-octadien-3-yl acetate; bergamol
CHEMICAL FORMULA: $C_{12}H_{20}O_2$
CAS NUMBER: 115-95-7
CLASSIFICATION: Acetate
OCCURRENCE: Bergamot, lavender, clary sage, petitgrain, neroli, and other oils
CHARACTERISTICS: *Form:* Liquid; *Color:* Colorless; *Odor:* Bergamot, lavender
PHYSICAL CONSTANTS: *Specific gravity:* 0.903–0.906; *Refractive index:* 1.4510–1.4530; *Optical rotation:* ± 0°15′; *Flash point:* 195 F
SOLUBILITY: Soluble in alcohol (≈ 3–4 parts/70%)
USES: Extensively used in numerous compositions, e.g., ylang ylang, lilac, jasmine, neroli, and other floral-type compounds

LINALYL BUTYRATE

SYNONYMS: 3,7-Dimethyl-1,6-octadien-3-yl butyrate
CHEMICAL FORMULA: $C_{14}H_{24}O_2$
CLASSIFICATION: Butyrate
OCCURRENCE: Lavender oil
CHARACTERISTICS: *Form:* Liquid; *Color:* Colorless to slightly yellow; *Odor:* Citrus, lavender
PHYSICAL CONSTANTS: *Specific gravity:* 0.893–0.904; *Refractive index:* 1.4510–

1.4560; *Flash point:* > 212 F
SOLUBILITY: Clearly soluble in alcohol (3 parts/80%)
USES: Lavender, cologne type; rose, jasmine; flavors

LINALYL CINNAMATE
CLASSIFICATION: Cinnamate
OCCURRENCE: Synthetic
CHARACTERISTICS: *Odor:* Lily
USES: Various types of perfumes; flavors

LINALYL FORMATE
SYNONYMS: 3,7-Dimethyl-1,6-octadien-3-yl formate
CHEMICAL FORMULA: $C_{11}H_{18}O_2$
CLASSIFICATION: Formate
OCCURRENCE: Synthetic
CHARACTERISTICS: *Form:* Liquid; *Color:* Colorless to slightly yellow; *Odor:* Bergamot, citrus, rosy
PHYSICAL CONSTANTS: *Specific gravity:* 0.915–0.924; *Refractive index:* 1.4550–1.4580; *Flash point:* 190 F
SOLUBILITY: Clearly soluble in alcohol (6 parts/70% or 1 part/80%)
USES: Colognes, lavender, rose, jasmine, and other floral compositions; flavors

LINALYL PROPIONATE
SYNONYMS: 3,7-Dimethyl-1,6-octadien-3-yl propionate
CHEMICAL FORMULA: $C_{13}H_{22}O_2$
CLASSIFICATION: Propionate
OCCURRENCE: Lavender oil
CHARACTERISTICS: *Form:* Liquid; *Color:* Colorless to slightly yellow; *Odor:* Bergamot, lily of the valley, coriander
PHYSICAL CONSTANTS: *Specific gravity:* 0.895–0.902; *Refractive index:* 1.4500–1.4550; *Flash point:* 196 F
SOLUBILITY: Clearly soluble in alcohol (8 parts/70% or 2 parts/80%)
USES: Clary sage, lavender, colognes, jasmine; flavors

LINALYL VALERIANATE
CLASSIFICATION: Valerate (valerianate)
OCCURRENCE: Synthetic
CHARACTERISTICS: *Odor:* Lavender
USES: Lavender, pine

MALIC ACID
CHEMICAL FORMULA: $C_4H_6O_5$
CAS NUMBER: 6915-15-7
CLASSIFICATION: Acid
OCCURRENCE: Unripe apples, cherries, raspberries, tomatoes, maple juice
CHARACTERISTICS: *Form:* Crystals; *Color:* Colorless; *Odor:* Sour

PHYSICAL CONSTANTS: *Specific gravity:* 1.601; *Melting point:* 128 C; *Boiling point:* 150 C
SOLUBILITY: Soluble in water, alcohol; slightly soluble in ether
USES: Esters; food acidulant; medicine; to age wine by removing tartrates

MENTHOL
CHEMICAL FORMULA: $C_{10}H_{20}O$
CAS NUMBER: 89-78-1
CLASSIFICATION: Alcohol
OCCURRENCE: Peppermint
CHARACTERISTICS: *Form:* Crystals; *Color:* White; *Odor:* Cool, characteristic
PHYSICAL CONSTANTS: *Optical rotation:* ±2; *Congealing point:* 27–32 C; *Flash point:* 200 F
SOLUBILITY: Soluble in alcohol (3 parts/70%)
USES: Cooling agent in cigarettes, colognes, pharmaceuticals, antiseptic, mouthwashes, dentifrices

MENTHONE
CHEMICAL FORMULA: $C_{10}H_{18}O$
CAS NUMBER: 1074-95-9
CLASSIFICATION: Ketone
OCCURRENCE: Peppermint, pennyroyal, geranium
CHARACTERISTICS: *Form:* Liquid; *Color:* Colorless; *Odor:* Peppermint
PHYSICAL CONSTANTS: *Specific gravity:* 0.888–0.895; *Refractive index;* 1.4480–1.4530; *Optical rotation:* –15 to +15; *Flash point:* 170 F
SOLUBILITY: Soluble in alcohol (3 parts/70%)
USES: Mint-type perfumes

MENTHYL ACETATE
SYNONYMS: Menthol acetic ester
CHEMICAL FORMULA: $C_{12}H_{22}O_2$
CAS NUMBER: 89-48-5
CLASSIFICATION: Acetate
OCCURRENCE: Peppermint oil
CHARACTERISTICS: *Form:* Liquid; *Color:* Colorless; *Odor:* Menthol-like; minty, rosy, herbaceous, sweetish
PHYSICAL CONSTANTS: *Specific gravity:* 0.922–0.927; *Refractive index:* 1.447; *Optical rotation:* –72°42′to –73°18′; *Boiling point:* 227–228 C
SOLUBILITY: Slightly soluble in water; miscible with alcohol and ether
USES: Citrus, lavender, used mostly in toilet soap water type; also used in flavors
WARNINGS AND CAUTION: Combustible; low toxicity

***p*-METHOXY PHENYLBUTYL ACETATE**
CLASSIFICATION: Acetate
OCCURRENCE: Synthetic
CHARACTERISTICS: *Odor:* Fruity, floral
USES: Jasmine, tuberose, gardenia, freesia, and others

METHYL ALCOHOL

SYNONYMS: Methanol; wood alcohol; carbinol; wood spirit
CHEMICAL FORMULA: CH_4O
CAS NUMBER: 67-56-1
CLASSIFICATION: Alcohol
OCCURRENCE: Destructive distillation of wood
CHARACTERISTICS: *Form:* Liquid; *Color:* Colorless; *Odor:* Woody
PHYSICAL CONSTANTS: *Specific gravity:* 0.7924; *Refractive index;* 1.329; *Congealing point:* –97.8 C; *Boiling point:* 64.5 C; *Flash point:* 54 F
SOLUBILITY: Miscible with water, alcohol, ether
USES: Preparation of formaldehyde, denaturant, synthesis
WARNINGS AND CAUTION: Highly toxic by ingestion. It causes blindness

METHYL ANISATE

SYNONYMS: Methyl *p*-methoxybenzoate
CHEMICAL FORMULA: $C_9H_{10}O_3$
CLASSIFICATION: Anisate
OCCURRENCE: Synthetic
CHARACTERISTICS: *Form:* Crystals; *Color:* White; *Odor:* Sweet, suggestive of new mown hay
SOLUBILITY: 1 g is clearly soluble in 10 ml 60% alcohol
USES: Mimosa, new mown hay, magnolia, hawthorn, linden, lime blossom; flavors; used in conjunction with anisic aldehyde (aubepine)

METHYL ANTHRANILATE

SYNONYMS: Methyl 2-aminobenzoate; methyl *o*-aminobenzoate
CHEMICAL FORMULA: $C_8H_9NO_2$
CAS NUMBER: 134-20-3
CLASSIFICATION: Anthranilate
OCCURRENCE: Citrus, jasmine, champaca, tuberose, ylang ylang, wallflower, gardenia oils
CHARACTERISTICS: *Form:* Liquid; *Color:* Colorless to pale yellow; *Odor:* Orange blossom and neroli
PHYSICAL CONSTANTS: *Specific gravity:* 1.162–1.167; *Refractive index:* 1.5820–1.5840; *Flash point:* > 212 F
SOLUBILITY: Clearly soluble in alcohol (4 parts/60%)
USES: Floral compositions and flavors

METHYL BENZOATE

SYNONYMS: Niobe oil; benzoic acid methyl ester; essence of niobe; oil of niobe
CHEMICAL FORMULA: $C_8H_8O_2$
CAS NUMBER: 93-58-3
CLASSIFICATION: Ester, benzoate
OCCURRENCE: Benzoic acid and methyl alcohol; ylang ylang, jonquil, tuberose, clove
CHARACTERISTICS: *Form:* Liquid; *Color:* Colorless, transparent; *Odor:* Pleasant,

fruity, ylang ylang
PHYSICAL CONSTANTS: *Specific gravity:* 1.085–1.088; *Refractive index;* 1.5150–1.5180; *Flash point:* 181 F; *Solidification point:* –15 C; *Boiling point:* 198 C, 200 C
SOLUBILITY: Clearly soluble in alcohol (4 parts/60%); soluble in ether, methanol
USES: Niobe essence, perfumery, eau d'espagne; cananga, ylang ylang, santal, musk, rose, geranium, labdanum, oakmoss, vetiver, floral types

METHYL BUTYRATE
CHEMICAL FORMULA: $C_5H_{10}O_2$
CAS NUMBER: 623-42-7
CLASSIFICATION: Ester
OCCURRENCE: Butyric acid and methyl alcohol
CHARACTERISTICS: *Form:* Liquid; *Color:* Colorless; *Odor:* Pleasant, rum-like
PHYSICAL CONSTANTS: *Specific gravity:* 0.898 (20 C); *Refractive index;* 1.3875; *Melting point:* –95 C; *Boiling point:* 102 C; *Flash point:* 57 F
SOLUBILITY: In 60 parts water; miscible in alcohol, ether
USES: Artificial rum, fruit essences
WARNINGS AND CAUTION: Flammable; dangerous fire risk; moderately toxic

METHYL CINNAMATE
SYNONYMS: Methyl 3-phenylpropenoate; methyl cinnamylate
CHEMICAL FORMULA: $C_{10}H_{10}O_2$
CAS NUMBER: 103-26-4
CLASSIFICATION: Cinnamate
OCCURRENCE: Galanga oil, and many others
CHARACTERISTICS: *Form:* Crystals; *Color:* White; *Odor:* Fruity, balsamic, strawberry-like
PHYSICAL CONSTANTS: *Specific gravity:* 1.0415; *Congealing point:* 33.8 C min.; *Boiling point:* 259.6 C
SOLUBILITY: Clearly soluble in alcohol (1 part/80%)
USES: Spicy, oriental-type perfumes, carnation, narcissus; flavors
WARNINGS AND CAUTION: Combustible; low toxicity

METHYL EUGENOL
SYNONYMS: 4-Allylveratrole; eugenyl methyl ether; 1-allyl-3,4-dimethoxybenzene
CHEMICAL FORMULA: $C_{11}H_{14}O_2$
CAS NUMBER: 93-15-2
CLASSIFICATION: Ether
OCCURRENCE: *Asarum pimento*, basil, ylang ylang, rose, hyacinth, coumarin
CHARACTERISTICS: *Form:* Liquid; *Color:* Colorless or yellowish; *Odor:* Carnation
PHYSICAL CONSTANTS: *Specific gravity:* 1.032–1.035; *Refractive index;* 1.5320–1.5360; *Flash point:* 240 F
SOLUBILITY: Soluble in alcohol (2 parts/70%)
USES: Carnation, lilac-type perfumes

METHYL HEXYL CARBINYL ACETATE

CLASSIFICATION: Acetate
OCCURRENCE: Synthetic
CHARACTERISTICS: *Odor:* Geranium
USES: Lavender, chypre, and others of herbaceous tone

METHYL PHENYL ACETATE

SYNONYMS: Methyl α-toluate
CHEMICAL FORMULA: $C_9H_{10}O_2$
CLASSIFICATION: Phenyl acetate
OCCURRENCE: Synthetic
CHARACTERISTICS: *Form:* Liquid; *Color:* Colorless; *Odor:* Honey, musky
PHYSICAL CONSTANTS: *Specific gravity:* 1.062–1.066; *Refractive index:* 1.5050–1.5080; *Flash point:* 193 F
SOLUBILITY: Clearly soluble in alcohol (7 parts/60% or 2 parts/70%)
USES: Rose, eglantine, soap perfumery; pharmaceuticals; flavors

METHYL SALICYLATE

SYNONYMS: Methyl *o*-hydroxybenzoate; oil of wintergreen synthetic; betula oil
CHEMICAL FORMULA: $C_8H_8O_3$
CAS NUMBER: 119-36-8
CLASSIFICATION: Salicylate
OCCURRENCE: Wintergreen oil, sweet birch, tuberose, carnation, ylang ylang, acacia, and many fruits such as apple, grape, raspberry, and cherry
CHARACTERISTICS: *Form:* Liquid; *Color:* Colorless; *Odor:* Wintergreen
PHYSICAL CONSTANTS: *Specific gravity:* 1.180–1.185; *Refractive index:* 1.5350–1.5380; *Flash point:* 210 F
SOLUBILITY: Slightly soluble in water; soluble in glacial acetic acid; clearly soluble in alcohol (7 parts/70%)
USES: Cassie, mimosa, tuberose, ylang ylang, gardenia, reseda, castoreum, spicy bouquet; flavor for toothpaste, mouthwashes, chewing gum

MUSK AMBRETTE

CHEMICAL FORMULA: $C_{12}H_{16}N_2O_5$
CLASSIFICATION: Nitro compound
OCCURRENCE: Synthetic
CHARACTERISTICS: *Form:* Powder; *Color:* Yellowish; *Odor:* Musky, ambrette seed-like
PHYSICAL CONSTANTS: *Melting point:* 83.4 C
SOLUBILITY: Soluble 3.3 g/100 ml 95% alcohol
USES: Heavy, sweet perfumes; blending

MUSK KETONE

CHEMICAL FORMULA: $C_{14}H_{18}N_2O_5$
CLASSIFICATION: Nitro compound
OCCURRENCE: Synthetic

CHARACTERISTICS: *Form:* Crystals; *Color:* Yellowish; *Odor:* Musky
PHYSICAL CONSTANTS: *Melting point:* 135 C
SOLUBILITY: Soluble 1.8 g/100 ml 95% alcohol
USES: Oriental, heavy, sweet perfumes

MUSK XYLOL
CHEMICAL FORMULA: $C_{12}H_{15}N_3O_6$
CLASSIFICATION: Nitro compound
OCCURRENCE: Synthetic
CHARACTERISTICS: *Form:* Crystals; *Color:* Yellowish; *Odor:* Sharp, musky
PHYSICAL CONSTANTS: *Melting point:* 112.5 C
SOLUBILITY: Soluble 0.88 g/100 ml 95% alcohol
USES: Fixative; sweetener; especially for soaps

MYRCENE
CHEMICAL FORMULA: $C_{10}H_{16}$
CLASSIFICATION: Aliphatic hydrocarbon
OCCURRENCE: Bay, verbena, hop
CHARACTERISTICS: *Form:* Liquid; *Color:* Yellow; *Odor:* Pleasant
PHYSICAL CONSTANTS: *Specific gravity:* 0.806 (15.5 C); *Refractive index:* 1.471; *Boiling point:* 67 C
SOLUBILITY: Alcohol, chloroform, ether, glacial acetic acid
USES: Perfumes, flavors

NEROL
CHEMICAL FORMULA: $C_{10}H_{18}O$
CAS NUMBER: 106-25-2
CLASSIFICATION: Alcohol
OCCURRENCE: Citrus, lemongrass, citronella, lavender, myrtle, rosewood, linaloe, tuberose, champaca, wallflower
CHARACTERISTICS: *Form:* Liquid; *Color:* Colorless; *Odor:* Fresh rose-like
PHYSICAL CONSTANTS: *Specific gravity:* 0.875–0.880; *Refractive index;* 1.4730–1.478; *Flash point:* 198 F
SOLUBILITY: Soluble in alcohol (9 parts/50%)
USES: Perfumes

NEROLIN
CHEMICAL FORMULA: $C_{12}H_{12}O$
CLASSIFICATION: Ether
OCCURRENCE: Synthetic
CHARACTERISTICS: *Form:* Crystals; *Color:* White; *Odor:* Orange blossom
PHYSICAL CONSTANTS: *Congealing point:* 35 C
SOLUBILITY: Soluble 1 gram in 7 ml 95% alcohol
USES: Orange blossom, cologne perfumes

NERYL ACETATE

SYNONYMS: *cis*-3,7-Dimethyl-2,6-octadien-1-yl acetate
CHEMICAL FORMULA: $C_{12}H_{20}O_2$
CLASSIFICATION: Acetate
OCCURRENCE: Neroli, petitgrain, lemon
CHARACTERISTICS: *Form:* Liquid; *Color:* Slightly yellow; *Odor:* Citrus, orange flower, sweet
PHYSICAL CONSTANTS: *Specific gravity:* 0.907–0.913; *Refractive index:* 1.4600–1.4650; *Flash point:* > 212 F
SOLUBILITY: Clearly soluble in alcohol (5 parts/70%)
USES: Rose, magnolia, neroli, jasmine

NONOIC ACID

SYNONYMS: Pelargonic acid; *n*-nonyl acid; *n*-nonanoic acid; *n*-nonylic acid
CHEMICAL FORMULA: $C_9H_{18}O_2$
CLASSIFICATION: Acid
OCCURRENCE: In geranium oil, or synthetically made
CHARACTERISTICS: *Form:* Liquid; *Color:* Colorless or yellowish; *Odor:* Characteristic
PHYSICAL CONSTANTS: *Specific gravity:* 0.903–0.906; *Refractive index;* 1.4322; *Melting point:* 9.0 C; *Boiling point:*254 C; *Flash point:* 212 F
SOLUBILITY: Soluble in alcohol, ether, chloroform
USES: Flavors, perfumes

γ-OCTA LACTONE

CHEMICAL FORMULA: $C_8H_{14}O_2$
CLASSIFICATION: Lactone
OCCURRENCE: Synthetic
CHARACTERISTICS: *Form:* Liquid; *Color:* Colorless or yellowish; *Odor:* Coconut
PHYSICAL CONSTANTS: *Specific gravity:* 0.970–0.980; *Refractive index;* 1.4430–1.4470; *Flash point:* 212 F
SOLUBILITY: Soluble in alcohol (3 parts/50%, 2 parts/60%, 1 part/70%)
USES: Floral, gardenia, tuberose-type perfumes

OCTYLENE

SYNONYMS: Octene; caprylene; 1-octylene; 1-caprylene
CHEMICAL FORMULA: C_8H_{16}
CLASSIFACTION: Aliphatic hydrocarbon
OCCURRENCE: Bergamot, lemon oils
CHARACTERISTICS: *Form:* Liquid; *Color:* Colorless; *Odor:* Citrus
PHYSICAL CONSTANTS: *Specific gravity:* 0.722; *Refractive index:* 1.4088; *Boiling point:* 123 C
SOLUBILITY: Alcohol, acetone, ether
USES: Perfumes

OCYMENE

CHEMICAL FORMULA: $C_{10}H_{16}$
CLASSIFACTION: Aliphatic hydrocarbon
OCCURRENCE: Sweet basil oil
CHARACTERISTICS: *Form:* Liquid; *Color:* Colorless; *Odor:* Basil
PHYSICAL CONSTANTS: Specific gravity: 0.8031; Boiling point: 81 C
SOLUBILITY: Alcohol, ether
USES: Flavors, perfumes

OXALIC ACID

CHEMICAL FORMULA: $C_2H_2O_4$
CAS NUMBER: 144-62-7
CLASSIFICATION: Acid
OCCURRENCE: Great number of plants and vegetables, mostly of oxalic and rumex families; prepared synthetically
CHARACTERISTICS: *Form:* Crystals; *Color:* Transparent, colorless
PHYSICAL CONSTANTS: *Specific gravity:* 1.653 (18.5 C); *Melting point:* 101–102 C
SOLUBILITY: Soluble in water, alcohol, ether
USES: Purifying agent in the manufacture of acids
WARNINGS AND CAUTION: Harmful if swallowed

PHENYL ACETALDEHYDE

SYNONYMS: Hyacinthin; α-tolualdehyde; benzeneacetaldehyde; α-toluic aldehyde
CHEMICAL FORMULA: C_8H_8O
CAS NUMBER: 122-78-1
CLASSIFICATION: Aldehyde
OCCURRENCE: Neroli oil
CHARACTERISTICS: *Form:* Liquid; *Color:* Colorless or yellowish; *Odor:* Fresh floral
PHYSICAL CONSTANTS: *Specific gravity:* 1.023–1.040; *Refractive index;* 1.5240–1.5320; *Flash point:* 188 F
SOLUBILITY: Soluble in alcohol (2 parts/80%)
USES: Hyacinth, lilac, jasmine, jonquil, lily, rose-type perfumes

PHENYL ACETIC ACID

CHEMICAL FORMULA: $C_8H_8O_2$
CAS NUMBER: 103-82-2
CLASSIFICATION: Acid
OCCURRENCE: Synthetic
CHARACTERISTICS: *Form:* Shiny crystals or plates
PHYSICAL CONSTANTS: *Freezing point:* 74.5–76.5 C; *Boiling point:*262 C
SOLUBILITY: Soluble in alcohol, ether; slightly soluble in water
USES: Perfumes, medicines

PHENYL ETHYL ACETATE

SYNONYMS: Phenethyl acetate; β-phenethyl acetate; benzylcarbinyl acetate
CHEMICAL FORMULA: $C_{10}H_{12}O_2$

CAS NUMBER: 103-45-7
CLASSIFICATION: Acetate
OCCURRENCE: Synthetic
CHARACTERISTICS: *Form:* Liquid; *Color:* Colorless; *Odor:* Sweet rosy-honey floral and peach
PHYSICAL CONSTANTS: *Specific gravity:* 1.030–1.034; *Refractive index:* 1.4970–1.5010; *Flash point:* > 212 F
SOLUBILITY: Clearly soluble in alcohol (2 parts/70%)
USES: Jasmine, hyacinth, mignonette, rose; also used in flavors

PHENYL ETHYL ALCOHOL
CHEMICAL FORMULA: $C_8H_{10}O$
CAS NUMBER: 60-12-8
CLASSIFICATION: Alcohol
OCCURRENCE: Rose, geranium, ylang ylang, champaca, narcissus, hyacinth, lily, tea leaf, neroli
CHARACTERISTICS: *Form:* Liquid; *Color:* Colorless; *Odor:* Rose-like, sweet
PHYSICAL CONSTANTS: *Specific gravity:* 1.017–1.020; *Refractive index;* 1.5310–1.5330; *Flash point:* 216 F
SOLUBILITY: Soluble in alcohol (2 parts/50% or 1 part/60%)
USES: Rose and all floral-type perfumes

PHENYL ETHYL ANTHRANILATE
SYNONYMS: Phenethyl anthranilate; benzylcarbinyl anthranilate; phenylethyl *o*-aminobenzoate
CHEMICAL FORMULA: $C_{15}H_{15}NO_2$
CAS NUMBER: 133-18-6
CLASSIFICATION: Anthranilate
OCCURRENCE: Synthetic
CHARACTERISTICS: *Form:* Fused solid; *Color:* Yellow to amber; *Odor:* Grape-orange; rosaceous
PHYSICAL CONSTANTS: *Specific gravity:* 0.991–0.994; *Refractive index:* 1.4880–1.4920; *Flash point:* 212 F
SOLUBILITY: Clearly soluble in alcohol (2 parts/80%, 1 part/90%)
USES: Honeysuckle, gardenia, orange blossom, violet; flavors

PHENYL ETHYL BUTYRATE
SYNONYMS: Phenethyl butyrate; benzylcarbinyl butyrate
CHEMICAL FORMULA: $C_{12}H_{16}O_2$
CLASSIFICATION: Butyrate
OCCURRENCE: Synthetic
CHARACTERISTICS: *Form:* Liquid; *Color:* Colorless; *Odor:* Sweet rosy, floral, leafy, honey
PHYSICAL CONSTANTS: *Specific gravity:* 0.991–0.994; *Refractive index:* 1.4880–1.4920; *Flash point:* 212 F
SOLUBILITY: Clearly soluble in alcohol (2 parts/80% or 1 part/90%)

USES: Jasmine, lily, magnolia, and other floral compositions; flavors

PHENYL ETHYL CINNAMATE

SYNONYMS: Phenethyl cinnamate; benzylcarbinyl cinnamate
CHEMICAL FORMULA: $C_{17}H_{16}O_2$
CLASSIFICATION: Cinnamate
OCCURRENCE: Synthetic
CHARACTERISTICS: *Form:* Crystalline powder; *Color:* White; *Odor:* Balsamic, heavy, rosaceous, honey, tolu balsam-like
PHYSICAL CONSTANTS: *Congealing point:* 54 C min.
SOLUBILITY: 1 g is soluble in 10 ml of 95% alcohol with a slight cloudiness
USES: Rose, muguet, lilac, hyacinth, sweet pea, garden; excellent fixative for floral-type perfumes

PHENYL ETHYL FORMATE

SYNONYMS: Phenethyl formate; benzylcarbinyl formate
CHEMICAL FORMULA: $C_9H_{10}O_2$
CLASSIFICATION: Formate
OCCURRENCE: Synthetic
CHARACTERISTICS: *Form:* Liquid; *Color:* Colorless to slightly yellow; *Odor:* Rosaceous, green, hyacinth
PHYSICAL CONSTANTS: *Specific gravity:* 1.056–1.062; *Refractive index:* 1.5060–1.5100; *Flash point:* 210 F
SOLUBILITY: Clearly soluble in alcohol (4 parts/70%)
USES: Lilac, rose, hyacinth, muguet, broom; flavors

PHENYL ETHYL PHENYL ACETATE

SYNONYMS: Phenethyl phenyl acetate; Phenyl ethyl α-toluate; benzylcarbinyl α-toluate
CHEMICAL FORMULA: $C_{16}H_{16}O_2$
CAS NUMBER: 102-20-5
CLASSIFICATION: Phenyl acetate
OCCURRENCE: Synthetic
CHARACTERISTICS: *Form:* Liquid; *Color:* Colorless to slightly yellow; *Odor:* Rose, hyacinth
PHYSICAL CONSTANTS: *Specific gravity:* 1.079–1.082; *Flash point:* > 212 F; *Congealing point:* 26 C min.
SOLUBILITY: Clearly soluble in alcohol (4 parts/90%)
USES: Rose, hyacinth, lily, jonquil, lilac, narcissus, jasmine; flavors

PHENYL ETHYL PROPIONATE

SYNONYMS: Phenethyl propionate; β-phenethyl propionate; benzylcarbinyl propionate
CHEMICAL FORMULA: $C_{11}H_{14}O_2$
CAS NUMBER: 120-45-6
CLASSIFICATION: Propionate

OCCURRENCE: Synthetic
CHARACTERISTICS: *Form:* Liquid; *Color:* Colorless to slightly yellow; *Odor:* Fruity, lily, rose
PHYSICAL CONSTANTS: *Specific gravity:* 1.010–1.014; *Refractive index:* 1.493–1.496; *Flash point:* 212 F
SOLUBILITY: Clearly soluble in alcohol (4 parts/70%)
USES: Modifier and fortifier for all types of floral compositions; flavors

PHENYL ETHYL SALICYLATE
SYNONYMS: Phenethyl salicylate; β-phenethyl salicylate; benzylcarbinyl salicylate
CHEMICAL FORMULA: $C_{15}H_{14}O_3$
CLASSIFICATION: Salicylate
OCCURRENCE: Synthetic
CHARACTERISTICS: *Form:* Crystalline; *Color:* White; *Odor:* Balsamic, rose
PHYSICAL CONSTANTS: *Congealing point:* 41.5 C
SOLUBILITY: 1 g is clearly soluble in 20 ml of 95% alcohol; soluble in 14 parts of 95% alcohol
USES: Rose, carnation, and many bouquets with a spicy, balsamic character
WARNINGS AND CAUTION: Combustible; low toxicity

PHENYL PROPYL ACETATE
SYNONYMS: Hydrocinnamyl acetate; 3-phenyl-1-propyl acetate
CHEMICAL FORMULA: $C_{11}H_{14}O_2$
CAS NUMBER: 122-72-5
CLASSIFICATION: Acetate
OCCURRENCE: Cassia oil
CHARACTERISTICS: *Form:* Liquid; *Color:* Colorless; *Odor:* Fresh balsamic, spicy and floral
PHYSICAL CONSTANTS: *Specific gravity:* 1.012–1.015; *Refractive index:* 1.4940–1.4970; *Flash point:* 212 F
SOLUBILITY: Clearly soluble in alcohol (3 parts/70%)
USES: Lilac, lily, and other floral bouquet oriental types

PHENYL PROPYL ALCOHOL
CHEMICAL FORMULA: $C_9H_{12}O$
CAS NUMBER: 122-97-4
CLASSIFICATION: Alcohol
OCCURRENCE: Peru balsam, Sumatra benzoin, storax
CHARACTERISTICS: *Form:* Liquid; *Color:* Colorless; *Odor:* Hyacinth-like
PHYSICAL CONSTANTS: *Specific gravity:* 0.997–1.001; *Refractive index;* 1.5240–1.5280; *Flash point:* 221 F
SOLUBILITY: Soluble in alcohol (4 parts/45% or 1 part/70%)
USES: Lilac, hyacinth, cyclamen, mignonette-type perfumes

PHENYL PROPYL BUTYRATE
CLASSIFICATION: Butyrate

OCCURRENCE: Synthetic
CHARACTERISTICS: *Odor:* Fruity, balsamic, heavy
USES: Narcissus, hyacinth, jasmine; apricot, peach, mango flavors

PHENYL PROPYL FORMATE
SYNONYMS: 3-Phenyl-1-propyl formate; hydrocinnamyl formate
CHEMICAL FORMULA: $C_{10}H_{12}O_2$
CLASSIFICATION: Formate
OCCURRENCE: Synthetic
CHARACTERISTICS: *Form:* Liquid; *Color:* Colorless to slightly yellow; *Odor:* Sweet honey, green, powerful floral character
PHYSICAL CONSTANTS: *Specific gravity:* 1.035–1.038; *Refractive index:* 1.5030–1.5060; *Flash point:* 212 F
SOLUBILITY: Clearly soluble in alcohol (2 parts/80%)
USES: Narcissus, hyacinth, chypre

PINENE
CHEMICAL FORMULA: $C_{10}H_{16}$
CLASSIFACTION: Terpene hydrocarbon
OCCURRENCE: Turpentine, savine, fir oils
CHARACTERISTICS: *Form:* Liquid; *Color:* Colorless; *Odor:* Aromatic
PHYSICAL CONSTANTS: *Specific gravity:* 0.859; *Refractive index;* 1.4655, 1.4670; *Boiling point:* 156 C, 160 C; *Congealing point:* –40 C; *Flash point:* 90 F
SOLUBILITY: Alcohol, ether, chloroform, glacial acetic acid
USES: Synthesis, camphene, camphor
WARNINGS AND CAUTION: Toxic by ingestion

PROPIONIC ACID
SYNONYMS: Methylacetic acid; propanoic acid; ethyl formic acid
CHEMICAL FORMULA: $C_3H_6O_2$
CAS NUMBER: 79-09-4
CLASSIFICATION: Acid
OCCURRENCE: Synthetic; in dairy products in small amount
CHARACTERISTICS: *Form:* Liquid; *Color:* Clear, colorless; *Odor:* Sharp
PHYSICAL CONSTANTS: *Specific gravity:* 0.9942 (20/4 C); *Refractive index:* 1.3862 (20 C); *Flash point:* 130 F; *Melting point:* –20.8 C; *Boiling point:* 140.7 C
SOLUBILITY: Soluble in water, alcohol, chloroform, ether
USES: Perfumes, flavors, pharmaceuticals
WARNINGS AND CAUTION: Low toxicity; flammable, moderate fire risk

PROPYL ALCOHOL
SYNONYMS: Propanol; 1-propanol; propylic alcohol; optal
CHEMICAL FORMULA: C_3H_8O
CAS NUMBER: 71-23-8
CLASSIFICATION: Alcohol
OCCURRENCE: Fusel oil

CHARACTERISTICS: *Form:* Liquid; *Color:* Colorless; *Odor:* Sharp
PHYSICAL CONSTANTS: *Specific gravity:* 0.804; *Refractive index;* 1.385; *Congealing point:* –127 C; *Boiling point:* 97.2 C; *Flash point:* 77 F
SOLUBILITY: Soluble in water, alcohol, ether
USES: Solvent, antiseptic, synthesis

PROPYL FORMATE
CHEMICAL FORMULA: $C_4H_8O_2$
CAS NUMBER: 110-74-7
CLASSIFICATION: Ester
OCCURRENCE: Formic acid and propyl alcohol
CHARACTERISTICS: *Form:* Liquid; *Color:* Colorless; *Odor:* Pleasant
PHYSICAL CONSTANTS: *Specific gravity:* 0.901 (20 C); *Refractive index;* 1.3771; *Melting point:* –93 C; *Boiling point:* 81–82 C; *Flash point:* –3 C
SOLUBILITY: In 45 parts water; miscible with alcohol, ether
USES: Flavors

PULEGONE
CHEMICAL FORMULA: $C_{10}H_{16}O$
CAS NUMBER: 89-82-7
CLASSIFICATION: Alcohol
OCCURRENCE: Pennyroyal, *Mentha pulegium*
CHARACTERISTICS: *Form:* Liquid; *Color:* Yellowish; *Odor:* Minty
PHYSICAL CONSTANTS: *Specific gravity:* 0.927–0.933; *Refractive index;* 1.4840–1.4870; *Flash point:* 192 F
SOLUBILITY: Soluble in alcohol (2 parts/70%)
USES: Industial odorants

PYROLIGNEOUS ACID
SYNONYMS: Wood vinegar; pyroligneous liquor; pyroligneous vinegar
CAS NUMBER: 8030-97-5
CLASSIFICATION: Acid
OCCURRENCE: Destructive distillation of wood
CHARACTERISTICS: *Form:* Liquid; *Color:* Yellow to red; *Odor:* Empyreumatic
PHYSICAL CONSTANTS: *Specific gravity:* 1.018–1.030
SOLUBILITY: Soluble in water, alcohol
USES: Smoking meat

RHODINOL
CHEMICAL FORMULA: $C_{10}H_{20}O$
CAS NUMBER: 6812-78-8
CLASSIFICATION: Alcohol
OCCURRENCE: Geranium
CHARACTERISTICS: *Form:* Liquid; *Color:* Colorless or yellowish; *Odor:* Rose-like
PHYSICAL CONSTANTS: *Specific gravity:* 0.860–0.880; *Refractive index;* 1.4630–1.4730; *Optical rotation:* –5 to –9; *Flash point:* 212 F

SOLUBILITY: Soluble in alcohol (5 parts/60%)
USES: Floral, especially rose

RHODINYL ACETATE

SYNONYMS: 3,7-Dimethyl-6-octen-1-yl acetate
CHEMICAL FORMULA: $C_{12}H_{22}O_2$
CLASSIFICATION: Acetate
OCCURRENCE: Geranium oil
CHARACTERISTICS: *Form:* Liquid; *Color:* Colorless to slightly yellow; *Odor:* Fruity, slightly green, fresh rose
PHYSICAL CONSTANTS: *Specific gravity:* 0.894–0.905; *Refractive index:* 1.4520–1.4580; *Flash point:* 212 F
SOLUBILITY: Clearly soluble in alcohol (2 parts/80%)
USES: Rose, carnation, muguet, toilet waters, soaps, and as a fixative

RHODINYL FORMATE

SYNONYMS: 3,7-Dimethyl-6-octen-1-yl formate
CHEMICAL FORMULA: $C_{12}H_{29}O_2$
CLASSIFICATION: Formate
OCCURRENCE: Geranium oil
CHARACTERISTICS: *Form:* Liquid; *Color:* Colorless to slightly yellow; *Odor:* Leaf, red rose
PHYSICAL CONSTANTS: *Specific gravity:* 0.901–0.906; *Refractive index:* 1.4530–1.4580; *Flash point:* $>$ 212 F
SOLUBILITY: Clearly soluble in alcohol (2 parts/80%)
USES: Rose and many floral types of perfume

SABINENE

CHEMICAL FORMULA: $C_{10}H_{16}$
CLASSIFACTION: Terpene hydrocarbon
OCCURRENCE: Savine, juniperus oils
CHARACTERISTICS: *Form:* Liquid; *Color:* Colorless; *Odor:* Pine-like
PHYSICAL CONSTANTS: *Specific gravity:* 0.840; *Boiling point:* 163 C
SOLUBILITY: Alcohol, ether, chloroform
USES: Geraniol, terpineol, perfumes

SAFROLE

CHEMICAL FORMULA: $C_{10}H_{10}O_2$
CAS NUMBER: 94-59-7
CLASSIFICATION: Ether
OCCURRENCE: Sassafras, camphor, nutmeg, star anise, cinnamon leaf, laurel
CHARACTERISTICS: *Form:* Liquid; *Color:* Colorless or yellowish; *Odor:* Sassafras root
PHYSICAL CONSTANTS: *Specific gravity:* 1.092–1.101; *Refractive index;* 1.5360–1.5385; *Optical rotation:* −1 to +1; *Flash point:* 212 F
SOLUBILITY: Soluble in alcohol (4 parts/90%)

USES: Source of heliotropine; soaps

SALICYLIC ACID

CHEMICAL FORMULA: $C_7H_6O_3$
CAS NUMBER: 69-72-7
CLASSIFICATION: Acid
OCCURRENCE: Leaves of wintergreen and bark of sweet birch; also synthetically made
CHARACTERISTICS: *Form:* Crystals, needles, or powder; *Color:* White
PHYSICAL CONSTANTS: *Specific gravity:* 1.443 (20/4 C); *Melting point:* 158–161 C; *Boiling point:* 211 C
SOLUBILITY: Soluble in acetone, alcohol, ether, benzene, turpentine
USES: Perfumes

SANTALENE

CHEMICAL FORMULA: $C_{15}H_{24}$
CLASSIFACTION: Sesquiterpene hydrocarbon
OCCURRENCE: Red cedar oil
CHARACTERISTICS: *Color:* Colorless or yellowish
PHYSICAL CONSTANTS: *Boiling point:* 120 C, 252 C
SOLUBILITY: Alcohol
USES: Perfumery

SANTALOL

CHEMICAL FORMULA: $C_{15}H_{24}O$
CAS NUMBER: α: 115-71-9; β: 77-42-9
CLASSIFICATION: Alcohol
OCCURRENCE: Sandalwood
CHARACTERISTICS: *Form:* Viscous liquid; *Color:* Colorless or yellowish; *Odor:* Woody
PHYSICAL CONSTANTS: *Specific gravity:* 0.970–0.974; *Refractive index;* 1.5050–1.5080; *Optical rotation:* 14–19; *Flash point:* 212 F
SOLUBILITY: Soluble in alcohol (4 parts/70%)
USES: Oriental-type perfumes with heavy fragrance

SANTALYL ACETATE

SYNONYMS: β-Santalyl acetate
CHEMICAL FORMULA: $C_{17}H_{26}O_2$
CLASSIFICATION: Acetate
OCCURRENCE: Synthetic
CHARACTERISTICS: *Form:* Liquid; *Color:* Colorless to slightly yellow; *Odor:* Sandalwood
PHYSICAL CONSTANTS: *Specific gravity:* 0.981–0.985; *Refractive index:* 1.4880–1.4910; *Flash point:* 212 F
SOLUBILITY: Clearly soluble in alcohol (9 parts/80% or 1 part/90%)
USES: Oriental-type and woody-lilac perfumes

SANTENE

CHEMICAL FORMULA: C_9H_{14}
CLASSIFACTION: Terpene hydrocarbon
OCCURRENCE: Various essential oils
CHARACTERISTICS: *Form:* Liquid; *Color:* Colorless; *Odor:* Aromatic
PHYSICAL CONSTANTS: *Boiling point:* 142 C
SOLUBILITY: Soluble in alcohol, ether, chloroform
USES: Perfumes

SEBACIC ACID

CHEMICAL FORMULA: $C_{10}H_{18}O_4$
CAS NUMBER: 111-20-6
CLASSIFICATION: Acid
OCCURRENCE: Synthetic
CHARACTERISTICS: *Form:* Leaflets; *Color:* White; *Odor:* Fatty acid
PHYSICAL CONSTANTS: *Specific gravity:* 1.110; *Refractive index;* 1.422; *Melting point:* 133 C; *Boiling point:* 295 C
SOLUBILITY: Soluble in alcohol, ether; slightly soluble in water
USES: Perfumes

SKATOLE

CHEMICAL FORMULA: C_9H_9N
CAS NUMBER: 83-34-1
CLASSIFICATION: Nitro compound
OCCURRENCE: Civet
CHARACTERISTICS: *Form:* Large crystals or fine powder; *Color:* Brownish; *Odor:* Civet
PHYSICAL CONSTANTS: *Melting point:* 93 C; *Boiling point:* 265 C
SOLUBILITY: Soluble 1 g/3 ml 95% alcohol
USES: Fixative for floral-type perfumes

STYRALYL ACETATE

SYNONYMS: Methyl phenyl carbinyl acetate; α-methylbenzyl acetate; *sec*-phenylethyl acetate
CHEMICAL FORMULA: $C_{10}H_{12}O_2$
CLASSIFICATION: Acetate
OCCURRENCE: Synthetic
CHARACTERISTICS: *Form:* Liquid; *Color:* Colorless; *Odor:* Strong floral
PHYSICAL CONSTANTS: *Specific gravity:* 1.023–1.026 (25/25 C); *Refractive index:* 1.4935–1.4960 (20 C); *Flash point:* 178 C
SOLUBILITY: Soluble in 70% alcohol, glycerin, and mineral oil; insoluble in water
USES: Tuberose, muguet, hyacinth, jasmine, gardenia; flavoring
WARNINGS AND CAUTION: Combustible; low toxicity

STYROL

SYNONYMS: Styrene; cinnamene; ethenylbenzene; styrolene; cinnamol; vinylbenzene

CHEMICAL FORMULA: C_8H_8
CLASSIFICATION: Aromatic resin
OCCURRENCE: Storax oil
CHARACTERISTICS: *Form:* Liquid; *Color:* Colorless to brownish; *Odor:* Aromatic penetrating
PHYSICAL CONSTANTS: *Specific gravity:* 0.959; *Refractive index;* 1.5463; *Boiling point:* 145–146 C; *Congealing point:* –30.6 C
SOLUBILITY: Soluble in alcohol, ether, acetone, carbon disulfide
USES: Organic synthesis
WARNINGS AND CAUTION: Toxic

SUCCINIC ACID
CHEMICAL FORMULA: $C_4H_6O_4$
CAS NUMBER: 110-15-6
CLASSIFICATION: Acid
OCCURRENCE: Fermentation of tartaric acid and synthetically
CHARACTERISTICS: *Form:* Crystals; *Color:* Colorless or white; *Odor:* Odorless
PHYSICAL CONSTANTS: *Specific gravity:* 1.552; *Melting point:* 185 C; *Boiling point:* 235 C
SOLUBILITY: Soluble in water; slightly soluble in alcohol, ether
USES: Esters for perfumes

TANNIC ACID
CHEMICAL FORMULA: $C_{76}H_{52}O_{46}$
CAS NUMBER: 1401-55-4
CLASSIFICATION: Acid
OCCURRENCE: Extaction with water and alcohol from nutgalls, barks, roots, leaves, etc. of sumac, oak, mangrove
CHARACTERISTICS: *Form:* Powder or flakes; *Color:* Yellowish to dark; *Odor:* Odorless
PHYSICAL CONSTANTS: *Specific gravity:* 1.0120; *Melting point:* 210 C
SOLUBILITY: Soluble in water, alcohol, acetone; insoluble in benzene, chloroform, ether
USES: Mordant, fixative; deodorizing agent for crude oils

TARTARIC ACID
CHEMICAL FORMULA: $C_4H_6O_6$
CAS NUMBER: 133-37-9
CLASSIFICATION: Acid
OCCURRENCE: From wine lees; exists in many plants, mainly in grape and tamarind juice
CHARACTERISTICS: *Form and Color:* Colorless transparent crystals or white granular; *Odor:* Odorless
PHYSICAL CONSTANTS: *Specific gravity:* 1.7598; *Melting point:* 170 C
SOLUBILITY: Soluble in alcohol, ether
USES: Effervescent beverages; fruit esters; acidulant for food; laxative

TERPINEOL

CHEMICAL FORMULA: $C_{10}H_{18}O$
CAS NUMBER: α-: 98-55-5
CLASSIFICATION: Alcohol
OCCURRENCE: Pine, cajuput, cardamom, nutmeg, cypress, cubeb, camphor, eucalyptus, rosewood, linaloe, citrus, jasmine
CHARACTERISTICS: *Form:* Viscous liquid; *Color:* Colorless; *Odor:* Lilac-like
PHYSICAL CONSTANTS: *Specific gravity:* 0.931–0.936; *Refractive index;* 1.4825–1.4850; *Flash point:* 195 F
SOLUBILITY: Soluble in alcohol (3 parts/60% or 2 parts/70%)
USES: Perfumes

TERPINYL ACETATE

CHEMICAL FORMULA: $C_{12}H_{20}O_2$
CAS NUMBER: 80-26-2
CLASSIFICATION: Acetate
OCCURRENCE: Cajuput, cardamom
CHARACTERISTICS: *Form:* Liquid; *Color:* Colorless; *Odor:* Bergamot, lavender
PHYSICAL CONSTANTS: *Specific gravity:* 0.952–0.960; *Refractive index:* 1.4640–1.4660; *Flash point:* 212 F
SOLUBILITY: Clearly soluble in alcohol (3–5 parts/70%)
USES: Lavender, bergamot, eau de cologne, soap

TERPINYL FORMATE

CLASSIFICATION: Formate
OCCURRENCE: Synthetic
CHARACTERISTICS: *Odor:* Bergamot, terpineol
USES: Woody, green, fern, chypre, cologne, lavender compositions

TERPINYL PROPIONATE

CHEMICAL FORMULA: $C_{13}H_{22}O_2$
CLASSIFICATION: Propionate
OCCURRENCE: Synthetic
CHARACTERISTICS: *Form:* Liquid; *Color:* Colorless to slightly yellow; *Odor:* Lavender, bergamot
PHYSICAL CONSTANTS: *Specific gravity:* 0.944–0.949; *Refractive index:* 1.4620–1.4660; *Flash point:* > 212 F
SOLUBILITY: Clearly soluble in alcohol (2 parts/80%)
USES: Lavender, bergamot, pine, eau de cologne, soap perfumes; bath crystal perfumes

THYMOL

CHEMICAL FORMULA: $C_{10}H_{14}O$
CAS NUMBER: 89-83-8
CLASSIFICATION: Phenol
OCCURRENCE: Thyme, origanum, monard oils

CHARACTERISTICS: *Form:* Crystalline; *Color:* White; *Odor:* Phenolic, herbaceous
PHYSICAL CONSTANTS: *Melting point:* 48.5–49.5 C; *Congealing point:* 49.3 C min. (fine crystals), 48 C min. (standard)
SOLUBILITY: Soluble 1 g/1000 ml water, 1 g/3 ml 80% alcohol, 1 g/1 ml 95% alcohol
USES: Antiseptic, germicide; soaps, creams; cosmetic stabilizer

TIGLIC ACID
CHEMICAL FORMULA: $C_5H_8O_2$
CAS NUMBER: 80-59-1
CLASSIFICATION: Acid
OCCURRENCE: Croton oil, Roman chamomile, geranium
CHARACTERISTICS: *Form and Color:* Thick syrup or colorless crystals; *Odor:* Spicy
PHYSICAL CONSTANTS: *Specific gravity:* 0.9641; *Melting point:* 65 C; *Boiling point:* 198.5 C
SOLUBILITY: Soluble in alcohol, ether; slightly soluble in water
USES: Esters in perfumes
WARNINGS AND CAUTION: Highly toxic by ingestion

TRICHLOROMETHYL PHENYL CARBINYL ACETATE
CHEMICAL FORMULA: $C_{10}H_9O_2Cl_3$
CAS NUMBER: 90-17-5
CLASSIFICATION: Acetate
OCCURRENCE: Synthetic
CHARACTERISTICS: *Form:* Crystalline; *Color:* White; *Odor:* Rose
PHYSICAL CONSTANTS: *Melting point:* 86–88 C
SOLUBILITY: Clearly soluble in alcohol (18 parts/95%)
USES: Powder-type rose perfumes (rose powder and crystals); fixative for essential oils and perfumes

UMBELLIFERONE
SYNONYMS: Hydroxy coumarin; 7-hydroxycoumarin; hydrangin; skimmetin
CHEMICAL FORMULA: $C_9H_6O_3$
CAS NUMBER: 93-35-6
CLASSIFICATION: Lactone
OCCURRENCE: Parsley, galbanum, and other Umbelliferae
CHARACTERISTICS: *Form:* Crystals; *Color:* Colorless; *Odor:* Coumarin on heating
PHYSICAL CONSTANTS: *Melting point:* 225–228 C
SOLUBILITY: Soluble 1 g/100 ml boiling water; soluble in alcohol, chloroform, acetic acid; sparingly soluble in ether
USES: Sunscreen lotion, creams, cosmetics

UNDECYLENIC ACID
CHEMICAL FORMULA: $C_{11}H_{20}O_2$
CAS NUMBER: 112-38-9
CLASSIFICATION: Acid

OCCURRENCE: Castor oil
CHARACTERISTICS: *Form and Color:* Clear liquid or crystals; *Odor:* Fruity, rose-like
PHYSICAL CONSTANTS: *Specific gravity:* 0.910–0.913; *Refractive index;* 1.4475–1.4485; *Freezing point:* 21 C
SOLUBILITY: Soluble in alcohol, ether, chloroform
USES: Perfumes, flavors; superficial fungus infection (zinc undecylenate)

VALERIANIC ACID
SYNONYMS: Valeric acid; *n*-pentanoic acid
CHEMICAL FORMULA: $C_5H_{10}O_2$
CAS NUMBER: 109-52-4
CLASSIFICATION: Acid
OCCURRENCE: Valerian
CHARACTERISTICS: *Form:* Liquid; *Color:* Clear, colorless; *Odor:* Unpleasant
PHYSICAL CONSTANTS: *Specific gravity:* 0.939; *Refractive index;* 1.4086; *Boiling point:* 187 C
SOLUBILITY: Soluble in alcohol, ether; slightly soluble in water
USES: Flavors, perfumes, medicines

VANILLIN
SYNONYMS: 3-Methoxy-4-hydroxybenzaldehyde; vanillic aldehyde; methyl ether protocatechuic aldehyde; protocatechualdehyde-3-methyl ether
CHEMICAL FORMULA: $C_8H_8O_3$
CAS NUMBER: 121-33-5
CLASSIFICATION: Aldehyde
OCCURRENCE: Vanilla beans, Peru and Tolu balsam, storax, benzoin, and in traces in essential oils containing eugenol
CHARACTERISTICS: *Form:* Crystalline needles; *Color:* White; *Odor:* Strong, sweet, characteristic
PHYSICAL CONSTANTS: *Specific gravity:* 1.056; *Melting point:* 81–83 C; *Boiling point:* 285 C
SOLUBILITY: Soluble in 125 parts water, in 20 parts glycerol, and in 2 parts 95% alcohol; soluble in chloroform and ether
USES: Fixative for perfumes; combines with heliotropin, coumarin, benzyl isoeugenol; flavoring; pharmaceuticals
WARNINGS AND CAUTION: Combustible; low toxicity

VETIVER ACETATE
SYNONYMS: Vetiveryl acetate; vetiverol acetate; vetivert acetate
CHEMICAL FORMULA: $C_{17}H_{26}O_2$
CLASSIFICATION: Acetate
OCCURRENCE: Synthetic
CHARACTERISTICS: *Form:* Viscous liquid; *Color:* Yellow; *Odor:* Woody-vetiver
PHYSICAL CONSTANTS: *Specific gravity:* 0.980–1.010; *Refractive index:* 1.5110–1.5190; *Flash point:* 210 F

SOLUBILITY: Clearly soluble in alcohol (7 parts/90%)
USES: Woody and oriental-type perfumes

YARA YARA

SYNONYMS: 2-Methoxynaphthalene; β-naphthol methyl ether; methyl β-naphthyl ether
CHEMICAL FORMULA: $C_{11}H_{10}O$
CLASSIFICATION: Ether
OCCURRENCE: Synthetic
CHARACTERISTICS: *Form:* Crystals; *Color:* White; *Odor:* Acacia, orange flower
PHYSICAL CONSTANTS: *Congealing point:* 71.5 C
SOLUBILITY: Soluble 1 g/25 ml 95% alcohol
USES: Soaps, perfumery, colognes

Chapter IV:

AROMATIC CHEMICALS

Aromatic Chemicals Used in Flavor and Perfume Compounds

ACETOPHENONE

SYNONYMS: Methyl phenyl ketone; phenyl methyl ketone; 1-phenylethanone; acetylbenzene; hypnone

CAS NUMBER: 98-86-2

CLASSIFICATION: Aromatic ketone

MOLECULAR FORMULA: C_8H_8O

MOLECULAR WEIGHT: 120.15

COMPONENTS PERCENTAGE: C: 79.97%, H: 6.71%, O: 13.32%

OCCURRENCE: Cistus and labdanum oils; green tea; orris; nettle; coal tar distillate; *Populus balsamifera L.*; *Stirlingia latifolia*

CHARACTERISTICS: *Form:* Liquid at room temperature; *Color:* Colorless; *Odor:* Harsh hawthorn; mimosa; sweet pungent; orange blossom in small amount; *Taste:* Bitter

PHYSICAL PROPERTIES: *Specific gravity:* 1.025–1.028 (25/25 C); *Refractive index:* 1.5330–1.5350 (20 C); *Optical rotation:* 1.033 (15 C); *Boiling point:* 202 C (760 mm) or 83.7 C (12 mm); *Freezing point:* 20.5 C; *Flash point:* 177 F (TCC); *Solubility:* Soluble in 5 parts 50% ethyl alcohol, essential oils, chloroform, ether, fatty oils, glycerol; insoluble in water

USES AND APPLICATIONS: *Flavors:* Strawberry (aldehyde C-16); ethyl methyl phenyl glycidate; *Perfumes:* Hawthorn; apple blossom; mimosa; enlivens lilac; neroli; new mown hay; syringa; fougere; *Other:* Solvent—tear gas by chlorinization

DERIVATION: (1) By Friedel-Crafts reaction with benzene and acetic anhydride, or acetyl chloride; (2) By-product from the oxidation of cumene; (3) Oxidation of ethylbenzene

METHOD OF PURIFICATION: Redistillation and crystallization

WARNING AND CAUTION: Narcotic in high concentration

SPECIAL NOTES: It forms laminar crystals at low temperature. By reduction it gives phenyl methyl carbinol.

AMYL CINNAMIC ALDEHYDE

SYNONYMS: α-Phenyl cinnamic aldehyde; α-amyl cinnamic aldehyde; α-*n*-amyl-β-phenyl acrolein; α-pentyl cinnamic aldehyde; jasmine aldehyde
CLASSIFICATION: Aromatic aldehyde
MOLECULAR FORMULA: $C_{14}H_{18}O$
MOLECULAR WEIGHT: 202.29
OCCURRENCE: Synthetic
CHARACTERISTICS: *Form:* Oily liquid; *Color:* Clear yellowish; *Odor:* Jasmine; lily
PHYSICAL PROPERTIES: *Specific gravity:* 0.920–0.968 (25/25 C); *Refractive index:* 1.554–1.559 (20 C); *Boiling point:* 153–154 C; *Flash point:* 221 F (TCC); *Solubility:* Soluble in 6 parts 80% ethyl alcohol and in almost all organic solvents
USES AND APPLICATIONS: *Flavors:* Flavoring; *Perfumes:* Jasmine; *Other:* Detergents
DERIVATION: (1) From heptaldehyde by condensation with benzaldehyde in presence of alkali; (2) From *n*-amyl aldehyde by condensation with cinnamic aldehyde
METHOD OF PURIFICATION: Redistillation and crystallization
WARNING AND CAUTION: Flammable—fire risk
SPECIAL NOTES: It decomposes on prolonged storage

AMYL SALICYLATE

SYNONYMS: Isoamyl salicylate; isopentyl salicylate; isoamyl-*o*-hydroxybenzoate
CAS NUMBER: 87-20-7
CLASSIFICATION: Aromatic salicylate
MOLECULAR FORMULA: $C_{12}H_{16}O_3$
MOLECULAR WEIGHT: 208.25
COMPONENTS PERCENTAGE: C: 69.21%, H: 7.74%, O: 23.05%
OCCURRENCE: Synthetic
CHARACTERISTICS: *Color:* Colorless; *Odor:* Orchid-like; herbaceous persistent; *Taste:* Bitter, strawberry reminiscent
PHYSICAL PROPERTIES: *Specific gravity:* 1.053–1.059 (15 C); *Refractive index:* 1.5050–1.5080 (20 C); *Optical rotation:* 0 to +2.30; *Boiling point:* 280 C; *Flash point:* 270 F (TCC); *Solubility:* Soluble in 4 parts 90% ethyl alcohol; ether; chloroform; insoluble in water and in glycerol
USES AND APPLICATIONS: *Perfumes:* Extensively used as the basis of all orchid and clover perfumes; in small amount as a modifier and a fixative
DERIVATION: Esterification of salicylic acid with amyl alcohol, in presence of hydrochloric acid
METHOD OF PURIFICATION: Redistillation

ANISIC ALDEHYDE

SYNONYMS: Anisaldehyde; aubepine; *p*-anisaldehyde; *p*-methoxybenzaldehyde
CAS NUMBER: 123-11-5
CLASSIFICATION: Aromatic aldehyde
MOLECULAR FORMULA: $C_8H_8O_2$
MOLECULAR WEIGHT: 136.14
COMPONENTS PERCENTAGE: C: 70.57%, H: 5.92%, O: 23.50%

OCCURRENCE: Anise and fennel oils; cassia; acacia; vanilla beans
CHARACTERISTICS: *Color:* Colorless to yellowish; *Odor:* Hawthorn; *Taste:* Pungent anise-like flavor, bitter
PHYSICAL PROPERTIES: *Specific gravity:* 1.119–1.123 (25/25 C); *Refractive index:* 1.5710–1.5740 (20 C); *Boiling point:* 248 C (760 mm) or 122 C (10 mm); *Freezing point:* 1.0 C; *Flash point:* 248 F (TCC); *Solubility:* Soluble in 1 part 70% ethyl alcohol; soluble in almost all organic solvents
USES AND APPLICATIONS: *Flavors:* In small amount for strawberry flavor; *Perfumes:* Acacia; cassie; new mown hay; heliotrope; lilac; *Other:* Cosmetic face powders
DERIVATION: Natural and synthetic sources, mostly anethole by oxidation with dichrome sulfuric acid
METHOD OF PURIFICATION: Redistillation
SPECIAL NOTES: It is used in small amounts in flavors because of its burning bitter taste

BENZALDEHYDE
SYNONYMS: Benzoic aldehyde; synthetic oil of bitter almond; artificial essential oil of almond
CAS NUMBER: 100-52-7
CLASSIFICATION: Aromatic aldehyde
MOLECULAR FORMULA: C_7H_6O
MOLECULAR WEIGHT: 106.13
COMPONENTS PERCENTAGE: C: 79.22%, H: 5.70%, O: 15.08%
OCCURRENCE: In 50 different natural oils: bitter almond, peach, apricot kernels; in small amount in neroli and acacia oils; rose, hyacinth, narcissus, rue, ylang ylang, cassia, cinnamon, cajeput, and various eucalyptus species
CHARACTERISTICS: *Form:* Liquid; *Color:* Colorless or yellowish; *Odor:* Bitter almond, fragrant; *Taste:* Aromatic bitter almond, burning
PHYSICAL PROPERTIES: *Specific gravity:* 1.041–1.046 (25/25 C); *Refractive index:* 1.5440–1.5465 (20 C); *Optical rotation:* 1.050 (15 C); *Boiling point:* 179 C; *Freezing point:* –56 C; *Flash point:* 148 F (TCC); *Solubility:* Soluble in 3 parts 60% ethyl alcohol; miscible with ether, oils
USES AND APPLICATIONS: *Flavors:* Flavoring compounds; *Perfumes:* Various perfumes, soaps; *Other:* Toilet preparation; manufacture of cinnamic acid and benzoic acid
DERIVATION: (1) Air oxidation of toluene with uranium, or molybdenum oxide as catalyst; (2) Chlorination of toluene with hydrolysis by acid or alkali; (3) Benzal chloride and lime
METHOD OF PURIFICATION: Redistillation
WARNING AND CAUTION: Narcotic in high concentrations; may cause dermatitis
SPECIAL NOTES: Benzaldehyde FFC indicates free from chlorine; it causes discoloration on soaps if it contains chlorine

BENZYL ACETATE
SYNONYMS: Phenyl methyl acetate; acetic acid phenyl methyl ester; acetic acid benzyl ester

CLASSIFICATION: Aromatic acetate ester
MOLECULAR FORMULA: $C_9H_{10}O_2$
MOLECULAR WEIGHT: 150.18
COMPONENTS PERCENTAGE: C: 71.98%, H: 6.71%, O: 21.31%
OCCURRENCE: Ylang ylang, cananga, neroli, jasmine, hyacinth, gardenia, tuberose; mainly in jasmine oil in which it is present up to 65%
CHARACTERISTICS: *Form:* Liquid; *Color:* Colorless; *Odor:* Fresh floral jasmine; *Taste:* Bitter and pungent pear-like
PHYSICAL PROPERTIES: *Specific gravity:* 1.052–1.056 (25/25 C); *Refractive index:* 1.5015–1.05035 (20 C); *Optical rotation:* 1.050 (25 C); *Boiling point:* 215.5–216.0 C; *Freezing point:* –51 C; *Flash point:* 216 F (TCC); *Solubility:* Soluble in 6 parts 60% ethyl alcohol, almost all organic solvents; slightly soluble in water
USES AND APPLICATIONS: *Flavors:* Flavoring; *Perfumes:* Soaps and detergents; basis for jasmine perfumes and component in rose, lilac, gardenia, lily, muguet; *Other:* Solvent for high boiler cellulose acetate and nitrate
DERIVATION: From benzyl alcohol with acetic acid or by heating benzyl chloride with potassium acetate at 180 C for a period of 10–12 h
METHOD OF PURIFICATION: Distillation
WARNING AND CAUTION: Irritating to the eyes, respiratory tract; ingestion causes vomiting and diarrhea

BENZYL ALCOHOL

SYNONYMS: α-Hydroxytoluene; phenyl methanol; phenyl carbinol; benzene methanol; α-hydroxytoluene primary
CAS NUMBER: 100-51-6
CLASSIFICATION: Aromatic alcohol
MOLECULAR FORMULA: C_7H_8O
MOLECULAR WEIGHT: 108.4
COMPONENTS PERCENTAGE: C: 77.75%, H: 7.46%, O: 14.80%
OCCURRENCE: Essential oils: acacia, champaca, clove buds, hyacinth, jasmine, neroli, orris, tea, tobacco, tuberose, violet, wallflowers, ylang ylang; castoreum; balsam Peru and tolu
CHARACTERISTICS: *Form:* Liquid; *Color:* Colorless; *Odor:* Pleasant, similar to benzaldehyde on aging; *Taste:* Sweet, sharp burning
PHYSICAL PROPERTIES: *Specific gravity:* 1.04927 (15 C), 1.041–1.046 (25 C); *Refractive index:* 1.54259 (15 C), 1.5385–1.5405 (20 C); *Boiling point:* 205.8 C (760 mm) or 98.2 C (14 mm); *Freezing point:* –15 to –19 C; *Flash point:* 96 C, 213 F (TCC), 220 F (open); *Solubility:* Soluble in 25 parts water, almost all organic solvents, 9 parts 30% ethyl alcohol, 2 parts 50% ethyl alcohol
USES AND APPLICATIONS: *Flavors:* In flavoring if free of chlorine (FFC); *Perfumes:* Floral compositions: jasmine, tuberose, ylang ylang; *Other:* Solvent for dyes, waxes, resins, gelatins, casein, shellac, cellulose acetate, textile, photographic; pharmaceutical aid
DERIVATION: By hydrolysis of benzyl chloride or benzyl acetate, sodium or potassium carbonate; from benzaldehyde by Cannizzaro method with potassium hydroxide

METHOD OF PURIFICATION: Distillation
WARNING AND CAUTION: Outignition at 817 F
SPECIAL NOTES: On prolonged standing and exposure odor becomes similar to benzaldehyde

BENZYL BENZOATE

SYNONYMS: Benzoic acid phenyl methyl ester; benzoic acid benzyl ester; benzyl benzene carboxylate; ascabin; ascabiol; benzylate; venzonate; vanzoate
CAS NUMBER: 120-51-4
CLASSIFICATION: Aromatic benzoate
MOLECULAR FORMULA: $C_{14}H_{12}O_2$
MOLECULAR WEIGHT: 212.25
COMPONENTS PERCENTAGE: C: 79.22%, H: 5.70%, O: 15.08%
OCCURRENCE: Peru and tolu balsam, cinnamon leaves, carnation, hyacinth, jonquil, tuberose, ylang ylang
CHARACTERISTICS: *Form:* Liquid or leaflets; *Color:* Colorless; *Odor:* Balsamic, reminiscent of benzaldehyde; *Taste:* Sharp pungent, sweet
PHYSICAL PROPERTIES: *Specific gravity:* 1.116–1.120 (25/25 C); *Refractive index:* 1.569 (20 C); *Boiling point:* 323–324 C (760 MM), 156 C (45 mm); *Melting point:* 18–19 C; *Solubility:* Soluble in ether, chloroform, 2 parts 90% ethyl alcohol; insoluble in water and glycerol
USES AND APPLICATIONS: *Flavor:* Chewing gum flavor; *Perfumes:* Solvent for musk; *Other:* Pharmaceuticals; medicine (external); plasticizers solvent for cellulose acetate and nitrocellulose; pesticides
DERIVATION: From benzaldehyde by oxidation with alkali; from benzyl alcohol and benzoic acid; from sodium benzoate with benzyl chloride; from sodium benzylate and benzaldehyde
METHOD OF PURIFICATION: Distillation and crystallization
WARNING AND CAUTION: Avoid contact with the eyes; causes skin irritation
SPECIAL NOTES: Should be free from chlorine (FFC); readily freezes

BENZYL CINNAMATE

SYNONYMS: Cinnamein; 3-phenyl-2-propenoic acid; phenyl methyl ester; *trans*-cinnamic acid benzyl ester
CLASSIFICATION: Aromatic cinnamate
MOLECULAR FORMULA: $C_{16}H_{14}O_2$
MOLECULAR WEIGHT: 238.29
COMPONENTS PERCENTAGE: C: 80.65%, H: 5.92%, O: 13.43%
OCCURRENCE: Peru and tolu balsam; styrax; copaiba balsam main constituent
CHARACTERISTICS: *Form:* Crystalline solid; *Color:* White pale and yellowish; *Odor:* Sweet balsamic; *Taste:* Honey-like
PHYSICAL PROPERTIES: *Specific gravity:* 1.109 (15 C); *Melting point:* 39 C; *Boiling point:* 228–230 C; *Freezing point:* 35–36 C or 39 C; *Flash point:* 212 F (TCC); *Solubility:* Soluble in ether, oils, 8 parts 90% ethyl alcohol; insoluble in water, propylene glycol, glycerin

USES AND APPLICATIONS: *Flavors:* Flavoring in artificial compounds, mainly as a fixative with heavy persistent aroma; used in oriental-type cosmetics face powder

BENZYLIDENE ACETONE

SYNONYMS: Benzalacetone; benzoyl acetone; cinnamic methyl ketone; 4-phenyl-3-buten-2-one; methyl styryl ketone
CLASSIFICATION: Aromatic ketone
MOLECULAR FORMULA: $C_{10}H_{10}O$
MOLECULAR WEIGHT: 146.19
COMPONENTS PERCENTAGE: C: 82.15%, H: 6.90%, O: 10.94%
OCCURRENCE: Synthetic
CHARACTERISTICS: *Form:* Crystals; *Color:* Colorless to yellowish; *Odor:* Coumarin; sweet pea; *Taste:* Sharp pungent
PHYSICAL PROPERTIES: *Specific gravity:* 1.0076 (47.3 C); *Refractive index:* 1.5824 (47.3 C); *Optical rotation:* 1.0377–1.0097; *Boiling point:* 260–262 C; *Freezing point:* 39 C; *Melting point:* 41–42 C; *Solubility:* Soluble in benzene, chloroform, 3 parts 60% ethyl alcohol; sparingly soluble in petroleum ether; insoluble in water
USES AND APPLICATIONS: *Perfumes:* Amber, chypre, heliotrope, sweet pea types; fixative for lavender compounds; organic synthesis
DERIVATION: By condensation of benzaldehyde and acetone in presence of alkali
METHOD OF PURIFICATION: Steam distillation
WARNING AND CAUTION: Irritating to the skin
SPECIAL NOTES: Protect from light; avoid heat and prolonged storage

BENZYL SALICYLATE

SYNONYMS: Benzyl-*o*-hydroxybenzoxybenzoate; 2-hydroxybenzoic acid phenyl methyl ester; salicylic acid benzyl ester
CLASSIFICATION: Aromatic salicylate; ester of benzyl alcohol
MOLECULAR FORMULA: $C_{14}H_{12}O_3$
MOLECULAR WEIGHT: 228.25
COMPONENTS PERCENTAGE: C: 73.67%, H: 5.30%, O: 21.03%
OCCURRENCE: In small amount in carnation and ylang ylang oil; in larger amount in *Primula auricula* oil
CHARACTERISTICS: *Form:* Liquid; *Color:* Colorless to slightly pink; *Odor:* Balsamic, faint sweet, pleasant; *Taste:* Currant-like rhubarb
PHYSICAL PROPERTIES: *Specific gravity:* 1.176–1.180 (25/25 C), 1.1799 (20 C); *Refractive index:* 1.5790–1.5820 (20 C); *Optical rotation:* 1.175; *Boiling point:* 208 C or 170–175 C; *Freezing point:* 23.5 C; *Melting point:* 24 C; *Flash point:* 212 F (TCC); *Solubility:* Soluble in 4 parts 95% ethyl alcohol; slightly soluble in water; miscible with ether
USES AND APPLICATIONS: *Perfumes:* Fixative; carnation, jasmine, lilac, lily, bouquet compounds; *Other:* Sunscreens, antisunburn oil, creams, lotion; synthetic musk solvent
DERIVATION: From sodium salicylate and benzyl chloride
SPECIAL NOTES: Solidifies at cool room temperature

BORNEOL

SYNONYMS: Bornyl alcohol; endo 2-camphanol; endo 2-hydroxy-camphane; endo-2-bornanol; endo-1,7,7-trimethyl bicyclo (2,2,1) heptane-2-ol; camphol
CAS NUMBER: 507-70-0
CLASSIFICATION: Aromatic alcohol
MOLECULAR FORMULA: $C_{10}H_{18}O$
MOLECULAR WEIGHT: 154.24
COMPONENTS PERCENTAGE: C: 77.86%, H: 11.76%, O: 10.37%
OCCURRENCE: Several essential oils, such as thyme oil
CHARACTERISTICS: *Form:* Translucent lumps; *Color:* White; *Odor:* Camphor-like, peculiar peppery; *Taste:* Burning, somewhat resembling that of mint
PHYSICAL PROPERTIES: *Specific gravity:* 1.011 (25/25 C); *Refractive index:* 37.7° (20 C); *Boiling point:* 212 C; *Melting point:* 203 C; *Flash point:* 150 F (closed cup); *Solubility:* Soluble in 95% ethyl alcohol, ether, toluene, acetone, decalin, tetralin; very slightly soluble in water
USES AND APPLICATIONS: *Perfumes:* As camphoraceous odor for rosemary, lavender; *Other:* Medicine; incense making
DERIVATION: Synthetically by reduction of camphor with hydrogen; from α-pinene (considered the best source); reduction of ordinary camphor to solid crystalline mass; from turpentine
WARNING AND CAUTION: Causes nausea, vomiting, dizziness, mental confusion, convulsion
SPECIAL NOTES: Flammable

BORNYL ACETATE

SYNONYMS: Bornyl acetic ether; 1,7,7 trimethyl bicyclo (2,2,1) heptan-2-ol acetate; borneol acetate
CLASSIFICATION: Aromatic acetate
MOLECULAR FORMULA: $C_{12}H_{20}O_2$
MOLECULAR WEIGHT: 196.28
COMPONENTS PERCENTAGE: C: 73.43%, H: 10.27%, O: 16.30%
OCCURRENCE: Found in levo and dextro rotatory forms in oils and leaves of many *Pinus abies* species; in coriander, valerian roots, spike lavender, rosemary, sage oils
CHARACTERISTICS: *Form:* Fused crystals melting at room temperature; *Color:* Colorless; *Odor:* Refreshing odor of pine; *Taste:* Persistent powerful piney and camphoraceous
PHYSICAL PROPERTIES: *Specific gravity:* 0.981–0.984 (25/25 C); *Refractive index:* 1.4620–1.4650 (20 C); *Optical rotation:* +40 to +44; *Boiling point:* 225–226 C; *Melting point:* 29 C; *Flash point:* 185 F (TCC); *Solubility:* Soluble in 3 parts 70% ethyl alcohol or 1 part 95% ethyl alcohol
USES AND APPLICATIONS: *Perfumes:* Lavender and fougere compounds; pine bouquet detergents; disinfectants; cleaning fluids; bath preparations; room sponges; *Other:* Nitrocellulose solvent; plasticizer
DERIVATION: By heating borneol with anhydrous acetic acid in presence of sulfuric acid or formic acid
SPECIAL NOTES: It is an intermediate in the manufacture of synthetic camphor

CINNAMIC ACID

SYNONYMS: β-Phenyl acrylic acid; 3-phenyl propenoic acid; cinnamyl acid
CAS NUMBER: 621-82-9
CLASSIFICATION: Aromatic acid
MOLECULAR FORMULA: $C_9H_8O_2$
MOLECULAR WEIGHT: 148.15
COMPONENTS PERCENTAGE: C: 72.96%, H: 5.44%, O: 21.60%
OCCURRENCE: In various essential oils, resins, storax, Peru and tolu balsam; coca leaves; cinnamon oil
CHARACTERISTICS: *Form:* Crystalline powder or scales; *Color:* White colorless; *Odor:* Reminiscent of strawberry odor; *Taste:* Burning taste; sweet, reminiscent of apricot taste
PHYSICAL PROPERTIES: *Specific gravity:* 1.245 (15 C), 1.285 (15.5 C); *Boiling point:* 300 C; *Freezing point:* –133 C; *Melting point:* 137 C; *Solubility:* Soluble in chloroform, acetone, essential oils, glacial acetic acid, carbon disulfide; slightly soluble in ethyl alcohol, benzene, ether; insoluble in water
USES AND APPLICATIONS: *Flavors:* Flavoring; *Perfumes:* Compounding; *Other:* Manufacture of methyl, ethyl, benzyl cinnamate esters
DERIVATION: By heating benzaldehyde with sodium or potassium acetate in presence of acetic anhydride; by heating benzyl chloride with sodium acetate; from oxalyl bromide and styrene; from acetylene and benzaldehyde; from benzaldehyde, anhydrous sodium acetate, acetic anhydride, pyridine (traces as catalyst); from benzaldehyde and ethyl acetate; from benzaldehyde and acetyl chloride; from benzylidene acetone and sodium hypochlorite

CINNAMIC ALCOHOL

SYNONYMS: Cinnamyl alcohol; 3-phenyl-2-propen-1-ol; styrone; styralyl carbinol; phenylallylic alcohol; styryl carbinol; γ-phenylallyl alcohol
CAS NUMBER: 104-54-1
CLASSIFICATION: Aromatic alcohol
MOLECULAR FORMULA: $C_9H_{10}O$
MOLECULAR WEIGHT: 134.17
COMPONENTS PERCENTAGE: C: 80.56%, H: 7.51%, O: 11.92%
OCCURRENCE: Styrax gum, Peru balsam; cassia cinnamon; hyacinth; narcissus daffodil flowers; cinnamon leaves
CHARACTERISTICS: *Form:* Needles or crystals; *Color:* White or yellowish; *Odor:* Mild pleasant floral, hyacinth-like; *Taste:* Bitter
PHYSICAL PROPERTIES: *Specific gravity:* 1.044 (20 C); *Refractive index:* 1.5890 (20 C); *Boiling point:* 257.5 C; *Freezing point:* 33 C (pure type), 31 C (prime), 15 C (styrax type); *Flash point:* 212 F (TCC); *Solubility:* Soluble in 1 part 70% ethyl alcohol, 3 parts 50% ethyl alcohol, and in almost all organic solvents
USES AND APPLICATIONS: *Flavors:* Flavoring; *Perfumes:* Carnation, jasmine, lilac, muguet, rose; fixative; *Other:* Detergents
DERIVATION: From oil of cassia or cinnamon with iron filling and acetic acid; from reduction of cinnamic aldehyde with sodium or potassium hydroxide; from styrax by alkaline hydrolysis; from cinnamic aldehyde with aluminum isopropoxide, by saponification of cinnamic cinnamate (styracin)

METHOD OF PURIFICATION: Recrystallization
SPECIAL NOTES: Oxidizes slowly on exposure to heat

CINNAMIC ALDEHYDE

SYNONYMS: Cinnamaldehyde; 3-phenyl-2-propenal; cinnamal; cinnamyl aldehyde; phenylacrolein
CAS NUMBER: 104-55-2
CLASSIFICATION: Aromatic aldehyde
MOLECULAR FORMULA: C_9H_8O
MOLECULAR WEIGHT: 132.15
COMPONENTS PERCENTAGE: C: 81.79%, H: 6.10%, O: 12.11%
OCCURRENCE: Cinnamon bark, roots, leaves, and oil; hyacinth, myrrh; narcissus, patchouli, rose (Bulgarian)
CHARACTERISTICS: *Form:* Oily liquid; *Color:* Greenish-yellowish; *Odor:* Spicy, cinnamon; *Taste:* Burning
PHYSICAL PROPERTIES: *Specific gravity:* 1.046–1.050 (25/25 C); *Refractive index:* 1.619–1.623 (20 C); *Boiling point:* 252 C; *Freezing point:* –8 C; *Flash point:* 268 F (TCC); *Solubility:* Completely soluble in sodium bisulfite; soluble in 5 parts 60% ethyl alcohol
USES AND APPLICATIONS: *Flavors:* Flavoring; *Perfumes:* Tuberose type
DERIVATION: From cinnamon oil by condensation of benzaldehyde and acetaldehyde in presence of sodium or calcium hydroxide; from 2-chloroallyl benzene by condensation of styrene with formyl methyl aniline in presence of phosphorus oxychloride; from oxidation of cinnamyl alcohol
METHOD OF PURIFICATION: Redistillation
SPECIAL NOTES: Avoid heat; polymerizes on long standing; discolors soaps

CITRAL

SYNONYMS: Coalein oil; geranial; geranialdehyde; 3-7-dimethyl-2-6 octadienal; *cis* and *trans*-3,7-dimethyl-2,6-octadiene-1-al; neral
CAS NUMBER: 5392-40-5
CLASSIFICATION: Aromatic aldehyde
MOLECULAR FORMULA: $C_{10}H_{16}O$
MOLECULAR WEIGHT: 152.24
COMPONENTS PERCENTAGE: C: 78.89%, H: 10.59%, O: 10.51%
OCCURRENCE: In nature in a mixture of two isomers: geranial and neral; in lemongrass; principle component (about 70–80%) of lemongrass, the main source; also occurs in 150 essential oils including citronella, lemon, lime, ginger root, verbena, melissa, orange, mandarin, lavender, pepper, bay
CHARACTERISTICS: *Form:* Mobile liquid; *Color:* Slightly yellowish; *Odor:* Powerful lemon-like odor; *Taste:* Bitter
PHYSICAL PROPERTIES: *Specific gravity:* 0.885–0.89 (25/25 C); *Refractive index:* 1.4860–1.4900 (20 C); *Boiling point:* 106–107 C; *Solubility:* Soluble in 5 parts 60% ethyl alcohol, almost all organic solvents, fixed and mineral oils; insoluble in water
USES AND APPLICATIONS: *Flavors:* Flavoring; *Perfumes:* Various types of perfume; *Other:* Manufacture of ionone and methyl ionone; intermediate for aromatic chemicals

DERIVATION: By fractional distillation of lemongrass; by oxidation of geraniol, nerol, linalool with chromic acid
SPECIAL NOTES: Unstable; strong tendency to discolor; it oxidizes and polymerizes

CITRONELLAL

SYNONYMS: 3,7-Dimethyl-6-octen-1-al; 3,7-dimethyloct-6- (or 7) enal; 3,7-dimethyl-6-octenal
CAS NUMBER: 8000-29-1
CLASSIFICATION: Aromatic aldehyde
MOLECULAR FORMULA: $C_{10}H_{18}O$
MOLECULAR WEIGHT: 154.25
COMPONENTS PERCENTAGE: C: 77.86%, H: 11.76%, O: 10.37%
OCCURRENCE: Citronella oil; various eucalyptus species; melissa
CHARACTERISTICS: *Form:* Liquid; *Color:* Colorless or slightly yellowish; *Odor:* Lemon-citronella, rose type; *Taste:* Strong
PHYSICAL PROPERTIES: *Specific gravity:* 0.848–0.856 (25/25 C); *Refractive index:* 1.4460–1.4520 (20 C); *Optical rotation:* +5 to +11 (inactive if from *Eucalyptus citriodora*); *Boiling point:* 205 C; *Flash point:* 178 F (TCC); *Solubility:* Soluble in 2 parts 70% ethyl alcohol, almost all organic solvents, fixed and mineral oils; slightly soluble in glycerol; miscible with 95% ethyl alcohol; insoluble in water
USES AND APPLICATIONS: *Perfumes:* Low class perfume types; *Other:* Detergents; hydroxycitronellal synthesis; insect repellent
DERIVATION: From citronella oil (about 30–40%)
SPECIAL NOTES: Citronellal is more stable in soap than citral

CITRONELLOL

SYNONYMS: 3,7-Dimethyl-6 (or 7)-octen-1-ol; 2,6-dimethyl-2-octen-8-ol; cephrol
CAS NUMBER: 106-22-9
CLASSIFICATION: Aromatic alcohol
MOLECULAR FORMULA: $C_{10}H_{20}O$
MOLECULAR WEIGHT: 156.27
COMPONENTS PERCENTAGE: C: 76.86%, H: 12.90%, O: 10.24%
OCCURRENCE: Hundreds of essential oils; main constituent of citronella, geranium, oak moss, palmarosa, Spanish verbena, and various eucalyptus
CHARACTERISTICS: *Form:* Liquid; *Color:* Colorless; *Odor:* Rose-like
PHYSICAL PROPERTIES: *Specific gravity:* 0.852–0.860 (25/25 C); *Refractive index:* 1.4530–1.4600 (20 C); *Optical rotation:* –1.30 to +3.0; *Boiling point:* 244 C; *Flash point:* >212 F (TCC); *Solubility:* Soluble in 2 parts 70% ethyl alcohol, almost all oils
USES AND APPLICATIONS: *Perfumes:* Rose-based odors; soaps; lily of the valley odor
DERIVATION: From reduction of citronellal with aluminum; from geraniol by hydrogenation with a nickel as a catalyst
SPECIAL NOTES: Avoid aluminum containers

COUMARIN

SYNONYMS: Benzopyrone; tonka beans camphor; lactone of *o*-hydroxy cinnamic acid; 2-H-1-benzopyran-2-one; 1,2-benzopyrone; coumarinic anhydride; *cis-o*-coumarianic acid lactone

CAS NUMBER: 91-64-5

CLASSIFICATION: Aromatic lactone

MOLECULAR FORMULA: $C_9H_6O_2$

MOLECULAR WEIGHT: 146.15

COMPONENTS PERCENTAGE: C: 73.96%, H: 4.14%, O: 21.90%

OCCURRENCE: Tonka beans constituent; cassia, lavender, lovage, orchid, vernal grass

CHARACTERISTICS: *Form:* Crystals, flakes, or powder; *Color:* Colorless; *Odor:* Vanilla-like; sweet hay-like; spicy note; *Taste:* Bitter aromatic burning; toxic

PHYSICAL PROPERTIES: *Boiling point:* 297–299 C; *Melting point:* 68–70 C; *Solubility:* Soluble in 10 parts 95% ethyl alcohol, chloroform, ether, boiling water, fixed and volatile oils

USES AND APPLICATIONS: *Perfumes:* Small amounts in chypre, fougere, lavender types; *Other:* Sweetener in both floral and nonfloral compounds giving grassy hay-like odor

DERIVATION: By heating salicylic aldehyde, sodium acetate, and acetic anhydride; from tonka beans

METHOD OF PURIFICATION: Redistillation and crystallization

WARNING AND CAUTION: Toxic; its use in food products is forbidden

SPECIAL NOTES: Used generally in the proportion of 1 g/l of perfume, mostly to enhance and fix the odor

p-CRESYL ACETATE

SYNONYMS: *p*-Tolyl acetate; acetyl-*p*-cresol; *p*-cresylic acetate; acetic acid *p*-cresol acetate; *p*-cresylic acetic acid ester; narceol

CLASSIFICATION: Aromatic acetate (ester)

MOLECULAR FORMULA: $C_9H_{10}O_2$

MOLECULAR WEIGHT: 150.18

COMPONENTS PERCENTAGE: C: 71.98%, H: 6.71%, O: 21.31%

OCCURRENCE: Derivative of *p*-cresol; constituent of cananga, ylang ylang essential oil and wallflower

CHARACTERISTICS: *Form:* Liquid; *Color:* Colorless; *Odor:* In extreme dilution has a strong floral odor (narcissus-like); *Taste:* Honey-like taste

PHYSICAL PROPERTIES: *Specific gravity:* 1.044–1.050 (25/25 C); *Refractive index:* 1.4990–1.5020 (20 C); *Boiling point:* 208–209 C; *Flash point:* 186 F (TCC); *Solubility:* Soluble in 2 parts 70% ethyl alcohol, almost all organic solvents, and hot water; insoluble in glycerol

USES AND APPLICATIONS: *Perfumes:* Used in small amount for narcissus and floral bouquet; *Other:* Antiseptic

DERIVATION: Refluxing cresol (from coal tar) with acetic anhydride

METHOD OF PURIFICATION: Redistillation

SPECIAL NOTES: It has a penetrating urine odor—has an odor reminiscent of narcissus only in very small amounts

p-CRESYL METHYL ETHER

SYNONYMS: p-Methylanisole; methyl p-cresol; methyl-tolyl ether; 4-methoxytoluene
CLASSIFICATION: Aromatic ether
MOLECULAR FORMULA: $C_8H_{10}O$
MOLECULAR WEIGHT: 122.17
COMPONENTS PERCENTAGE: C: 71.98%, H: 6.71%, O: 21.31%
OCCURRENCE: From p-cresol; champaca, wallflower, ylang ylang flowers
CHARACTERISTICS: *Form:* Liquid; *Color:* Colorless; *Odor:* Pungent, ylang ylang-like
PHYSICAL PROPERTIES: *Specific gravity:* 0.966–0.970 (25/25 C); *Refractive index:* 1.510–1.513 (20 C); *Boiling point:* 175 C; *Flash point:* 151 F (TCC); *Solubility:* Soluble in 3 parts 80% ethyl alcohol, almost all organic solvents
USES AND APPLICATIONS: *Perfumes:* Hyacinth, jonquil, narcissus, wallflower, ylang ylang; soap in combination with bromostyrol
DERIVATION: Refluxing cresol (from coal tar) with methanol
SPECIAL NOTES: Used mostly in soap perfumes

CYCLAMEN ALDEHYDE

SYNONYMS: Cyclamal; alpine violet; p-isopropyl-α-methylhydrocinnamic aldehyde; p-isopropyl-α-methyl phenylpropyl aldehyde; aldehyde B
CAS NUMBER: 103-95-7
CLASSIFICATION: Aromatic aldehyde
MOLECULAR FORMULA: $C_{13}H_{18}O$
MOLECULAR WEIGHT: 190.28
OCCURRENCE: Synthetic
CHARACTERISTICS: *Form:* Liquid; *Color:* Colorless to yellowish; *Odor:* Strong flowery, cyclamen, lily of the valley, lilac
PHYSICAL PROPERTIES: *Specific gravity:* 0.949–0.959 (25/25 C); *Refractive index:* 1.507–1.520 (20 C); *Boiling point:* 270 C (760 mm), 127 C (9 mm); *Flash point:* 205 F (TCC); *Solubility:* Soluble in 1 part 80% ethyl alcohol, 3 parts of all grades of ethyl alcohol, and in almost all oils
USES AND APPLICATIONS: *Perfumes:* Lily of the valley type and other sweet floral compositions
DERIVATION: From cumin aldehyde, ethyl alcohol, and potassium hydroxide with addition of propionic aldehyde, acetic acid, and p-isopropyl α-methyl cinnamic aldehyde
METHOD OF PURIFICATION: Redistillation

DIPHENYL KETONE

SYNONYMS: Benzophenone; benzoyl benzene; diphenyl methanone
CAS NUMBER: 119-61-9
CLASSIFICATION: Aromatic ketone
MOLECULAR FORMULA: $C_{13}H_{10}O$
MOLECULAR WEIGHT: 182.22
COMPONENTS PERCENTAGE: C: 85.69%, H: 5.53%, O: 8.78%
OCCURRENCE: Synthetic

CHARACTERISTICS: *Form:* Rhombic crystalline flakes or solid; *Color:* White; *Odor:* Soft rose, geranium rose-like
PHYSICAL PROPERTIES: *Specific gravity:* 1.0496; *Refractive index:* 1.5893 (45 C); *Boiling point:* 305.4 C; *Freezing point:* 48.5 C; *Solubility:* Soluble in 10 parts 80% ethyl alcohol, ether, acetone, acetic acid; insoluble in water
USES AND APPLICATIONS: *Perfumes:* Fixative with lasting sweet note for many types (oriental, rose, geranium, sweet pea, mimosa, lily of the valley); *Other:* Polymerization inhibitor; organic synthesis; insecticides
DERIVATION: From benzene and benzoic chloride in presence of aluminum chloride; decarboxylation of *o*-benzoyl benzoic acid in presence of copper catalyst; from calcium benzoate by distillation
METHOD OF PURIFICATION: Crystallization from alcohol

DIPHENYL OXIDE
SYNONYMS: Geranium crystals; phenyl ether; diphenyl ether; phenoxybenzene; 1,1-oxybisbenzene
CAS NUMBER: 101-84-8
CLASSIFICATION: Aromatic ether
MOLECULAR FORMULA: $C_{12}H_{10}O$
MOLECULAR WEIGHT: 170.21
COMPONENTS PERCENTAGE: C: 84.68%, H: 5.92%, O: 9.40%
OCCURRENCE: Synthetic
CHARACTERISTICS: *Form:* Liquid at room temperature; *Color:* Nearly colorless; *Odor:* Geranium leaves, harsh
PHYSICAL PROPERTIES: *Specific gravity:* 1.072–1.074 (25/25 C); *Refractive index:* 1.5780–1.5790 (20 C); *Boiling point:* 259 C; *Freezing point:* –26.7 C; *Flash point:* 239 F or 115 C (TCC); *Solubility:* Soluble in 5 parts 95% ethyl alcohol, benzene, ether, glacial acetic acid; insoluble in water
USES AND APPLICATIONS: *Perfumes:* Floral as foin coupé; bouquet compounds; *Other:* General toiletries; detergents; organic synthesis
DERIVATION: From phenol and zinc or aluminum chloride; from bromobenzene and sodium phenate heated under pressure; by heating sodium phenolate with chlorobenzene in presence of catalyst
SPECIAL NOTES: Its odor is ten times that of bourbon oil

EUGENOL
SYNONYMS: 4-Allyl-2-methoxyphenol; eugenic acid; 4-allyl guaiacol; caryophyllic acid
CAS NUMBER: 97-53-0
CLASSIFICATION: Aromatic phenol
MOLECULAR FORMULA: $C_{10}H_{12}O_2$
MOLECULAR WEIGHT: 164.20
COMPONENTS PERCENTAGE: C: 73.14%, H: 7.37%, O: 19.49%
OCCURRENCE: In many essential oils; in clove buds, leaves, oil; pimento leaf and berry; bay and cinnamon leaf oil; cinnamon bark; laurel; nutmeg; acacia; carnation; hyacinth; orange flower; tuberose; violet

CHARACTERISTICS: *Form:* Oily liquid; *Color:* Colorless to yellowish with tendency to darken on exposure; *Odor:* Strongly carnation; *Taste:* Pungent spicy, pleasant, characteristic of cloves

PHYSICAL PROPERTIES: *Specific gravity:* 1.064–1.070 (25/25 C); *Refractive index:* 1.5400–1.5420 (20 C); *Optical rotation:* –1.30; *Boiling point:* 253 C; *Freezing point:* –9 C; *Flash point:* 230 F (TCC); *Solubility:* Soluble in 1 part 60% ethyl alcohol, 2 parts glacial acetic acid, in almost all organic solvents, in alkali hydroxide solutions

USES AND APPLICATIONS: *Flavors:* Flavoring; *Perfumes:* Carnation type; *Other:* Production of vanillin; germicide

DERIVATION: By extraction from clove oil with potassium hydroxide, acid, and rectification in a stream of carbon dioxide; from guaiacol-*o*-carboxylic acid; mostly from essential oils containing high percentage of eugenol: clove oil (80–85%), cinnamon leaf oil (80–95%), pimento oil (80%), bay oil (50%)

WARNING AND CAUTION: Irritating to the skin

SPECIAL NOTES: Discolors soap and cosmetics; avoid iron containers

GERANIOL

SYNONYMS: *trans*-3,7-Dimethyl-2,6-octadien-1-ol; 2,6-dimethyl-2,6-octadien-8-ol; lemonol

CLASSIFICATION: Aromatic alcohol

MOLECULAR FORMULA: $C_{10}H_{18}O$

MOLECULAR WEIGHT: 154.25

COMPONENTS PERCENTAGE: C: 77.86%, H: 11.76%, O: 10.37%

OCCURRENCE: Constituent of palmarosa, rose, geranium, citronella, lemongrass, rosewood, linaloe, petitgrain oils; the palmarosa oil contains the highest amount (80–95%); about 160 essential oils contain geraniol

CHARACTERISTICS: *Form:* Liquid; *Color:* Colorless to pale yellowish; *Odor:* Rose-like; *Taste:* Sweet

PHYSICAL PROPERTIES: *Specific gravity:* 0.870–0.890 (25/25 C), 0.873 (20 C); *Refractive index:* 1.4710–1.4780 (20 C); *Optical rotation:* –2 to +2; *Boiling point:* 230 C; *Flash point:* 217 F (TCC); *Solubility:* Soluble in 2 parts 70% ethyl alcohol, in almost all organic solvents, fixed and mineral oils; insoluble in water and in glycerol

USES AND APPLICATIONS: *Perfumes:* Used extensively in all floral rose-type perfumes; *Other:* Detergents

DERIVATION: From geranium oil, citronella oil, palmarosa oil by forming double compound with calcium carbonate; separated from citronella oil by fractional distillation at 230 C; synthetically from pinene

METHOD OF PURIFICATION: Redistillation

SPECIAL NOTES: It is catalytically oxidized to citral and employed in the manufacture of ionones; citral can be obtained by chromic acid oxidation

HELIOTROPIN

SYNONYMS: Piperonal; pipernol; 3,4-methylenedioxybenzaldehyde; piperonyl aldehyde; protocatechuic aldehyde methylene ether; piperonyl aldehyde; 1,3-benzodioxide-5-carboxaldehyde; dioxymethylene protocatechuic aldehyde

CLASSIFICATION: Aromatic aldehyde
MOLECULAR FORMULA: $C_8H_6O_3$
MOLECULAR WEIGHT: 150.14
COMPONENTS PERCENTAGE: C: 63.95%, H: 4.03%, O: 31.97%
OCCURRENCE: In small amount in a few essential oils: Brazilian sassafras oil, violet, vanilla
CHARACTERISTICS: *Form:* Lustrous crystalline; *Color:* White becoming yellowish or light to red brown on exposure; *Odor:* Sweet heliotrope flower, persistent; *Taste:* Bitter
PHYSICAL PROPERTIES: *Boiling point:* 263 C; *Melting point:* 37 C
USES AND APPLICATIONS: *Flavors:* Limited to use in cherry and vanilla types due to its bitter taste; *Perfumes:* Lilac, violet, and spice-type perfumes; honeysuckle, lily of the valley, carnation, sweet pea; *Other:* Organic synthesis
DERIVATION: From black pepper (5–9%) piperine; from hydrolysis of piperine and piperic acid and further to piperonal; from sassafras and camphor oil oxidation; by oxidation of 3,4-(methylcrudioxy) benzyl alcohol with chromium oxide-pyridine; by reaction of 4-bromo-1,2-methylenedioxybenzene
SPECIAL NOTES: Not advisable for cosmetics and soap because of its changing color

HYDROXYCITRONELLAL
SYNONYMS: Citronellal hydrate; 7-hydroxy-3,7-dimethyloctan-1-al; 3,7-dimethyl-7-hydroxyoctanal; laurine
CAS NUMBER: 107-75-5
CLASSIFICATION: Aromatic aldehyde
MOLECULAR FORMULA: $C_{10}H_{20}O_2$
MOLECULAR WEIGHT: 172.27
OCCURRENCE: Synthetic
CHARACTERISTICS: *Form:* Viscous liquid; *Color:* Colorless or slightly yellowish; *Odor:* Lily of the valley, intense; *Taste:* Sweet
PHYSICAL PROPERTIES: *Specific gravity:* 0.925–0.930 (15 C); *Refractive index:* 1.448–1.450 (20 C); *Optical rotation:* +9 to +10 (30 C); *Boiling point:* 94–96 C; *Flash point:* 270 F (TCC); *Solubility:* Soluble in 1 part 50% ethyl alcohol, in essential oils and all organic solvents, vegetable oils; slightly soluble in water
USES AND APPLICATIONS: *Flavors:* Flavoring; *Perfumes:* Fixative; jasmine, lily, lilac, magnolia, hyacinth compounds; basis for lily of the valley and linden flower-type perfumes
DERIVATION: From citronellal (citronella or *Eucalyptus citriodora*)
SPECIAL NOTES: Avoid heat

INDOLE
SYNONYMS: Benzopyrrole; 1-benzazole; 2,3-benzopyrrole
CAS NUMBER: 120-72-9
CLASSIFICATION: Aromatic cyclic nitrogen compound
MOLECULAR FORMULA: C_8H_7N
MOLECULAR WEIGHT: 117.15
COMPONENTS PERCENTAGE: C: 82.02%, H: 6.02%, N: 11.96%
OCCURRENCE: In jasmine oil (2.5%); neroli, jonquil, wallflower, citrus oil

CHARACTERISTICS: *Form and Color:* Pearl lustrous white crystalline flakes or yellowish scales turning red on exposure; *Odor:* Slightly floral odor if purified and extremely diluted

PHYSICAL PROPERTIES: *Specific gravity:* 1.0643 (25 C); *Refractive index:* 1.0609 (20 C); *Boiling point:* 253–254 C; *Melting point:* 52 C; *Solubility:* Soluble in 2 parts 70% ethyl alcohol, in almost all organic solvents; slightly soluble in water; insoluble in mineral oils and in glycerol

USES AND APPLICATIONS: *Perfumes:* Fixative

DERIVATION: From indigo by hydrogenation; from coal tar at 220–260 C fractions; by heating sodium phenyl glycine-*o*-carboxylate with sodium hydroxide, saturating the aqueous solution with carbon dioxide, and reducing with sodium amalgam

WARNING AND CAUTION: Carcinogenic

SPECIAL NOTES: Unstable; causes discoloration

IONONE

SYNONYMS: α or β-Cyclocitrylideneacetone; 4-(2,6,6-trimethyl-2-cyclohexenyl-1-yl)-3-buten-2-one; β-ionone; irisone

CAS NUMBER: 8013-90-9

CLASSIFICATION: Aromatic ketone

MOLECULAR FORMULA: $C_{13}H_{20}O$

MOLECULAR WEIGHT: 192.30

COMPONENTS PERCENTAGE: C: 81.20%, H: 10.48%, O: 8.32%

OCCURRENCE: Synthetic; raspberry, violet moss, costus root, boronia negastima new

CHARACTERISTICS: *Form:* Liquid; *Color:* Colorless to yellowish; *Odor:* Cedar wood-like; when diluted in alcoholic solution, it is violet-like in odor

PHYSICAL PROPERTIES: *Specific gravity:* 0.941–0.943 (25/25 C); *Refractive index:* 1.5195–1.5215 (20 C); *Boiling point:* 128–129 C; *Flash point:* 212 F (TCC); *Solubility:* Soluble in 3 parts 70% ethyl alcohol, ether, mineral oils, propylene glycol; insoluble in water and in glycerin

USES AND APPLICATIONS: *Flavors:* Flavoring; *Perfumes:* Violet bouquet, lily of the valley, jasmine, rose, tuberose, and for all fancy perfume compositions

DERIVATION: By condensation of citral or lemongrass with acetone in presence of sodium hydroxide, yielding α and β-ionone; from oil of costus root, violet moss, boronia megastima; from isobutylene and vinyl methyl ketone; by cyclation of pseudo-ionone with sulfuric acid (yielding α-ionone) or phosphoric acid (yielding β-ionone)

LINALOOL

SYNONYMS: 3,7-Dimethyl-1,6-octadien-3-ol; 2,6-dimethyl-2,7-octadien-6-ol; linalol

CAS NUMBER: 78-70-6

CLASSIFICATION: Aromatic alcohol

MOLECULAR FORMULA: $C_{10}H_{18}O$

MOLECULAR WEIGHT: 154.25

COMPONENTS PERCENTAGE: C: 77.87%, H: 11.76%, O: 10.37%

OCCURRENCE: Main constituent of Brazilian rosewood (90%) and coriander (70%); in several hundred essential oils including bergamot, petitgrain, rosewood, lavender, lavandin, clary sage, neroli, sweet orange, tangerine, jasmine, geranium, sweet pea, muguet, lilac, cinnamon (Sri Lanka), sassafras

CHARACTERISTICS: *Form:* Liquid; *Color:* Colorless; *Odor:* Pleasant floral, sweet intense

PHYSICAL PROPERTIES: *Specific gravity:* 0.859–0.867 (25 C); *Refractive index:* 1.4610–1.4640 (20 C); *Optical rotation:* –2 to +2; *Boiling point:* 195–199 C; *Flash point:* 175 F (TCC); *Solubility:* Soluble in 4 parts 60% ethyl alcohol, ether, and in fixed oils; insoluble in water

USES AND APPLICATIONS: *Perfumes:* As topnote for lily, lilac, honeysuckle, sweet pea, neroli, rose; detergents

DERIVATION: From many essential oils, particularly from rosewood, petitgrain, linaloe wood, bergamot; synthetically from geraniol, from mircene via acetate

METHOD OF PURIFICATION: Rectification

SPECIAL NOTES: Linalol can be converted to terpineol, geraniol, and citral and employed in the preparation of citronellol, ionones, and farnesol

LINALYL ACETATE

SYNONYMS: 3,7-Dimethyl-1,6-octadiene-3-yl acetate; bergamol

CAS NUMBER: 115-95-7

CLASSIFICATION: Aromatic acetate

MOLECULAR FORMULA: $C_{12}H_{20}O_2$

MOLECULAR WEIGHT: 196.29

COMPONENTS PERCENTAGE: C: 73.43%, H: 10.27%, O: 16.30%

OCCURRENCE: Bergamot, lavender, lavandin, clary sage, petitgrain, sassafras, neroli, lemon, lime, jasmine, orange, *Mentha arvensis*, and in small amount in many other essential oils

CHARACTERISTICS: *Form:* Oily liquid; *Color:* Colorless to yellowish; *Odor:* Strong bergamot-lavender odor, pleasant

PHYSICAL PROPERTIES: *Natural: Specific gravity:* 0.908–0.920; *Refractive index:* 1.450–1.458; *Optical rotation:* –1 to +1; *Boiling point:* 108–110 C; *Flash point:* 85 C (TCC); *Solubility:* Soluble in 4 parts 70% ethyl alcohol, ether, diethyl phthalate, benzyl benzoate, mineral oils, fixed oils; slightly soluble in propylene glycol; insoluble in water and in glycerin; *Synthetic: Specific gravity:* 0.895–0.905 (25/25 C); *Refractive index:* 1.4495–1.4512 (20 C)

USES AND APPLICATIONS: *Perfumes:* Used extensively in perfumery for fine perfumes, extracts, toilet waters, cosmetics, and soaps; it provides a lavender note in the composition of cologne water and floral compounds

DERIVATION: From linalol and acetic anhydride, in presence of sulfuric acid; from bergamot and other essential oils; from myrcene hydrochloride and anhydrous sodium acetate, acetic anhydride in presence of a catalyst, or anhydrous sodium acetate

METHOD OF PURIFICATION: Rectification

METHYL ANTHRANILATE

SYNONYMS: Methyl-2-aminobenzoate; methyl-*o*-aminobenzoate; 2-aminobenzoic acid methyl ether; neroli oil, artificial

CAS NUMBER: 134-20-3

CLASSIFICATION: Aromatic anthranilate
MOLECULAR FORMULA: $C_8H_9NO_2$
MOLECULAR WEIGHT: 151.17
COMPONENTS PERCENTAGE: C: 63.56%, H: 6.00%, N: 9.27%, O: 21.17%
OCCURRENCE: Neroli oil, jasmine, acacia, tuberose, gardenia, hyacinth, ylang ylang; citrus oil: mandarin, orange, petitgrain, lemon, bergamot; champaca, wallflower
CHARACTERISTICS: *Form:* Liquid; *Color:* Colorless to yellowish with a bluish fluorescence; *Odor:* Orange blossom, neroli; also grape type; *Taste:* Slight bitter, pungent
PHYSICAL PROPERTIES: *Specific gravity:* 1.162–1.167 (25/25 C); *Refractive index:* 1.5820–1.5840 (20 C); *Boiling point:* 132 C; *Freezing point:* 23.8 C; *Flash point:* 212 F (TCC); *Solubility:* Soluble in 2 parts 60% ethyl alcohol, in almost all organic solvents, in fixed oils, propylene glycol, volatile oils; slightly soluble in water, mineral oils; insoluble in glycerin
USES AND APPLICATIONS: *Flavors:* Synthetic grapefruit; *Perfumes:* In small amount in fancy floral perfumes; *Other:* Powerful aromatic for soaps, deodorants
DERIVATION: By heating anthranilic acid and methyl alcohol in presence of sulfuric acid or hydrochloric acid and further distilling; by condensation with hydroxycitronellal producing "aurantiol," a greenish-yellow viscous liquid

METHYL HEPTYNE CARBONATE

SYNONYMS: Methyl-2-octynoate; heptyne carboxyl acid methyl ester
CAS NUMBER: 111-12-6
CLASSIFICATION: Aromatic acetylenic
MOLECULAR FORMULA: $C_9H_{14}O_2$
MOLECULAR WEIGHT: 154.21
OCCURRENCE: Synthetic
CHARACTERISTICS: *Form:* Liquid; *Color:* Colorless to yellowish; *Odor:* Green sharp, heavy melon-cucumber-like odor which becomes violet-like in large dilution
PHYSICAL PROPERTIES: *Specific gravity:* 0.919–0.924 (25/25 C); *Refractive index:* 1.4460–1.4490 (20 C); *Boiling point:* 215–217 C; *Flash point:* 192 F (TCC); *Solubility:* Soluble in 6 parts 70% ethyl alcohol, 2 parts 80% ethyl alcohol, in almost all fixed oils and mineral oils; insoluble in water
USES AND APPLICATIONS: *Flavors:* In small amount to give a fruit and berry-type flavor; *Perfumes:* Intense green fresh violet odor; fixative particularly for violet-type odors
DERIVATION: From heptaldehyde; from destructive distillation of castor oil through heptyne carboxylic acid

p-METHYL QUINOLINE

SYNONYMS: 6-Methyl quinoline; lepidine; quinaldine; cincholepidine
CLASSIFICATION: Aromatic cyclic nitrogen compound
MOLECULAR FORMULA: $C_{10}H_9N$
MOLECULAR WEIGHT: 143.19
COMPONENTS PERCENTAGE: C: 83.88%, H: 6.34%, N: 9.78%
OCCURRENCE: Synthetic; occurs in coal tar

CHARACTERISTICS: *Form:* Liquid; *Color:* Colorless or brownish-yellow which darkens on exposure; *Odor:* Very pungent, powerful civet-like odor

PHYSICAL PROPERTIES: *Specific gravity:* 1.063–1.067 (25/25 C); *Refractive index:* 1.6120–1.6160 (20 C); *Optical rotation:* 1.0826; *Boiling point:* 261–263 C; *Flash point:* > 212 F (TCC); *Solubility:* Slightly soluble in water; miscible with ethyl alcohol, ether, benzene

USES AND APPLICATIONS: *Flavors:* In small amount to enhance the note; *Perfumes:* In small amount for floral bouquet and oriental types

DERIVATION: From aniline acetaldehyde and hydrochloride; from ethylacetanilide

METHYL SALICYLATE

SYNONYMS: 2-Hydroxybenzoic acid methyl ester; wintergreen artificial; methyl-*o*-hydroxybenzoate; wintergreen synthetic; teaberry oil; gaultheria oil; wintergreen oil; betula oil; sweet birch oil

CAS NUMBER: 119-36-8

CLASSIFICATION: Aromatic salicylate

MOLECULAR FORMULA: $C_8H_8O_3$

MOLECULAR WEIGHT: 152.14

COMPONENTS PERCENTAGE: C: 63.15%, H: 5.30%, O: 31.55%

OCCURRENCE: Wintergreen oil (sweet birch); *Betula lenta*; cassie, spice wood, rue, tuberose, viola tricolor roots, cherry, grape, apple, raspberry, carnation, ylang ylang, acacia

CHARACTERISTICS: *Form:* Liquid; *Color:* Colorless or reddish; *Odor:* Wintergreen; *Taste:* Gaultheria

PHYSICAL PROPERTIES: *Specific gravity:* 1.180–1.185 (25 C); *Refractive index:* 1.535–1.538 (20 C); *Optical rotation:* Inactive (natural), –1.5 angular rotation (synthetic); *Boiling point:* 222–223 C; *Melting point:* –8.3 C; *Flash point:* 210 F (TCC); *Solubility:* Soluble in 7 parts 70% ethyl alcohol, in almost all organic solvents, glacial acetic acid; sparingly soluble in water

USES AND APPLICATIONS: *Flavors:* Flavoring agent for dental preparations, toothpaste in small amount; *Perfumes:* Ylang ylang odor; cassie, tuberose, chypre, mimosa types; *Other:* Suntan preparations

DERIVATION: By heating methanol and salicylic acid in presence of sulfuric acid; by distillation from leaves of *Gaultheri procumbens*; by distillation from bark of *Betula lenta*

METHOD OF PURIFICATION: Rectification

SPECIAL NOTES: Discolors in presence of iron

MUSK AMBRETTE

SYNONYMS: 6-*t*-Butyl-3-methyl-2,4-dinitroanisole; 2,4-dinitro-3-methyl-6-*t*-butylanisole; 2,6-dinitro-3-methoxy-4-*t*-butyl toluene; trinitro-butyl-*m*-cresyl methyl ether

CLASSIFICATION: Aromatic nitrogen compound

MOLECULAR FORMULA: $C_{12}H_{16}N_2O_5$

MOLECULAR WEIGHT: 268.27

OCCURRENCE: Synthetic

CHARACTERISTICS: *Form:* Granular crystalline powder; *Color:* Pale yellow; *Odor:*

Musk ambrette seed
PHYSICAL PROPERTIES: *Melting point:* 83.4 C; *Solubility:* Soluble in all solvents, in fixed oils and mineral oils; sparingly soluble in ethyl alcohol; insoluble in water and in glycerin
USES AND APPLICATIONS: *Perfumes:* Fixative in perfumes and cosmetics for face powder
DERIVATION: From *t*-butyl-3-methoxy toluene, acetic anhdyride in presence of nitric acid and sodium bicarbonate
METHOD OF PURIFICATION: Redistillation and crystallization
SPECIAL NOTES: Discolors on exposure

MUSK KETONE
SYNONYMS: Musk malman; 4-*t*-butyl-3,5-dinitro-2,6-dimethyl acetophenone; 2,6-dinitro-3,5-dimethyl-4-aceto-*t*-butylbenzene; 3,5-dinitro-2,6-dimethyl-4-*t*-butyl acetophenone; dinitro-pseudo-butyl-xylyl ketone
CLASSIFICATION: Aromatic ketone
MOLECULAR FORMULA: $C_{14}H_{18}N_2O_5$
MOLECULAR WEIGHT: 294.30
OCCURRENCE: Synthetic
CHARACTERISTICS: *Form:* Platelets or fine crystalline powder; *Color:* White or yellow; *Odor:* Musk-like, sweet
PHYSICAL PROPERTIES: *Melting point:* 134.5–136 C; *Solubility:* Soluble in all solvents, in fixed oils, in 2 parts 95% ethyl alcohol; slightly soluble in mineral oils; insoluble in water, glycerin, propylene glycol
USES AND APPLICATIONS: *Perfumes:* Fixative for oriental and heavy compositions and fine perfumery
DERIVATION: From butyl xylene, aluminum chloride, acetyl chloride, carbon disulfide, sodium bicarbonate in presence of nitric acid
METHOD OF PURIFICATION: Redistillation and crystallization
SPECIAL NOTES: Discolors

MUSK XYLENE
SYNONYMS: Musk xylol; 2,4,6-trinitro-1,3-dimethyl-5-*t*-butyl benzene; 2,4,6-trinitro-*t*-butyl-*m*-xylene; butyl-2,4,6-trinitro-*m*-xylene; trinitro-butyl xylene
CLASSIFICATION: Aromatic nitrogen compound
MOLECULAR FORMULA: $C_{12}H_{15}N_3O_6$
MOLECULAR WEIGHT: 297.27
OCCURRENCE: Synthetic
CHARACTERISTICS: *Form:* Crystalline powder or needle-like; *Color:* Yellow; *Odor:* Musk
PHYSICAL PROPERTIES: *Melting point:* 112.5 C; *Solubility:* Soluble in 1 part 95% ethyl alcohol, fixed oils, mineral oils, and almost all solvents; insoluble in water, glycerin, propylene glycol
USES AND APPLICATIONS: *Perfumes:* Fixative; *Other:* It blends well with almost all raw materials in soap manufacturing
DERIVATION: From *t*-butyl-*m*-xylene, sulfuric and nitric acids
METHOD OF PURIFICATION: Redistillation

SPECIAL NOTES: Discolors on exposure

NEROL

SYNONYMS: *cis*-3,7-Dimethyl-2,6-octadien-1-ol; 2,6-dimethyl-2,6-octadien-8-ol
CAS NUMBER: 106-25-2
CLASSIFICATION: Aromatic alcohol
MOLECULAR FORMULA: $C_{10}H_{18}O$
MOLECULAR WEIGHT: 154.25
COMPONENTS PERCENTAGE: C: 77.86%, H: 11.76%, O: 10.73%
OCCURRENCE: Mainly in nerol oil and lemongrass, citronella, ylang ylang, champaca, bergamot, lemon, sweet orange, clary sage, lavender, lavandin, myrrh, jasmine, myrtle, rosewood, linalol, grapefruit, tuberose, robinia, wallflower. *Helicrysum angustfoleum* contains about 30–35% of nerol
CHARACTERISTICS: *Form:* Liquid; *Color:* Colorless; *Odor:* Fresh lemon-like, sweet odor
PHYSICAL PROPERTIES: *Specific gravity:* 0.875–0.880 (25/25 C); *Refractive index:* 1.4730–1.4780 (20 C); *Boiling point:* 225–226 C; *Flash point:* 198 F (TCC); *Solubility:* Soluble in 9 parts 50% ethyl alcohol and in almost all organic solvents; insoluble in water
USES AND APPLICATIONS: *Perfumes:* Basically for orange-blossom and rose compounds; characteristically for magnolia perfume
DERIVATION: Synthetically from pinene; by iodization of geraniol with hydriodic acid and alcoholic sodium

γ-NONALACTONE

SYNONYMS: γ-Nonyl lactone; coconut aldehyde; aldehyde C-18; 4-hydroxynonanoic acid lactone; γ-lactone; γ-*n*-amyl butyrolactone nonanolide-1,4
CLASSIFICATION: Aromatic lactone
MOLECULAR FORMULA: $C_9H_{16}O_2$
MOLECULAR WEIGHT: 156.23
OCCURRENCE: In peaches, apricots, coconut
CHARACTERISTICS: *Form:* Liquid; *Color:* Colorless or yellowish; *Odor:* Coconut; *Taste:* Coconut
PHYSICAL PROPERTIES: *Specific gravity:* 0.958–0.966 (25/25 C); *Refractive index:* 1.4460–1.4500 (20 C); *Boiling point:* 243 C or 136 C (13 mm); *Flash point:* 212 F (100 C) (TCC); *Solubility:* Soluble in 5 parts 50% ethyl alcohol, 2 parts 60% ethyl alcohol, in almost all organic solvents; insoluble in water
USES AND APPLICATIONS: *Flavors:* Flavoring; *Perfumes:* Gardenia, jasmine, tuberose, and heavy floral compounds
DERIVATION: From nonenoic acid; by condensing heptaldehyde with malonic acid in presence of sodium or potassium hydroxide

PHENYLACETALDEHYDE

SYNONYMS: Hyacinthin; α-toluic aldehyde; α-tolualdehyde; benzeneacetaldehyde
CAS NUMBER: 122-78-1
CLASSIFICATION: Aromatic aldehyde
MOLECULAR FORMULA: C_8H_8O

MOLECULAR WEIGHT: 120.14
COMPONENTS PERCENTAGE: C: 79.97%, H: 6.71%, O: 13.32%
OCCURRENCE: In neroli oil, in about a dozen essential oils, and in some fruits in a smaller amount
CHARACTERISTICS: *Form:* Liquid which polymerizes and becomes viscous on aging; *Color:* Colorless to yellowish; *Taste:* Unpleasant, pungent, bitter flavor which becomes sweet and fruit-like at low level of dilution
PHYSICAL PROPERTIES: *Specific gravity:* 1.025–1.035 (25/25 C); *Refractive index:* 1.524–1.532 (20 C); *Boiling point:* 193–194 C; *Freezing point:* 33–34 C; *Flash point:* 188 F (TCC); *Solubility:* Soluble in 2 parts 80% ethyl alcohol, ether, benzyl benzoate, diethyl phthalate, fixed oils, propylene glycol; slightly soluble in water; insoluble in glycerol and mineral oils
USES AND APPLICATIONS: *Perfumes:* Basic in bouquet to give a green top note; hyacinth, jonquil, narcissus, lilac, lily, jasmine, sweet pea, lilac, and in small amount for rose-type perfumes
DERIVATION: From phenyl-α-chloroacetic acid by action of alkali; by oxidation of phenylethyl alcohol with chromic acid

PHENYL ACETIC ACID

SYNONYMS: α-Toluic acid; benzeneacetic acid
CAS NUMBER: 103-82-2
CLASSIFICATION: Aromatic acid
MOLECULAR FORMULA: $C_8H_8O_2$
MOLECULAR WEIGHT: 136.15
COMPONENTS PERCENTAGE: C: 70.75%, H: 5.92%, O: 23.50%
OCCURRENCE: In neroli oil, rose oil, tobacco leaf
CHARACTERISTICS: *Form:* Crystalline solid; *Color:* Shiny white; discolors on prolonged storage; *Odor:* Honey-like odor which in large dilution is like that of civet
PHYSICAL PROPERTIES: *Specific gravity:* 1.0809 (25/25 C); *Optical rotation*: 1091; *Boiling point:* 265.5 C; *Freezing point:* 74.0 C; *Melting point:* 76.78 C; *Solubility:* Soluble in hot water, alcohol, ether, propylene glycol, and 2% in cold water
USES AND APPLICATIONS: *Perfumes:* Fixative: acacia, treflé, neroli, jasmine, lilac; *Other:* Toiletries lotions; blends well with indole
DERIVATION: By refluxing benzyl cyanide with diluted sulfuric acid or hydrochloric acid
METHOD OF PURIFICATION: Redistillation and crystallization
WARNING AND CAUTION: Probably toxic

PHENYL ETHYL ACETATE

SYNONYMS: Ethyl-α-toluate; benzeneacetic acid ethyl ester; phenethyl acetate; β-phenylethyl acetate; benzylcarbinyl acetate
CAS NUMBER: 103-45-7
CLASSIFICATION: Aromatic acetate
MOLECULAR FORMULA: $C_{10}H_{12}O_2$
MOLECULAR WEIGHT: 164.21
COMPONENTS PERCENTAGE: C: 73.14%, H: 7.37%, O: 19.49%
OCCURRENCE: Synthetic

CHARACTERISTICS: *Form:* Liquid; *Color:* Colorless; *Odor:* Sweet honey-rose; peach-like

PHYSICAL PROPERTIES: *Specific gravity:* 1.030–1.034 (25/25 C); *Refractive index:* 1.497–1.501 (20 C); *Optical rotation:* 1.0333; *Boiling point:* 226 C; *Freezing point:* 22 C; *Flash point:* 212 F (TCC); *Solubility:* Soluble in 8 parts 60% ethyl alcohol, ether, and almost all fixed oils; insoluble in water

USES AND APPLICATIONS: *Flavors:* Basis for tobacco flavor; *Perfumes:* Artificial otto rose, orange blossom, honey, sweet pea

DERIVATION: By esterification of phenyl acetic acid and sulfuric acid; by interaction of acetic anhydride and phenylethyl alcohol in the presence of sodium acetate; by interaction of ethyl acetate and aluminum phenyl ethylate

PHENYL ETHYL ALCOHOL

SYNONYMS: β-Phenylethyl alcohol; benzyl carbinol; 2-phenyl ethanol; β-hydroxyethylbenzene; phenethyl alcohol

CAS NUMBER: 60-12-8

CLASSIFICATION: Aromatic alcohol

MOLECULAR FORMULA: $C_8H_{10}O$

MOLECULAR WEIGHT: 122.17

COMPONENTS PERCENTAGE: C: 78.65%, H: 8.25%, O: 13.10%

OCCURRENCE: In many essential oils in small quantity: otto rose, geranium, bitter orange, carnation, champaca, hyacinth, ylang ylang, lily, tea leaf, orange blossom

CHARACTERISTICS: *Form:* Viscous liquid; *Color:* Colorless; *Odor:* Mild, pleasant and persistent rose odor; *Taste:* Sharp, slightly bitter taste, peach-like

PHYSICAL PROPERTIES: *Specific gravity:* 1.017–1.020 (25/25 C); *Refractive index:* 1.5310–1.5330 (20 C); *Boiling point:* 220–222 C; *Freezing point:* –27 C; *Flash point:* 216 F (TCC); *Solubility:* Soluble in 2 parts 50% ethyl alcohol, in almost all organic solvents, fixed oils, and mineral oils

USES AND APPLICATIONS: *Perfumes:* Enhances the odors of a variety of perfume compositions; used extensively in synthetic rose, orange blossom, neroli, jasmine, lilac

DERIVATION: By reduction of phenylacetic ethyl ester by sodium in 95% ethyl alcohol; by the action of ethylene oxide on phenyl magnesium bromide and hydrolysis; by the hydrogenation of phenyl acetaldehyde in presence of nickel catalyst

SPECIAL NOTES: Avoid aluminum containers

ROSE CRYSTALS

SYNONYMS: Trichloromethyl phenyl carbinyl acetate; α-(trichloromethyl) benzyl acetate; rosacetol

MOLECULAR FORMULA: $C_{10}H_9Cl_3O_2$

MOLECULAR WEIGHT: 267.55

OCCURRENCE: Synthetic

CHARACTERISTICS: *Form:* Crystalline; *Color:* White

PHYSICAL PROPERTIES: *Boiling point:* 280–282 C; *Melting point:* 86–88 C; *Solubility:* Soluble in 18 parts 95% ethyl alcohol

USES AND APPLICATIONS: *Perfumes:* Talcum powder; bath salts; fixative for

essential oils and perfumes
DERIVATION: By crystallization of trichloromethyl phenyl carbinyl acetate with acetyl chloride

ROSE OXIDE

OCCURRENCE: Bulgarian otto rose and geranium bourbon; synthetic
PHYSICAL PROPERTIES: *Refractive index:* 1.4566; *Optical rotation:* 41.5; *Boiling point:* 70 C
USES AND APPLICATIONS: *Perfumes:* In small amount for rose and geranium compositions; enhances effect in soap and perfumery
DERIVATION: By reaction of citronellol or citronellyl acetate with allylic oxidizing agent

TERPINEOL

SYNONYMS: α-Terpineol; β-terpineol; γ-terpineol; α: *p*-1 menthen-8-ol; 1-methyl-4-isopropyl-1-cyclohexen-8-ol; β: *p*-8 menthen-1-ol; 1-methyl-4-isopropenyl-cyclohexan-1-ol
CAS NUMBER: 98-55-5 (α)
CLASSIFICATION: Aromatic alcohol
MOLECULAR FORMULA: $C_{10}H_{18}O$
MOLECULAR WEIGHT: 154.25
COMPONENTS PERCENTAGE: C: 77.86%, H: 11.76%, O: 10.37%
OCCURRENCE: In 150 essential oils in small amount; in large quantity in pine oil (70%), cajeput, maouli, cardamom, marjoram, nutmeg, juniper, cypress, cubebe, camphora, rosewood, linaloe, sweet orange, neroli, lime, jasmine, and various eucalyptus species
CHARACTERISTICS: *Form and Color:* Colorless viscous liquid at room temperature or low melting transparent crystals; *Odor:* Sweet lilac odor; *Taste:* Sweet taste which is peach-like on dilution
PHYSICAL PROPERTIES: *α-: Specific gravity:* 0.930–0.936 (25/25 C); *Boiling point:* 218 C; *β-: Specific gravity:* 0.923–0.924 (25/25 C); *Boiling point:* 210 C; *γ-: Specific gravity:* 0.936–0.941 (25/25 C); *Boiling point:* 35 C; *All: Refractive index:* 1.4825–1.4850 (20 C); *Flash point:* 195 F (TCC); *Solubility:* Soluble in 2 parts 70% ethyl alcohol, 4 parts 60% ethyl alcohol, 8 parts 50% ethyl alcohol, and in propylene glycol; slightly soluble in water
USES AND APPLICATIONS: *Perfumes:* Lilac type; extensively applied to floral and woody types; *Other:* Soaps, detergents; blends well with hydroxycitronellal, linalol, and ylang ylang; solvent for resins, gums, waxes, esters
DERIVATION: From turpentine oil (the most economic); by heating terpin hydrate with phosphoric acid or dilute sulfuric acid, separating, and distilling; from α-pinene
SPECIAL NOTES: Avoid aluminum containers

γ-UNDELACTONE

SYNONYMS: γ-Undecalactone; peach aldehyde; aldehyde C-14 pure; persicol; 4-hydroxyundecanoic acid lactone; γ-*n*-heptylbutyrolactone; undecanolide-1,4; γ-undecyl lactone; γ-lactone
CAS NUMBER: 710-04-3

CLASSIFICATION: Aromatic lactone
MOLECULAR FORMULA: $C_{11}H_{20}O_2$
MOLECULAR WEIGHT: 184.28
COMPONENTS PERCENTAGE: C: 71.69%, H: 10.94%, O: 17.36%
OCCURRENCE: Synthetic
CHARACTERISTICS: *Form:* Viscous liquid; *Color:* Colorless to yellowish; *Odor:* Peach odor; *Taste:* Strong peach-like, pungent
PHYSICAL PROPERTIES: *Specific gravity:* 0.941–0.944 (25/25 C); *Refractive index:* 1.450–1.454 (20 C); *Boiling point:* 297 C; *Flash point:* 212 F (100 C) (TCC); *Solubility:* Soluble in 5 parts 60% ethyl alcohol, 2 parts 70% ethyl alcohol, in almost all organic solvents and fixed oils; insoluble in water
USES AND APPLICATIONS: *Flavors:* Flavoring; *Perfumes:* In small amount for jasmine, lilac, rose types
DERIVATION: By heating undecylenic acid in presence of sulfuric acid

VANILLIN

SYNONYMS: 4-Hydroxy-3-methoxy benzaldehyde; methoxy protocatechuic aldehyde; protocatechualdehyde-3-methyl ether; vanillic aldehyde; methyl protocatechuic aldehyde
CAS NUMBER: 121-33-5
CLASSIFICATION: Aromatic aldehyde
MOLECULAR FORMULA: $C_8H_8O_3$
MOLECULAR WEIGHT: 152.15
COMPONENTS PERCENTAGE: C: 63.15%, H: 5.30%, O: 31.55%
OCCURRENCE: Vanilla bean pods; citronella, benzoin, Peru and tolu balsam, clove buds oil, storax; in traces in many essential oils containing eugenol
CHARACTERISTICS: *Form:* Crystalline needles or powder; *Color:* White to yellowish; *Odor:* Characteristic strong vanilla-like; *Taste:* Very sweet
PHYSICAL PROPERTIES: *Specific gravity:* 1.056 (liquid); *Boiling point:* 284–285 C with decomposition; *Melting point:* 81–83 C; sublimes when heated; *Solubility:* Soluble in 3 parts 70% ethyl alcohol, 2 parts 90% ethyl alcohol, in ether, chloroform, carbon disulfide, glacial acetic acid, pyridine, oils, and alkali hydroxide solutions; miscible with water
USES AND APPLICATIONS: *Flavors:* Primarily for flavoring; *Perfumes:* Fixative; combines with heliotropin, benzyl isoeugenol; musk; *Other:* Face powder, deodorants
DERIVATION: From eugenol by direct oxidation (nitrobenzene method); from safrole obtained from camphor by conversion to isosafrole through methylation and oxidation; from guaiacol; as a by-product of the paper-pulp industry from waste of sulfite liquor upon heating with alkali and air oxidation
SPECIAL NOTES: Avoid iron containers; 1 part vanillin equals 400 parts vanilla beans

Chapter V:

PERFUMES

Natural Odors Simulated with Aromatic Chemicals

BALSAMIC

DESCRIPTION: Chemicals with a penetrating, pleasant odor similar to the fragrant resin or oleoresin flowing from various plants containing benzoic or cinnamic acid.

COMMON VARIETIES: Peru Balsam, from Central America; Tolu Balsam, from Colombia; Copaiba Balsam, from Brazil and Venezuela; Balm of Gilead, shrub, Middle East, Africa; Canada Balsam, North America fir tree; Benzoin, from Styrax tree in Southeast Asia and Sumatra.

CHEMICALS FOR SCENT MATCHING: (1) Benzyl benzoate; (2) Benzyl cinnamate; (3) Cinnamic alcohol; (4) Cinnamyl acetate; (5) Cinnamyl anthranilate; (6) Cinnamyl butyrate; (7) Cinnamyl isobutyrate; (8) Isobutyl cinnamate; (9) Phenyl ethyl salicylate; (10) Phenyl propyl cinnamate

CITRUS

DESCRIPTION: Chemicals with odor similar to the citrus trees and shrubs flowers (*Aurantiaceae*). Citrus is a generic name referring to a group of trees and shrubs of the *Rutaceae* whose fruits are edible, with juice, rinds, oils, and acids, all useful.

Citrus trees are thorny, evergreen, with long shiny, pointed leaves. The leaves and the flowers are fragrant. Citrus plants grow in warm climates where there is no frost or wind. They contain large amounts of vitamins and minerals and are high in Vitamin C. Ripe citrus fruits are yellow to orange-red in color.

Bergamot is only used in perfumery and as a histological clearing agent.

COMMON VARIETIES: *Citrus aurantium*, sweet orange; *Citrus aurantium*, var. *Bigaradia*, bitter orange; *Citrus medica*, citron; *Citrus medica*, var. *Limonum*, lemon; *Citrus medica*, var. *Acida*, lime; *Citrus decumana*, grapefruit (shaddock); *Citrus bergamia*, bergamot

CHEMICALS FOR SCENT MATCHING: (1) Acetate C-12; (2) Alcohol C-7; (3) Alcohol C-8; (4) Alcohol C-9; (5) Alcohol C-11, undecylenic; (6) Alcohol C-11, undecylic; (7) Aldehyde C-8; (8) Citral; (9) Linalyl butyrate; (10) Methyl heptenone, pure; (11) Methyl nonyl ketone; (12) Neryl acetate

FATTY

DESCRIPTION: Chemicals with a fatty odor
CHEMICALS FOR SCENT MATCHING: (1) Benzyl laurate; (2) Nonoic acid

FLOWERY

DESCRIPTION: Chemicals with a floral odor
CHEMICALS FOR SCENT MATCHING: (1) Acetanisole; (2) Acetate C-9; (3) Acetate C-11; (4) α-Amyl cinnamic alcohol; (5) Anisyl alcohol; (6) Benzyl isovalerate; (7) Benzyl propionate; (8) Cinnamic alcohol; (9) Cinnamyl acetate; (10) Cinnamyl propionate; (11) Ethyl laurate; (12) Hydroxycitronellal dimethyl acetal; (13) Linalool; (14) *p*-Methyl acetophenone; (15) Methyl phenyl carbinol; (16) Methyl phenyl propionate; (17) Phenyl acetaldehyde; (18) Phenyl acetic acid; (19) Phenyl propyl acetate; (20) Phenyl propyl cinnamate; (21) Phenyl propyl formate

GRASSY

DESCRIPTION: Chemicals with a grassy odor
CHEMICALS FOR SCENT MATCHING: (1) Isocyclocitral

GREEN-FLORAL

DESCRIPTION: Chemicals with green top note and floral background odor
CHEMICALS FOR SCENT MATCHING: (1) Methyl heptyne carbonate; (2) Methyl octine carbonate; (3) Methyl phenyl carbinol; (4) Phenyl acetaldehyde

HARSH-PUNGENT

DESCRIPTION: Chemicals with a harsh-pungent-penetrating odor
CHEMICALS FOR SCENT MATCHING: (1) Aldehyde C-7; (2) Methyl quinoline

HERB-LIKE

DESCRIPTION: Chemicals with an herb-like odor
CHEMICALS FOR SCENT MATCHING: (1) α-Phellandrene

LEAF-GREEN

DESCRIPTION: Chemicals with an odor similar to green leaves
CHEMICALS FOR SCENT MATCHING: (1) Acetal R; (2) *p*-Methyl hydratropic aldehyde; (3) Phenyl acetaldehyde dimethyl acetal; (4) Phenyl acetaldehyde ethylene acetal; (5) Phenyl ethyl acetal; (6) *n*-Propyl acetal

MUSKY

DESCRIPTION: Chemicals with a persistent odor similar to musk
CHEMICALS FOR SCENT MATCHING: (1) Civettal; (2) Skatole

ODORLESS-FAINT

DESCRIPTION: Chemicals with an almost imperceptible odor

CHEMICALS FOR SCENT MATCHING: (1) Benzyl alcohol; (2) Cetyl alcohol

WAXY

DESCRIPTION: Chemicals with a waxy odor
CHEMICALS FOR SCENT MATCHING: (1) Myristic alcohol

WOODY

DESCRIPTION: Chemicals with an odor similar to wood
CHEMICALS FOR SCENT MATCHING: (1) Dimethyl benzyl carbinol; (2) Isobutyl quinoline; (3) Isopropyl quinoline; (4) Vetacetyl

Simulated Flower Scents

ACACIA

BOTANICAL: *Family: Leguminosae; Genus: Acacia; Species: Greggii*
OCCURRENCE: About 450 kinds of acacia grow in tropical regions and lands close to the tropics. Twelve varieties grow in the U.S., mostly in Texas and California.
DESCRIPTION: The flowers are bright yellow with a sweet odor. In some plants they cluster together forming balls. Others have white flowers.
CHEMICALS FOR SCENT MATCHING: (1) Anisic aldehyde; (2) Isobutyl benzoate; (3) Methyl anthranilate; (4) Phenyl acetic aldehyde; (5) Yara yara
*Basis**: (1) Alcohol C-9; (2) Alcohol C-10; (3) Aldehyde C-9; (4) Aldehyde C-10

BERGAMOT

BOTANICAL: *Family: Rutaceae; Genus: Citrus; Species: Bergamia; Subspecies: Risso, Poiteau*
CHEMICALS FOR SCENT MATCHING: (1) Citronellyl acetate; (2) Limonene; (3) Linalool; (4) Linalyl acetate; (5) Linalyl formate; (6) Linalyl propionate; (7) Menthanyl acetate; (8) Terpinyl acetate

CARNATION

BOTANICAL: *Family: Caryophyllaceae; Genus: Dianthus; Species: Caryophyllus* (common garden)
DESCRIPTION: There are pink, purple, red, white, and yellow carnation flowers
CHEMICALS FOR SCENT MATCHING: (1) Acetyl isoeugenol; (2) Benzyl isoeugenol; (3) Coumarin; (4) Eugenol; (5) Methyl eugenol; (6) Methyl isoeugenol; (7) Nerol; (8) Terpineol; (9) Vanillin
Basis: (1) Alcohol C-9; (2) Aldehyde C-8; (3) Aldehyde C-9

---

* Basis: The chief or most stable component of any material; fundamental ingredient.

CASSIA

BOTANICAL: *Family: Leguminosae; Genus: Cassia; Species: Acutifolia, Angustifolia* (Indian), *Matilandia* (wild Surna), *Fasciculate* (partridge peas); There are more than 400 species of cassia

CHEMICALS FOR SCENT MATCHING: (1) Anisic aldehyde; (2) Anisyl acetate; (3) Ionone; (4) Methyl acetophenone

Basis: (1) Aldehyde C-8; (2) Aldehyde C-9; (3) Aldehyde C-10; (4) Aldehyde C-12

CHRYSANTHEMUM

BOTANICAL: *Family: Compositae; Genus: Chrysanthemum*

DESCRIPTION: A strong-scented shrubby herb growing in temperate regions worldwide. The name is from the Greek word meaning "golden flower." Because of its beautiful and abundant blooms, it is extensively cultivated. The flowers are white, yellow, pink, or red.

CHEMICALS FOR SCENT MATCHING: (1) Phenylethyl formate

CLOVE

SYNONYMS: *Eugenia caryophyllata*

BOTANICAL: *Family: Myrtaceae; Genus: Caryophyllus; Species: Aromaticus*

OCCURRENCE: The tree grows wild in the Moluccas (also called Spice Islands), in Sumatra, Jamaica, West Indies, and Brazil

DESCRIPTION: The name clove refers to the dried flowers (buds) of a tropical tree. The buds are picked before they open to become a flower. They are used as a spice and are called cloves.

An oil distilled from the dried buds and stems is widely used in the flavor and perfumery industry.

CHEMICALS FOR SCENT MATCHING: (1) Caryophyllene; (2) Eugenol; (3) Eugenol acetate; (4) Isoeugenol phenyl acetate

CLOVER

SYNONYMS: New mown hay; Foin coupe

BOTANICAL: *Family: Leguminosae; Genus and Species:* See Common Varieties

COMMON VARIETIES: *Trifolium pratense* (red clover); *Trifolium repens, hybridum, crimson, incarnatum, alsike* (white clover); *Melilotus alba* (white sweet clover); *Melilotus officinalis* (yellow sweet clover); *Melilotus indica* (sour clover)

DESCRIPTION: About 300 different kinds of clover plants exist, growing wild in fields, lawns, and along roadsides. Some species are cultivated for livestock food.

Red clover provides pasture for farm animals and enriches the soil because of its high nitrogen content. It is also the main source of hay. *White clover*, in addition to being a valuable pasture corp, provides its blossom nectar to bees for the making of superior honey. *Alsike clover*, also called Swedish clover, is white or pink in color. *Crimson clover* has a variety of colors: red, white, yellow, scarlet. It is also called "Italian-type clover." *Sweet clover* is called "Melilot" from the Latin word "miele" (honey). *Sour clover* is primarily used for improving the soil.

Clover generally has three leaves. According to superstition, four-leaved clover brings luck while five- or six-leaved clovers bring misfortune.

CHEMICALS FOR SCENT MATCHING: (1) Benzylidene acetone; (2) Benzyl salicylate; (3) Coumarin; (4) Linalyl acetate; (5) Methyl salicylate

CYCLAMEN

BOTANICAL: *Family: Primulaceae* (primrose); *Genus: Cyclamen*

CHEMICALS FOR SCENT MATCHING: (1) Cyclamen aldehyde; (2) Hydroxycitronellal; (3) Ionone; (4) Rhodinol

Basis: (1) Alcohol C-9; (2) Aldehyde C-9; (3) Aldehyde C-10; (4) Aldehyde C-12

FERN

SYNONYMS: Fougere

BOTANICAL: The ferns are classified into 12 families.

The most common and widely distributed family is: *Family: Polypodiaceae* which includes several genera; *Genus: Pteridium* (the bracken), *Adiantum* (maidenhair), *Dryopteris* (woodfern), *Asplenium* (spleenworts), *Polypodium* (polypody), *Comptosorus* (walking-leaf), *Onoclea* (sensitive fern), *Polystichum* (holly ferns).

Other families include: *Family: Trichomanes* (filmy fern), *Lygodium* (climbing fern), *Ophioglossum* (adder's tongue), *Botrychium* (rattlesnake fern)

OCCURRENCE: Ferns grow worldwide but more commonly in the tropics. About 300 varieties grow in the U.S.

DESCRIPTION: There are about 10,000 kinds of ferns in different sizes and shapes, from moss-like to 40-foot tall trees. The fern is a flowerless plant.

The basic "fougere" perfume is made by simple blending of oakmoss, coumarin, and amyl salicylate, or just oakmoss and amyl salicylate.

CHEMICALS FOR SCENT MATCHING: (1) Ethyl phenyl acetate; (2) Isobutyl salicylate; (3) Linalyl acetate

Basis: (1) Alcohol C-8; (2) Alcohol C-9; (3) Aldehyde C-8; (4) Aldehyde C-9; (5) Aldehyde C-10; (6) Aldehyde C-11; (7) Aldehyde C-12 MNA

FRANGIPANI

BOTANICAL: *Family: Apocynaceae; Genus: Plumeria; Species: Acutifolia* (yellowish), *Alba* (white), *Rubra* (pink)

OCCURRENCE: The plant grows extensively in all tropical areas, particularly in the eastern part of central Africa.

DESCRIPTION: Frangipani is one of the most beautiful and pleasantly scented flowers. Like other tropical fragrant flowers, frangipani is more fragrant at night than during the day. It is a decorative plant, especially in India. Since no synthetic imitation can really match the exceptionally pleasant fragrance of the frangipani, it is obtained using an odorless solvent such as hexane, or by enfleurage.

CHEMICALS FOR SCENT MATCHING: (1) Cinnamic aldehyde; (2) Citral; (3) Coumarin; (4) Eugenol; (5) Ionone; (6) Linalyl acetate; (7) Rhodinyl butyrate; (8) Terpineol; (9) Vetiverol

GARDENIA

BOTANICAL: *Family: Rubiaceae; Genus: Jasminoides*

DESCRIPTION: The name gardenia was given to this plant in honor of Alexander Garden, a Scottish naturalist, who collected plants in South Carolina before the Revolutionary War.

Gardenia is an ornamental plant in subtropical warm temperate areas. The flower has a very outstanding fragrance.

It's essential oil occurs in a very minimal amount (1 × 5000). Therefore, it's fragrance is synthetically imitated.

CHEMICALS FOR SCENT MATCHING: (1) Ethyl acetate; (2) Methyl phenyl carbinyl acetate

Basis: (1) Aldehyde C-8; (2) Aldehyde C-10; (3) Aldehyde C-12; (4) Aldehyde C-14

GERANIUM

BOTANICAL: *Family: Geraniaceae; Genus: Pelargonium; Species: Graveolens* (rose geranium), *Domesticus* (Lady Washington), *Robertianum* (herb Robert, red robin), *Erodium cicutarium* (Alfilaria, red stem filareae), *Peltatum* (ivy geranium)

DESCRIPTION: It grows widely in home and gardens. Leaves of the rose geranium are used to flavor jellies and for the extraction of geranium rose essential oil, particularly that of African origin. Alfilaria or red stem filareae is grown for forage in western and southwestern U.S. Herb Robert or red robin has been used in medicine.

CHEMICALS FOR SCENT MATCHING: (1) Benzophenone; (2) Diphenyl methane; (3) Diphenyl oxide; (4) Isobutyl benzoate; (5) Isopulegol extra

HAWTHORN

BOTANICAL: *Family: Rosaceae; Genus: Crataegus; Species: Oxyacantha* (English), *Mollis* (downy hawthorn), *Crus-galli* (cockspur thorn)

DESCRIPTION: Its fruit called "haw" looks like a small apple. The flowers are white and bloom in May with a fragrant rose-like odor. In Autumn, the small leaves have a brilliant color.

CHEMICALS FOR SCENT MATCHING: (1) Acetophenone; (2) Anisic aldehyde; (3) Anisyl acetate; (4) Citral

Basis: (1) Alcohol C-9; (2) Aldehyde C-9; (3) Aldehyde C-10

HELIOTROPE

BOTANICAL: *Family: Boraginaceae; Genus: Heliotropium; Species: Arborescence* (Peruvian type)

DESCRIPTION: The plant has beautiful flowers with a vanilla-honey fragrance and a delicate bitter almond scent. It is also known as a "cherry-pie blossom."

CHEMICALS FOR SCENT MATCHING: (1) Coumarin; (2) Heliotropin; (3) Hydroxycitronellal; (4) Vanillin

HONEYSUCKLE

SYNONYMS: Chevrefeuille

BOTANICAL: *Family: Caprifoliaceae; Genus: Lonicera; Species: Caprifolium, Sempervirens* (coral type or trumpet), *Peryclymenum* (woodbine), *Tatarica* (landscaping type), *Fragrantissima* (landscaping type), *Nitida* (box evergreen), *Pileata* (privet)

DESCRIPTION: Honeysuckle is also called "woodbine." The bush honeysuckle attracts bees. It has yellow blossoms. The coral or trumpet honeysuckle has a blossom which is red outside and orange-yellow inside. Honeysuckle produces trumpet-shaped flowers. Some people believe that it was the "trusted eglantine" referred to in the poems of Milton.

CHEMICALS FOR SCENT MATCHING: (1) Benzyl acetate; (2) Cresyl acetate; (3) Rhodinol; (4) Vanillin

Basis: (1) Alcohol C-9; (2) Aldehyde C-9 MNA (methyl nonyl acetaldehyde)

HYACINTH

SYNONYMS: Jacynth

BOTANICAL: *Family: Liliaceae; Genus: Hyacinthus; Species: Orientalis*

DESCRIPTION: Hyacinth flowers have a variety of colors from white, pink, blue, yellow to purple, with a characteristic delicate fragrance.

CHEMICALS FOR SCENT MATCHING: (1) Cinnamic alcohol; (2) Bromystyrol; (3) Hydratropic aldehyde; (4) Phenyl acetaldehyde; (5) Phenyl ethyl formate; (6) Phenyl ethyl phenyl acetate; (7) Phenyl propyl alcohol; (8) Phenyl propyl aldehyde

Basis: (1) Alcohol C-8; (2) Aldehyde C-8; (3) Aldehyde C-10

IRIS

BOTANICAL: *Family: Iridiceae; Genus: Iris* (yellow flag iris); *Species: Pseudacorus* (blue flag), *Versicolor* (blue flag), *Kaempferi* (Japanese iris), *Sibirica* (Siberian iris), *Spuria* (butterfly iris), *Pumila* (dwarf bearded iris); *Genus: Freesia; Species: Refracta*

DESCRIPTION: Iris has a faint violet-like odor. The name "iris" comes from the Greek word "rainbow." The roots of iris (orris roots) are dried and employed in perfumes, cosmetics, and medicine. The French name "fleur de lis" (flower of the lily) is also applied in the manufacture of specific perfumes with a characteristic iris odor.

CHEMICALS FOR SCENT MATCHING: (1) Anisic aldehyde; (2) Cuminic aldehyde; (3) Methyl ionone; (4) Irone

Basis: (1) Alcohol C-9; (2) Alcohol C-10; (3) Aldehyde C-9; (4) Aldehyde C-10; (5) Aldehyde C-12

JASMINE

BOTANICAL: *Family: Oleaceae; Genus: Jasminum; Species: Officinalis* or *Officinale, Grandiflorum* (Spanish)

CHEMICALS FOR SCENT MATCHING: (1) Acetate C-8; (2) Amyl cinnamic aldehyde; (3) α-Amyl cinnamic aldehyde; (4) α-Amyl cinnamic aldehyde dimethyl acetal; (5) Benzyl acetate; (6) Benzyl butyrate; (7) Benzyl isobutyrate; (8) Hexyl cinnamic aldehyde; (9) Indole; (10) Ionone; (11) Isojasmone; (12) Linalool; (13) Methyl anthranilate

Basis: (1) Alcohol C-10; (2) Aldehyde C-8; (3) Aldehyde C-10

JONQUIL

SYNONYMS: Narcissus jounquil

BOTANICAL: *Family: Amaryllidaceae; Genus: Narcissus odorous*

DESCRIPTION: It is the name of several yellow narcissus. The jonquil fragrance, sweet scented, is that of the common jonquil, classified as *Narcissus odorous*. The name jonquil is from the Latin word "juncus" meaning "rush."

CHEMICALS FOR SCENT MATCHING: (1) Benzyl acetate; (2) Cinnamic alcohol; (3) Hydratropic aldehyde; (4) Hydroxycitronellal; (5) Indole; (6) Isoeugenol; (7) Linalool; (8) Musk ambrette; (9) Phenyl acetate; (10) Terpineol

Basis: (1) Alcohol C-9; (2) Aldehyde C-9

LAVENDER

BOTANICAL: *Family: Labiatae; Genus: Lavandula; Species: Vera, Officinalis*

DESCRIPTION: The name "lavender" comes from the Latin word "lavo" meaning "to wash" as the Romans used the leaves and flowers of this plant when they were bathing. Traditionally "lavender" represents "purity." The expression "lavender" is also used with reference to someone with gentle manners. The fragrance of the lavender lasts even after the plant is totally dry.

CHEMICALS FOR SCENT MATCHING: (1) Citronellyl butyrate; (2) Geranyl acetate; (3) Linalyl acetate; (4) Linalyl butyrate; (5) Menthanyl acetate; (6) Perpinyl acetate; (7) Terpinyl propionate

Basis: (1) Alcohol C-9; (2) Aldehyde C-10

LILAC

BOTANICAL: *Family: Oleaceae; Genus: Syringa; Species: Vulgaris*

DESCRIPTION: Lilac has white or purple flowers with a peculiar fresh green fragrance. It is one of the odors imitated and synthesized for multiple purposes in perfuming.

CHEMICALS FOR SCENT MATCHING: (1) Anisyl acetate; (2) Anisic alcohol; (3) Cinnamic alcohol; (4) Dimethyl acetophenone; (5) Heliotropin; (6) Hydroxycitronellal; (7) Indole; (8) Isoeugenol; (9) Phenyl ethyl alcohol; (10) Terpineol

Basis: (1) Alcohol C-9; (2) Aldehyde C-9; (3) Aldehyde C-10; (4) Aldehyde C-12 MNA

LILY OF THE VALLEY

SYNONYMS: Muguet

BOTANICAL: *Family: Lilaceae; Genus: Convallaria; Species: Majalis, Montana*

DESCRIPTION: In Germany it is also called "mayflower" because it is one of the special flowers of the month of May. It has one of the most delightful fragrances. A toilet water imitating its odor, a fresh rosy-lemon note of distinct greenness, is called "eau d'oro" (golden water) by the French.

CHEMICALS FOR SCENT MATCHING: (1) Amyl cinnamic aldehyde; (2) Cinnamyl acetate; (3) Cyclamen aldehyde; (4) Ethyl phenyl acetate; (5) Hydroxycitronellal; (6) Ionone; (7) Linalool; (8) Linalyl propionate; (9) Phenyl ethyl propionate; (10) Tetrahydro linalool

Basis: (1) Alcohol C-9; (2) Alcohol C-10; (3) Alcohol C-11; (4) Aldehyde C-9; (5) Aldehyde C-10; (6) Aldehyde C-12; (7) Aldehyde C-16

LINDEN

SYNONYMS: Basswood

BOTANICAL: *Family: Tiliaceae; Genus: Tilia; Species: Americana, Platy phyllos, Lacimata* (European cut-leaf linden), *Cordata* (little-leaf linden)

DESCRIPTION: It is a graceful cone-shaped tree, growing in many areas of the world. It is also called "lime tree" or basswood. The flowers are small, white or yellowish with fragrant lime odor. The European "cut leaf" linden and the "little leaf" linden are extensively planted as ornamentals. The nectar of its fragrant flowers is a source of honey.

CHEMICALS FOR SCENT MATCHING: (1) Benzyl benzoate; (2) Farnesol; (3) Hydroxycitronellal; (4) Methyl anthranilate; (5) Verdantol

MAGNOLIA

BOTANICAL: *Family: Magnoliaceae; Genus: Magnolia; Species: Grandiflora* (southern type), *Virginiana* (sweet bay, swamp magnolia), *Tripetala* (umbrella tree), *Macrophylla* (big leaf magnolia), *Acuminata* (cucumber tree)

DESCRIPTION: There are 35 kinds of magnolia trees. Eight varieties grow widely in the eastern part of the U.S. The southern magnolia (*grandiflora*) is popular because of the beauty and fragrance of its large whitish flowers. Its flowers have an extremely delicate, sweet fragrance of rose, violet, and orange flowers.

CHEMICALS FOR SCENT MATCHING: (1) Amyl cinnamic aldehyde; (2) Anisic aldehyde; (3) Benzyl acetate; (4) Citral; (5) Heliotropin; (6) Hydroxycitronellal; (7) Linalool; (8) Linalyl acetate; (9) Methyl ionone; (10) Musk ketone

Basis: Aldehyde C-10

MIGNONETTE

SYNONYMS: Reseda

BOTANICAL: *Family: Resedaceae; Genus: Reseda; Species: Odorata*

DESCRIPTION: The name comes from the French word "mignonette" which means "little darling." Mignonette has a very pleasant fragrance, particularly from small flowers.

CHEMICALS FOR SCENT MATCHING: (1) Benzyl acetate; (2) Cinnamic alcohol; (3) Ethyl laurinate; (4) Geraniol; (5) Guaiacol acetate; (6) Linalool; (7) α-Ionone; (8) Methyl heptyne carbonate; (9) Methyl ionone; (10) Methyl nonyl ketone; (11) Phenyl ethyl acetate; (12) Phenyl propyl acetate; (13) Santolol or cedrol; (14) Terpineol; (15) Vetiverol

Basis: (1) Alcohol C-9; (2) Aldehyde C-10; (3) Aldehyde C-12

MIMOSA

BOTANICAL: *Family: Leguminosae; Genus: Mimosa*

OCCURRENCE: Mimosa is a plant growing mostly in tropical lands and in warm areas worldwide.

DESCRIPTION: It is similar to acacia. Its flowers are small and yellow, pink, lavender, or purple. The fragrance of mimosa is very strong.

CHEMICALS FOR SCENT MATCHING: (1) Acetophenone; (2) Dimethyl acetophenone; (3) Hydroxycitronellal; (4) Terpineol

Basis: (1) Alcohol C-10; (2) Alcohol C-11; (3) Aldehyde C-10; (4) Aldehyde C-11

MOON FLOWER

BOTANICAL: *Family: Convolvulaceae; Genus: Calonyction; Species: Aculeatum*

DESCRIPTION: The scent is very delicate. It is also of the morning glory flower family.

CHEMICALS FOR SCENT MATCHING: (1) Benzo dihydropyrone; (2) Coumarin; (3) Dimethyl hydroquinone; (4) Methyl anisate

MORNING GLORY

BOTANICAL: *Family: Convolvulaceae; Genus: Ipomoeae; Species: Purpurea*

DESCRIPTION: It is a climbing plant with a funnel-like flower with a mixture of purple, blue, red, pink, and white colors. The fragrant flower opens in the morning and closes later in the evening.

CHEMICALS FOR SCENT MATCHING: (1) Benzo dihydropyrone; (2) Coumarin; (3) Dimethyl hydroquinone; (4) Methyl anisate

MOSS

BOTANICAL: *Family: Lichens; Genus: Evernia; Species: Prunastri* (oak moss), *Furfuraceae* (tree moss); *Genus: Urnea; Species: Barbata* (tree moss)

DESCRIPTION: *E. prunastri* grows mostly on oak trees and is called "oak moss." the *furfuraceae* and the *barbata* species grow on spruce and fir trees and are called "tree moss."

CHEMICALS FOR SCENT MATCHING: (1) Cinnamic alcohol; (2) Coumarin; (3) Benzyl benzoate; (4) Benzyl cinnamate; (5) Heliotropin; (6) Ionone; (7) Linalool; (8) Linalyl acetate; (9) Musk; (10) Vetiverol

MUSK

DESCRIPTION: It is an oily substance with a strong, persistent odor. It is from a gland of the male musk deer. The finest quality is from China and is called "tog king." Artificial musk, however, is used more often in the manufacture of perfumes to give a more permanent odor than the natural musk.

The musk deer is a small animal about 2 feet tall. It lives in the Himalaya mountains and in the high regions of the northern hemisphere at an altitude of 8000–12,000 feet. It lives alone contrary to habits of deer in herds. It feeds on lichens, grass, roots, and twigs of shrubs and comes out only at night.

The musk product derives from a globe-shaped gland in the skin of the male deer abdomen.

CHEMICALS FOR SCENT MATCHING: (1) Musk ambrette; (2) Musk ketone; (3) Musk tibetene; (4) Musk xylol

NARCISSUS

SYNONYMS: Daffodil

BOTANICAL: *Family: Amaryllidaceae; Genus: Narcissus; Species: Pseudo-narcissus* (daffodil), *Poeticus, Tazetta, Poet's Poeticus* (hybrid of tazetta), *Polyanthus*

DESCRIPTION: Narcissus flowers are white or yellow and have a very delicate, fragrant odor similar to that of hyacinth

CHEMICALS FOR SCENT MATCHING: (1) Cinnamic alcohol; (2) *p*-Cresyl acetate; (3) *p*-Cresyl phenyl acetate; (4) Phenyl ethyl alcohol

Basis: (1) Alcohol C-9; (2) Aldehyde C-9

ORANGE BLOSSOM

SYNONYMS: Neroli

BOTANICAL: *Family: Rutaceae; Genus: Citrus; Species: Sinensis, Aurantium* (bitter orange); *Subspecies: Amara*

DESCRIPTION: Neroli is extracted from fresh picked flowers of the bitter orange (*Citrus aurantium amara*) whose leaves and twigs are also the source of petitgrain.

CHEMICALS FOR SCENT MATCHING: (1) Dimethyl anthranilate; (2) Ethyl anthranilate; (3) Methyl anthranilate; (4) Methyl β-naphthyl ketone; (5) Nerolin; (6) Neryl acetate; (7) Yara yara

Basis: (1) Alcohol C-9; (2) Alcohol C-10; (3) Alcohol C-12; (4) Aldehyde C-9; (5) Aldehyde C-12

ORCHID

BOTANICAL: *Family: Orchidaceae; Genus: Cypripedium* (peristeria dove), *Arethusa, Calypso, Calopogon, Habernaria, Elata* (dove plant).

DESCRIPTION: There are more than 6000 species of orchids, one of which furnishes vanilla.

CHEMICALS FOR SCENT MATCHING: (1) Amyl salicylate; (2) Isobutyl salicylate; (3) Isoeugenol; (4) Linalool; (5) Nerolin; (6) Terpineol

PATCHOULI

BOTANICAL: *Family: Labiatae; Genus: Pogostemon; Species: Hyeneanus*

OCCURRENCE: India; also widely cultivated in the Philippines and Malaya.

DESCRIPTION: The patchouli plant is 2 or 3 feet high with a purple flower or small white spikes. The oil from the leaves has a musty odor. It is used in tropical Asia.

CHEMICALS FOR SCENT MATCHING: (1) Benzyl salicylate; (2) Cinnamic alcohol; (3) Cinnamic aldehyde; (4) Coumarin; (5) Geraniol; (6) Heliotropin; (7) Methyl salicylate; (8) Musk xylene; (9) Phenyl ethyl alcohol; (10) Rhodinol; (11) Vanillin

PINE (NEEDLES)

BOTANICAL: *Family: Pinaceae; Genus: Pinus; Species: Strobus* (white pine), *Lambertiana* (sugar pine), *Banksiana* (jack pine), *Palustris* (longleaf pine), *Ponderosa* (Ponderosa)

DESCRIPTION: The common name "pine" refers to the largest and most important group of conifers, cone-bearing trees. Among these are larch, spruce, hemlock, and fir. These differ from the trees of the pine genus which comprises about 80 different kinds of pine, growing mostly in the northern hemisphere. Of these, 35 species grow in the U.S.

Pinus are evergreen trees. They are mostly used for timber and for the extraction of the resin which provides turpentine and sub-derivatives through distillation. A pure essential oil employed in perfumery and flavors in small amounts is also extracted from the pine needles. Turpentine, obtained chiefly by steam distillation of pine palustris resin, is extensively used in blending with rosemary oil, camphene, isobornyl acetate, coumarin, oakmoss, etc. and for the fractional distillation of its many components: terpineol, estragole, fenchone, fenchyl alcohol, borneol. Turpentine is an excellent solvent, particularly in the paint industry.

CHEMICALS FOR SCENT MATCHING: (1) Bornyl acetate; (2) Isobornyl acetate

ROSE

BOTANICAL: *Family: Rosaceae; Genus: Rosa; Species: Centifolia; Variety: Muscosa, Setigera* (climbing type), *Damascena* (rose, otto)

DESCRIPTION: Attar, oil from rose petals, is used to make toilet water perfumes. In the rose family there are about 2000 species of trees, shrubs, and herbs. These include apple, apricot, berries, cherries,peach, pear, plum, quince, and strawberry.

CHEMICALS FOR SCENT MATCHING: (1) Acetate C-10; (2) Acetate C-12; (3) Anisic aldehyde; (4) Benzophenone; (5) Benzyl butyrate; (6) Benzyl isoeugenol; (7) Butyl phenyl acetate; (8) Cinnamic isovalerate; (9) Citronellal; (10) Citronellol; (11) Citronellyl acetate; (12) Citronellyl butyrate; (13) Citronellyl formate; (14) Citronellyl isobutyrate; (15) Citronellyl propionate; (16) Citronellyl oxycetaldehyde; (17) Dimethyl octanol; (18) Ethyl pelargonate; (19) Ethyl phenyl acetate; (20) Geraniol; (21) Geranyl acetate; (22) Geranyl butyrate; (23) Geranyl formate; (24) Geranyl phenyl acetate; (25) Geranyl propionate; (26) Guaiacwood acetate; (27) Hydroxycitronellal; (28) Isobutyl benzoate; (29) Isobutyl phenyl acetate; (30) Isopulegol extra; (31) Linalyl formate; (32) Methyl acetate, racemic; (33) Methyl diphenyl ether; (34) Nerol; (35) Nerolidol; (36) Phenoxy isobutyrate; (37) Phenyl ethyl acetate; (38) Phenyl ethyl alcohol; (39) Phenyl ethyl benzoate; (40) Phenyl ethyl butyrate; (41) Phenyl ethyl cinnamate; (42) Phenyl ethyl isobutyrate; (43) Phenyl ethyl phenyl acetate; (44) Phenyl ethyl propionate; (45) Phenyl ethyl salicylate; (46) Rhodinol extra; (47) Rhodinyl acetate; (48) Rhodinyl butyrate; (49) Rhodinyl formate; (50) Rhodinyl phenyl acetate; (51) Rosacetol; (52) Tetrahydrolinalool

Basis: Rosa centifolia: (1) Alcohol C-9; (2) Aldehyde C-9; (3) Aldehyde C-11; (4) Aldehyde C-16; Rose blanche (white): (1) Alcohol C-8; (2) Aldehyde C-8; Rose rouge (red): (1) Alcohol C-9; (2) Alcohol C-11; Rose d'oriente: (1) Alcohol C-9; (2) Aldehyde C-11

SWEET PEA

BOTANICAL: *Family: Leguminosae; Genus: Lathyrus; Species: Odoratus, Latifolius*

DESCRIPTION: More than 1000 species of sweet peas exist in two types: (1) dwarf, only a few inches high; (2) climbing, growing along strings or trellises. The fragrance of sweet pea is very pleasant.

CHEMICALS FOR SCENT MATCHING: (1) Amyl cinnamic aldehyde; (2) Benzyl acetate; (3) Benzylidene acetone; (4) Cinnamic alcohol; (5) Dimethyl benzyl carbinol acetate; (6) Heliotropin; (7) Hydroxycitronellal; (8) α-Ionone; (9) Isobutyl phenyl acetate; (10) Linalool; (11) Methyl anthranilate; (12) Methyl naphthyl ketone; (13) Methyl nonyl acetic acid; (14) Musk ambrette; (15) Phenyl acetic aldehyde; (16) Phenyl ethyl acetate; (17) Phenyl ethyl alcohol; (18) Rhodinol; (19) Terpineol; (20) Vanillin

Basis: (1) Alcohol C-10; (2) Aldehyde C-9; (3) Aldehyde C-10; (4) Aldehyde C-12

SYRINGA

SYNONYMS: Mock orange

BOTANICAL: *Family: Saxifragraceae; Genus: Philadelphus; Species: Virginalis, Coronarius*

DESCRIPTION: The syringa is a flower with white-ivory color and a strong lilac-orange blossom-type fragrance. It is used mostly as a border around lawns and gardens. The *Philadelphus virginalis* type is among the best and most fragrant of the mock orange.

CHEMICALS FOR SCENT MATCHING: (1) Anisyl formate; (2) Hydroxycitronellal; (3) Isobutyl anthranilate; (4) Isobutyl benzoate

TOBACCO

BOTANICAL: *Family: Solanaceae; Genus: Nicotiana; Species: Tabacum, Petunoids, Affinis*

DESCRIPTION: The fragrance of the tobacco flowers is extremely delicate, sweet, spice-like, and reminiscent of fresh carnation. Phenyl acetic acid is its major constituent.

CHEMICALS FOR SCENT MATCHING: (1) Heliotropin; (2) Methyl ionone; (3) Methyl phenyl acetate; (4) Musk ketone; (5) Phenyl acetic acid; (6) γ-Valerolactone; (7) Vanillin; (8) Vetiverol

TREFLÉ

SYNONYMS: Trefoil

BOTANICAL: *Family: Leguminosae; Genus: Lotus* (bird's foot as it bears clusters of pods resembling a croce's foot)*; Species: Corniculatus, Uliginous, Bertholeti* (coralgem deervetch)

DESCRIPTION: Treflé or trefoil means "three lead." It is applied to plants having compound leaves with three leaflets, e.g., clover. Any of several trifoliate leguminous herbs.

CHEMICALS FOR SCENT MATCHING: (1) Amyl cinnamic aldehyde; (2) Ethyl salicylate; (3) Heliotropin; (4) Isobutyl phenyl acetate; (5) Isoeugenol; (6) Musk ketone; (7) Rhodinol; (8) Vanillin

Basis: (1) Aldehyde C-9; (2) Aldehyde C-11; (3) Aldehyde C-12; (4) Aldehyde C-12 MNA

TUBEROSE

BOTANICAL: *Family: Amaryllidaceae; Genus: Polianthes; Species: Tuberosa*

DESCRIPTION: Tuberose has been described as a "lump of cloying sweetness." It has a heavy fragrance. More than 100,000 pounds of tuberose flowers are employed each year for essential oil production.

CHEMICALS FOR SCENT MATCHING: (1) Benzyl acetate; (2) Butyl benzyl oxide; (3) Butyl phenyl acetate; (4) Hydroxycitronellal; (5) Methyl benzoate; (6) Methyl nonyl acetaldehyde; (7) Methyl salicylate; (8) Propyl phenyl alcohol

Basis: (1) Alcohol C-10; (2) Alcohol C-12; (3) Aldehyde C-10; (4) Aldehyde C-12

VERBENA

SYNONYMS: Eau de verveine

BOTANICAL: *Family: Verbenaceae; Genus: Verbena; Species: Hybrida, Erinoides* (moss verbena), *Lippia citriodora*

DESCRIPTION: The verbena flowers are pink, purple, red, white, and other colors except yellow. Their fragrance is citrus-lilac-like.

CHEMICALS FOR SCENT MATCHING: (1) Benzyl isoeugenol; (2) Citral; (3) Cyclamen aldehyde; (4) Hydroxycitronellal; (5) Isobutyl benzoate; (6) Linalool; (7) Linalyl acetate; (8) Neroli

Basis: (1) Aldehyde C-8; (2) Aldehyde C-10

VIOLET

BOTANICAL: *Family: Violaceae; Genus: Viola; Species: Papilionaceae* (the bird's foot violet), *Tricolor* (pansy violet), *Canina* (dog violet), *Odorata* (Victoria variety)

DESCRIPTION: More than 300 species of violets are grown worldwide with about 100 in the U.S. Some have white and yellow flowers. The blue and purple types are more abundant. The dog violet has no fragrance. The pansy is a cultivated species.

CHEMICALS FOR SCENT MATCHING: (1) Benzyl acetate; (2) Ethyl myristate; (3) Heliotropin; (4) Ionone; (5) α-Ionone; (6) β-Ionone; (7) α-Irone; (8) α-Isoamyl ionone; (9) *α*-Isomethyl ionone; (10) Methyl heptyne carbonate; (11) γ-Methyl ionone; (12) Methyl-2-nonanoate; (13) Methyl octine carbonate

Basis: (1) Alcohol C-9; (2) Alcohol C-10; (3) Alcohol C-12; (4) Aldehyde C-9; (5) Aldehyde C-10; (6) Aldehyde C-11, undecylenic; (7) Aldehyde C-12, lauric; (8) Aldehyde C-14, myristic

WALLFLOWER

SYNONYMS: Goldenlack, Germany

BOTANICAL: *Family: Cruciferae; Genus: Cheiranthus; Species: Cheiri*

DESCRIPTION: The name comes from the fact that it grows on walls over strong cliffs and supporting places. It is a plant related to the mustard. It has a purple flower with a lilac-violet-jasmine-orange flower-ylang ylang-narcissus-carnation-like fragrance with green top note.

CHEMICALS FOR SCENT MATCHING: (1) Anisic aldehyde; (2) Heliotropin; (3) Hydroxycitronellal; (4) Ionone; (5) Isoeugenol; (6) Methyl-*p*-cresol; (7) Methyl β-naphthyl ketone

Basis: (1) Alcohol C-9; (2) Aldehyde C-9

WISTERIA

BOTANICAL: *Family: Leguminosae; Genus: Wisteria; Species: Sinensis*

OCCURRENCE: It is a native of China. It is often seen around homes in the U.S.

DESCRIPTION: Wisteria is a climbing plant with beautiful clusters of bluish-lavender blossom flowers similar to pea blossom. This plant grows fast and covers large areas with its branches. It is one of the most attractive vining plants.

CHEMICALS FOR SCENT MATCHING: *Basis:* (1) Alcohol C-8; (2) Aldehyde C-8; (3) Aldehyde C-12

WINTERGREEN

BOTANICAL: *Family: Ericaceae; Genus: Gaultheria; Species: Procumbens*

DESCRIPTION: The name of this plant refers to its leaves which remain green all winter. Its berries have a pleasant smell and their oil is used in chewing gum, tooth paste and powder, and medicine because of the agreeable flavor.

It is a low-growing shrub with creeping or subterranean stems. The berries are bright red. The flowers, which are like urns, are covered by the leaves.

CHEMICALS FOR SCENT MATCHING: (1) Ethyl benzoate; (2) Ethyl salicylate; (3) Methyl salicylate

YLANG YLANG

SYNONYMS: *Cananga odorata*

BOTANICAL: *Family: Anonaceae; Genus: Anona odoratissima; Species: Uvaria odorata, Cananga odorata*

DESCRIPTION: Ylang ylang is employed as a base in muguet-type perfumes: gardenia, honeysuckle, hyacinth, lilac, lily, narcissus, peonia freesia, sweet pea, and many other delicate floral compositions of oriental type such as sandalwood, opopanax, and spice. It is also used in flavors such as peach, apricot, and sweet types.

CHEMICALS FOR SCENT MATCHING: (1) *m*-Cresyl phenyl acetate; (2) Ethyl acetate; (3) Geranyl benzoate; (4) Methyl benzoate; (5) Methyl-*p*-cresol

Basis: (1) Alcohol C-9; (2) Aldehyde C-9

Simulated Marine Scents (Algae)

SEAWEED (ALGAE)

BOTANICAL: *Phyla: Algae; Family: Thallophyta*

Genus: Macrocystis; Species: Pyrifera

Genus: Phylum; Species: Phacophyta (brown algae)

Genus: Sargassum (gulfweed); *Species: Bacciferum*

Genus: Phylum; Species: Rodophyta (red algae)

Genus: Chondrus; Species: Crispus (Irish moss)

Genus: Phylum; Species: Cyanophyta (blue-green)

Genus: Phylum; Species: Chlorophyta (green)

DESCRIPTION: The seaweeds of cold water are mostly brown algae. Those of the tropics are mainly red algae. Seaweeds contain large amounts of iodine as well as algin which is used in cream for its nonfoaming capacity to hold different liquids together in milk. Agar and carrageen, from seaweeds, are also employed in foods and drugs.

Seaweeds reach more than 200 feet, particularly in the South Pacific, and occur in large masses in the Sargasso Sea, floating in the Atlantic Ocean east of Florida. Agar-agar is a gelatinous substance from seaweeds particularly from the algae classified as *Gelidium*. It occurs in tropical Asia and along the Pacific coast of America.

CHEMICALS FOR SCENT MATCHING: (1) Acetaldehyde; (2) Alcohol C-7; (3) Butyraldehyde; (4) Butyric acid; (5) Propionic acid; (6) Valeraldehyde

Suggested New Perfumes

The creation of the following perfumes is suggested:

1. Adonis, a mythological subject
2. Forsythia, the golden spring bell of the U.S.
3. Fringe, the botanical splendor of the southern U.S.

ADONIS

BOTANICAL: *Family: Ranunculaceae; Genus: Adonis, Anemone* (wind flower); *Species: Quinquifolia*

DESCRIPTION: A group of plants native to Europe and Asia, they also grow in North America. The flowers may be yellow or red with 5–16 petals.

According to Greek mythology, the petals were stained by the blood of Adonis. Adonis was a very handsome youth with whom Venus was in love. Venus was the goddess of love and beauty in Roman mythology. The Greeks called her Aphrodite. Adonis loved hunting and was killed by a wild boar. Venus, in her grief, changed Adonis' blood to a flower, called anemone or wind flower from the Greek word meaning "wind." Many poets have written about this love including Shakespeare who wrote a long poem called "Venus and Adonis."

Even though this plant has no fragrance it stimulates the fantasy in compounding a fine perfume.

COMPONENTS: *Basis:* (1) Benzyl acetate; (2) Hydroxycitronellal; (3) Isobutyl phenyl acetate

FORSYTHIA

SYNONYMS: Golden bell

BOTANICAL: *Family: Oleaceae; Genus: Forsythia; Species: Suspensa, Spectabilis, Viridissima, Intermedia*

DESCRIPTION: Forsythia is a shrub about nine feet high. Because the flowers have a beautiful golden color, they are called "golden bells" and "spring garden flowers."

In early spring forsythia blossoms are the earliest sign of flowers. The leaves

grow to about 3 inches long and are egg shaped.
The name is from the English botanist William Forsyth (1737–1804).
Forsythia flowers have no fragrance, but as it is the first beautiful flower in the beginning of spring, it invokes agreeable feelings. Therefore, the creation of a special perfume with the "forsythia" name would certainly be appreciated.

FRINGE TREE

BOTANICAL: *Family: Oleaceae; Genus: Chionanthus; Species: Virginicus*

DESCRIPTION: It is a fragrant, small tree, sometimes reaching 30 feet high, with delicate white flowers with four slim petals blooming in early spring. It is native to the middle and southern U.S. from southern Pennsylvania to Florida, and also in the West Brazos River in Texas.

A perfume similar to the "fringe" would be valued.

Fixatives for Perfumes

The formulation of a well compounded perfume is usually based on three basic odors: the one first perceived with its peculiar tonality; the second floral portion well in harmony with the tonality; and the third longer lasting fixative. Consequently, the fixative is the most difficult part of preparing a perfume in the search to harmonize all elements for a very pleasant and lasting scent.

There are perfumes which contain 50–100 different compounds, each compound itself containing other compounds. In fact, as many as 300 ingredients may be employed in a perfume. There are about 500 natural and 3000 synthetic oils available for the production of perfumes.

Two of the preferred fixatives are ambergris and musk, both of natural origin.

AMBERGRIS

DESCRIPTION: Ambergris is a wax-like substance occurring in the sperm whale's intestine. It is found floating on the oceans or seashores as waste. It has a disagreeable odor when inside the whale's intestines but, on exposure to air, it acquires a sweet earthy smell and combines very well in the manufacture of perfumes.

COMPONENTS: *Basis:* (1) Aldehyde C-8; (2) Aldehyde C-9; (3) Aldehyde C-10

MUSK

DESCRIPTION: See page 166.

Chapter VI:
BASIC FLAVORING MATERIALS

Introduction

The esters of amyl, benzyl, butyl, ethyl, methyl, and propyl alcohols with acetic, butyric, cinnamic, formic, oenanthic, propionic, salicylic, and valeric acids are extensively used in synthetic compounding of flavors. Pure aldehyde C-14 (peach) and aldehyde C-16 (strawberry) are also extensively employed. Ethyl vanillin is used in the preparation of flavors for beverages, ice creams, cakes, cookies, etc.

The esters are listed by similarity of flavor and odor to each specific natural product. Esters much closer in flavor and odor to the natural product are indicated by an asterisk (*). They may be categorized as:

Fruity—Esters with a generic fruity flavor and odor
Fresh fruits—Esters specifically similar in flavor and odor to each fruit
Tropical fruits—Esters specifically similar in flavor and odor to each fruit
Dry fruits—Esters specifically similar in flavor and odor to each fruit
Naturally sweet products—Esters specifically similar in flavor and odor to each product
Daily beverages—Esters specifically similar in flavor and odor to each product
Alcoholic beverages—Esters specifically similar in flavor and odor to each product
Dairy products—Esters specifically similar in flavor and odor to each product
Culinary additives—Esters specifically similar in flavor and odor to each product
Stabilizers—Esters specifically similar in flavor and odor to each product

During compounding, the quantity of each ester or other chemical is determined by the individual's taste and olfactory sense in matching the flavor and odor of each natural product. These are reported as a general orientation for the compounding of flavors and perfumes.

Natural Flavors Simulated with Synthetic Chemicals

FRUITY

FRUITY

CHEMICALS FOR FLAVOR MATCHING: (1) Acetate C-8; (2) Acetate C-9; (3) Aldehyde C-7; (4) Allyl pelargonate; (5) Amyl benzoate; (6) Amyl butyrate; (7) Benzyl butyrate; (8) Benzyl isoamyl ether; (9) Benzyl isovalerate; (10) Cinnamyl anthranilate; (11) Cinnamyl butyrate; (12) Cinnamyl isobutyrate; (13) Cinnamyl propionate; (14) Ethyl acetate; (15) Ethyl amyl ketone); (16) Ethyl laurate; (17) Ethyl pelargonate; (18) Ethyl propionate; (19) Ethyl sebacate; (20) Linalyl butyrate; (21) Linalyl isobutyrate; (22) *p*-Methyl acetophenone; (23) Methyl phenyl propionate; (24) Phenyl ethyl isobutyrate; (25) Phenyl ethyl isovalerate; (26) Phenyl ethyl propionate; (27) Octyl butyrate; (28) Octyl formate; (29) Rhodinyl butyrate; (30) Santalyl phenyl acetate; (31) Terpinyl propionate

FRESH FRUIT

APPLE

BOTANICAL: *Family: Rosaceae; Genus: Malus; Species: Pumila* (cultivated); Wild: *(Malus sylvestris, Malus baccata)*

OCCURRENCE: There are about 30 varieties of wild apples worldwide; seven are found in the U.S.A.

CHEMICALS FOR FLAVOR MATCHING: (1) Acetaldehyde; (2) Aldehyde C-11 (undecylenic); (3) Aldehyde C-14, pure; (4) Aldehyde C-16; (5) Amyl acetate; (6) Amyl butyrate; (7) Amyl propionate*; (8) Amyl valerianate*; (9) Citronellol; (10) Ethyl acetate; (11) Ethyl butyrate; (12) Ethyl malonate; (13) Ethyl nitrate; (14) Ethyl phenyl glycidate; (15) Geranyl butyrate; (16) Isoamyl butyrate; (17) Isoamyl valerianate; (18) Isovaleraldehyde*; (19) Malic acid; (20) Nerolidol; (21) Tartaric acid

APRICOT

BOTANICAL: *Family: Rosaceae; Genus: Prunus; Species: Armeniaca*

CHEMICALS FOR FLAVOR MATCHING: (1) Aldehyde C-9; (2) Aldehyde C-14, pure; (3) Amyl acetate; (4) Amyl butyrate; (5) Amyl propionate*; (6) Benzyl acetate; (7) Benzyl butyrate; (8) Benzyl cinnamate; (9) Benzyl propionate; (10) Cinnamyl alcohol; (11) Citronellol; (12) Ethyl acetate; (13) Ethyl benzoate; (14) Ethyl butyrate; (15) Ethyl cinnamate; (16) Ethyl formate; (17) Ethyl oenanthate; (18) Ethyl salicylate; (19) Ethyl valerianate; (20) Eugenol; (21) Heliotropin; (22) Isoamyl butyrate; (23) Phenyl ethyl acetate; (24) Phenyl ethyl alcohol

BARBERRY

BOTANICAL: *Family: Berbindaceae; Genus: Berberis; Species: Vulgaris; Thunbergie* (Japanese); *Julianae* (Wintergreen)

---

* Closer in flavor and odor to the natural product

OCCURRENCE: Grows in Europe and western Asia
CHEMICALS FOR FLAVOR MATCHING: (1) Aldehyde C-10; (2) Amyl acetate; (3) Amyl butyrate; (4) Ethyl acetate; (5) Ethyl benzoate; (6) Ethyl butyrate; (7) Ethyl formate; (8) Ethyl oenanthate; (9) Ethyl salicylate; (10) Tartaric acid
USES AND NOTES: The berries can be eaten. Beverages: wine "berberi" through fermentation, with honey "hydromele"; Syrups, jams, and jellies

BILBERRY
BOTANICAL: *Family: Ericaceae; Genus: Vaccinium; Species: Corymbosium; Variety: Scandinavian*
CHEMICALS FOR FLAVOR MATCHING: (1) Amyl butyrate; (2) Ethyl acetate; (3) Ethyl benzoate; (4) Ethyl salicylate; (5) Rhodinyl butyrate

BLACKBERRY
BOTANICAL: *Family: Rosaceae; Genus: Rubus; Species: Occidentalis*
CHEMICALS FOR FLAVOR MATCHING: (1) Anisaldehyde; (2) Diphenyl oxide; (3) Ethyl oenanthate; (4) Heliotropin; (5) Ionone; (6) Methyl anthranilate; (7) Methyl ionone; (8) Neryl isovalerate; (9) Rhodinyl butyrate; (10) Vanillin

BLACK CURRANT
BOTANICAL: *Family: Saxifrage; Genus: Ribes; Species: Nigrum*
CHEMICALS FOR FLAVOR MATCHING: (1) Amyl formate*; (2) Ethyl benzoate; (3) Isoamyl formate; (4) Linalyl isobutyrate; (5) Linalyl propionate; (6) Methyl propionate
USES AND NOTES: Black currant has a sharper flavor than the red currant. It is more popular in Canada and in Europe than in the U.S. where the red currant (*Ribes rubrum*) is used to make jellies, jams, wines, and pies.

The golden currant (*Ribes odoratum*) or Missouri flowering currant grows wild in North America. White and yellowish currants are usually eaten as a fresh dessert.

BLUEBERRY
BOTANICAL: *Family: Ericaceae; Genus: Vaccinium; Species: Corymbosium* (high blueberry), *Pennsylvanium* (low blueberry)
CHEMICALS FOR FLAVOR MATCHING: (1) Amyl propionate; (2) Methyl ionone; (3) Rhodinyl butyrate
USES AND NOTES: Desserts, creams, pastries, pies

CHERRY (SWEET AND SOUR)
BOTANICAL: *Family: Roseaceae; Genus: Prunus* (sweet); *Species: Avium, Cerasus* (sour)
CHEMICALS FOR FLAVOR MATCHING: (1) Allyl benzoate; (2) Allyl isovalerate; (3) Amyl cinnamate; (4) Amyl formate; (5) Anisaldehyde; (6) Anisyl acetate; (7) Anisyl propionate; (8) Benzaldehyde, pure; (9) Benzyl acetate; (10) Cinnamaldehyde;

---

* Closer in flavor and odor to the natural product

(11) Ethyl acetate; (12) Ethyl benzoate; (13) Ethyl butyrate; (14) Ethyl oenanthate; (15) Methyl benzyl propionate; (16) Rhodinyl formate; (17) Rhodinyl isovalerate; (18) *p*-Tolyl acetaldehyde; (19) Tolyl aldehyde; (20) Vanillin

USES AND NOTES: Several kinds of cherry trees are planted for ornamental reasons. Japanese cherry trees are world famous for their beauty

CRANBERRY

BOTANICAL: *Family: Ericaceae; Genus: Vaccinium; Species: Macrocarpon, Oxycoccus* (European)

CHEMICALS FOR FLAVOR MATCHING: (1) Alcohol C-8; (2) Alcohol C-10; (3) Aldehyde C-10; (4) Acetophenone; (5) Amyl alcohol; (6) Benzaldehyde, pure; (7) Benzyl acetae; (8) Benzyl alcohol; (9) Benzyl formate; (10) Ethyl acetate; (11) Ethyl benzoate; (12) Ethyl isovalerate; (13) Ethyl salicylate; (14) Eucalyptol; (15) Furfural; (16) Isoamyl acetate; (17) Isoamyl alcohol; (18) Isoamyl butyrate; (19) Isobutyl alcohol; (20) Linalool; (21) Phenyl ethyl alcohol; (22) α-Terpineol; (23) Valeraldehyde; (24) Vanillin

USES AND NOTES: Sauces, jellies, and juices

DATE

BOTANICAL: *Family: Palmaceae; Genus: Phoenix; Species: Dactylifera*

CHEMICALS FOR FLAVOR MATCHING: (1) Aldehyde C-14, pure; (2) Cinnamic aldehyde; (3) Isoamyl acetae; (4) Isoamyl butyrate; (5) Isobutyl phenyl acetate; (6) Eugenol

USES AND NOTES: A tall palm with pinnate leaves yielding dates. Dates are generally marketed dried. A liquor called "arrack" is made from dates. Ground dates yield oil; roasted ground dates can substitute for coffee

FIG

BOTANICAL: *Family: Moraceae; Genus: Ficus; Species: Carica*

CHEMICALS FOR FLAVOR MATCHING: (1) Maltol; (2) Ethyl cinnamate

GOOSEBERRY

BOTANICAL: *Family: Saxifragaceae; Genus: Ribes; Species: Hirtillum* (American), *Grossularia* (European)

CHEMICALS FOR FLAVOR MATCHING: (1) Aldehyde C-14; (2) Ethyl acetate; (3) Ethyl benzoate; (4) Ethyl oenanthate

USES AND NOTES: Gooseberries are related to the currants. They may have prickly, hairy, or smooth surfaces. They are used in preserves and pies.

GRAPE

BOTANICAL: *Family: Vitaceae; Genus: Vitis; Species: Vinifera*

OCCURRENCE: There are various species of grapes in America: Labrusca or fox; Aestivalis, Norton, Delaware, Vulpina, Rotundifloria, or Muscadine; Catawba, red (winemaking); Concord, purple black; Niagara, green; Scuppernong

CHEMICALS FOR FLAVOR MATCHING: (1) Aldehyde C-14; (2) Amyl butyrate; (3) Cinnamyl propionate; (4) Ethyl acetate; (5) Ethyl formate; (6) Ethyl oenanthate; (7) Ethyl pelargonate; (8) Ethyl salicylate; (9) Eugenol; (10) Isoeugenol; (11) Methyl anthranilate; (12) Methyl β-naphthyl ketone; (13) Phenyl ethyl anthranilate*; (14) Tartaric acid; (15) Seedless raisin (unbleached); (16) Lees (dregs) extract (sediment of wine during fermentation)

GRAPEFRUIT

BOTANICAL: *Family: Rutaceae; Genus: Citrus; Species: Paradisi, Decumana; Maxima* (Shaddoh or pomelo)

CHEMICALS FOR FLAVOR MATCHING: (1) Ethyl acetate; (2) Citral; (3) Limonene; (4) Linalool; (5) Linalyl acetate

USES AND NOTES: Some grapefruits have no seeds but their taste is not as good as those with seeds. Commercial seedless grapefruits include the marsh variety, as well as ruby and Thompson varieties, the popular pink grapefruits. No difference in taste is detectable between the pale-yellowish and the pink-fleshed grapefruit. Grapefruit and tangerine trees produce a fruit called tangelo.

HOP

BOTANICAL: *Family: Cannabinaceae; Genus: Humulus; Species: Lupulus* (European), *Americanus* (wild, American), *Scandens* (Japanese)

CHEMICALS FOR FLAVOR MATCHING: (1) Anisaldehyde; (2) Butyric acid; (3) Capraldehyde; (4) Cinnamic aldehyde; (5) Ethyl acetate; (6) Ethyl isovalerate; (7) Ethyl oenanthate; (8) Ethyl pelargonate; (9) Eugenol; (10) Heliotropin; (11) Limonene; (12) Phenyl ethyl acetate

USES AND NOTES: Hops are used to make beer

HUCKLEBERRY

BOTANICAL: *Family: Ericaceae; Genus: Gaylussacia; Species: Baccata*

CHEMICALS FOR FLAVOR MATCHING: (1) Anethole; (2) Ethyl acetate; (3) Isoamyl acetate; (4) Isoamyl butyrate; (5) Ethyl benzoate; (6) Linalool

USES AND NOTES: The berries have a sweet juice. They are blue-black.

LEMON

BOTANICAL: *Family: Rutaceae; Genus: Citrus; Species: Limonia*

CHEMICALS FOR FLAVOR MATCHING: (1) Acetaldehyde; (2) Alcohol C-8; (3) Aldehyde C-8; (4) Aldehyde C-9; (5) Amyl valerianate; (6) Citral; (7) Citral dimethyl acetal extra; (8) Ethyl acetate; (9) Ethyl nitrate; (10) Geraniol; (11) Geranyl acetate; (12) Linalyl acetate

LIME

BOTANICAL: *Family: Rutaceae; Genus: Citrus; Species: Aurantifolia*

---

* Closer in flavor and odor to the natural product

CHEMICALS FOR FLAVOR MATCHING: (1) Amyl acetate; (2) Amyl butyrate; (3) *p*-Cymene; (4) Dipentene; (5) Ethyl acetate; (6) Hydroxycitronellal; (7) Linalyl acetate; (8) Methyl nonyl acetaldehyde; (9) Terpineol

LOGANBERRY

BOTANICAL: *Family: Rosaceae; Genus: Rubus; Species: Ursinus*

CHEMICALS FOR FLAVOR MATCHING: (1) Aldehyde C-9; (2) Benzoic acid; (3) Amyl acetate; (4) Ethyl acetate; (5) Ethyl benzoate; (6) Ethyl butyrate; (7) Ethyl formate; (8) Ethyl oenanthate; (9) Tartaric acid

USES AND NOTES: The flavor of loganberry is sharp. On cooking, however, it improves and is used for canned jams, juices, or dried.

MANDARIN

BOTANICAL: *Family: Rutaceae; Genus: Citrus; Species: Nobilis; Variety: Deliciosa*

CHEMICALS FOR FLAVOR MATCHING: (1) Aldehyde C-8; (2) Aldehyde C-9; (3) Aldehyde C-10; (4) Amyl acetate; (5) Citral; (6) Ethyl anthranilate; (7) Ethyl formate; (8) Ethyl salicylate; (9) Linalool; (10) Tartaric acid

MELON (WATERMELON)

BOTANICAL: *Family: Cucurbitaceae; Genus: Citrullus; Species: Vulgaris*

CHEMICALS FOR FLAVOR MATCHING: (1) Acetaldehyde; (2) Alcohol C-7; (3) Aldehyde C-14, pure; (4) Aldehyde C-14, myristic; (5) Aldehyde C-18; (6) Amyl valerianate; (7) Benzyl acetate; (8) Citrulline; (9) Cuminic aldehyde; (10) Ethyl acetate; (11) Ethyl butyrate; (12) Ethyl formate; (13) Ethyl laurate; (14) Ethyl nitrate; (15) Ethyl sebacate; (16) Ethyl valerianate; (17) α-Ionone; (18) β-Ionone; (19) Methyl heptenone; (20) Methyl heptyne carbonate; (21) Sebacic acid

USES AND NOTES: There are several types of melons: casaba, musk melon, watermelon, gourd. The gourds include pumpkins, squashes, cucumbers, cantaloupe. The melons are diuretic.

MULBERRY

BOTANICAL: *Family: Moraceae; Genus: Morus; Species: Alba* (white), *Rubra* (red), *Nigra* (black)

CHEMICALS FOR FLAVOR MATCHING: (1) Acetate C-10; (2) Benzaldehyde, pure; (3) Benzyl acetate; (4) Benzyl pelargonate; (5) Ethyl acetate; (6) Ethyl butyrate; (7) Ethyl formate; (8) Ethyl oenanthate; (9) Ionone; (10) Isoamyl acetate

USES AND NOTES: The white mulberry from China, with its bright green leaves, provides nourishment to silkworms. The worm spins a cocoon of fine silk fibers after eating the leaves. These fibers are collected and woven into silk fabrics

ORANGE

BOTANICAL: *Family: Rutaceae; Genus: Citrus; Species: Aurantium* (bitter), *Sinensis* (sweet)

CHEMICALS FOR FLAVOR MATCHING: (1) Acetaldehyde; (2) Acetate C-10; (3) Alcohol C-9; (4) Alcohol C-10; (5) Aldehyde C-8; (6) Aldehyde C-9; (7) Aldehyde C-10; (8) Aldehyde C-11, undecylic; (9) Amyl acetate; (10) Citric acid; (11) Ethyl acetate; (12) Ethyl benzoate; (13) Ethyl butyrate; (14) Ethyl formate; (15) Ethyl oenanthate; (16) Ethyl salicylate; (17) Linalyl acetate; (18) Tartaric acid

BITTER ORANGE: (1) Acetaldehyde; (2) Amyl acetate; (3) Amyl butyrate; (4) *p*-Cymene; (5) Ethyl acetate; (6) α-Ionone; (7) Linalool; (8) Linalyl acetate; (9) Methyl anthranilate

SWEET ORANGE: (1) Aldehyde C-10; (2) Amyl acetate; (3) Amyl anthranilate; (4) Amyl butyrate; (5) Cinnamyl butyrate; (6) Ethyl anthranilate; (7) Linalyl anthranilate; (8) Methyl nonyl acetaldehyde

PEACH (FREESTONE, CLINGSTONE, NECTARINE)

BOTANICAL: *Family: Rosaceae; Genus: Prunus; Species; Persica*

CHEMICALS FOR FLAVOR MATCHING: (1) Aldehyde C-14, pure*; (2) Aldehyde C-16; (3) Amyl acetate; (4) Amyl valerianate; (5) Benzyl acetate; (6) Ethyl acetate; (7) Ethyl butyrate; (8) Ethyl formate; (9) Ethyl oenanthate; (10) Ethyl salicylate; (11) Ethyl sebacate; (12) Ethyl valerianate; (13) Geraniol; (14) Geranyl acetate; (15) Isoamyl butyrate; (16) Phenylethyl acetate*; (17) Phenylethyl propionate; (18) Rhodinol; (19) Rhodinyl acetate; (20) Sebacic acid

USES AND NOTES: There are many varieties of peaches. The freestone type, "Elberta," is the best known variety. It is softer than clingstone. However, some clingstones are very mellow with fine aroma and excellent texture. Clingstone varieties include: Fortuna, Paloro, Johnson, Gaume, Sims.

Nectarines are also a variety of peaches of the *genus Prunus species Persica.*

Peaches are dried or frozen, used in pastries and preserves, or used to make juices. Clingstone varieties are usually canned.

PEAR

BOTANICAL: *Family: Rosaceae; Genus: Pyrus; Species: Communis, Pyrifolia* (Japanese and Chinese), *Usuriensis* (Ussurian pear), *Calleryana* (cullery pear)

CHEMICALS FOR FLAVOR MATCHING: (1) Amyl acetate*; (2) Amyl butyrate; (3) Ethyl acetate; (4) Ethyl butyrate; (5) Ethyl formate; (6) Ethyl nitrate; (7) Geranyl butyrate; (8) Isoamyl acetate; (9) Isobutyl acetate; (10) Sebacic acid

USES AND NOTES: Among the many varieties of pears the Bartlett is the most appreciated

PLUM (PRUNES)

BOTANICAL: *Family: Rosaceae; Genus: Prunus* (European); *Species: Domestica* (European), *Salicina* (Japanese), *Americana, Insititia* (Damson), *Cerasifera* (Myrobalan), *Ornamental* (Myrobalan)

CHEMICALS FOR FLAVOR MATCHING: (1) Aldehyde C-16; (2) Amyl formate*; (3) Ethyl acetate; (4) Ethyl butyrate; (5) Ethyl formate; (6) Ethyl oenanthate

---

* Closer in flavor and odor to the natural product

USES AND NOTES: About 2000 varieties of plums are known. They are classified as European, Japanese, American, Damson, ornamental, and, when dried, as prunes (sun-dried plums).

Plums have many uses as food. They are eaten fresh, used to make jelly, preserves, plum butter, jam, or dried to make prunes.

The prunes are dipped in hot alkali solutions, in order to unwrinkle the skins and to speed the evaporation. They are further washed and spread on drying trays under the sun for about five days. The dried fruit is then washed in cold water, and again with nearly boiling water. They are shaken over a shaker drainer, then weighed and packaged.

Prunes have a high iron content and vitamin value, more than any other dried fruits.

POMEGRANATE

BOTANICAL: *Family: Punicaceae; Genus: Punica; Species: Granatum*

CHEMICALS FOR FLAVOR MATCHING: (1) Aldehyde C-20; (2) Citric acid; (3) Tartaric acid

USES AND NOTES: A soft beverage called "grenadine" is made from the juice of the seeds of pomegranate.

QUINCE

BOTANICAL: *Family: Rosaceae; Genus: Cydonia; Species: Oblonga*

CHEMICALS FOR FLAVOR MATCHING: (1) Benzaldehyde, pure; (2) Ethyl butyrate; (3) Ethyl oenanthate; (4) Ethyl pelargonate; (5) Eugenol; (6) Isoamyl acetate; (7) Isoamyl valerate; (8) Linalyl acetate; (9) Phenylethyl alcohol

USES AND NOTES: The quince has a fragrant smell. It is used to make marmalades, preserves, and jelly.

RASPBERRY

BOTANICAL: *Family: Rosaceae; Genus: Rubus* (European); *Species: Idacus* (red, American), *Strigosus* (red, American), *Occidentalis* (black, American), *Neglectus* (purple)

CHEMICALS FOR FLAVOR MATCHING: (1) Acetate C-8; (2) Alcohol C-7; (3) Aldehyde C-16; (4) Aldehyde C-20; (5) Amyl acetate; (6) Benzoic acid; (7) Ethyl acetate; (8) Ethyl benzoate; (9) Ethyl butyrate; (10) Ethyl formate; (11) Ethyl oenanthate; (12) Ethyl salicylate; (13) Ethyl valeraniate; (14) Isoamyl acetate; (15) Isoamyl butyrate; (16) Isobutyl acetate; (17) Sebacic acid

USES AND NOTES: Raspberries are used for canning, pies, jams, desserts

RED CURRANT

BOTANICAL: *Family: Saxifragaceae; Genus: Ribes; Species: Rubrum*

CHEMICALS FOR FLAVOR MATCHING: (1) Alcohol C-7; (2) Benzyl salicylate; (3) Ethyl acetate; (4) Ethyl formate; (5) Isobutyl cinnamate

STRAWBERRY

BOTANICAL: *Family: Rosaceae; Genus: Fragaria; Species: Virginiana, Chiloensis*

CHEMICALS FOR FLAVOR MATCHING: (1) Aldehyde C-9; (2) Aldehyde C-10; (3) Aldehyde C-14, pure; (4) Aldehyde C-16*; (5) Aldehyde C-20; (6) Amyl acetate; (7) Amyl butyrate; (8) Amyl formate; (9) Amyl valerate; (10) Anethole; (11) Anisaldehyde; (12) Benzaldehyde, pure; (13) Benzyl acetate; (14) Benzyl butyrate; (15) Benzyl propionate; (16) Butyric acid; (17) Cinnamyl butyrate; (18) Cinnamyl isobutyrate; (19) Cinnamyl isovalerate; (20) Citral; (21) Citronellol; (22) Citronellyl acetate; (23) Citronellyl formate; (24) Ethyl acetate; (25) Ethyl cinnamate*; (26) Ethyl formate; (27) Ethyl lactate; (28) Ethyl nitrate; (29) Ethyl oenanthate; (30) Ethylphenyl glycidate*; (31) Ethyl salicylate; (32) Ethyl vanillin; (33) Eugenol; (34) Geraniol; (35) Ionone; (36) Lactic acid; (37) Maltol; (38) Methyl acetophenone; (39) Methyl anthranilate; (40) Methyl cinnamate*; (41) Methyl heptyne carbonate; (42) Nerolin; (43) Phenylethyl acetate; (44) Phenylethyl anthranilate; (45) Phenylethyl butyrate; (46) Phenylethyl propionate; (47) Rhodinol; (48) Rhodinyl butyrate; (49) Valeric acid

USES AND NOTES: Strawberries are used as frozen berries, in ice cream, pastries, jellies, and the juice is used in alcoholic beverages.

TROPICAL FRUITS

AVOCADO

BOTANICAL: *Family: Lauraceae; Genus: Persea; Species: Americana*

CHEMICALS FOR FLAVOR MATCHING: (1) Acetal; (2) Aldehyde C-10; (3) Amyl phenyl acetate

USES AND NOTES: Guacamole, a popular Mexican and Cuban salad, is made from avocado, hot pepper, tomato, onion, and other ingredients.

Avocado has a butter-nutty flavor.

BANANA

BOTANICAL: *Family: Musaceae; Genus: Musa; Species: Sapientum* (sweet, yellow), *Paradisiaca* (plantain)

CHEMICALS FOR FLAVOR MATCHING: (1) Acetoin; (2) Alcohol C-7; (3) Amyl acetate*; (4) Benzyl butyrate; (5) Bornyl acetate; (6) Cinnamyl isobutyrate; (7) Citral; (8) Ethyl acetate; (9) Ethyl butyrate; (10) Isoamyl acetate*; (11) Isoamyl butyrate; (12) Isoamyl valerate; (13) Isovaleraldehyde

USES AND NOTES: The banana oil is a compound of amyl alcohol and acetic acid. It is colorless. Because of its strong banana-like odor it is improperly called "banana oil." It is used as a solvent for cellulose substances, to make celluloid and rayon, and in flavoring.

CHERIMOYA

BOTANICAL: *Family: Annonaceae; Genus: Annona; Species: Cherimoya*

---

* Closer in flavor and odor to the natural product

OCCURRENCE: A small tree of tropical America growing in high elevation
CHEMICALS FOR FLAVOR MATCHING: (1) Aldehyde C-10; (2) Aldehyde C-14, pure; (3) Allyl caproate; (4) Amyl acetate; (5) Amyl butyrate; (6) Benzyl acetate; (7) Ethyl butyrate; (8) Ethyl valerianate; (9) Geraniol; (10) Isobutyl butyrate; (11) Phenylethyl alcohol; (12) Vanillin
USES AND NOTES: The taste of the fruit is similar to a combintion of banana and pineapple

COCONUT
BOTANICAL: *Family: Palmaceae; Genus: Cocos; Species: Nucifera*
CHEMICALS FOR FLAVOR MATCHING: (1) Alcohol C-7; (2) Alcohol C-11; (3) Aldehyde C-18; (4) γ-Lactone
USES AND NOTES: The coconut meat, called copra, is used for making soaps, cooking fats, and margarine. Dry copra is used in baking goods, biscuits, and pastries.

GUAVA
BOTANICAL: *Family: Myrtaceae; Genus: Psidium; Species: Gujava, Lemon guava* (California), *Strawberry, Brazil, Castilianum*
CHEMICALS FOR FLAVOR MATCHING: (1) Geranyl phenyl acetate; (2) Isobutyl phenyl acetate
USES AND NOTES: Guava has a musk-like odor and flavor. It is a popular dessert. A jelly is also made with it.

MANGO
BOTANICAL: *Family: Anacardiaceae; Genus: Mangifera; Species: Indica*
CHEMICALS FOR FLAVOR MATCHING: (1) Citral; (2) Heliotropin; (3) Hydrocinnamic aldehyde
USES AND NOTES: There are about 500 species of mangos, a tropical tree. Mango has a very delicious, peculiar taste which is very difficult to imitate due to its complexity.

PAPAYA
BOTANICAL: *Family: Caricaceae; Genus: Carica; Species: Papaya*
CHEMICALS FOR FLAVOR MATCHING: (1) Aldehyde C-14; (2) Amyl phenyl acetate; (3) Maltol
USES AND NOTES: Papaya is the source of papain, an enzyme similar to pepsin which helps the digestion of foods. It is also used as a remedy in dispepsia. It is utilized in making meat tender before cooking.

PINEAPPLE (ANANAS)
BOTANICAL: *Family: Bronuliaceae; Genus: Ariaria; Species: Comosus*
CHEMICALS FOR FLAVOR MATCHING: (1) Acetaldehyde; (2) Acetate PA*; (3)

* Closer in flavor and odor to the natural product

Allyl caproate*; (4) Allyl-α-ionone; (5) Amyl acetate; (6) Amyl butyrate; (7) Amyl propionate*; (8) Butyric acid; (9) Citric acid; (10) Ethyl acetate; (11) Ethyl butyrate*; (12) Ethyl caprylate*; (13) Ethyl formate; (14) Ethyl pelargonate; (15) Ethyl propionate*; (16) Ethyl valerianate; (17) Isoamyl acetate; (18) Isoamyl butyrate; (19) Isoamyl valerianate; (20) Phenylethyl acetate

USES AND NOTES: The citrus-honey-like flavor of the pineapple makes it a favorite dessert and salad fruit.

DRY FRUITS

ALMOND, BITTER

BOTANICAL: *Family: Rosaceae; Genus: Prunus; Species: Communis*

CHEMICALS FOR FLAVOR MATCHING: (1) Amyl cinnamate; (2) Benzaldehyde, pure; (3) Benzyl alcohol; (4) Dibenzyl ketone*†; (5) Ethyl acetate; (6) Ethyl benzoate; (7) Ethyl formate; (8) Hydrocinnamic aldehyde; (9) Isoamyl acetate; (10) *p*-Methyl benzaldehyde, pure*†; (11) Rhodinyl propionate; (12) Salicylic aldehyde*†; (13) *p*-Tolyl acetaldehyde*†; (14) Tolyl aldehyde*†; (15) Vanillin

USES AND NOTES: There are two kinds of almond: sweet and bitter. The oil of the bitter almond contains the poisonous hydroprussic or prussic acid. After its removal, the oil can be used in flavoring compounds.

BRAZIL NUT (CREAM NUT, BUTTER NUT, PURA NUT, SHENUT)

BOTANICAL: *Family: Lecythidaceae; Genus: Bertholletea; Species: Excelsa*

OCCURRENCE: The tree grows in the large evergreen forests near the Amazon River.

USES AND NOTES: The kernels of Brazil nut have an agreeable taste and oil which is used in salad.

CASHEW NUT

BOTANICAL: *Family: Anacardiaceae; Genus: Anacardium; Species: Occidentale*

USES AND NOTES: The cashew tree, which is a tropical plant, is somewhat related to the poison ivy plant. People are sometimes poisoned by touching the tree. The poison is removed from the kernels by roasting the nuts before they are put on the market.

CHESTNUT

BOTANICAL: *Family: Fagageae; Genus: Castaneae; Species: Dentata, Pumila* (Chinquapin)

USES AND NOTES: The chestnut is a common food in Europe. The flavor is pleasant, particularly when the nuts are roasted. A flour is also made from the chestnut and is used in making pastries.

---

* Closer in flavor and odor to the natural product

† All products with bitter almond odor must be evaluated for purity from hydrocyanic (prussic) acid.

HAZELNUT (COBNUTS, FILBERT)

BOTANICAL: *Family: Betulaceae; Genus: Corylus* (American), *Avilla* (European)
USES AND NOTES: Stories report of divining rods made of hazel. It is believed that with hazel rods, water and valuable minerals can be found.

MACADAMIA (QUEENSLAND NUT)

BOTANICAL: *Family: Proteaceae; Genus: Macadamia; Species: Ternifolia*
OCCURRENCE: Macadamia is native to Australia. Hawaii has made it a major commercial crop.
USES AND NOTES: The flavor of macadamia is much like that of Brazil nut.

PEANUT

BOTANICAL: *Family: Leguminosae; Genus: Arachis; Species: Hypogaea*
USES AND NOTES: The peanut contains more edible oil than any other commercially grown crop. The oil is extracted by pressure or with solvent after roasting.

PECAN

BOTANICAL: *Family: Juglandaceae; Genus: Carya; Species: Pecan*
OCCURRENCE: The tree grows in the southern U.S.A, particularly in the Mississippi area
USES AND NOTES: Pecan is a type of hickory. The wood of the pecan tree is used for smoking meats.

PISTACHIO

BOTANICAL: *Family: Anacardiaceae; Genus: Pistacia; Species: Vera*
USES AND NOTES: The pistachio tree is in the same family as cashew. Its fruits have an agreeable flavor. The kernels are ground and used as a flavoring and coloring for food, particularly ice cream and candy. With pressure the kernels yield an oil which is used in the eastern Mediterranean regions.

WALNUT

BOTANICAL: *Family: Juglandaceae; Genus: Juglans* (English); *Species: Regia, Nigra* (black walnut), *Cinerea* (butternut), *Hindsii* (California)
CHEMICALS FOR FLAVOR MATCHING: *Note:* For all nine types of nuts the following esters may be utilized in simulating their flavors: (1) Aldehyde C-14; (2) Amyl formate; (3) Benzaldehyde, pure; (4) Butyl laurate; (5) Ethyl oenanthate; (6) Ethylphenyl acetate; (7) Furfural; (8) Maltol; (9) Tolyl aldehyde
USES AND NOTES: The English type is the most valuable for its flavor.

NATURALLY SWEET PRODUCTS

HONEY

CHEMICALS FOR FLAVOR MATCHING: (1) Amyl acetate; (2) Amyl butyrate; (3) Amyl phenyl acetate*; (4) Benzyl acetate; (5) Benzyl phenyl acetate*; (6) Benzyl propionate*; (7) Butyl phenyl acetate*; (8) Ethyl cinnamate*; (9) Ethyl phenyl acetate*; (10) Geranyl phenyl acetate*; (11) Homoquinoline*; (12) Isobutyl phenyl acetate*; (13) Isoeugenol phenyl acetate*; (14) Methyl acetophenone; (15) Methyl phenyl acetate*; (16) Phenoxy ethyl isobutyrate*; (17) Phenyl acetaldehyde ethylene acetal*; (18) Phenyl acetic acid*; (19) Phenylethyl acetate*; (20) Phenylethyl benzoate*; (21) Phenylethyl phenyl acetate*; (22) Phenyl propyl formate*; (23) Rhodinyl phenyl acetate*; (24) Santalyl phenyl acetate*

USES AND NOTES: The flavor and color of honey depends on the kind of flowers producing the nectar. The most common source of nectar is alfalfa, alsike clover, sweet clover, and white clover. Nectar may come from other sources such as sage, orange blossom, tupelo, mesquite, sourwood, galbery, etc.

Chemically honey differs from cane sugar. Honey contains mineral salts and other materials useful in the human body.

In addition to being used in baked goods, it is also employed in medicine for cough remedies and laxatives.

LICORICE

BOTANICAL: *Family: Leguminosae; Genus: Glycyrrhiza; Species: Glabra* (southern Europe), *Lipidata* (North America)

CHEMICALS FOR FLAVOR MATCHING: (1) Dihydroanethole; (2) Ethyl cinnamate; (3) Isoeugenol ethyl ether; (4) Phenyl acetaldehyde ethylene acetal; (5) Phenyl acetic acid; (6) Phenylethyl phenyl acetate; (7) Santalyl phenyl acetate

USES AND NOTES: Licorice extract is made by boiling the roots and then evaporating after filtration of the extract. It is used to flavor tobacco, cigars, cigarettes, soft drinks, candies, and chewing gum. In medicine it improves the flavor of disagreeable drugs, and is mainly used for anticough preparations.

MAPLE

BOTANICAL: *Family: Aceraceae; Genus: Acer* (sugar rock or hard maple); *Species: Saccharinum* (silver maple), *Macrophyllum* (big leaf maple, Oregon), *Pennsylvanicum* (striped maple), *Spicatum* (mountain maple), *Rubrum* (red maple), *Pseudo platanus* (sycamore, European), *Platanoides* (Norway maple), *Palmatum* (Japanese maple)

CHEMICALS FOR FLAVOR MATCHING: (1) Carob (St. John's bread) tincture; (2) Corn syrup; (3) Ethyl oenanthate; (4) Fenugreek tincture; (5) Isoeugenol ethyl ether; (6) Maltol

USES AND NOTES: The sugar maple is the most important of all maple trees, not only for its sap but also for its hard wood used as fuel and pulp used for paper.

---

* Closer in flavor and odor to the natural product

VANILLA BEANS

BOTANICAL: *Family: Orchidaceae; Genus: Vanilla; Species: Planifolia*

CHEMICALS FOR FLAVOR MATCHING: (1) Cinnamic acid; (2) Ethyl vanillin*; (3) Heliotropin; (4) Methyl isoeugenol; (5) Propenyl guaethol*; (6) Vanillin*

USES AND NOTES: Vanilla extract, obtained by chopping the beans in small pieces and macerating with pure alcohol and water, is far more delicate than any synthetic. Its flavor is used in first-quality ice cream, chocolate, and candies.

Vanillin is a constituent of the vanilla bean and of many balsams and resins. It is commercially produced from the lignin contained in sulfite waste pulp liquor.

WOODRUFF

BOTANICAL: *Family: Madder; Genus: Asperula; Species: Odorata*

CHEMICALS FOR FLAVOR MATCHING: (1) Benzyl acetate; (2) Ethyl acetate; (3) Ethyl oenanthate; (4) Ethyl pelargonate; (5) Isoamyl butyrate; (6) Vanillin

USES AND NOTES: A small European sweet-scented herb employed in perfumery and wine flavoring.

DAILY BEVERAGES

COCOA—CHOCOLATE

BOTANICAL: *Family: Sterculiaceae; Genus: Theobroma; Species: Cacao*

CHEMICALS FOR FLAVOR MATCHING: (1) Aldehyde C-12, lauric; (2) Amyl phenyl acetate; (3) Benzyl alcohol; (4) Butyl phenyl acetate; (5) Cinnamic aldehyde; (6) Ethyl acetate; (7) Ethyl oenanthate; (8) Eugenol; (9) Isoamyl acetate; (10) Isoamyl butyrate; (11) Isobutyl caproate*; (12) Methyl ethyl diketone*; (13) Vanillin

USES AND NOTES: The beans of cacao provide chocolate and butter cocoa used in ice cream, baked foods, pastries, biscuits, and candies.

The word "chocolate" comes from the Mayan indians. It means "warm" beverage and bitter juice.

COFFEE

BOTANICAL: *Family: Rubiaceae; Genus: Coffea; Species: Arabica*

CHEMICALS FOR FLAVOR MATCHING: (1) Furfuryl mercaptan; (2) Ethyl oenanthate

USES AND NOTES: The aroma of coffee develops on roasting. Instant coffee is made by brewing the roasted and powdered coffee, then evaporating the water. The remaining powdered crystals are ready to become coffee again by adding water (soluble coffee).

Coffee is originally from Ethiopia. Goatherds noticed that their goats, after feeding on coffee berries and leaves, stayed awake. The aroma was accidentally discovered on burning the berries.

---

* Closer in flavor and odor to the natural product

KOLA

BOTANICAL: *Family: Sterculaceae; Genus: Cola; Species: Acuminata*

USES AND NOTES: Kola nuts contain twice the amount of caffeine as coffee beans. They are widely employed in soft drinks and in medicine.

TEA

BOTANICAL: *Family: Theaceae; Genus: Camellia; Species: Sinensis*

CHEMICALS FOR FLAVOR MATCHING: (1) Benzyl acetate; (2) Ethyl acetate; (3) Ethyl formate; (4) Ethyl oenanthate; (5) Ethyl pelargonate; (6) Isoamyl butyrate; (7) Phenylethyl alcohol; (8) Vanillin

USES AND NOTES: Tea is classified as black, fermented, or green unfermented. The formosa tea (*oolonga* species) is considered among the best in quality.

ALCOHOLIC BEVERAGES

Liqueur—A sweetened alcoholic beverage flavored with fruits or herb extracts. It is a combination of alcohol, sugar, and an herb, such as "crème de menthe," a green liqueur flavored exclusively with peppermint; "crème de cacao" flavored with cacao and vanilla; "curaçao" flavored with orange peels of Curaçao Island; "maraschino" flavored with marasca cherries of Dalmatia; and "chartreuse," originally made in a monastery near Grenoble, France, and which contains peppermint, orange peels, and spices.

EXAMPLES: (1) Crème de menthe; (2) Curaçao; (3) Maraschino; (4) Chartreuse

Liquor—A distilled alcoholic beverage

BEER

USES AND NOTES: A beverage containing 3–7% alcohol, it is a fermented infusion or decoction of malted barley with hops. A process called brewing, which involves a complex series of enzymatic reactions, also includes the production of "ale" and malt liquors in which starch is converted to malt and further fermented with yeast. Ale is specifically a fermented liquor brewed with rapid fermentation from an infusion of malt and hops.

EXAMPLES: (1) Pilsner from Pilsen, Bohemia; (2) Munchner from Munich, Germany; (3) Carlsberg from Denmark

BITTERS

USES AND NOTES: This term is assigned to some beverages made with essences from bitter herbs, leaves, barks, roots, or flower heads. They are mostly used as aperitifs, to stimulate the appetite.

EXAMPLES: (1) Angostura; (2) Cincona; (3) Gentian

COGNAC

CHEMICALS FOR FLAVOR MATCHING: (1) Aldehyde C-7; (2) Almond, shales broken; (3) Amyl acetate; (4) Amyl butyrate; (5) Benzaldehyde, pure; (6) Ethyl acetate; (7) Ethyl oenanthate; (8) Ethyl pelargonate; (9) Licorice; (10) Neroli; (11) Orris root, granulated; (12) Peach kernels, broken; (13) Plums, dried; (14) Sassafras, wood

USES AND NOTES: Obtained by distillation of wine, it is considered a brandy. Brandy is made from fermented fruits aged in wooden casks. Other brandies include: armagnac, applejack, kirsch (cherry), slivovitz, mirabelle (plum); those made from blackberries, peaches, apricots, and melons; and benedictine, made with sugar and aromatic herbs.

FERMENTED DRINKS

EXAMPLES: (1) ***Akwavit or Aquavit*** is the favorite distilled beverage of Scandinavian countries. It is made from grain or fermented potato mash and flavored with orange or lemon peels and caraway.

(2) ***Cordial*** is made from a variety of fruits with alcohol from wine and sugar.

(3) ***Gin*** is distilled from a mash of rye, corn, and other grains with essential oil of juniper berries in a special kind of still called "pot still"

(4) ***Pulque***, the national drink of Mexico, is made from the juice of the agave plant, or ***Mezial***, originally made by the Aztecs.

(5) ***Sake***, a fermented liquor with 14–16% alcohol made from rice by the Japanese.

(6) ***Vodka***, a Russian beverage distilled from potatoes or a fermented mash of rye, barley, and corn without any other ingredient.

FORTIFIED BEVERAGES

USES AND NOTES: The alcohol content is not less than 21%. They include products named for their area of origin.

EXAMPLES: (1) Madeira; (2) Malaga; (3) Marsala

LIGHT OR STILL

USES AND NOTES: Wine from any place worldwide.

EXAMPLES: (1) Alsatian; (2) Barbera; (3) Barolo; (4) Bordeaux; (5) Chablis; (6) Chianti; (7) Claret; (8) Rhine; (9) Sauterne; (10) Tokay; (11) Zinfandel

RUM

CHEMICALS FOR FLAVOR MATCHING: (1) Acetic acid; (2) Amyl formate; (3) Birch tar; (4) Butyric acid; (5) Clove oil; (6) Ethyl butyrate; (7) Ethyl formate; (8) Ethyl oenanthate; (9) Ethyl propionate; (10) Lemon oil; (11) Peru balsam; (12) Pyrolegnous acid (tar-free); (13) Styrax

USES AND NOTES: It is distilled from sugar cane or rice and from a fermented mash of sugar cane or molasses.

SPARKLING WINES

USES AND NOTES: Characterized by the bubbles and fizzes when they are poured, the sparkling is due to the carbon dioxide content.

EXAMPLES: (1) Asti spumanti; (2) Burgundy; (3) Catawba; (4) Champagne; (5) Moselle; (6) Sawmur

VERMOUTH

CHEMICALS FOR FLAVOR MATCHING: (1) Absinthe; (2) Acetic acid; (3)

Angelic root; (4) Cardamom; (5) Cardo benedict herb; (6) Calamus; (7) Cinnamon; (8) Elecampane root; (9) Gentian root; (10) Germandice; (11) Kino; (12) Little centaury; (13) Nutmeg; (14) Orange peels, dried; (15) Raisin; (16) Wine, sweet red and white

USES AND NOTES: It is made with many aromatic herbs and spices with a special wine of 15–20% alcohol content.

WHISKEY

CHEMICALS FOR FLAVOR MATCHING: (1) Ethyl caprate; (2) Ethyl caproate; (3) Phenylethyl anthranilate

USES AND NOTES: It is distilled from a fermented mash of corn, rye, barley, or wheat, and aged in wood barrels. Irish whiskey, made from malt, barley, and other grains is the oldest and most famous. Scotch whiskey is made mainly from barley. Bourbon whiskey was originally made from corn in Bourbon County, Kentucky.

DAIRY PRODUCTS

BUTTER

CHEMICALS FOR FLAVOR MATCHING: (1) Alcohol C-7; (2) Acetyl butyryl; (3) Acetyl caproyl; (4) Acetyl isobutyryl; (5) Acetyl isovaleryl; (6) Acetyl propionyl; (7) Benzylidene acetone; (8) Butyl isoacetate; (9) Butyl isoundecanoate; (10) Butyric acetate; (11) Butyric acid; (12) Capric acid; (13) Caproaldehyde; (14) Caproic acid; (15) Caprylic acid; (16) γ-Decalactone; (17) γ-Dodelactone; (18) Diisobutyryl; (19) Dipropionyl butyryl; (20) Ethyl formate; (21) Ethyl myristate; (22) Ethyl oenanthate; (23) Ethyl pelargonate; (24) Isoamyl acetate; (25) Isobutyl acetate; (26) Lactic acid; (27) Valeric acid

USES AND NOTES: Butter is made from the milk of cows, goats, sheep, or buffalo. The milk is vigorously agitated and, at an appropriate temperature when it becomes creamy, it is separated. The cream is then heated quickly to a temperature of 180–185 F and then cooled below 50 F. This pasteurization can also be made in vacuum at 200 F and cooled in stages.

The cream is churned as a sweet cream, or soured by adding lactic acid. The buttermilk is drained from the churn and the butter is washed in cold water and salted. The natural color of butter is either white or golden. The color of the butter is deeper when the animal is fed in pasture instead of in the barn with dry feed. Butter is also artificially colored gold with legally approved color. Butter is one of the richest foods as a source of heat and energy with a large amount of vitamin A.

Butter, which is the oily portion of milk, is composed of glycerides of oleic, stearic, and palmitic acids and smaller amounts of glyceric, butyric, caproic, caprylic, and capric acids.

The specific gravity is 0.910–0.914. Cow milk has about 4% butterfat.

CHEESE

CHEMICALS FOR FLAVOR MATCHING: (1) Acetoin; (2) Butyric acid; (3) Caproic acid; (4) Butyryl lactate; (5) Ethyl butyrate; (6) Lactic acid; (7) Methyl amyl ketone; (8) Isovaleric acid, pure

USES AND NOTES: The flavor of cheese depends on the quantity of ingredients, salt, temperature, moisture, and length of curing.

The kind of mold or bacteria culture added to some cheeses provides a distinct flavor, e.g., blue cheese, Roquefort, or Gorgonzola which obtain the veined blue, marbled appearance and sharp taste from a penicillin mold.

Curing requires different lengths of time. The American cheddar cheese requires from 60 days to 2 years. The longer curing periods produce cheese with a much sharper taste and crumbly, dry texture. Cottage cheese and ricotta are among the simplest varieties of cheese. They are very soft and not cured.

There are more than 400 kinds of cheese with many different names. Some are named for the country, town, or community in which they are manufactured, e.g., Swiss cheese, Bel paese (Italy). However, they are generally divided according to texture (soft, medium, hard), or flavor (medium or sharp). Various flavors and textures are produced by mixing milk from several animals, e.g., goats, sheep, buffalo, reindeer, camels, ewes.

MILK

USES AND NOTES: Milk is a complex mixture of 3.8% fat, 3% casein, 5% lactose, traces of calcium, phosphorus, potassium compounds, lactalbumin, and several vitamins. The remaining material (about 87%) is water.

The casein coagulates when the lactose is converted into lactic acid by heat or bacteria.

Human milk has only one-third the protein of cow milk but its smaller percentage of lactose facilitates its digestion by infants.

Powdered milk is made by dehydrating the whole milk. Pasteurization is made by heating to 160 F for at least $^1/_2$ hour to destroy the bacteria and rapidly cooling it below 50 F.

The flavor components of milk are the same as those for butter and cheese but in a lesser amount.

YOGURT

CHEMICALS FOR FLAVOR MATCHING: (1) Acetaldehyde; (2) Butyric acid; (3) Capric acid; (4) Valeric acid

USES AND NOTES: The name yogurt refers to a Turkish fermented, slightly acidic and semisolid milk from cows, goats, and other cud-chewing mammals. It is an important dietary product largely used by the people of Turkey, the Balkans, Armenia, and Iran.

Yogurt is fermented by the bacteria *Lactobacillus bulgaricus* and *Streptococcus thermophilus* which changes fresh milk into yogurt.

Yogurt, which has the same nutritional elements as milk, has fewer calories (about 15%) and it is, therefore, considered very useful to people on low-calorie diets.

CULINARY ADDITIVES

CAPSICUM

BOTANICAL: *Family: Solanaceae; Genus: Capsicum; Species: Annum, frutescens*

CHEMICALS FOR FLAVOR MATCHING: (1) Benzyl formate; (2) Carvacol; (3) Cinnamyl isovalerate; (4) Isoeugenol; (5) Isoeugenol acetate; (6) Methyl isoeugenol; (7) Phenyl propyl acetate

CUCUMBER

BOTANICAL: *Family: Cucurbitaceae; Genus: Cucumus; Species: Sativus*

USES AND NOTES: (1) Acetaldehyde; (2) Aldehyde C-12, lauric; (3) Amyl propionate; (4) Amyl valerate; (5) α-Ionone; (6) β-Ionone; (7) Irone; (8) Methyl heptyne carbonate

GARLIC

BOTANICAL: *Family: Amaryllidaceae; Genus: Allicum; Species: Sativum*

CHEMICALS FOR FLAVOR MATCHING: (1) Allyl sulfide

USES AND NOTES: Garlic is used whole, ground, powdered, or its juice extract or oil is used. It has a strong pungent characteristic flavor, widely employed in culinary preparation.

WARNINGS AND CAUTION: Allyl sulfide is highly toxic by ingestion and inhalation, strongly irritant to eyes and skin. It is a component of garlic oil in small amounts.

HICKORY

BOTANICAL: *Family: Juglandaceae; Genus: Carya; Species: Ovata* (shagbark), *Laciniosa* (shellbark), *Alba* (mockernut), *Glabra* (pignut), *Aquatica* (water)

USES AND NOTES: Hickory is considered an excellent fuel wood because it produces much heat. It also yields a high quality charcoal. It is used for smoking meat, bacon, ham, and fish producing an excellent flavor.

MUSTARD

BOTANICAL: *Family: Cruciferae; Genus: Brassica; Species: Alba* (white), *Juncea* (green), *Nigra* (black)

CHEMICALS FOR FLAVOR MATCHING: (1) Allyl isothiocyanate

USES AND NOTES: A powder made from the seeds of some mustards is used in salad dressing, to flavor meat, pickles, and some fish. The seeds of the black mustard are used in commercial mustard products. The oil of the mustard seeds is the main source of mustard flavor.

Mustard greens are a source of vitamins A, B, and C.

Mustard is used in medicine as a stimulant, diuretic, emetic, and counterirritant, and as a plaster (ointment) to relieve pain. Mixed with warm water it causes vomiting (emetic).

WARNINGS AND CAUTION: Allyl isothiocyanate is highly toxic by inhalation and is also flammable. It is a component of black mustard seeds in small amounts.

ONION

BOTANICAL: *Family: Liliaceae; Genus: Allium; Species: Cepa*
CHEMICALS FOR FLAVOR MATCHING: (1) Allyl mercaptan
USES AND NOTES: The odor of onion is due to its oil content which forms vapor immediately on cutting and peeling the onion. The vapors are extremely irritating to the eyes and cause tearing.

Onions are classified into two types: (1) American, strong onions; (2) Foreign, mild onions. The strong onion type includes the yellow globe and the flatter "Ebenezer" type. Other types of onions are: red globe, flat bermuda, pale yellow Spanish (prizetaker), small green onions, brown Spanish, Danvers with yellow skin and white flesh.

WARNINGS AND CAUTION: Allyl mercaptan is highly toxic by ingestion and inhalation. It is a component of onion oil in small amounts.

PAPRIKA

BOTANICAL: *Family: Solanaceae; Genus: Capsicum; Species: Tetragonum*

SAFFRON

BOTANICAL: Spring type: *Family: Iridaceae; Genus: Crocus; Species: Susianus;* Autumn type: *Family: Liliaceae; Genus: Colchicum*
USES AND NOTES: Saffron has a sweet odor but its taste is bitter. It was once used extensively as a yellow dye to color food and as a spice. It is now replaced by aniline dye. Four thousand flowers of saffron yield only one ounce of color. It is preferred over aniline in cooking, flavoring, and coloring candies

SMOKE

CHEMICALS FOR FLAVOR MATCHING: ***Smoke:*** (1) Tar oil; (2) Hickory (*Carya ovata*) oil; ***Smoked meat:*** (1) Cade oil; (2) Capsicum oleoresin; (3) Black pepper oil
USES AND NOTES: Smoke from special kinds of wood, such as hickory or maple, is used to cure ham, fish, meat, etc. Smoking the food changes its flavor and odor but does not ruin it. The smoking preserves meat and fish, particularly if it is combined with salting and drying.

TARRAGON

BOTANICAL: *Family: Compositae; Genus: Artemisia; Species: Dracunculus*
USES AND NOTES: The leaves from the plant are used to flavor pickles and vinegar. Some of the *Compositae* family are poisonous.

TOMATO

BOTANICAL: *Family: Solanaceae; Genus: Lycopersicum; Species: Esculentum*
CHEMICALS FOR FLAVOR MATCHING: (1) Acetaldehyde; (2) Aldehyde C-12, lauric; (3) Benzaldehyde, pure; (4) Citral; (5) Citronellyl butryate; (6) Citronellyl propionate; (7) Ethyl acetate; (8) Ethyl propionate; (9) Ethyl salicylate; (10) Geranyl acetate; (11) Geranyl butyrate; (12) Isoamyl butyrate; (13) Linalyl acetate
USES AND NOTES: As a culinary additive, tomatoes are used especially in making ketchup which consists of tomato pulp, sugar, mustard, vinegar, and spices. Its

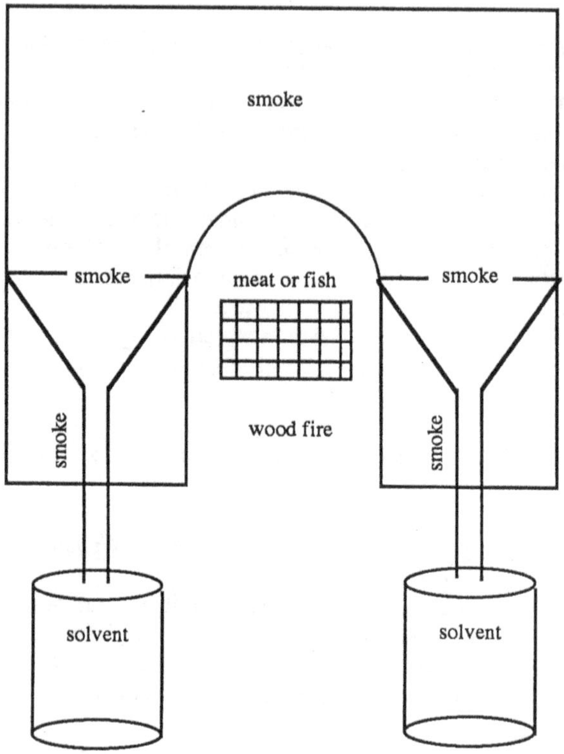

solvent: propylene glycol

LIQUID SMOKED FLAVOR

preparation is not standard even though it is classified by: (1) Ketchup grade A, U.S.A. Agriculture Department, as a ketchup grade fancy; (2) Ketchup Grade C, as a ketchup grade standard. These grades are based on color, consistency, flavor, and purity of components.

TURMERIC

BOTANICAL: *Family: Zinziberaceae; Genus: Curcuma; Species: Longa*

USES AND NOTES: It is employed in the pickling industry due to its strong aromatic odor and pungent taste.

Aromatic Chemicals Used in Flavor Compounding

ALDEHYDE C-18

CHEMICAL FORMULA: $C_9H_{16}O_2$

PHYSICAL PROPERTIES: *Specific gravity:* 0.958–0.965 (15 C); *Refractive index:* 1.4460–1.4500 (20 C)

CHARACTERISTICS AND USES: Coconut

ANETHOLE

CHEMICAL FORMULA: $C_{10}H_{12}O$

DERIVATION: By crystallization from anise or fennel oil; synthetically from *p*-cresol

PHYSICAL PROPERTIES: *Specific gravity:* 0.984–0.987 (15 C); *Refractive index:* 1.5570–1.5610 (20 C); *Boiling point:* 233–234 C; *Melting point:*22.5–23 C

CHARACTERISTICS AND USES: Anise

ANISALDEHYDE

SYNONYMS: Aubepine

CAS NUMBER: 123-11-5

CHEMICAL FORMULA: $C_8H_8O_2$

DERIVATION: From anethole or anisole by oxidation (anisole is obtained from sodium phenate, methyl chloride, heating phenol with methyl alcohol)

PHYSICAL PROPERTIES: *Specific gravity:* 1.119–1.123 (25/25 C); *Refractive index:* 1.570–1.574 (20 C); *Boiling point:* 245–249 C; *Melting point:* 0 to –4 C

CHARACTERISTICS AND USES: Cherry, anise

BENZALDEHYDE

CHEMICAL FORMULA: C_7H_6O

CAS NUMBER: 100-52-7

DERIVATION: (a) Air oxidation of toluene with uranium or molybdenum oxides as catalysts; (b) Chlorination of toluene with further hydrolysis by acid or alkali

PHYSICAL PROPERTIES: *Specific gravity:* 1.041–1.046 (25/25 C); *Refractive index:* 1.5440–1.5465 (20 C); *Boiling point:* 179.5 C

CHARACTERISTICS AND USES: Bitter almond

BENZYL BUTYRATE

CHEMICAL FORMULA: $C_{11}H_{14}O_2$

PHYSICAL PROPERTIES: *Specific gravity:* 1.006–1.009 (25/25 C); *Refractive index:* 1.4920–1.4960 (20 C); *Boiling point:* 242 C

CHARACTERISTICS AND USES: Rose, apricot

BOURBONAL

SYNONYMS: Ethyl vanillin

CAS NUMBER: 121-32-4

CHEMICAL FORMULA: $C_9H_{10}O_3$

DERIVATION: From vanilla beans

PHYSICAL PROPERTIES: *Melting point:* 76.5–78 C
CHARACTERISTICS AND USES: Vanilla

CARVONE
CAS NUMBER: 99-49-0
CHEMICAL FORMULA: $C_{10}H_{14}O$
DERIVATION: *d*-form main component of caraway and dill oils; *l*-form occurs in spearmint, synthetically from *d*-limonene and rectified
PHYSICAL PROPERTIES: *Specific gravity:* 0.960–0.964 (15 C); *Refractive index:* 1.4995–1.1502 (20 C); *Boiling point:* 225–231 C
CHARACTERISTICS AND USES: Caraway

CINNAMIC ALDEHYDE
CAS NUMBER: 104-55-2
CHEMICAL FORMULA: C_9H_8O
DERIVATION: (a) From Ceylon and Chinese cinnamon oils; (b) By condensation of benzaldehyde and acetaldehyde
PHYSICAL PROPERTIES: *Specific gravity:* 1.047–1.051 (25/25 C); *Refractive index:* 1.6200–1.6230 (20 C); *Boiling point:* 118–120 C
CHARACTERISTICS AND USES: Cinnamon

CINNAMYL ALCOHOL
CAS NUMBER: 104-54-1
CHEMICAL FORMULA: $C_9H_{10}O$
DERIVATION: (a) From cassia oil or cinnamon oil; (b) By reduction of cinnamic aldehyde
PHYSICAL PROPERTIES: *Specific gravity:* 1.029–1.034 (30 C); *Refractive index:* 1.572–1.577 (30 C); *Boiling point:* 256.6 C; *Melting point:* 32–34 C
CHARACTERISTICS AND USES: Rose

CINNAMYL BUTYRATE
CHEMICAL FORMULA: $C_{13}H_{16}O_2$
PHYSICAL PROPERTIES: *Specific gravity:* 1.010–1.015 (25/25 C); *Refractive index:* 1.5250–1.5280 (20 C); *Boiling point:* 262 C
CHARACTERISTICS AND USES: Rose, fruits

CINNAMYL PROPIONATE
CHEMICAL FORMULA: $C_{12}H_{14}O_2$
PHYSICAL PROPERTIES: *Specific gravity:* 1.029–1.033 (25/25 C); *Refractive index:* 1.5320–1.5370 (20 C)
CHARACTERISTICS AND USES: Grape

CITRAL
CAS NUMBER: 5392-40-5
CHEMICAL FORMULA: $C_{10}H_{16}O$
DERIVATION: (a) Isolated by fractional distillation of lemongrass; (b) Synthetically

by oxidation of geraniol, neroli, or linalool by chromic acid
PHYSICAL PROPERTIES: *Specific gravity:* 0.881–0.889 (25/25 C); *Refractive index:* 1.4820–1.4910 (20 C); *Boiling point:* 228–229 C
CHARACTERISTICS AND USES: Lemon

CITRONELLOL
CAS NUMBER: 106-22-9
CHEMICAL FORMULA: $C_{10}H_{20}O$
DERIVATION: (a) From citronella oil, geranium oil, savin oil; (b) Reduction of citronella or geraniol
PHYSICAL PROPERTIES: *Specific gravity:* 0.852–0.860 (25/25 C); *Refractive index:* 1.4530–1.4600 (20 C); *Boiling point:* 224.4 C
CHARACTERISTICS AND USES: Rose

COUMARIN
CAS NUMBER: 91-64-5
CHEMICAL FORMULA: $C_9H_6O_2$
DERIVATION: (a) By heating salicylic aldehyde, sodium acetate, and acetic anhydride; (b) Isolated from tonka beans
PHYSICAL PROPERTIES: *Boiling point:* 301.7 C; *Melting point:* 68–70.5 C
CHARACTERISTICS AND USES: Caramel

CUMIC ALDEHYDE
CAS NUMBER: 122-03-2
CHEMICAL FORMULA: $C_{10}H_{12}O$
PHYSICAL PROPERTIES: *Specific gravity:* 0.976–0.980 (25/25 C); *Refractive index:* 1.530–1.5340 (20 C); *Boiling point:* 235–237 C
CHARACTERISTICS AND USES: Violet

DECYL ACETATE
SYNONYMS: Acetate C-10
CHEMICAL FORMULA: $C_{12}H_{24}O_2$
DERIVATION: By gently boiling capric aldehyde and glacial acetic acid (for several hours together) in presence of zinc dust or powder, precipitating with water, and distilling under reduced pressure
PHYSICAL PROPERTIES: *Specific gravity:* 0.862–0.866 (25/25 C); *Refractive index:* 1.4250–1.4300; *Boiling point:* 103–104 C
CHARACTERISTICS AND USES: Fruits, rose

***n*-DECYL ALCOHOL**
SYNONYMS: Alcohol C-10; 1-decanol
CHEMICAL FORMULA: $C_{10}H_{22}O$
DERIVATION: Reduction of coconut oil fatty acids; from C_9 olefin and gas synthesis by otto process
PHYSICAL PROPERTIES: *Specific gravity:* 0.826–0.832 (25/25 C); *Refractive index:* 1.4350–1.4390 (20 C); *Boiling point:* 231 C
CHARACTERISTICS AND USES: Rose, neroli

n-DECYL ALDEHYDE

SYNONYMS: Aldehyde C-10; *n*-decanal
CHEMICAL FORMULA: $C_{10}H_{20}O$
DERIVATION: Occurs in lemongrass, citronella, orange, and many other oils; Synthetically by oxidation of alcohol C-10 or reduction of decanoic acid (capric acid). Capric acid is obtained by fractional distillation of coconut fatty acids
PHYSICAL PROPERTIES: *Specific gravity:* 0.822–0.830 (25/25 C); *Refractive index:* 1.4270–1.4300 (20 C); *Boiling point:* 207–209 C
CHARACTERISTICS AND USES: Orange, violet

DODECYL ALDEHYDE

SYNONYMS: Aldehyde C-12 MNA; lauric aldehyde; lauryl aldehyde
CAS NUMBER: 112-54-9
CHEMICAL FORMULA: $C_{12}H_{24}O$
PHYSICAL PROPERTIES: *Specific gravity:* 0.822–0.830 (25/25 C); *Refractive index:* 1.4310–1.4360 (20 C); *Boiling point:* 184–185 C
CHARACTERISTICS AND USES: Violet

ETHYL ACETATE

CAS NUMBER: 141-78-6
CHEMICAL FORMULA: $C_4H_8O_2$
DERIVATION: By heating acetic acid and ethyl alcohol in presence of sulfuric acid and distilling
PHYSICAL PROPERTIES: *Specific gravity:* 0.905 (15 C); *Refractive index:* 1.3726 (20 C); *Boiling point:* 75.7–78 C
CHARACTERISTICS AND USES: Cognac, fruity

ETHYL ACETOACETATE

CHEMICAL FORMULA: $C_6H_{10}O_3$
DERIVATION: By the reaction of metallic sodium on ethyl acetate and distilling
PHYSICAL PROPERTIES: *Specific gravity:* 1.026 (15 C); *Boiling point:* 181 C
CHARACTERISTICS AND USES: Apple, pineapple

ETHYL BENZOATE

CAS NUMBER: 93-89-0
CHEMICAL FORMULA: $C_9H_{10}O_2$
DERIVATION: By heating ethyl alcohol and benzoic acid in presence of sulfuric acid and distilling
PHYSICAL PROPERTIES: *Specific gravity:* 1.043–1.046 (25/25 C); *Refractive index:* 1.5030–1.5060 (20 C); *Boiling point:* 260 C
CHARACTERISTICS AND USES: Black currant

ETHYL BUTYRATE

CAS NUMBER: 105-54-4
CHEMICAL FORMULA: $C_6H_{12}O_2$
DERIVATION: By heating ethyl alcohol and butyric acid in presence of sulfuric acid

and distilling
PHYSICAL PROPERTIES: *Specific gravity:* 0.881–0.886 (15 C); *Refractive index:* 1.396–1.492 (20 C); *Boiling point:* 120–125 C
CHARACTERISTICS AND USES: Pineapple

ETHYL MALONATE
CAS NUMBER: 105-53-3
CHEMICAL FORMULA: $C_6H_{10}O_4$
DERIVATION: By passing hydrogen chloride into cyanoacetic acid dissolved in absolute alcohol and distilling
PHYSICAL PROPERTIES: *Specific gravity:* 1.055 (15 C); *Boiling point:* 198.4 C
CHARACTERISTICS AND USES: Apple

ETHYL MYRISTATE
SYNONYMS: Ethyl tetradecanoate
CHEMICAL FORMULA: $C_{16}H_{32}O_2$
PHYSICAL PROPERTIES: *Boiling point:* 295 C; *Melting point:* 10–11 C
CHARACTERISTICS AND USES: Butter

ETHYL OENANTHATE
SYNONYMS: Ethyl heptanoate; cognac oil
CHEMICAL FORMULA: $C_9H_{18}O_2$
DERIVATION: By heating oenanthic acid and ethyl alcohol in presence of sulfuric acid, and distilling (oenanthic acid is obtained by oxidizing heptanol with potassium dichromate and sulfuric acid)
PHYSICAL PROPERTIES: *Specific gravity:* 0.871–0.872 (15 C); *Refractive index:* 1.414 (20 C); *Boiling point:* 187–189 C
CHARACTERISTICS AND USES: Cognac, wine, fruity soft drinks (apricot, cherry, currant, gooseberry, grape, artificial essence of bourbon, etc.)

ETHYL PELARGONATE
SYNONYMS: Ethyl nonylate
CHEMICAL FORMULA: $C_{11}H_{22}O_2$
DERIVATION: From alcoholic solutions of various essences
PHYSICAL PROPERTIES: *Specific gravity:* 0.863–0.865 (25/25 C); *Refractive index:* 1.421–1.426 (20 C); *Boiling point:* 227–231 C
CHARACTERISTICS AND USES: Wine, cognac

ETHYL PROPIONATE
CAS NUMBER: 105-37-3
CHEMICAL FORMULA: $C_5H_{10}O_2$
DERIVATION: By treating ethyl alcohol with propionic acid (propionic acid is obtained by reaction of ethyl alcohol and carbon monoxide in presence of boron trifluoride as a catalyst; also by the reaction of carbon monoxide with hydrogen and olefins or alcohols)
PHYSICAL PROPERTIES: *Specific gravity:* 0.8904–0.8967 (15 C); *Refractive index:*

1.3847 (20 C); *Boiling point:* 96–100 C
CHARACTERISTICS AND USES: Fruity

ETHYL SEBACATE
CHEMICAL FORMULA: $C_{14}H_{26}O_4$
PHYSICAL PROPERTIES: *Specific gravity:* 0.957–0.9675 (15 C); *Refractive index:* 1.4365–1.4375 (20 C); *Boiling point:* 307–308 C
CHARACTERISTICS AND USES: Fruity

ETHYL VALERATE
SYNONYMS: Ethyl isovalerate
CAS NUMBER: 108-64-5
CHEMICAL FORMULA: $C_7H_{14}O_2$
DERIVATION: By heating sodium valerate and ethyl alcohol in presence of sulfuric acid or hydrochloric acid and distilling
PHYSICAL PROPERTIES: *Specific gravity:* 0.876 (15 C); *Refractive index:* 1.3975 (20 C); *Boiling point:* 142–144.6 C
CHARACTERISTICS AND USES: Pineapple, fruity

EUGENOL
CAS NUMBER: 97-53-0
CHEMICAL FORMULA: $C_{10}H_{12}O_2$
DERIVATION: By extraction of clove oil with aqueous potassium hydroxide, separation of acid and distillation in a stream of carbon dioxide
PHYSICAL PROPERTIES: *Specific gravity:* 1.064–1.068 (25/25 C); *Refractive index:* 1.5400–1.5420 (20 C); *Boiling point:* 251–256 C
CHARACTERISTICS AND USES: Clove

GERANIOL
CHEMICAL FORMULA: $C_{10}H_{18}O$
DERIVATION: From geranium oil, citronella oil, or palmarosa oil with calcium chloride
PHYSICAL PROPERTIES: *Specific gravity:* 0.870–0.880 (25/25 C); *Refractive index:* 1.4710–1.4760 (20 C); *Boiling point:* 229 C
CHARACTERISTICS AND USES: Rose

GERANYL ACETATE
CAS NUMBER: 105-87-3
CHEMICAL FORMULA: $C_{12}H_{20}O$
DERIVATION: By heating geraniol and sodium acetate with acetic anhydride
PHYSICAL PROPERTIES: *Specific gravity:* 0.900–0.910 (25/25 C); *Refractive index:* 1.4570–1.4620 (20 C); *Boiling point:* 242–245 C
CHARACTERISTICS AND USES: Rose

GERANYL *n*-BUTYRATE
CHEMICAL FORMULA: $C_{14}H_{24}O_2$

PHYSICAL PROPERTIES: *Specific gravity:* 0.8924 (15 C); *Refractive index:* 1.455 (20 C); *Boiling point:* 142–143 C
CHARACTERISTICS AND USES: Pear, apple, rose

HELIOTROPIN
SYNONYMS: Piperonal
CHEMICAL FORMULA: $C_8H_6O_3$
DERIVATION: By oxidation of isosafrole
PHYSICAL PROPERTIES: *Boiling point:* 263–264 C; *Melting point:* 36–37 C
CHARACTERISTICS AND USES: Heliotrope

HEPTYLIC ALDEHYDE
SYNONYMS: Aldehyde C-7; oenanthol
CAS NUMBER: 111-71-7
CHEMICAL FORMULA: $C_7H_{14}O$
DERIVATION: From castor oil by decomposition of the ricinoleic acid glyceride (see ethyl oenanthate)
PHYSICAL PROPERTIES: *Specific gravity:* 0.8226 (15 C); *Refractive index:* 1.415–1.4257 (20 C); *Boiling point:* 152–155 C
CHARACTERISTICS AND USES: Fruity

HYDROCINNAMIC ALDEHYDE
SYNONYMS: Phenyl propyl aldehyde
CAS NUMBER: 104-53-0
CHEMICAL FORMULA: $C_9H_{10}O$
DERIVATION: From reduction of cinnamic acid with sodium amalgam
PHYSICAL PROPERTIES: *Specific gravity:* 1.0175–1.095 (15 C); *Refractive index:* 1.5207–1.5253 (20 C); *Boiling point:* 221–224 C
CHARACTERISTICS AND USES: Cinnamon

HYDROXYCITRONELLAL
CAS NUMBER: 107-75-5
CHEMICAL FORMULA: $C_{10}H_{20}O_2$
DERIVATION: From citronella, java, or *Eucalyptus citriodora*
PHYSICAL PROPERTIES: *Specific gravity:* 0.917–0.921 (25/25 C); *Refractive index:* 1.4470–1.4500 (20 C); *Boiling point:* 124 C
CHARACTERISTICS AND USES: Orange blossom, other citrus

IONONE
CAS NUMBER: 8013-90-9
CHEMICAL FORMULA: $C_{13}H_{20}O$
DERIVATION: Synthetically by condensation of citral with acetone and phosphoric, formic, or sulfuric acid as a catalyst; from violet moss, *Boronia mejastigma*, or costus root
PHYSICAL PROPERTIES: α-: *Specific gravity:* 0.930–0.936 (25/25 C); *Refractive index:* 1.5030–1.5090 (20 C); *Boiling point:* 132 C; β-: *Specific gravity:* 0.946–0.952

(15 C); *Refractive index:* 1.515–1.5198; *Boiling point:* 138.5 C
CHARACTERISTICS AND USES: Violet

IRONE

CAS NUMBER: α-: 79-69-6; β-: 79-70-9; γ-: 79-68-5
CHEMICAL FORMULA: $C_{14}H_{22}O$
PHYSICAL PROPERTIES: *Specific gravity:* 0.932–0.936 (25/25 C); *Refractive index:* 1.5020–1.5030 (20 C); *Boiling point:* 146 C
CHARACTERISTICS AND USES: Orris

ISOAMYL ACETATE

CHEMICAL FORMULA: $C_7H_{14}O_2$
DERIVATION: Rectification of commercial amyl acetate
PHYSICAL PROPERTIES: *Specific gravity:* 0.875, 0.876 (15 C); *Refractive index:* 1.3999 (20 C); *Boiling point:* 138.5 C, 139 C
CHARACTERISTICS AND USES: Pear, banana

ISOAMYL BUTYRATE

CHEMICAL FORMULA: $C_9H_{18}O_2$
DERIVATION: By treating isoamyl alcohol with butyric acid and distilling
PHYSICAL PROPERTIES: *Specific gravity:* 0.863, 0.869 (15 C); *Refractive index:* 1.407, 1.411 (20 C); *Boiling point:* 169.8 C, 178.6 C
CHARACTERISTICS AND USES: Apricot, apple, pineapple, pear, plum

ISOAMYL VALERATE

CHEMICAL FORMULA: $C_{10}H_{20}O_2$
DERIVATION: By adding sulfuric acid to a mixture of amyl alcohol and valeric acid and distilling
PHYSICAL PROPERTIES: *Specific gravity:* 0.866, 0.876 (15 C); *Refractive index:* 1.412 (20 C); *Boiling point:* 189 C, 190 C
CHARACTERISTICS AND USES: Apple, banana

ISOBUTYL ACETATE

CHEMICAL FORMULA: $C_6H_{12}O_2$
DERIVATION: By treating isobutyl alcohol with acetic acid in the presence of a catalyst
PHYSICAL PROPERTIES: *Specific gravity:* 0.871–0.875 (15 C); *Refractive index:* 1.392 (20 C); *Boiling point:* 116–118 C
CHARACTERISTICS AND USES: Raspberry, pear, rose

ISOBUTYL BUTYRATE

CHEMICAL FORMULA: $C_8H_{16}O_2$
PHYSICAL PROPERTIES: *Specific gravity:* 0.864 (15 C); *Refractive index:* 1.403 (20 C); *Boiling point:* 156.9 C
CHARACTERISTICS AND USES: Rum

ISOEUGENOL
CAS NUMBER: 97-54-1
CHEMICAL FORMULA: $C_{10}H_{12}O_2$
DERIVATION: From eugenol by isomerization with potassium hydroxide
PHYSICAL PROPERTIES: *Specific gravity:* 1.079–1.085 (25/25 C); *Refractive index:* 1.5720–1.5770 (20 C); *Boiling point:* 266.5 C; *Melting point:* 32 C
CHARACTERISTICS AND USES: Carnation

LINALOOL
SYNONYMS: Boi de rose
CAS NUMBER: 78-70-6
CHEMICAL FORMULA: $C_{10}H_{18}O$
DERIVATION: From rosewood, petitgrain, linaloe wood, bergamot, etc.; synthetically from geraniol
PHYSICAL PROPERTIES: *Specific gravity:* 0.859–0.867 (25/25 C); *Refractive index:* 1.4610–1.4640 (20 C); *Boiling point:* 197–199 C
CHARACTERISTICS AND USES: Neroli

LINALYL ACETATE
CAS NUMBER: 115-95-7
CHEMICAL FORMULA: $C_{12}H_{20}O_2$
DERIVATION: By the reaction of acetic anhydride on linalool in presence of sulfuric acid; by fractional distillation of citrus oils
PHYSICAL PROPERTIES: *Specific gravity:* 0.903–0.906 (25/25 C); *Refractive index:* 1.4510–1.4530 (20 C); *Boiling point:* 105–106 C
CHARACTERISTICS AND USES: Bergamot, lavender

LINALYL BUTYRATE
CHEMICAL FORMULA: $C_{14}H_{24}O$
PHYSICAL PROPERTIES: *Specific gravity:* 0.893–0.904 (25/25 C); *Refractive index:* 1.4510–1.4560 (20 C); *Boiling point:* 105–106 C
CHARACTERISTICS AND USES: Bergamot, fruity

MENTHOL
CAS NUMBER: 89-78-1
CHEMICAL FORMULA: $C_{10}H_{20}O$
DERIVATION: By freezing peppermint oil; synthetically from citronellal
PHYSICAL PROPERTIES: *Specific gravity:* 0.890 (15 C); *Refractive index:* 1.4505 (45 C); *Boiling point:* 215 C; *Melting point:* 43 C
CHARACTERISTICS AND USES: Peppermint

METHYL ANTHRANILATE
CAS NUMBER: 134-20-3
CHEMICAL FORMULA: $C_8H_9NO_2$
DERIVATION: By heating anthranilic acid and methyl alcohol in presence of sulfuric acid, and distilling

PHYSICAL PROPERTIES: *Specific gravity:* 1.162–1.167 (25/25 C); *Refractive index:* 1.5820–1.5840 (20 C); *Boiling point:* 132 C; *Melting point:* 24–25 C
CHARACTERISTICS AND USES: Honey, neroli

METHYL *m*-ANTHRANILATE
CHEMICAL FORMULA: $C_{10}H_9NO_2$
DERIVATION: By heating anthranilic acid and methyl alcohol in presence of sulfuric acid, and distilling
PHYSICAL PROPERTIES: *Specific gravity:* 1.120–1.134 (15 C); *Refractive index:* 1.5796 (20 C); *Boiling point:* 130.5 C; *Melting point:* 18.5–19.5 C
CHARACTERISTICS AND USES: Tangerine

METHYL EUGENOL
CAS NUMBER: 93-15-2
CHEMICAL FORMULA: $C_{11}H_{14}O_2$
PHYSICAL PROPERTIES: *Specific gravity:* 1.032–1.035 (25/25 C); *Refractive index:* 1.5320–1.5360 (20 C); *Boiling point:* 248–251 C; *Melting point:* 20–24 C
CHARACTERISTICS AND USES: Grape

METHYL HEPTYNE CARBONATE
SYNONYMS: Methyl octine carbonate
CAS NUMBER: 111-12-6
CHEMICAL FORMULA: $C_9H_{14}O_2$
DERIVATION: From heptaldehyde
PHYSICAL PROPERTIES: *Specific gravity:* 0.919–0.924 (25/25 C); *Refractive index:* 1.4460–1.4490 (20 C)
CHARACTERISTICS AND USES: Violet, melon, cucumber

METHYL ISOEUGENOL
SYNONYMS: Propenyl guaiacol
CAS NUMBER: 93-16-3
CHEMICAL FORMULA: $C_{11}H_{14}O$
PHYSICAL PROPERTIES: *Specific gravity:* 1.047–1.053 (25/25 C); *Refractive index:* 1.5650–1.5690 (20 C); *Boiling point:* 260–263 C
CHARACTERISTICS AND USES: Grape

METHYLNONYL ACETALDEHYDE
SYNONYMS: Aldehyde C-12 MNA
CHEMICAL FORMULA: $C_{12}H_{24}O$
PHYSICAL PROPERTIES: *Specific gravity:* 0.8279–0.8460 (15 C); *Refractive index:* 1.4312–1.4455 (20 C)
CHARACTERISTICS AND USES: Citrus

METHYL PHENYL ACETATE
CHEMICAL FORMULA: $C_9H_{10}O_2$
PHYSICAL PROPERTIES: *Specific gravity:* 1.062–1.066 (25/25 C); *Refractive index:*

1.5050–1.5080 (20 C); *Boiling point:* 215–220 C
CHARACTERISTICS AND USES: Honey

METHYL PHENYL GLYCIDATE
SYNONYMS: Aldehyde C-16; ethyl methyl phenyl glycidate
CHEMICAL FORMULA: $C_{12}H_{14}O$
PHYSICAL PROPERTIES: *Specific gravity:* 1.0887–1.0920 (25/25 C); *Refractive index:* 1.534–1.537 (20 C)
CHARACTERISTICS AND USES: Strawberry

β-NAPHTHOL ISOBUTYL
SYNONYMS: Fragarol
CHEMICAL FORMULA: $C_{12}H_{12}O$
DERIVATION: By reaction of β-naphthol acid and isobutyl alcohol in presence of sulfuric acid
PHYSICAL PROPERTIES: *Melting point:* 32–34 C
CHARACTERISTICS AND USES: Neroli, strawberry

β-NAPHTHYL ETHYL ETHER
SYNONYMS: Nerolin
CHEMICAL FORMULA: $C_{12}H_{12}O$
DERIVATION: By the reaction of β-naphthol and ethyl alcohol in presence of sulfuric acid
PHYSICAL PROPERTIES: *Specific gravity:* 1.064 (20 C); *Refractive index:* 1.5975 (36 C); *Boiling point:* 282 C; *Melting point:* 35–37 C
CHARACTERISTICS AND USES: Neroli, strawberry

NEROL
CAS NUMBER: 106-25-2
CHEMICAL FORMULA: $C_{10}H_{18}O$
DERIVATION: By iodization of geraniol with hydriodic acid, and alcoholic sodium
PHYSICAL PROPERTIES: *Specific gravity:* 0.875–0.880 (25/25 C); *Refractive index:* 1.4730–1.4780 (20 C); *Boiling point:* 225–227 C
CHARACTERISTICS AND USES: Rose, neroli

***n*-NONYL ALCOHOL**
SYNONYMS: Alcohol C-9; nonanol
CAS NUMBER: 143-08-8
CHEMICAL FORMULA: $C_9H_{20}O$
PHYSICAL PROPERTIES: *Specific gravity:* 0.824–0.830 (25/25 C); *Refractive index:* 1.4310–1.4350 (20 C); *Boiling point:* 213.5 C
CHARACTERISTICS AND USES: Orange, neroli, rose

NONYL ALDEHYDE
SYNONYMS: Aldehyde C-9; nonanal
CHEMICAL FORMULA: $C_9H_{18}O$

PHYSICAL PROPERTIES: *Specific gravity:* 0.820–0.828 (25/25 C); *Refractive index:* 1.422–1.426 (20 C); *Boiling point:* 80 C
CHARACTERISTICS AND USES: Orange, lemon, rose

OCTYL ACETATE
SYNONYMS: Acetate C-8; caprylyl acetate
CAS NUMBER: 103-09-3
CHEMICAL FORMULA: $C_{10}H_{20}O$
PHYSICAL PROPERTIES: *Specific gravity:* 0.865–0.868 (25/25 C); *Refractive index:* 1.4180–1.4210 (20 C); *Boiling point:* 82–84 C
CHARACTERISTICS AND USES: Raspberry

***n*-OCTYL ALCOHOL**
SYNONYMS: Alcohol C-8
CAS NUMBER: 111-87-5
CHEMICAL FORMULA: $C_8H_{18}O$
DERIVATION: By reduction of caprylic acid; by distilling sodium ricinoleate with an excess of sodium hydroxide
PHYSICAL PROPERTIES: *Specific gravity:* 0.822–0.828 (25/25 C); *Refractive index:* 1.4280–1.4310; *Boiling point:* 195–197 C
CHARACTERISTICS AND USES: Rose, lemon

***n*-OCTYL ALDEHYDE**
SYNONYMS: Aldehyde C-8; caprylic aldehyde
CAS NUMBER: 124-13-0
CHEMICAL FORMULA: $C_8H_{16}O$
PHYSICAL PROPERTIES: *Specific gravity:* 0.818–0.825 (25/25 C); *Refractive index:* 1.4180–1.4220 (20 C); *Boiling point:* 175 C
CHARACTERISTICS AND USES: Lemon, orange

OCTYL BUTYRATE
CHEMICAL FORMULA: $C_{10}H_{20}O$
PHYSICAL PROPERTIES: *Specific gravity:* 0.8688–0.8692 (15 C); *Refractive index:* 1.421 (20 C); *Boiling point:* 244–245 C
CHARACTERISTICS AND USES: Fruity

PHENYL ETHYL ACETATE
CAS NUMBER: 103-45-7
CHEMICAL FORMULA: $C_{10}H_{12}O$
DERIVATION: By reaction of ethyl acetate and aluminum phenyl ethylate; from acetic anhydride and phenyl alcohol in presence of sodium acetate
PHYSICAL PROPERTIES: *Specific gravity:* 1.030–1.034 (25/25 C); *Refractive index:* 1.4970–1.5010 (20 C); *Boiling point:* 232 C
CHARACTERISTICS AND USES: Peach, rose

PHENYL ETHYL ALCOHOL

SYNONYMS: Phenethyl alcohol
CAS NUMBER: 60-12-8
CHEMICAL FORMULA: $C_8H_{10}O$
DERIVATION: By reduction of phenylacetic ethyl ester with sodium in absolute alcohol; by reaction of ethylene oxide and phenyl magnesium bromide with further hydrolysis
PHYSICAL PROPERTIES: *Specific gravity:* 1.017–1.020 (25/25 C); *Refractive index:* 1.5310–1.5330 (20 C); *Boiling point:* 222 C
CHARACTERISTICS AND USES: Honey, rose

PHENYL ETHYL PROPIONATE

CAS NUMBER: 120-45-6
CHEMICAL FORMULA: $C_{11}H_{14}O$
PHYSICAL PROPERTIES: *Specific gravity:* 1.010–1.014 (25/25 C); *Refractive index:* 1.493–1.496 (20 C); *Boiling point:* 244 C
CHARACTERISTICS AND USES: Rose

RHODINOL

CAS NUMBER: 6812-78-8
CHEMICAL FORMULA: $C_{10}H_{20}O$
DERIVATION: By fractional distillation of citronellol
PHYSICAL PROPERTIES: *Specific gravity:* 0.860–0.880 (25/25 C); *Refractive index:* 1.4630–1.4730 (20 C)
CHARACTERISTICS AND USES: Rose

RHODINYL ACETATE

CHEMICAL FORMULA: $C_{12}H_{22}O_2$
DERIVATION: By reaction of rhodinol and acetic anhydride in presence of sodium acetate
PHYSICAL PROPERTIES: *Specific gravity:* 0.894–0.905 (25/25 C); *Refractive index:* 1.4520–1.4580 (20 C); *Boiling point:* 115 C
CHARACTERISTICS AND USES: Rose

RHODINYL BUTYRATE

CHEMICAL FORMULA: $C_{14}H_{26}O_2$
PHYSICAL PROPERTIES: *Specific gravity:* 0.886–0.890 (25/25 C); *Refractive index:* 1.4510–1.4550 (20 C); *Boiling point:* 260–268 C
CHARACTERISTICS AND USES: Fruity

α-TERPINEOL

CAS NUMBER: 98-55-5
CHEMICAL FORMULA: $C_{10}H_{18}O$
DERIVATION: By heating terpin hydrate with phosphoric acid and distilling or with dilute sulfuric acid and separating on a different boiling point; by fractional distillation of pine oil

PHYSICAL PROPERTIES: *Specific gravity:* 0.931–0.936 (25/25 C); *Refractive index:* 1.4825–1.4850 (20 C); *Boiling point:* 217–219 C
CHARACTERISTICS AND USES: Many uses

TERPINYL PROPIONATE
CHEMICAL FORMULA: $C_{13}H_{22}O$
DERIVATION: By heating terpineol with oleofin in presence of sulfuric acid and further distilling
PHYSICAL PROPERTIES: *Specific gravity:* 0.944–0.949 (25/25 C); *Refractive index:* 1.4620–1.4660 (20 C)
CHARACTERISTICS AND USES: Lavender

***p*-TOLUYL ALDEHYDE**
CAS NUMBER: 1334-78-7
CHEMICAL FORMULA: C_8H_8O
PHYSICAL PROPERTIES: *Specific gravity:* 1.015–1.023 (25/25 C); *Refractive index:* 1.5390–1.5440 (14 C); *Boiling point:* 204–205 C
CHARACTERISTICS AND USES: Cherry

***n*-γ-UNDELACTONE**
SYNONYMS: Aldehyde C-14
CHEMICAL FORMULA: $C_{11}H_{20}O$
DERIVATION: By heating undecylenic acid in the presence of sulfuric acid (undecylenic acid obtained by destructive distillation of castor oil)
PHYSICAL PROPERTIES: *Specific gravity:* 0.940–0.944 (25/25 C); *Refractive index:* 1.4500–1.4540 (20 C)
CHARACTERISTICS AND USES: Peach, rose

UNDECYLENIC ALDEHYDE
SYNONYMS: Aldehyde C-11; undecenal
CHEMICAL FORMULA: $C_{11}H_{20}O$
PHYSICAL PROPERTIES: *Specific gravity:* 0.840–0.841 (25/25 C); *Refractive index:* 1.4410–1.4460 (20 C); *Boiling point:* 116 C; *Melting point:* –4 C
CHARACTERISTICS AND USES: Violet, rose

VANILLIN
CAS NUMBER: 121-33-5
CHEMICAL FORMULA: $C_8H_8O_3$
DERIVATION: By extraction from vanilla beans; from sulfite waste of pulp liquor upon heating with alkali, air oxidation, and further crystallization (by-product of the paper-pulp industry)
PHYSICAL PROPERTIES: *Boiling point:* 285 C; *Melting point:* 81–82 C
CHARACTERISTICS AND USES: Vanilla

Chapter VII:

SOLVENTS

Introduction

Solvents are liquids which dissolve other substances (solute), generally a solid, without any change in the chemical composition (solution).

The proportion of the substances in a solution depends on the solvent solubility, which is limited to a certain quantity at a given temperature and pressure. The solution, when a maximum of solute is dissolved, is termed "saturated." A supersaturated solution can be created but may be turbid and may further precipitate.

Solvents are classified by their dissolving capacity. The aromatic hydrocarbon solvents have a higher solvent capacity than the aliphatic type. The organic solvents are classified in groups based on their chemical composition and are given with some examples:

1. ***Hydrocarbons, aliphatic:*** Naphtha and its fractions
   Hydrocarbons, aromatic: Benzene, toluene, xylene
2. ***Alcohols:*** Ethyl alcohol, ethylene, methyl alcohol
3. ***Ethers:*** Dimethyl ether, ethylene glycol monoethyl ether
4. ***Ketones:*** Acetone, methyl ethyl ketone, methyl isobutyl ketone
5. ***Esters:*** Butyl acetates, butyl lactate, ethyl acetate
6. ***Chlorinated:*** Chloroform, tetrachloroethane, monochlorobenzene
7. ***Nitrated:*** Nitroethane, nitromethane, 1-nitropropane, 2-nitropropane, nitrobenzene
8. ***Amines:*** Monoethanolamine, diethanolamine, pyridine
9. ***Liquefied gases:*** Ammonia, sulfur dioxide

Solvents Commonly Used for Flavors and Perfumes

ACETONE

SYNONYMS: Dimethyl ketone; 2-propanone; β-ketopropane; pyroacetic ether
CAS NUMBER: 67-64-1
CHEMICAL FORMULA: C_3H_6O

MOLECULAR WEIGHT: 58.08
DERIVATION: Oxidation of cumene or butane or oxidation of isopropyl alcohol with a metallic catalyst; by-product of synthetically produced glycerol
CHARACTERISTICS: *Form:* Volatile liquid; *Color:* Colorless; *Odor:* Sweetish
PHYSICAL PROPERTIES: *Specific gravity:* 0.792; *Refractive index:* 1.3591; *Boiling point;* 56.2 C; *Flash point:* 15 F; *Solubility:* Miscible with water, alcohol, ether, chloroform, and most oils
USES AND NOTES: General solvent (not for flavors)
WARNING AND CAUTION: Toxic; fire risk

BENZENE
SYNONYMS: Benzol cyclohexatriene
CAS NUMBER: 71-43-2
CHEMICAL FORMULA: C_6H_6
MOLECULAR WEIGHT: 78.11
DERIVATION: Fractional distillation of coal tar; catalytic reforming of petroleum
CHARACTERISTICS: *Form:* Liquid; *Color:* Colorless or yellowish; *Odor:* Aromatic
PHYSICAL PROPERTIES: *Specific gravity:* 0.8790 (20/4 C); *Refractive index:* 1.50110; *Flash point:* 12 F; *Solubility:* Miscible with alcohol, ether, acetone, carbon tetrachloride; slightly soluble in water
USES AND NOTES: General solvent (not for flavors)
WARNINGS AND CAUTION: Toxic; fire risk

CORN OIL
SYNONYMS: Maize oil; mazola oil; maydol
BOTANICAL: *Family: Graminaceae; Genus: Zea; Species: Mays*
CHARACTERISTICS: *Form:* Oil; *Color:* Yellowish or brownish; *Odor:* Faintly oily
PHYSICAL PROPERTIES: *Specific gravity:* 0.914–0.921; *Refractive index:* 1.464–1.468; *Flash point:* 610 F; *Solubility:* Soluble in chloroform, ether; slightly soluble in alcohol
USES AND NOTES: Food, pharmaceuticals

COTTONSEED OIL
BOTANICAL: *Family: Malvaceae; Genus: Gossypium; Species: Herbaceum* oil
CHARACTERISTICS: *Form:* Oil; *Color:* Yellowish; *Odor:* Odorless
PHYSICAL PROPERTIES: *Specific gravity:* 0.915–0.921; *Refractive index:* 1.4645–1.4655; *Solubility:* Slightly soluble in alcohol; soluble in ether, chloroform, carbon disulfide
USES AND NOTES: Cosmetics, soaps, foods

CYCLOHEXANE
SYNONYMS: Hexamethylene; hexanaphthene; hexahydrobenzene
CAS NUMBER: 110-87-7
CHEMICAL FORMULA: C_6H_{12}
MOLECULAR WEIGHT: 84.16
DERIVATION: From crude petroleum; catalytic hydrogenation of benzene

CHARACTERISTICS: *Form:* Mobile liquid; *Color:* Colorless; *Odor:* Pungent
PHYSICAL PROPERTIES: *Specific gravity:* 0.779 (20/4 C); *Refractive index:* 1.4264 (20 C); *Boiling point;* 80.7 C; *Flash point:* –1 F; *Solubility:* Insoluble in water; soluble in alcohol
USES AND NOTES: Essential oils extraction; solvent for resins, fats, oils
WARNINGS AND CAUTION: Fire risk

DIETHYL PHTHALATE
SYNONYMS: Ethyl phthalate; 1,2-benzenedicarboxylic acid diethyl ether
CAS NUMBER: 84-66-2
CHEMICAL FORMULA: $C_{12}H_{14}O$
MOLECULAR WEIGHT: 222.23
DERIVATION: Reaction of phthalic anhydride with ethyl alcohol
CHARACTERISTICS: *Form:* Liquid; *Color:* Colorless; *Odor:* Odorless
PHYSICAL PROPERTIES: *Specific gravity:* 1.120; *Refractive index:* 1.5002 (25 C); *Flash point:* 325 F; *Solubility:* Insoluble in water; miscible with almost all esters and hydrocarbons
USES AND NOTES: Perfumery; solvent; fixative; denaturant
WARNINGS AND CAUTION: Toxic

ETHYL ACETATE
SYNONYMS: Acetic ether; acetic ester; acetic acid ethyl ester; vinegar naphtha
CAS NUMBER: 141-78-6
CHEMICAL FORMULA: $C_4H_8O_2$
MOLECULAR WEIGHT: 88.10
DERIVATION: By heating acetic acid and ethyl alcohol in presence of sulfuric acid and distilling
CHARACTERISTICS: *Form:* Liquid; *Color:* Colorless; *Odor:* Fragrant
PHYSICAL PROPERTIES: *Specific gravity:* 0.8945; *Boiling point;* 77 C; *Flash point:* 24 F; *Solubility:* Slightly soluble in water; soluble in alcohol, ether, chloroform
USES AND NOTES: Flavors, pharmaceuticals
WARNINGS AND CAUTION: Toxic; fire risk

ETHYL ALCOHOL
SYNONYMS: Grain alcohol; ethanol
CAS NUMBER: 64-17-5
CHEMICAL FORMULA: C_2H_6O
MOLECULAR WEIGHT: 46.07
DERIVATION: Wine from grapes; molasses; from ethylene
CHARACTERISTICS: *Form:* Volatile liquid; *Color:* Colorless; *Odor:* Pleasant
PHYSICAL PROPERTIES: *Specific gravity:* 0.816 (15.56 C); *Refractive index:* 1.3651; *Boiling point;* 78 C; *Flash point:* 55 F; *Solubility:* Miscible with water, ether, chloroform, acetone
USES AND NOTES: Solvent for essential oils, flavors, perfumes, beverages, medicine
WARNINGS AND CAUTION: Fire risk

GLYCEROL

SYNONYMS: Glycerin; glycyl alcohol; 1,2,3-propanetriol; trihydroxy propane
CAS NUMBER: 56-81-5
CHEMICAL FORMULA: $C_3H_8O_3$
MOLECULAR WEIGHT: 92.09
DERIVATION: By-product of soap; from propylene and chlorine
CHARACTERISTICS: *Form:* Syrupy liquid; *Color:* Colorless; *Odor:* Odorless
PHYSICAL PROPERTIES: *Specific gravity:* 1.2620; *Boiling point;* 290 C; *Flash point:* 320 F; *Solubility:* Soluble in water, alcohol; insoluble in ether, benzene, chloroform
USES AND NOTES: Perfumery, cosmetics, liqueurs, flavors

GLYCERYL TRIACETATE

SYNONYMS: Triacetin; 1,2,3-propanetriol triacetate; triacetyl glycerin; enzactin
CAS NUMBER: 102-76-1
CHEMICAL FORMULA: $C_9H_{14}O_6$
MOLECULAR WEIGHT: 218.20
DERIVATION: From glycerol and acetic acid
CHARACTERISTICS: *Form:* Liquid; *Color:* Colorless; *Odor:* Fatty
PHYSICAL PROPERTIES: *Specific gravity:* 1.160 (20 C); *Refractive index:* 1.4312 (20 C); *Boiling point;* 258–260 C; *Flash point:* 300 F; *Solubility:* Slightly soluble in water; soluble in alcohol, ether
USES AND NOTES: Perfumery, cosmetics, flavors, medicine

***n*-HEXANE**

CAS NUMBER: 100-54-3
CHEMICAL FORMULA: C_6H_{14}
MOLECULAR WEIGHT: 86.17
DERIVATION: Fractional distillation from petroleum (molecular sieve process)
CHARACTERISTICS: *Form:* Liquid; *Color:* Colorless; *Odor:* Faint
PHYSICAL PROPERTIES: *Specific gravity:* 0.65937 (20/4 C); *Refractive index:* 1.37486 (20 C); *Boiling point;* 68.742 C; *Flash point:* –9 F; *Solubility:* Insoluble in water; soluble in alcohol, acetone, ether
USES AND NOTES: Solvent for vegetable oils
WARNINGS AND CAUTION: Toxic; fire risk

ISOPROPYL ALCOHOL

SYNONYMS: Isopropanol; dimethyl carbinol; 2-propanol; petrohol
CAS NUMBER: 67-63-0
CHEMICAL FORMULA: C_3H_8O
MOLECULAR WEIGHT: 60.09
DERIVATION: From propylene and sulfuric acid with hydrolyzing
CHARACTERISTICS: *Form:* Liquid; *Color:* Colorless; *Odor:* Fragrant
PHYSICAL PROPERTIES: *Specific gravity:* 0.7863 (20/20 C); *Refractive index:* 1.3756 (20 C); *Boiling point;* 82.4 C; *Flash point:* 59 F; *Solubility:* Soluble in water, alcohol, ether
USES AND NOTES: Solvent for essential oils, flavors, perfumes
WARNINGS AND CAUTION: Toxic, fire risk

POLYSORBATE 80

SYNONYMS: POE (20) sorbitan oleate; "Tween" 80
CAS NUMBER: 9005-65-6 (generic)
DERIVATION: Condensation of ethylene glycol or ethylene oxide and water
CHARACTERISTICS: *Form:* Viscous liquid; *Color:* Yellowish
PHYSICAL PROPERTIES: *Solubility:* Soluble in water and almost all solvents
USES AND NOTES: Cosmetics, flavors, pharmaceuticals

PROPYLENE GLYCOL

SYNONYMS: Methyl glycol; 1,2-propanediol; 1,2-dihydroxypropane methylethylene glycol
CAS NUMBER: 57-55-6
CHEMICAL FORMULA: $C_3H_8O_2$
MOLECULAR WEIGHT: 76.09
DERIVATION: Hydration of propylene oxide
CHARACTERISTICS: *Form:* Viscous liquid; *Color:* Colorless; *Odor:* Odorless
PHYSICAL PROPERTIES: *Specific gravity:* 1.0381 (20/20 C); *Refractive index:* 1.4293 (27 C); *Boiling point:* 187.3 C; *Flash point:* 210 F; *Solubility:* Soluble in water, alcohol, and almost all solvents
USES AND NOTES: Flavors, perfumes, syrups, soft drinks

SOYBEAN OIL

SYNONYMS: Soya bean oil; soy oil; Chinese bean oil
BOTANICAL: *Family: Leguminosae; Genus: Soya; Species: Hispida* oil
CHARACTERISTICS: *Form:* Oil; *Color:* Yellowish or brownish; *Odor:* Characteristic
PHYSICAL PROPERTIES: *Specific gravity:* 0.924–0.929; *Refractive index:* 1.4760–1.4775; *Flashpoint:* 540 F; *Solubility:* Soluble in alcohol, ether, chloroform, carbon disulfide
USES AND NOTES: Foods

WATER, DISTILLED

SYNONYMS: Hydrogen oxide
CHARACTERISTICS: *Color:* Colorless; *Odor:* Odorless
PHYSICAL PROPERTIES: *Specific gravity:* 0.997; *Refractive index:* 1.333; *Boiling point;* 100 C
USES AND NOTES: Universal solvent

Chapter VIII: COLORANTS FOR FLAVORS AND PERFUMES

Natural Colors

ALKANET

SOURCE/COLOR: Alkanet root, red

BOTANICAL: *Family: Boraginaceae; Genus: Alkanna; Anchusa; Species: Tinctoria*

USES AND NOTES: The color red is prepared from its roots (alkannin). It is employed for coloring wines, cosmetics, and fats, and as an astringent.

ANNATTO

SOURCE/COLOR: Annatto, yellowish-red

BOTANICAL: *Family: Bixaceae; Genus: Bixia; Species: Orellana*

USES AND NOTES: The color is made from the pulp around the seeds of this tropical tree (bixion). It is employed in coloring butter, margarine, cheese, oils, ice cream, ice cream cones, sausage casing, bakery goods, and spices. It is also used in combination with turmeric.

β-APO-8′-CAROTENAL

SOURCE/COLOR: β-Apo-8′-carotenal, orange 6

USES AND NOTES: It is an aldehydic carotenoid found in spinach, oranges, grass, tangerine, and marigold. It is used in coloring fat products such as cheese, margarine, and oils.

BEET

SOURCE/COLOR: Beets (dehydrated powder), dark red

BOTANICAL: *Family: Chenopodiaceae* (goosefoot); *Genus: Beta; Species: Vulgaris*

USES AND NOTES: The beet roots contain red pigments (betacyanins) and yellow pigments (betaxanthins) collectively classified as "betalains." Of the betacyanins 75–95% is betanin, which is the main colorant of the beet.

The colorant is employed in candies, yogurts, ice creams, cakes, powdered drinks, soft drinks, gelatin dessert, meat substitutes. Much of the world's sugar comes from the sugar beet.

BUCKTHORN

SOURCE/COLOR: Buckthorn, yellow

BOTANICAL: *Family: Rhamnaceae, Sapodilla; Genus: Rhamnus, Brumelia; Species: Cathartica, Lycioides*

USES AND NOTES: Native to Eurasia with small greenish flowers, black berries

CAMPEACHY

SOURCE/COLOR: Campeachy wood (longwood), blue

BOTANICAL: *Family: Leguminosae; Genus: Haematoxylon; Species: Campeachianum*

USES AND NOTES: A crystalline phenolic compound is also in the logwood and employed mainly as a biological stain.

CANTHAXANTHIN

SOURCE/COLOR: Canthaxanthin, orange

BOTANICAL: *Family: Thallophyta; Genus: Cantharellus; Species: Cinnabarinus*

USES AND NOTES: Initially isolated from an edible mushroom (*Cantharellus cinnabarinus*) and also found in marine algae, in sea trout, daphnia, salmon, brine shrimps, and several species of flamingo.

Canthaxantin is available as a dry powder and used as a colorant (orange 8) for tomato, fruit drinks, baked goods, sausage products.

CARAMEL

SOURCE/COLOR: Caramel, dark brown

USES AND NOTES: Caramel is a burned sugar, generally made from liquid corn syrup. The major use for caramel is in soft drinks, particularly root beer and cola. Other uses include the coloring of syrups, rum, candies, preserves, canned meat products, cough syrups, and pharmaceuticals.

CATECHU

SOURCE/COLOR: Catechu, brown

BOTANICAL: *Family: Acacia; Genus: Catechu; Species: Gambier*

USES AND NOTES: It is obtained from a tropical Asiatic plant. It is used in dyeing and tanning, and in medicines. Catechu makes brown dyes used in coloring leather. It is also used to dye and print cotton cloth, such as calico.

CHLOROPHYLL

SOURCE/COLOR: Chlorophyll, green

USES AND NOTES: The extraction is made with strong alcohol from green plants. It is employed as a coloring agent and deodorant. The solution is blue-green with a deep red fluorescence. The extract, which is waxy, is soluble in alcohol, ether, chloroform, acetone, carbon disulfide, and benzene. As a green colorant, it is used mostly for soaps, oils, fats, waxes, liquors, preserves, cosmetics, toothpaste, medicine.

COCHINEAL

SOURCE/COLOR: Cochineal, carmine, red 4

ZOOLOGICAL: *Family: Cochinilla; Genus: Dactylopius; Species: Coccus; Variety: Cacti*

USES AND NOTES: A red dyestuff made from the dried bodies of the female cochineal insects which feed on cactus (*Coccus cacti*).

It is used in candies, pill coating, and as a biological stain and indicator.

CUD BEAR

SOURCE/COLOR: Cud bear, yellow

BOTANICAL: *Family: Lichens; Genus: Lecano raceal; Species: Rocellaceae*

USES AND NOTES: A reddish-purple powder colorant from lichens. It is used for coloring syrups, elixirs, etc.

CURCUMA

SOURCE/COLOR: Curcuma root, yellow

BOTANICAL: *Family: Zingiberaceae; Genus: Curcuma; Species: Longa*

USES AND NOTES: See Turmeric

ERYTHROSINE

SOURCE/COLOR: Erythrosine, brown

USES AND NOTES: Brown powder forming cherry-red solution in water. It is employed for coloring foods.

GUANINE

SOURCE/COLOR: Guanine, iridescent

USES AND NOTES: A crystalline substance obtained from fish scales, consisting of two purines, guanine and hypoxanthine. The colorant content of guanine is about 75–97% while that of hypoxanthine is about 3–25% depending on fish type and respective tissue. Fishes providing this material include herrings, alewives, and menhades.

The material is not a colorant but a pearly white, silvery iridescent employed in lipsticks, nail polishes, and eye makeup.

HUCKLEBERRY

SOURCE/COLOR: Huckleberry, black-red

BOTANICAL: *Family: Ericaceae; Genus: Gaylussacia; Species: Baccata*

USES AND NOTES: American shrubs, related to the blueberries and bearing edible fruits

INDIGOTIN

SOURCE/COLOR: Indigotin, indigo, blue

BOTANICAL: *Family: Leguminosae; Genus: Indigofera; Species: Indigo*

USES AND NOTES: A tropical plant growing mostly in Bengal, Java, and Guatemala. Indigotin is a dark blue crystalline powder with coppery luster. It is insoluble in water, alcohol, and ether and soluble in chloroform, glacial acetic acid, and nitrobenzene.

Indigotin is also produced synthetically from aniline and chloroacetic acid. The resultant phenyl glycine is further fused with alkali and sodium amide.

KINO

SOURCE/COLOR: Kino, red

BOTANICAL: *Family: Leguminosae; Genus: Pterocarpus; Species: Marsupium*

USES AND NOTES: Kino is a plant which grows in western Africa, East India, and Sri Lanka. It is used as an astringent.

MALLOW FLOWERS

BOTANICAL: *Family: Malvaceae; Genus: Malva, Arborea; Species: Silvestris, Rotundifolia*

USES AND NOTES: It is used mostly in coloring vinegar and food products.

PAPRIKA

SOURCE/COLOR: Paprika and paprika oleoresins, red

BOTANICAL: *Family: Solanaceae; Genus: Capsicum; Species: Tetragonum*

USES AND NOTES: Paprika has a brighter red color and a sweeter taste than the red cayenne pepper. Both paprika and its oleoresin have a good tinctorial capacity in producing orange to bright red color.

PERNAMBUCO

SOURCE/COLOR: Pernambuco wood, red

BOTANICAL: *Family: Leguminosae; Genus: Caesalpina; Species: Echinata*

USES AND NOTES: A wood from Lima, Peru and Nicaragua used as a dye.

POKEBERRY

SOURCE/COLOR: Pokeberry, red, or pockeweed

BOTANICAL: *Family: Phytolaccaceae; Genus: Phytolaceae; Species: Americana*

USES AND NOTES: The pokeweed plant has dark purple, juicy berries and white flowers. Its roots are poisonous.

SAFFLOWER

SOURCE/COLOR: Safflower, yellow

BOTANICAL: *Family: Compositae; Genus: Carthamus; Species: Tinctorius*

USES AND NOTES: An edible drying oil is obtained from the seeds of this herb which has orange or red flowers. The color is prepared from the flower's heads.

SAFFRON

SOURCE/COLOR: Saffron, yellow

BOTANICAL: *Family: Iridaceae; Genus: Crocus; Species: Sativus*

USES AND NOTES: Saffron has a sweet scent and taste. It is a brilliant yellow dye. Four thousand flowers of saffron make about one ounce of commercial saffron which is used in flavoring and coloring candy and in cooking.

SANDALWOOD

SOURCE/COLOR: Sandalwood, red

BOTANICAL: *Family: Santalaceae; Genus: Santalum; Species: Album*

USES AND NOTES: A kind of scented wood from a tropical tree, the sandalwood oil is pressed out and used for perfume, cosmetics, and medicine

TARTRAZINE

SOURCE/COLOR: Tartrazine, yellow 5

USES AND NOTES: A bright orange-yellow powder. It is employed as a color additive in foods, drugs, and cosmetics. It is freely soluble in water.

TITANIUM DIOXIDE

SOURCE/COLOR: Titanium dioxide, white

USES AND NOTES: It is found in nature in three crystalline forms: anatase, brookite, and rutile. Anatase exhibits stability toward light. Titanium dioxide may be prepared by direct combination of titanium with oxygen. It is employed in cosmetics such as lipsticks, nail enamels, face powders, eye makeup, and rouges.

TURMERIC

SOURCE/COLOR: Turmeric and turmeric oleoresin, yellow 3

BOTANICAL: *Family: Zingiberaceae; Genus: Curcuma; Species: Longa*

USES AND NOTES: Turmeric is an East Indian perennial herb. The roots are cleaned, boiled for some hours, dried in an oven, and then ground. The resulting yellowish powder has a strong, aromatic odor and a strong, pungent taste. It is used as a colorant and spice for food, especially to color mustard. It is also used for making test papers in combination with alkali.

ULTRAMARINE

SOURCE/COLOR: Ultramarine, green 24; blue 29; violet 15; red

USES AND NOTES: Ultramarine designates the color produced from the naturally occurring semiprecious gem lazurite (lapis lazuli). Ultramarines are prepared synthetically in the following manner:

(1) Use kaolin (china clay), silica, sulfur, soda ash, sodium sulfate, and carbonaceous reducing agent such as rosin or charcoal pitch. Heat from 700–800 C for about 150 h. Cool. Produces ultramarine, green 24.

(2) Add sulfur and reheat. Produces ultramarine, blue 29.

(3) Add 5% ammonium chloride and heat for 4 days at 200–250 C. Produces ultramarine, violet 15.

(4) Add gaseous hydrochloric acid and heat at 70–200 C. Produces ultramarine, red.

Ultramarines are used mostly in the cosmetics industry to manufacture mascara, eyebrow pencils, and soaps.

YELLOWWOOD

SOURCE/COLOR: Yellowwood, yellow

BOTANICAL: *Family: Leguminosae; Genus: Cladrastis; Species: Lutea*

USES AND NOTES: This plant has fragrant white flowers.

ZINC OXIDE

SOURCE/COLOR: Zinc oxide, white 4

USES AND NOTES: A white or yellowish-white amorphous, odorless powder. It is insoluble in water, and soluble in ammonia, dilute acetic acid, alkali hydroxide, and mineral acids. It is used for face powder, rouge, and eye makeup.

Colors of Common Flavors and Perfumes

Apple, fruit	Green
Apple, preserve	Yellow
Apricot	Yellow-orange
Blackberry	Dark bluish red
Brandy	Golden brown
Butter	Canary to reddish yellow
Butterscotch	Golden brown
Candy	Any color, including black
Caramel	Tan to dark brown
Cheese	Light dull yellow, off-white
Cherry	Bright bluish red
Chocolate (cocoa)	Dark reddish brown
Coffee	Tan (liquid); dark brown (beans)
Cream sauce, food	Pastel brown to off-white
Currant	Light dull red, slightly bluish
Egg	Strong reddish yellow
Elderberry	Dark bluish red
Grape	Reddish purple
Honey	Golden yellow
Icing, food	Most pastel except gray
Juleps	Mint green
Ketchup (catsup)	Bright (tomato) red
Leaves	Leaf green
Lemon	Greenish or canary yellow
Licorice	Dark blackish brown
Lime	Bright, strong; slight bluish green
Maple	Golden brown
Mayonnaise	Slight dull or creamy yellow
Mint	Yellow green
Nut	Walnut to golden brown
Orangeade	Bright yellow orange
Orange, fruit	Bright, red orange

Peach	Light, dull gold, dull red
Pistachio	Bright green
Plum	Reddish navy
Prune, fruit	Dark navy
Prune, preserve	Red brown
Quince, fruit	Green, brown (ripe)
Quince, preserve	Dull, orange red
Raspberry	Bright bluish red
Root beer	Golden brown
Sage	Dark bluish green
Sarsaparilla	Golden brown
Sauce, food	Dark (gravy) brown
Strawberry	Bright, bluish pink
Vanilla, concentrated	Dark, yellow brown
Wine	Dark, bluish red, red violet
Whiskey	Golden brown

Chapter IX

STABILIZERS

Stabilizers are substances which are added to another substance to prevent or retard any alteration. Those utilized in compounding flavors and perfumes are of vegetal origin occurring as natural gums.

Gums occur as exudations from various trees and shrubs in tropical areas. They differ from natural resins in their chemical composition and solubility properties. Some contain acidic components, while others are neutral. Their main use is as protective colloids and emulsifying agents in food products and pharmaceuticals, as sizing agents for textiles, and in the electrolytic deposition of metals. They are insoluble in alcohol and other solvents, but are generally soluble, or dispersible, in water.

Seaweeds of cold water, especially brown algae, are also used as stabilizers.

AGAR-AGAR

BOTANICAL: *Family: Rhodophyceae; Genus: Gelidium, Gracilaria, Gigartina; Species: Corneum, Lichenoides, Speciosa*

DERIVATION: Agar is a dried, gelatinous substance obtained by concentration and decoction of seaweeds or marine algae.

Derived from red algae, mostly from the *Gelidium* and *Gracilaria*, they occur in tropical Asia and along the Pacific coast of the U.S. There are four kinds of algae: brown, red, green, and blue-green. Blue-green algae are toxic to fish and other aquatic life. Algae range in size from single cell to giant (over 200 ft) and include many kinds of seaweeds.

Algae are employed as food supplements, soil conditioners, animal feeds, and as a source of iodine.

PROPERTIES: Agar-agar is translucent or pale powder. It is strongly hydrophilic, absorbing 20 times more than its weight of cold water, and forming hard gel at about 40 C

USES: Agar-agar is used in confectionery, meat and poultry, desserts, beverages, ice cream, foods, laxatives, pharmaceuticals, dental impressions, laboratory reagents, photographic emulsions.

ARABIC GUM

SYNONYMS: Acacia gum

BOTANICAL: *Family: Leguminosae; Genus: Acacia; Species: Senegal*

DERIVATION: Exudes from the stems of *Acacia senegal* and other related species
PROPERTIES: Thin flakes, powder, or granules; white or yellowish; almost odorless with a mucilaginous taste; soluble in water, yielding a viscous solution; insoluble in alcohol
USES: Arabic gum is used in food preparation as a thickening agent and colloidal stabilizer; adhesive for multipurpose use in textile, printing, ink, pharmaceuticals, and cosmetics

BEAN GUMS, LOCUST

BOTANICAL: *Family: Leguminosae; Genus: Robinia* (black); *Species: Pseudoacacia; Kelseyi; Neomexican* (New Mexico); *Viscosa* (clammy)
DERIVATION: From the long locust pods which are filled with wax-coated seeds
PROPERTIES: It swells in cold water with increasing viscosity on heating; insoluble in organic solvents
USES: Food stabilizer, thickener, emulsifier; cosmetics; sizing and finishes for textiles; pharmaceuticals; paints.

CARRAGEEN

SYNONYMS: Irish moss
BOTANICAL: *Family: Gigartinaceae; Genus: Chondrus; Species: Crispus*
DERIVATION: Extracted from a phycocolloid (algae) called "carrageen" or "Irish moss" in the red algae (*Chondrus* and several species). Growing in rocky places off Great Britain, Ireland, east coast of southern Canada, New England, and southern New Jersey.
PROPERTIES: It is hydrophilic and readily absorbs water
USES: Emulsifier in food products, especially chocolate milk; toothpastes; cosmetics; pharmaceuticals

GUAR GUM

BOTANICAL: *Family: Leguminosae; Genus: Cyamopsis; Species: Tetragonoloba*
DERIVATION: From the *Cyamopsis tetragonoloba*, cultivated in Pakistan for livestock feeding.

The water-soluble part of the flowers (85%) is called "guaran," which consists of 35% galactose and 63% mannose.

PROPERTIES: White or yellowish powder. It is soluble in water with a thickening power 5–8 times greater than starch.
USES: The seeds contain a chemical compound called "mannolagactan" used in foods, cosmetics, pharmaceuticals; thickener; emulsifier; paper manufacture.

KARAYA GUM

SYNONYMS: Sterculia gum; Indian tragacanth
BOTANICAL: *Family: Sterculiaceae; Genus: Sterculia; Species: Urens*
DERIVATION: Exudes from Indian trees of the genus *Sterculia*
PROPERTIES: White to dark brown or black. Its viscosity decreases over six months storage. It forms a translucent colloidal gel in water.
USES: Ice cream and other food products; adhesives; thickener; emulsifier; toothpastes.

PECTIN

DESCRIPTION: From "pektos," a Greek word meaning "congealed." Pectin is a substance found in many fruits and vegetables which yield pectin when boiled. It is a white amorphous carbohydrate substance that forms a gelatinous mass in the cooking of fruits or vegetables, causing gelation.

EXTRACTION: *Extraction Method from Juice:* (1) Use filtered clear juice; (2) Add double volume of alcohol 95%; (3) Precipitate in a gelatinous mass; (4) Filter through linen or canvas; (5) Press; (6) Dry; (7) Dissolve in distilled water; (8) Filter several times; (9) Add hydrochloric acid*; (10) Precipitate again with alcohol 95%.

Extraction from Dry Peels of Fruits: (1) Use raw shredded or dry stored peels; (2) Add distilled water; (3) Boil in a stainless steel vessel; (4) Add diluted hydrochloric acid or sulfuric acid*; (5) Heat at 93–100 C for one hour; (6) Yields water-soluble pectin.

Pectic Acid Extraction: (1) Use ripe fruit washed with a sodium hydroxide solution; (2) Dry; (3) Wash with isopropyl alcohol; (4) Dry; (5) Add hydrogen chloride alcoholic solution (10%); (6) Dry; (7) Wash again with isopropyl alcohol; (8) Dry.

Extraction of Pectin from Lemon Fruit: (1) Use lemon rinds, boiling in several changes of alcohol; (2) Heat in an autoclave for one hour at 110 C in presence of distilled water; (3) Filter; (4) Precipitate using double volume of acidified alcohol; (5) Remove acidity by washing with alcohol or ether; (6) Dry in a vacuum dessicator over sulfuric acid.

Extraction of Pectin from Orange Fruit: (1) Boil oranges in a reflux condenser, eight times for 20 min each time; (2) Add 6 liters of alcohol 95%; (3) Press the mass between each boiling; (4) Add 3 liters of distilled water to the final press cake; (5) Heat the mixture in autoclave for one hour at 110 C; (6) Press; (7) Filter until clear; (8) Add double volume of alcohol 95% with 7 ml of concentrated hydrochloric acid* per liter; (9) Press the coagulum in a cloth; (10) Wash the pectin with ether; (11) Dry in a vacuum dessicator over sulfuric acid; Yield: 20% of pectin

Pectin General Preparation: (A) (1) Use mass; (2) Add hot diluted acid (Cu, Al metal salts) at 70–90 C; (3) Precipitate by adding ethyl or isopropyl alcohol; (4) Wash with distilled water to remove the metal; (5) Dry; (6) Pulverize.

(B) (1) Use mass; (2) Add hot distilled water (acidified); (3) Precipitate by adding Al salts; (4) Dry at low temperature; (5) Pulverize.

(C) (1) Use mass; (2) Add water; (3) Filter; (4) Concentrate; (5) Precipitate by adding alcohol; (6) Recover alcohol.

(D) (1) Use mass; (2) Add diluted acid; (3) Dehydrate by evaporation; (4) Precipitate by adding alcohol or acetone.

---

* The acidification by concentrated hydrochloric or sulfuric acid should be 7 ml of either acid per liter of alcohol used. The adding of acids, particularly the sulfuric, must be done slowly, in small amounts, with stirring. Protection of hands and eyes is necessary.

TRAGACANTH GUM

SYNONYMS: Gum dragon

BOTANICAL: *Family: Leguminosae; Genus: Astragalus; Species: Gummifer*

OCCURRENCE: Southwestern Europe, Greece, Turkey, Iran

DERIVATION: Exudes from the stems of the *Astragalus gummifer* and other *Astragalus* genus plants

PROPERTIES: Dull white, translucent plates or yellowish powder. Strongly hydrophilic. It swells in water. It contains bassorin, pectin, and starch.

USES: Emulsifying agent; thickener for food, ice cream, desserts; toothpastes; soap chips and powders; hair wave preparations; adhesives; leather dressing; textile printing and sizing; pharmaceutical emulsions; cigar making.

Chapter X:

FORMULARY OF PERFUMES

NOTE:

A. All formulas are specified by the name of each perfume. If the formula is prevalently made with natural products, such as essential oils, it is called "imitation." If the formula is prevalently made with chemical products, it is called "synthetic."

B. The amount of each ingredient in all formulas is by weight (g).

C. All formulas are alphabetically listed, including their ingredients. The solvents (ethyl alcohol—95% and distilled water) are included at the end of each formula.

D. Ingredients denoted by an asterisk (*) are formulas which may be found in this book.

E. The polysolvent for the perfumes is:

1.	Propylene Glycol	500
2.	Triton	250
3.	Tween	250
		1000

ACACIA

1.	Acetophenone	50
2.	Alcohol C-9	12
3.	Alcohol C-10	5
4.	Alcohol C-11	5
5.	Aldehyde C-9	13
6.	Aldehyde C-10	5
7.	Aldehyde C-14	5
8.	Aldehyde C-18	5
9.	Anethole	125
10.	Anisaldehyde	125
11.	Bergamot, Oil	50
12.	Bromostyrol	10
13.	Geranium, Oil	100
14.	Hydroxycinnamic Aldehyde	10
15.	Ionone	25
16.	Isobutyl Benzoate	200
17.	Jasmine, Oil	25
18.	Linalool	25
19.	Methyl Anthranilate	25
20.	Musk Ketone	30
21.	Musk Xylene	30
22.	β-Naphthol Methyl Ether	10
23.	Nerolin	15
24.	Phenyl Acetic Aldehyde	15
25.	Styrax	15
26.	Terpineol	50
27.	Vanillin	5
28.	Vetiverol, Oil	10
		1000

ACETIC ACID, TINCTURE

1.	Glacial Acetic Acid	10
2.	Ethyl Alcohol 95%	990
		1000

ALPESTRINE, PERFUME

1.	Lavender, Oil	30
2.	Lavandin, Oil	50
3.	Rosemary, Oil	40
4.	Sage, Oil	30
5.	Spike, Oil	50
6.	Ethyl Alcohol 95%	400
7.	Distilled Water	400
		1000

AMBER, BASE

1.	Aldehyde C-8	60
2.	Aldehyde C-9	200
3.	Aldehyde C-10	150
4.	Aldehyde C-12	90
5.	Ethyl Alcohol 95%	500
		1000

AMBER, CONCRETE (FIXATIVE)

1.	Balsam Tolu	100
2.	Benzyl Benzoate	500
3.	Jasmine, Oil	10
4.	Labdanum, Resinoid	250
5.	Musk Ambrette	40
6.	Oakmoss, Oil	50
7.	Vanillin	50
		1000

AMBER, LIQUID (CHYPRE BASIS)

1.	Benzyl Benzoate	500
2.	Clary Sage	175
3.	Musk Ambrette	125
4.	Musk Xylol	50
5.	Oakmoss, Oil	150
		1000

* Formulas which appear in this book

AMBERGRIS, PERFUME IMITATION NO. 1

1.	Amber, Base*	70
2.	Ambergris, Tincture*	500
3.	Musk Ambrette	100
4.	Rose, Oil	20
5.	Vanilla, Oil	10
6.	Ethyl Alcohol 95%	300
		1000

AMBERGRIS, PERFUME IMITATION NO. 2

1.	Benzoin	125
2.	Castor, Oil	125
3.	Civet	125
4.	Jasmine, Oil	10
5.	Labdanum, Oil	50
6.	Musk	125
7.	Oakmoss, Oil	50
8.	Peru Balsam	125
9.	Rose, Oil	10
10.	Storax	125
11.	Tolu Balsam	125
12.	Vanillin	5
		1000

AMBERGRIS, TINCTURE

1.	Ambergris	100
2.	Ethyl Alcohol 95%	900
		1000

Macerate for a three-month period. Filter.

BERGAMMONIA, DISINFECTANT

1.	Ammonia	100
2.	Bergamot	500
3.	Limonene	100
4.	Terpineyl Acetate	100
5.	Ethyl Alcohol 95%	200
		1000

BERGAMOT, ESSENCE (NATURAL) NO. 1

1.	Bergamot, Oil	300
2.	Limonene	300
3.	Linalool	60
4.	Linalyl Acetate	300
5.	Terpinyl Acetate	40
		1000

BERGAMOT, ESSENCE (NATURAL) NO. 2

1.	Bergamot, Oil	430
2.	Bois de Rose, Oil	80
3.	Geranyl Acetate	30
4.	Linalyl Acetate	150
5.	Nerolin	10
6.	Petitgrain, Paraguay	20
7.	Terpineol	190
8.	Terpinyl Acetate	90
		1000

BOUQUET, NO. 1 (FOR SOAP)

1.	Bergamot, Oil	325
2.	Clove, Oil	25
3.	Geranium, Oil	200
4.	Gingergrass, Oil	150
5.	Lemongrass, Oil	75
6.	Methyl Anthranilate	60
7.	Musk Xylene	40
8.	Patchouli, Oil	75
9.	Styrax	50
		1000

BOUQUET, NO. 2 (FOR SOAP)

1.	Aldehyde C-10 (10% sol'n.)	25
2.	Linalool	300
3.	Linalyl Acetate	100
4.	Methyl Anthranilate	100
5.	Orange (Sweet), Oil	125
6.	Phenyl Ethyl Alcohol	350
		1000

BOUVARDIA

1.	Acetyl Isoeugenol	5
2.	Alcohol C-9	2
3.	Aldehyde C-9	5
4.	Aldehyde C-10	6
5.	Aldehyde C-12	3
6.	Hydroxycitronellal	20
7.	Jasmine, Oil	6
8.	Linalool	50
9.	Methyl Heptyne Carbonate	4
10.	Methyl Ionone	5
11.	Ethyl Alcohol 95%	894
		1000

CALAMUS, IMITATION NO. 1

1.	Benzyl Alcohol (10% sol'n.)	300
2.	Eucalyptol	100
3.	Limonene (10% sol'n.)	300
4.	Phellandrene	50
5.	α-Pinene	50
6.	Terpinyl Acetate	200
		1000

CALAMUS, IMITATION NO. 2

1.	Calamus	800
2.	Calamus, Oil	200
		1000

CAMPHOR, TINCTURE

1.	Camphor	10
2.	Ethyl Alcohol 95%	990
		1000

CANANGA (FOR SOAP)

1.	Bromostyrene	25
2.	Cedarwood, Oil	75
3.	*p*-Cresyl Methyl Ether	25
4.	Geranium Palmarosa, Oil	375
5.	Methyl Anthranilate	50
6.	Musk Xylene	50
7.	Sassafras, Oil	25
8.	Terpineol	375
		1000

CAPSICUM

1.	Capsicum, Oleoresin (10% sol'n.)	750
2.	Cotton Seeds, Oil	200
3.	Paprika, Oleoresin	50
		1000

CARNATION, IMITATION NO. 1

1.	Cinnamon, Oil	55
2.	Clary Sage	30
3.	Eugenol	100
4.	Heliotropin	50
5.	Hydroxycitronellal	30
6.	α-Ionone	20
7.	Isoeugenol (10% sol'n.)	400
8.	Methyl Isoeugenol	100
9.	Musk	50
10.	Neroli, Oil	50
11.	Pimento, Oil	50
12.	Rose, Oil	30
13.	Vanillin	5
14.	Ylang Ylang, Oil	30
		1000

CARNATION, IMITATION NO. 2

1.	Cinnamon, Oil	10
2.	Clary Sage, Oil	40
3.	Eugenol	150
4.	Heliotropin	100
5.	Hydroxycitronellal	40
6.	α-Ionone	10
7.	Isoeugenol	150
8.	Methyl Isoeugenol	150
9.	Neroli, Oil	100
10.	Pimento, Oil	150
11.	Rose, Oil (10% sol'n.)	60
12.	Ylang Ylang, Oil	40
		1000

CARNATION (FOR SOAP)

1.	Benzyl Acetate	75
2.	Benzyl Benzoate	30
3.	Cananga, Oil	250
4.	Cinnamon, Oil	10
5.	Eugenol	500
6.	Heliotropin	20
7.	Nutmeg, Concrete	20
8.	Nutmeg, Oil	20
9.	Orris, Absolute	50
10.	Rose, Oil	5
11.	Ylang Ylang, Oil	20
		1000

CARNATION, PINK (PERFUME)

1.	Alcohol C-7	2
2.	Alcohol C-9	2
3.	Aldehyde C-8	1
4.	Aldehyde C-9	1
5.	Amyl Salicylate	1
6.	Bay, Oil	5
7.	Benzyl Isoeugenol	5
8.	Cinnamon, Oil	1
9.	Clary Sage, Oil	2
10.	Coumarin	5
11.	Heliotropin	5
12.	Hydroxycitronellal	2
13.	α-Ionone	1
14.	Isobutyl Phenyl Acetate	1
15.	Isoeugenol	45
16.	Musk Ambrette	4
17.	Neroli, Oil	5
18.	Rose, Oil	3
19.	Terpineol	45
20.	Vanillin	2
21.	Ylang ylang	2
22.	Ethyl Alcohol 95%	860
		1000

CASTOR, TINCTURE NO. 1

1.	Castor, Brown (finely cut)	80
2.	Ethyl Alcohol 95%	920
		1000

CASTOR, TINCTURE NO. 2

1.	Castor, Brown (finely cut)	486
2.	Ethyl Alcohol 95%	514
		1000

CEDRELA, "WOOD TYPE"

1.	Cedarwood, Oil	5
2.	Geranium, Oil	2
3.	Patchouli, Oil	1
4.	Sandalwood, Oil	2
5.	Ethyl Alcohol 95%	990
		1000

CITRONELLA (FOR SOAP)

1.	Benzaldehyde	25
2.	Bergamot, Oil	200
3.	Caraway, Oil	225
4.	Citronella, Oil	275
5.	Geranium Palmarosa, Oil	225
6.	Musk Xylene	25
7.	Terpineol	25
		1000

COCONUT, EXTRACT (NATURAL)

1.	Coconut, Rasped (pulp fresh, not rancid)	10	kg
2.	Ethyl Alcohol 95%	30	l

Macerate for 10 days, stirring each day for 1 h. Collect, without pressure,20 l of extract. To the residue add:

3.	Distilled Water	20	l

Let stand for another 3 days, and add:

4.	Aldehyde C-18	1	ml
5.	Amyl Formate	45	ml
6.	Ethyl Oenanthate	24	ml
7.	Vanilla Beans, Tincture	100	ml

Distill altogether.
Yield: 40 liters

COCONUT, PASTE

1.	Coconut (desiccated fine powder	4	kg
2.	Corn Syrup	3	kg
3.	Creme, Fondant (80% sugar + 20% distilled water)	2	kg
4.	Milk, Condensed Sweet	2	kg
5.	Sugar	10	kg

Mix milk and syrup (#2 and 3) hot. Stir with desiccated powdered coconut. Cool.

COLOGNE

1.	Bergamot, Oil	200
2.	Lemon, Oil	100
3.	Musk Ambrette	1
4.	Neroli, Oil	20
5.	Orange, Oil	50
6.	Rosemary, Oil	1
7.	Ethyl Alcohol 95%	314
8.	Distilled Water	314
		1000

COLOR BASE STANDARD FORMULA NO. 1

1.	Distilled Water	847	ml
2.	Dyestuff	50	g
3.	Glycerin (28 Bé)	100	ml
4.	Sodium Benzoate	3	g

Heat to 100 C. Dissolve well. Cool. Filter.

COLOR BASE STANDARD FORMULA NO. 2

1.	Color	10	g
2.	Ethyl Alcohol 95%	190	ml
3.	Distilled Water	800	ml

COLOR MIXTURE

		Dye**	g
1.	Cherry	Blue	2.5
		Red	97.5
2.	Green	Blue	10.0
		Yellow	90.0
3.	Orange	Red	10.0
		Yellow	90.0

** The dye, as per the specified amount, must be dissolved as in Color Base Standard Formula No. 2.

4.	Peach	Orange	75.0
		Yellow	25.0
5.	Pineapple	Brown	50.0
	(Ananas)	Peach	50.0
6.	Pomegranate	Red	97.5
		Yellow	2.5
7.	Raspberry	Red	90.0
		Yellow	10.0

COLORS (NATURAL DYES)

1.	Blue	Indigo
2.	Brown	Burnt sugar
3.	Green	Chlorophyll
4.	Red	Malva arborea; berries; cochineal
5.	Yellow	Bixa orellana
6.	Violet	Indigo; cochineal

COVER ODOR, PERFUME NO. 1

1.	Almond, Oil	100
2.	Apricot, Oil	100
3.	Formaldehyde	100
4.	Peach, Oil	100
5.	Propylene Glycol	600
		1000

COVER ODOR, PERFUME NO. 2

1.	Ambergris	20
2.	Castor, Oil	40
3.	Hyacinth, Oil	100
4.	Jasmine, Absolute	100
5.	Lilac, Oil	100
6.	Neroli, Oil	100
7.	Rose, Bulgarian Absolute	100
8.	Tuberose, Oil	100
9.	Violet, Oil	100
10.	Zibet, Oil	40
11.	Ethyl Alcohol 95%	100
12.	Distilled Water	100
		1000

COVER ODOR, PERFUME NO. 3

1.	Anisic Alcohol	15
2.	Benzyl Acetate	15
3.	Benzyl Formate	30
4.	Cinnamic Alcohol	15
5.	Coumarin	84
6.	Ethyl Vanillin	110
7.	Heliotropin	105
8.	Hydroxycitronellal	42
9.	Ionone	6
10.	Linalool	90
11.	Methyl Anthranilate	30
12.	Phenyl Acetic Aldehyde	18
13.	Phenyl Ethyl Alcohol	60
14.	Rhodinol	10
15.	Terpineol	240
16.	Ethyl Alcohol 95%	130
		1000

CYCLAMEN, BASE (SYNTHETIC)

1.	Alcohol C-9	1
2.	Aldehyde C-9	1
3.	Aldehyde C-10	1
4.	Aldehyde C-11	1
5.	Aldehyde C-12	1
6.	Hydroxycitronellal	20
7.	Ionone	25
9.	α-Methyl Benzyl Acetate (garden)	25
10.	Ethyl Alcohol 95%	463
11.	Distilled Water	462
		1000

CYCLAMEN (FOR SOAP)

1.	Amyl Cinnamic Aldehyde	65
2.	Anisaldehyde	85
3.	Cananga, Oil	85
4.	Cyclamen Aldehyde	100
5.	Geraniol	150
6.	Hydroxycitronellal	100
7.	Ionone	85
8.	Musk Xylene	25
9.	Phenyl Acetic Acid	25

10.	Rosewood, Oil	65
11.	Styrax, Resinoid	65
12.	Terpineol	150
		1000

DEODORANT FOR CREAM

1.	Clove, Oil	6
2.	Ethyl Acetate	6
3.	Rose, Oil	28
4.	Ethyl Alcohol 95%	500
5.	Distilled Water	460
		1000

DEODORANT FOR VESSELS

1.	Potatoes, Raw Smashed (amount depends on the size of the vessel)	1/3
2.	Hot Water (to fill the vessel)	2/3

Let stand for 1 h. Repeat if necessary.

DEODORANT FOR WATER

1.	Magnesia Oxide	30
2.	Rose, Tincture	120
3.	Distilled Water, Warm	4000

Filter.

DEODORANTS (MASKING AGENT)

1.	Eucalyptus, Citriodora, Oil	60
2.	Formaldehyde 40%	120
3.	Lemon, Oil	60
4.	Ethyl Alcohol 95%	760
		1000

DEODORANTS (MASKING AGENT) FOR HEAVY ODORS

1.	Pine, Oil	30
2.	Potassium Permanganate	16
3.	Spike Lavender	30
4.	Thymol	160
5.	Isopropyl Alcohol 95%	700
6.	Distilled Water	64
		1000

DEODORANTS (MASKING AGENT) GRASSY ODORS

1.	Ammonia	1
2.	Bergamot, Oil	40
3.	Cineol	20
4.	Citronellol	40
5.	Lemon, Oil	40
6.	Lemongrass, Oil	10
7.	Menthol	20
8.	Thymol	10
9.	Ethyl Alcohol 95%	819
		1000

DIACETYL, TINCTURE

1.	Diacetyl	10
2.	Ethyl Alcohol 95%	990
		1000

EAU DE COLOGNE

1.	Bergamot, Oil	500
2.	Lavender, Oil	40
3.	Lemon, Oil	250
4.	Melissa, Oil	40
5.	Neroli, Oil	40
6.	Ethyl Alcohol 95%	130
		1000

EAU DE COLOGNE (FOR SOAP)

1.	Cedarwood, Oil	100
2.	Cinnamyl Butyrate	30
3.	Citronella, Oil	100
4.	Clove, Oil	50
5.	Diphenyl Oxide	100
6.	Lavender, Oil	100
7.	Linalyl Acetate	50

8.	Musk Xylene	30
9.	Rosewood, Oil	200
10.	Styrax, Resinoid	20
11.	Terpineol	200
12.	Thyme, Oil	20
		1000

EGLANTINE (WILD ROSE)

1.	Anisaldehyde	30
2.	Geraniol	40
3.	Isobutyl Phenyl Acetate	30
4.	Ethyl Alcohol 95%	450
5.	Distilled Water	450
		1000

ESTERS, GENERAL BASE

1.	Amyl Acetate	225
2.	Amyl Butyrate	75
3.	Ethyl Acetate	385
4.	Ethyl Formate	225
5.	Ethyl Alcohol 95%	90
		1000

FENUGREEK, TINCTURE

1.	Fenugreek, Powdered after Roasting	100
2.	Propylene Glycol	225
3.	Ethyl Alcohol 95%	450
4.	Distilled Water	225
		1000

Filter.

FERN (FOR SOAP)

1.	Benzoin, Resinoid	65
2.	Bergamot, Oil	125
3.	Bornyl Acetate	25
4.	Coumarin	125
5.	Geranyl Acetate	85
6.	Lavender	150
7.	Linalool	125
8.	Musk Ketone	125
9.	Oakmoss, Resinoid	65
10.	Patchouli, Oil	25
11.	Terpenyl Isobutyrate	85
		1000

FLORAL FRAGRANCE (FOR SOAP)

1.	Carnation (for Soap)*	100
2.	Jasmine, Oil	100
3.	Lilac, Imitation No. 1*	366
4.	Muguet (Lily of the Valley) Imitation No. 2*	234
5.	Rose, Imitation No. 6*	200
		1000

FLORAL, IMITATION NO. 1

1.	Jasmine, Absolute	100
2.	Muguet, Absolute	200
3.	Orange Flower, Absolute	100
4.	Rose, Absolute (10% sol'n.)	450
5.	Violet, Leaf, Absolute	150
		1000

FLORAL, IMITATION NO. 2

1.	Jonquil, Absolute (10% sol'n.)	500
2.	Muguet, Absolute	200
3.	Rose, Petals	100
4.	Violet, Leaf, Absolute	200
		1000

Note: For Floral, Imitation No. 1 and No. 2, add to each double the amount of ethyl alcohol 95% (1000) and distilled water (1000). Macerate for 5 days and distill over 1800 cc.

FOUGÈRE

1.	Aldehyde C-14 Myristic	30
2.	Bergamot, Oil	75
3.	Labdanum, Resinoid	70
4.	Lavender, Oil	70
5.	Lavender Spike, Oil	240
6.	Oakmoss, Resin	50
7.	Vanillin	30

* Formulas which appear in this book

8.	Ethyl Alcohol 95%	225
9.	Distilled Water	210
		1000

FOUGÈRE, BASE (FERN)

1.	Alcohol C-8	10
2.	Alcohol C-9	30
3.	Aldehyde C-8	5
4.	Aldehyde C-9	5
5.	Aldehyde C-10	5
6.	Aldehyde C-11	50
7.	Aldehyde C-12	25
8.	Ethyl Phenyl Acetate	25
9.	Isobutyl Acetate	15
10.	Lavender	50
11.	Musk Xylene	10
12.	Ethyl Alcohol 95%	770
		1000

FRANGIPANNI, IMITATION NO. 1 (ACUTIFOLIA, ALBA, RUBRA)

1.	Balsam Peru	25
2.	Bergamot, Oil	125
3.	Carnation	125
4.	Cinnamic Alcohol	25
5.	Coumarin	25
6.	Lemon, Oil	125
7.	Lily of the Valley	125
8.	Orange Flower, Oil	125
9.	Terpineol	175
10.	Tuberose	125
		1000

FRANGIPANNI, IMITATION NO. 2

1.	Gardenia	100
2.	Honeysuckle	50
3.	Jasmine	300
4.	Lilac	100
5.	Mimosa	100
6.	Muguet	100
7.	Orange Flowers, Oil	50
8.	Tuberose	100
9.	Ylang Ylang	100
		1000

FRANGIPANNI, IMITATION NO. 3

1.	Ambergris	8
2.	Jasmine, Oil (10% sol'n.)	100
3.	Musk Ambrette	15
4.	Neroli, Oil	1
5.	Orris, Powder	750
6.	Rose, Oil	1
7.	Sandalwood, Oil	1
8.	Sandalwood, Powder	62
9.	Vetiver, Powder	62
		1000

FRANGIPANNI, IMITATION NO. 4

1.	Bergamot, Oil	30
2.	Cassia, Oil	174
3.	Civet	45
4.	Geranium, Palmarosa	40
5.	Musk Ambrette	70
6.	Neroli, Oil	36
7.	Orange, Oil	140
8.	Rose Otto, Tincture (10% sol'n.)	320
9.	Sandalwood, Oil	5
10.	Tonquin, Musk	70
11.	Vanillin	70
		1000

FRESHENER, PERFUME

1.	Eucalyptol, Oil	200
2.	Eugenol, Oil	10
3.	Formaldehyde	70
4.	Methyl Eugenol	20
5.	Ethyl Alcohol 95%	350
6.	Distilled Water	350
		1000

GARDENIA, BASE

1.	Acetate C-9	1
2.	Alcohol C-9	2
3.	Aldehyde C-8	1
4.	Aldehyde C-10	1
5.	Aldehyde C-12	1
6.	Aldehyde C-14 (pure)	2
7.	Aldehyde C-18	2
8.	Amyl Cinnamic Aldehyde	30
9.	Anisyl Acetate	30
10.	Benzyl Acetate	50
11.	Isoamyl Benzyl Ether	10
12.	Linalyl Benzoate	50
13.	Methyl Anthranilate	45
14.	Methyl Heptyne Carbonate	5
15.	Methyl Phenyl Carbinyl Acetate	50
16.	Phenyl Ethyl Acetate	50
17.	Ethyl Alcohol 95%	670
		1000

GERANIUM

1.	Bois De Rose, Oil	250
2.	Geranium Bourbon, Oil	250
3.	Ethyl Alcohol 95%	250
4.	Distilled Water	250
		1000

GERANIUM, IMITATION (FOR SOAP)

1.	Cedarwood, Oil	150
2.	Citronella, Oil	150
3.	Clove, Oil	25
4.	Diphenyl Oxide	75
5.	Linalyl Acetate	75
6.	Musk Xylene	25
7.	Rosewood, Oil	150
8.	Spike Lavender, Oil	150
9.	Styrax, Resinoid	25
10.	Terpineol	150
11.	Thyme	25
		1000

GERANIUM, SYNTHETIC

1.	Citronellol	250
2.	Diphenyl Oxide	100
3.	Geraniol	300
4.	Phenyl Ethyl Alcohol	175
5.	Rosewood, Oil (Bois de Rose)	175
		1000

GINGERGRASS (FOR SOAP)

1.	Cassia, Oil	75
2.	Cedarwood, Oil	150
3.	Clove, Oil	75
4.	Geranium Palmarosa, Oil	225
5.	Gingergrass, Oil	275
6.	Musk Xylene	25
7.	Spike Lavender, Oil	150
8.	Styrax, Resinoid	25
		1000

GIROFLÉ, IMITATION NO. 1

1.	Amyl Salicylate (10% sol'n.)	250
2.	Isobutyl Salicylate (10% sol'n.)	250
3.	Methyl Salicylate (10% sol'n.)	250
4.	Vanillin (10% sol'n.)	250
		1000

GIROFLÉ, IMITATION NO. 2

1.	Amyl Salicylate (10% sol'n.)	150
2.	Benzyl Isoeugenol	50
3.	Benzylidene Acetone	50
4.	Clary Sage	50
5.	Isobutyl Salicylate (10% sol'n.)	150
6.	Linalyl Acetate	50
7.	Methyl Salicylate (10% sol'n.)	150
8.	Musk Ambrette	50
9.	Oak Moss, Resin	50
10.	Vanillin (10% sol'n.)	100
11.	Ylang Ylang, Oil	150
		1000

HALO, SEA SALT ODOR

1.	Aldehyde C-20	20
2.	Coumarin	10
3.	Geranyl Acetate	100

4.	Geranyl Formate	10
5.	Lavender, Oil	450
6.	Linalool, Ex Bois de Rose	120
7.	Linalyl Acetate	230
8.	Musk Xylene	10
9.	Sage, Oil	50
		1000

HAWTHORN

1.	Acetophenone	68
2.	Alcohol C-9	20
3.	Aldehyde C-9	4
4.	Aldehyde C-10	1
5.	Anisaldehyde	200
6.	Benzaldehyde (pure)	2
7.	Benzyl Benzoate	165
8.	Citral	5
9.	Geraniol	400
10.	Methyl Ionone	50
11.	Methyl *p*-Tolyl Ketone	80
12.	Rose, Oil	5
		1000

HAWTHORN (FOR SOAP)

1.	Acetophenone	25
2.	Anisaldehyde	300
3.	Benzaldehyde	1
4.	Benzoin, Resinoid	123
5.	Methyl Ionone	100
6.	Mimosa, Absolute	30
7.	Musk Ambrette	25
8.	Petitgrain	71
9.	Rhodinol	300
10.	Rose, Oil	25
		1000

HELIOTROPE (FOR SOAP)

1.	Aldehyde C-18	5
2.	Anisaldehyde	5
3.	Anisic Alcohol	45
4.	Benzyl Acetate	45
5.	Cinnamic Alcohol	50
6.	Coumarin	40
7.	Heliotropin	175
8.	Hydroxycitronellal	5
9.	α-Ionone	80
10.	Methoxy Acetophenone	5
11.	Musk Ketone	30
12.	Phenyl Ethyl Alcohol	150
13.	Rhodinol	150
14.	Vanillin	175
15.	Ylang Ylang, Oil	40
		1000

HERBAL BASE, "GOLD WATER"

1.	Angelic Root, Oil	16
2.	Basil, Oil	34
3.	Caraway, Oil	34
4.	Cherry, Essence (Natural)*	115
5.	Cinnamon, Oil	34
6.	Clove Flowers, Oil	34
7.	Coriander, Oil	34
8.	Fennel Seeds, Oil	34
9.	Lemon, Oil	16
10.	Mandarin, Oil	34
11.	Marjoram, Oil	50
12.	Orange (Bitter), Oil	50
13.	Peppermint, Oil	16
14.	Rose, Oil	16
15.	Star Anise, Oil	150
16.	Sugar	100
17.	Ethyl Alcohol 95%	233
		1000

HIP, EXTRACT (NATURAL)

1.	Hips, Crushed	10 kg
2.	Ethyl Alcohol 95%	10 l
3.	Distilled Water	10 l

Macerate for 3 days. Express, and to the residue add:

4.	Distilled Water	20 l

Let stand for another 3 days. Add:

5.	Amyl Valerianate	5 ml
6.	Ethyl Acetate	45 ml

Distill altogether.
Yield: 40 liters

* Formulas which appear in this book

HIP, IMITATION NO. 1

1.	Amyl Acetate	240
2.	Amyl Butyrate	250
3.	Anisaldehyde	5
4.	Butyric Acid	6
5.	Clove, Oil	3
6.	Ethyl Acetate	240
7.	Ethyl Valerianate	250
8.	Heliotropin	5
9.	Rose, Oil	1
		1000

HONEY, SYNTHETIC (FOR PERFUME)

1.	Acetophenone	10
2.	Diisobutyl Pyrocatechol Ketal (10% sol'n.)	750
3.	Methyl Ionone	60
4.	Phenyl Acetic Acid (10% sol'n.)	30
5.	Rose Oil (1% sol'n.)	150
		1000

HONEYSUCKLE

1.	Alcohol C-9	5
2.	Aldehyde C-9	10
3.	Aldehyde C-12, MNA	20
4.	Amyl Cinnamic Aldehyde	10
5.	Benzyl Acetate	100
6.	Citronellyl Propionate	15
7.	Dimethyl Benzyl Carbinyl Acetate	15
8.	Geraniol	200
9.	Heliotropin	10
10.	Hydroxycitronellal	100
11.	Jasmine (10% sol'n.)	50
12.	Linalool	100
13.	Linalyl Acetate	50
14.	Methyl Anthranilate	100
15.	Methyl Heptyne Carbonate	1
16.	Narcissus, Absolute	50
17.	Phenyl Ethyl Alcohol	34
18.	Phenyl Ethyl Isobutyrate	15
19.	Rhodinol	100
20.	Rose Oil (10% sol'n.)	10
21.	Vanillin	5
		1000

HYACINTH

1.	Alcohol C-8	10
2.	Aldehyde C-8	5
3.	Aldehyde C-10	5
4.	Benzyl Alcohol	100
5.	Bromostyrol	25
6.	Cinnamic Alcohol	25
7.	Phenyl Acetic Aldehyde	150
8.	Phenyl Ethyl Formate	25
9.	Phenyl Propyl Alcohol	50
10.	Terpineol	25
11.	Ethyl Alcohol 95%	290
12.	Distilled Water	290
		1000

IONONE

1.	Acetone	500
2.	Citral or Lemongrass	250
3.	Sodium Hydroxide	250
		1000

Stir for 72 h. Let stand. Separate the liquid's layers. Distill the reddish-brown layer.

IRIS

1.	Orris, Concrete	50
2.	Orris, Oil	100
3.	Methylionone (10% sol'n.)	840
4.	Santalyl Acetate	10
		1000

IRIS, SYNTHETIC

1.	Alcohol C-9	10
2.	Alcohol C-10	10
3.	Aldehyde C-9	10
4.	Aldehyde C-10	5
5.	Aldehyde C-12	5
6.	Anisaldehyde	25
7.	Cuminic Aldehyde	25
8.	α-Irone	60
9.	Methyl Ionone	100
10.	Ethyl Alcohol 95%	375
11.	Distilled Water	375
		1000

JASMINE (FOR BRILLIANTINE)

1.	α-Amylcinnamic Aldehyde (10% sol'n.)	380
2.	Benzyl Acetate (10% sol'n.)	250
3.	Benzyl Propionate	20
4.	Cinnamic Alcohol	100
5.	Cyclamen, Oil	20
6.	Jasmine, Concrete	20
7.	Linalool	50
8.	Musk Ambrette	30
9.	Neroli, Oil	50
10.	Orange Flower, Oil	30
11.	Terpineol	50
		1000

JASMINE "GRANDIFLORA"

1.	Acetate C-8	5
2.	Acetate C-10	5
3.	Alcohol C-7	5
4.	Alcohol C-8	5
5.	Alcohol C-9	5
6.	Aldehyde C-8	5
7.	Aldehyde C-10	5
8.	Aldehyde C-11	5
9.	Amyl Cinnamic Aldehyde	5
10.	Amyl Alcohol	50
11.	Benzyl Acetate	160
12.	Benzyl Alcohol	100
13.	Benzyl Butyrate	160
14.	Benzyl Formate	50
15.	Benzyl Isobutyrate	50
16.	Benzyl Propionate	50
17.	Citral	21
18.	Dimethyl Benzyl Carbinol	50
19.	Dimethyl Benzyl Carbinyl Acetate	50
20.	Ethyl Anthranilate	27
21.	Hexyl Cinnamic Aldehyde	5
22.	Hydroxycitronellal	5
23.	Indole	5
24.	Isojasmone	12
25.	Linalool	12
26.	Linalyl Acetate	12
27.	Methyl Anthranilate	15
28.	Methyl Benzoate	12
29.	Methyl-*p*-Cresol	12
30.	Phenoxy Ethyl Isobutyrate	12
31.	Phenyl Ethyl Alcohol	25
32.	Phenyl Ethyl Isobutyrate	12
33.	Phenyl Ethyl Phenyl Acetate	12
34.	Phenyl Propyl Acetate	12
35.	Phenyl Propyl Alcohol	12
36.	Phenyl Propyl Aldehyde	12
		1000

* Formulas which appear in this book

JASMINE, IMITATION NO. 1

1.	α-Amylcinnamic Aldehyde	200
2.	Benzyl Acetate	300
3.	Benzyl Alcohol	100
4.	Benzyl Chloroacetate	100
5.	Benzyl Formate	30
6.	Benzyl Propionate	20
7.	Methyl Anthranilate	50
8.	Phenyl Allylic Alcohol	100
9.	Phenyl Ethyl Acetate	100
		1000

JASMINE, IMITATION NO. 2

1.	Jasmine, Absolute (10% sol'n.)	500
2.	Jasmine, Imitation No. 1*	500
		1000

JASMINE, IMITATION NO. 3 (FOR SOAP)

1.	Amyl Cinnamic Aldehyde	75
2.	Benzyl Acetate	250
3.	Benzyl Phenyl Acetate	75
4.	Hydroxycitronellal	250
5.	Indole	15
6.	Jasmine, Absolute	50
7.	Methyl Ionone	75
8.	Orris, Concrete	10
9.	Phenyl Ethyl Alcohol	125
10.	Ylang Ylang, Oil	75
		1000

JASMINE, INFUSION

1.	Jasmine, Fresh Flowers	1 kg
2.	Ethyl Alcohol 95%	500 ml

3.	Distilled Water	500 ml
4.	Indole (10% sol'n.)	10 ml

Let stand until the odor is well developed. Express and filter.

Yield: 1 liter

JASMINE, SYNTHETIC NO. 1

1.	Alcohol C-8	30
2.	Alcohol C-10	25
3.	Aldehyde C-10	40
4.	Benzyl Acetate	25
5.	Benzyl Butyrate	25
6.	Linalool	25
7.	Indole	10
8.	Ionone	5
9.	Methyl Anthranilate	25
10.	Ethyl Alcohol 95%	395
11.	Distilled Water	395
		1000

JASMINE, SYNTHETIC NO. 2

1.	Alcohol C-10	10
2.	Aldehyde C-10	12
3.	Amyl Cinnamic Aldehyde	40
4.	Benzyl Acetate	25
5.	Benzyl Propionate	2
6.	Cinnamic Alcohol	10
7.	Cyclamen Aldehyde	10
8.	Linalool	5
9.	Musk Ambrette	3
10.	Neroli, Oil	3
11.	Terpineol	5
12.	Ethyl Alcohol 95%	438
13.	Distilled Water	437
		1000

JASMINE, SYNTHETIC NO. 3

1.	Benzyl Acetate	650
2.	Benzyl Alcohol	60
3.	Indole	30
4.	Linalool	150
5.	Linalyl Acetate	70
6.	Methyl Anthranilate	10
7.	Phenyl Ethyl Alcohol	30
		1000

JASMINE, SYNTHETIC NO. 4

1.	Benzyl Acetate	300
2.	Benzyl Alcohol	300
3.	Benzyl Formate	150
4.	Benzyl Propionate	150
5.	Geraniol	25
6.	Linalool	35
7.	Menthyl Anthranilate	20
8.	Musk Ketone	10
9.	Paracresol	10
		1000

JASMINE, SYNTHETIC NO. 5

1.	β-Acetophenone	50
2.	α-Amyl Cinnamic Aldehyde Dimethyl Acetal	200
3.	Benzyl Acetate	300
4.	Benzyl Salicylate	20
5.	Cinnamic Alcohol	30
6.	Hydroxycitronellal	60
7.	Indole (10% sol'n.)	50
8.	Linalool	100
9.	Linalyl Acetate	30
10.	Methyl Amyl Pyrocatechol Ketal	60
11.	Phenyl Ethyl Alcohol	100
		1000

JASMINE, SYNTHETIC NO. 6

1.	α-Amyl Cinnamic Aldehyde	100
2.	Benzyl Acetate	150
3.	Benzyl Alcohol	100
4.	Benzyl Formate	20
5.	Benzyl Propionate	20
6.	α-Ionone	20
7.	Methyl Anthranilate	30
8.	Phenyl Ethyl Acetate	30
9.	Phenyl Ethyl Alcohol	30
10.	Rhodinol	10
11.	Ethyl Alcohol 95%	245
12.	Distilled Water	245
		1000

JONQUIL (DAFFODIL), IMITATION

1.	Alcohol C-9	8
2.	Aldehyde C-8	3
3.	Aldehyde C-9	7
4.	Benzyl Salicylate	75
5.	Cinnamic Alcohol	25
6.	Coumarin	25
7.	Hydroxycitronellal	32
8.	Jasmine, Oil	125
9.	Lilac, Imitation	25
10.	Linalool	25
11.	Methyl Ionone	12
12.	Methyl Isoeugenol	8
13.	Musk Ketone	33
14.	Nerol	25
15.	Neroli, Oil	25
16.	Patchouli, Oil	12
17.	Phenyl Acetaldehyde Dimethyl Acetal	15
18.	Phenyl Ethyl Acetate	125
19.	Phenyl Ethyl Alcohol	75
20.	Sandalwood, Oil	30
21.	Styrax, Resinoid	13
22.	Ylang Ylang, Oil	35
23.	Ethyl Alcohol 95%	242
		1000

JONQUIL (DAFFODIL), SYNTHETIC

1.	Benzyl Benzoate	150
2.	Cinnamic Acid	150
3.	Indole (10% sol'n.)	100
4.	Linalool	100
5.	Methyl Anthranilate	100
6.	Methyl Benzoate	150
7.	Methyl Cinnamate	150
8.	Phenyl Acetaldehyde Dimethyl Acetal	50
9.	Phenyl Ethyl Phenyl Acetal	50
		1000

LAVENDER, ESSENCE (NATURAL)

1.	Bergamot, Oil	150
2.	Clove, Oil	10
3.	Lavender, Oil	800
4.	Linalyl Acetate	10
5.	Neroli, Oil	10
6.	Patchouli, Oil	10
7.	Rose, Oil	10
		1000

LAVENDER, IMITATION NO. 1

1.	Citronellol	190
2.	Geraniol	150
3.	Geranyl Acetate	70
4.	Heptyl Alcohol (Alcohol C-7)	10
5.	Lavendin (40% sol'n.)	500
6.	Linalyl Acetate (75% sol'n.)	80
		1000

LAVENDER, IMITATION NO. 2

1.	Bergamot, Oil	150
2.	Clary Sage, Oil	5
3.	Clove, Oil	7
4.	Geranyl Benzoate	5
5.	Lavender, Oil (10% sol'n.)	800
6.	Linalool	5
7.	Linalyl Acetate	5
8.	Linalyl Butyrate	5
9.	Methyl Amyl Ketone	5
10.	Neroli, Oil	3
11.	Patchouli, Oil	3
12.	Rose, Oil	7
		1000

LAVENDER, IMITATION NO. 3

1.	Cedarwood, Oil (10% sol'n.)	460
2.	Lavender, Oil (10% sol'n.)	500
3.	Musk Ambrette	20

4.	Musk Xylol	10
5.	Oak Moss, Resin Extract	10
		1000

LAVENDER, IMITATION NO. 4

1.	Citronellyl Acetate	30
2.	Lavandin (10% sol'n.)	270
3.	Lavender 40/42 (10% sol'n.)	440
4.	Linalyl Acetate (10% sol'n.)	230
5.	Octyl Acetate	30
		1000

LAVENDER, IMITATION NO. 5

1.	Citronellyl Acetate	180
2.	Geraniol	70
3.	Lavandin (10% sol'n.)	750
		1000

LAVENDER, IMITATION NO. 6

1.	Aspic (*Lavandula spica*)	60
2.	Lavandin (10% sol'n.)	250
3.	Marjoram	30
4.	Musk Xylene	10
5.	Petitgrain	10
6.	Sage	30
7.	Terpinolene (10% sol'n.)	300
8.	Vanillin (10% sol'n.)	10
9.	Ethyl Alcohol 95%	300
		1000

LAVENDER, IMITATION NO. 7

1.	Citronellyl Acetate	60
2.	Lavender 40/42 (10% sol'n.)	520
3.	Linalyl Acetate	130
4.	Spike, Oil	160
5.	Terpinyl Acetate	130
		1000

* Formulas which appear in this book

LAVENDER, IMITATION NO. 8

1.	Geranyl Acetate	200
2.	Heliotropine	70
3.	Isobornyl Acetate	20
4.	Lavender (10% sol'n.)	300
5.	Linalyl Acetate	150
6.	Linalyl Formate	30
7.	Musk Ambrette	40
8.	Terpineol	100
9.	Terpinyl Acetate	80
10.	Vanillin (10% sol'n.)	10
		1000

LAVENDER, IMITATION NO. 9

1.	Geranyl Acetate (10% sol'n.)	250
2.	Geranyl Formate	15
3.	Linalool (10% sol'n.)	220
4.	Linalyl Acetate (10% sol'n.)	500
5.	Nonyl Acetate	5
6.	Vanillin (10% sol'n.)	10
		1000

LAVENDER, IMITATION NO. 10

1.	Lavender, Imitation No. 8*	475
2.	Lavender, Imitation No. 9*	375
3.	Musk Xylol (10% sol'n.)	150
		1000

LAVENDER, IMITATION NO. 11

1.	Alcohol C-9	25
2.	Aldehyde C-10	25
3.	Clary Sage, Oil	200
4.	Coumarin	50
5.	Geranyl Acetate	100
6.	Geranyl Benzoate	100
7.	Linalool	100
8.	Linalyl Acetate	100
9.	Linalyl Butyrate	100
10.	Terpinyl Acetate	100
11.	Terpinyl Propionate	100
		1000

LAVENDER, IMITATION NO. 12 (FOR SOAP)

1.	Benzyl Acetate	40
2.	Bergamot, Oil	125
3.	Borneol	30
4.	Coumarin	30
5.	Geranium, Oil	200
6.	Lavender, Oil	200
7.	Musk Xylene	25
8.	Patchouli, Oil	40
9.	Rosemary, Oil	60
10.	Spike, Oil	200
11.	Thyme, Oil	50
		1000

LAVENDER, SWEET

1.	Bergamot, Oil	110
2.	Citral	10
3.	Coumarin	10
4.	Geranyl Acetate	20
5.	α-Ionone	20
6.	Isobornyl Acetate	50
7.	Lavender, Oil	110
8.	Linalyl Acetate	50
9.	Musk Ketone	10
10.	Pine, White Oil	10
11.	Terpinyl Acetate	10
12.	Ethyl Alcohol 95%	295
13.	Distilled Water	295
		1000

LEATHER

1.	Amyl Salicylate	50
2.	Balsam Peru	100
3.	Birch Tar Rectified	100
4.	Coumarin	30
5.	Methyl Salicylate	50
6.	Ethyl Alcohol 95%	335
7.	Distilled Water	335
		1000

LILAC, IMITATION NO. 1

1.	Anisic Aldehyde	10
2.	Benzyl Acetate	30
3.	Benzyl Alcohol	40
4.	Benzyl Formate	10
5.	Benzyl Salicylate	10
6.	Cananga, Oil	40
7.	Cinnamic Alcohol	100
8.	*p*-Cresyl Acetate	10
9.	Cuminic Aldehyde	10
10.	Decyl Alcohol	10
11.	Farnesol	10
12.	Heliotropin	60
13.	Hydroxycitronellal	150
14.	Isoeugenol	10
15.	Methyl Anthranilate	10
16.	Linalool	40
17.	Phenylacetaldehyde	10
18.	Phenyl Ethyl Acetate	50
19.	Phenyl Ethyl Alcohol	150
20.	Phenylpropyl Acetate	40
21.	Rose, Oil	10
22.	Terpineol	150
23.	*p*-Tolyl Aldehyde	10
24.	Tuberose, Oil	20
25.	Vanillin (10% sol'n.)	10
		1000

LILAC, IMITATION NO. 2

1.	Anisic Aldehyde	140
2.	Benzyl Alcohol	110
3.	Citronellol	150
4.	α-Ionone	10
5.	Musk Ketone	10
6.	Phenylacetaldehyde	10
7.	Phenyl Ethyl Alcohol (10% sol'n.)	200
8.	Terpineol	350
9.	Tuberose, Oil	10
10.	Vanillin (10% sol'n.)	10
		1000

LILAC, IMITATION NO. 3

1.	Anisic Alcohol	40
2.	Benzaldehyde (pure, 10% sol'n.)	10
3.	Cananga, Oil	20
4.	Cinnamic Alcohol	150

5.	Heliotropin	50
6.	Hydroxycitronellal (10% sol'n.)	230
7.	Neroli	100
8.	Phenyl Ethyl Alcohol (10% sol'n.)	250
9.	Terpineol	150
		1000

LILAC, IMITATION NO. 4

1.	Benzyl Benzoate (10% sol'n.)	275
2.	Benzyl Formate (10% sol'n.)	275
3.	Cananga, Oil	30
4.	Cinnamic Alcohol	30
5.	Hydroxycitronellal	100
6.	Linalool	120
7.	Phenyl Ethyl Alcohol	100
8.	Terpineol	70
		1000

LILAC, IMITATION NO. 5

1.	Benzoin	100
2.	Cananga, Oil	80
3.	Hydroxycitronellal	150
4.	Musk Ketone	20
5.	Terpineol (10% sol'n.)	600
6.	Vanillin (10% sol'n.)	50
		1000

LILAC, IMITATION NO. 6

1.	Benzyl Benzoate	150
2.	Lilac, Imitation No 1*	140
3.	Lilac, Imitation No. 2*	140
4.	Lilac, Imitation No. 3*	140
5.	Lilac, Imitation No. 4*	140
6.	Lilac, Imitation No. 5	140
7.	Terpineol	150
		1000

LILAC, IMITATION NO. 7

1.	Dimethyl Benzyl Carbinol	50
2.	Heliotropin	10
3.	Hydroxycitronellal	100
4.	Phenyl Ethyl Alcohol	350
5.	Terpineol	200
6.	Vanillin	5
7.	Ylang Ylang, Oil	285
		1000

* Formulas which appear in this book

LILAC, IMITATION NO. 8

1.	Benzoin	50
2.	Heliotropin	10
3.	Jasmine, Absolute	55
4.	Musk Ketone	30
5.	Phenyl Ethyl Alcohol	350
6.	Rosewood, Oil	300
7.	Terpineol	200
8.	Vanillin	5
		1000

LILAC, IMITATION NO. 9 (FOR SOAP)

1.	Amyl Cinnamic Aldehyde	30
2.	Anisic Aldehyde	75
3.	Benzyl Acetate	40
4.	Cyclamen Aldehyde	30
5.	Hydroxycitronellal	75
6.	Methyl Anthranilate	75
7.	Musk Xylene	40
8.	Petitgrain, Oil	40
9.	Phenyl Ethyl Alcohol	275
10.	Terpineol	275
11.	Tolu Balsam	45
		1000

LILAC, SYNTHETIC NO. 1 (FOR SOAP)

1.	Heliotropin	100
2.	Hydroxycitronellal	150
3.	Methyl Anthranilate	50
4.	Musk Ketone	50
5.	Phenyl Ethyl Acohol	350
6.	Terpineol	300
		1000

LILAC, SYNTHETIC NO. 2 (FOR SOAP)

1.	Alcohol C-9	5
2.	Aldehyde C-9	5
3.	Aldehyde C-10	5
4.	Aldehyde C-12, MNA	10
5.	Aldehyde C-14 (pure)	15
6.	Anisic Alcohol	50
7.	Cinnamic Alcohol	70
8.	Heliotropin	150
9.	Hydroxycitronellal	200
10.	Indole	10
11.	Isoeugenol	30
12.	Phenyl Ethyl Alcohol	250
13.	Terpineol	200
		1000

LILY, BASE

1.	Hydroxycitronellal	400
2.	Linalool	300
3.	Terpineol	300
		1000

MAGNOLIA

1.	Cinnamic Alcohol	75
2.	Hydroxycitronellal	225
3.	Isoeugenol	5
4.	Jasmine, Oil	150
5.	Lemon, Oil	75
6.	Musk Ketone	30
7.	Nerol	225
8.	Vanilla, Oil	15
9.	Ylang Ylang, Oil	200
		1000

MIGNONETTE (RESEDA)

1.	Alcohol C-9	10
2.	Aldehyde C-12 (lauric)	10
3.	Cassia, Absolute	20
4.	Clary Sage, Oil	20
5.	Jasmine, Absolute	20
6.	Methyl Ionone	10
7.	Tolu Balsam	10
8.	Ethyl Alcohol 95%	450
9.	Distilled Water	450
		1000

MIMOSA, IMITATION

1.	Hydroxycitronellal	150
2.	Jasmine, Concrete	60
3.	Methyl Acetophenone	30
4.	Methyl Heptyne Carbonate	10
5.	Peru Balsam	50
6.	Styrax, Resinoid	50
7.	Terpineol	150
8.	Ethyl Alcohol 95%	250
9.	Distilled Water	250
		1000

MIMOSA, SYNTHETIC

1.	Alcohol C-10	20
2.	Alcohol C-12	10
3.	Aldehyde C-10	50
4.	Aldehyde C-11	20
5.	Hydroxycitronellal	150
6.	Methyl Acetophenone	150
7.	Terpineol	100
8.	Ethyl Alcohol 95%	250
9.	Distilled Water	250
		1000

MOSS

1.	Ambergris, Tincture	50
2.	Benzyl Acetate	100
3.	Cinnamic Alcohol	100
4.	Coumarin	25
5.	Heliotropin	100
6.	Ionone	50
7.	Linalool	100
8.	Linalyl Acetate	100
9.	Musk Ambrette	25
10.	Patchouli, Oil	100
11.	Peru Balsam	25
12.	Vetiverol	25
13.	Ethyl Alcohol 95%	100
14.	Distilled Water	100
		1000

MUGUET (LILY OF THE VALLEY), IMITATION NO. 1

1.	Civet	10
2.	Jasmine, Oil	75
3.	Lime, Oil	25
4.	Linalool	150
5.	Musk Ambrette	15
6.	Rose, Oil	10
7.	Terpineol	150
8.	Ylang Ylang, Oil	25
9.	Ethyl Alcohol 95%	270
10.	Distilled Water	270
		1000

MUGUET (LILY OF THE VALLEY), IMITATION NO. 2

1.	Aldehyde C-11 (undecylenic)	5
2.	Aldehyde C-12 (lauric)	5
3.	Aldehyde C-14 (myristic)	5
4.	Almond (Bitter), Oil (pure)	10
5.	Cassie, Oil	20
6.	Jasmine, Oil	40
7.	Orange Flowers, Oil	45
8.	Rose, Oil	10
9.	Tuberose, Oil	45
10.	Vanilla Beans, Oil	15
11.	Ethyl Alcohol 95%	400
12.	Distilled Water	400
		1000

MUGUET (LILY OF THE VALLEY), IMITATION NO. 3 (FOR SOAP)

1.	Benzyl Acetate	50
2.	Civet, Absolute	5
3.	Geranium Palmarosa, Oil	325
4.	Hydroxycitronellal	325
5.	Jasmine, Absolute	20
6.	Linalool	75
7.	Terpineol	75
8.	Ylang Ylang, Oil	125
		1000

MUGUET (LILY OF THE VALLEY), SYNTHETIC NO. 1

1.	Benzyl Acetate	200
2.	Cinnamic Alcohol	200
3.	Hydroxycitronellol (10% sol'n.)	300
4.	Musk Ambrette	50
5.	Phenyl Ethyl Alcohol	100
6.	Terpineol	100
7.	Ylang Ylang, Oil	50
		1000

MUGUET (LILY OF THE VALLEY), SYNTHETIC NO. 2

1.	Alcohol C-9	6
2.	Alcohol C-10	1
3.	Alcohol C-11 (undecylenic)	5
4.	Aldehyde C-9	4
5.	Aldehyde C-10	3
6.	Aldehyde C-12	4
7.	Aldehyde C-16	2
8.	Cinnamyl Acetate	150
9.	Ethyl Phenyl Acetate	150
10.	Hydroxycitronellal	150
11.	Ionone	25
12.	Linalool	150
13.	Ethyl Alcohol 95%	175
14.	Distilled Water	175
		1000

MUSK

1.	Ambergris	50
2.	Bergamot, Oil	250
3.	Benzyl Salicylate (10% sol'n.)	50
4.	Heliotropin	150
5.	Linalool	150
6.	Orris, Oil	50
7.	Vanillin (10% sol'n.)	150
8.	Vetiverol	150
		1000

MUSK, IMITATION NO. 1 (FOR POWDER)

1.	Amyl Benzoate	250
2.	Cassia, Oil	55

3.	Clary Sage, Oil	5
4.	Ionone	50
5.	Musk Ambrette	300
6.	Rhodinol	300
7.	Sandalwood, Oil	25
8.	Vetiver, Oil	15
		1000

MUSK, IMITATION NO. 2 (FOR SOAP)

1.	Benzyl Acetate	50
2.	Cassia, Oil	50
3.	Castor, Tincture	150
4.	Cedarwood, Oil	100
5.	Civet	5
6.	Clove, Oil	75
7.	Geranium Palmarosa, Oil	300
8.	Lemon, Oil	75
9.	Musk Ambrette	55
10.	Musk Xylene	100
11.	Sandalwood, Oil	25
12.	Vetiver, Oil	15
		1000

NARCISSUS, IMITATION NO. 1 (FOR POWDER)

1.	Hydroxycitronellal	150
2.	Jasmine, Oil	70
3.	Linalool	50
4.	Methyl Anthranilate	150
5.	Methyl Ionone	25
6.	Musk Ketone	5
7.	Neroli, Oil	10
8.	Phenyl Ethyl Acetate	2
9.	Styrax, Resinoid	150
10.	Ylang Ylang, Oil	25
11.	Ethyl Alcohol 95%	363
		1000

NARCISSUS, IMITATION NO. 2 (FOR COLOGNE)

1.	Aldehyde C-10	4
2.	Aldehyde C-11	6
3.	Civet, Tincture	10
4.	Coumarin	3
5.	Jasmine, Oil	20
6.	Methyl Naphthyl Ketone	3
7.	Musk Ketone	5
8.	Orange (Sweet), Oil	10
9.	Orange Flowers, Oil	50
10.	Rose Otto, Oil	4
11.	Sandalwood, Oil	2
12.	Vanillin	3
13.	Ethyl Alcohol 95%	440
14.	Distilled Water	440
		1000

NARCISSUS, IMITATION NO. 3 (FOR COLOGNE)

1.	Aldehyde C-16	9
2.	Amyl Salicylate	10
3.	Geraniol	40
4.	Geranyl Formate	15
5.	Hydroxycitronellal	40
6.	Linalool	15
7.	Musk Ketone	15
8.	Neroli, Oil	86
9.	Phenyl Ethyl Alcohol	70
10.	Rhodinol	100
11.	Styrax, Resinoid	5
12.	Ylang Ylang, Oil	75
13.	Ethyl Alcohol 95%	260
14.	Distilled Water	260
		1000

NARCISSUS, IMITATION NO. 4 "POETICUS" (FOR COLOGNE)

1.	Alcohol C-9	10
2.	Aldehyde C-8	10
3.	Aldehyde C-10	10
4.	Ambergris	10
5.	Benzoin	10
6.	Chamomile, Oil	10
7.	Cinnamic Alcohol	50
8.	Clary Sage	10
9.	Honey, Synthetic No. 1*	110
10.	Hydratropic Aldehyde	50
11.	Jasmine, Oil	50

* Formulas which appear in this book

12.	Orange Flower, Imitation No. 1*	50
13.	Phenyl Acetaldehyde	50
14.	Phenyl Acetaldehyde Dimethyl Acetal	50
15.	Phenyl Ethyl Acetate	50
16.	Phenyl Ethyl Alcohol	30
17.	Rose, Oil	50
18.	Terpineol	250
19.	Tolu Balsam	20
20.	Vanillin	10
21.	Ethyl Alcohol 95%	110
		1000

NARCISSUS, IMITATION NO. 5 (FOR SOAP)

1.	Anisaldehyde	110
2.	Isoeugenol	110
3.	Linalool	250
4.	Methyl-*p*-Cresol	15
5.	Petitgrain, Oil	115
6.	Phenyl Acetaldehyde	100
7.	Rose, Absolute	25
8.	Terpineol	250
9.	Tuberose, Absolute	25
		1000

NARCISSUS, SYNTHETIC NO. 1

1.	Alcohol C-9	20
2.	Aldehyde C-9	15
3.	Benzyl Benzoate	150
4.	Benzyl Cinnamate	50
5.	Cinnamic Alcohol	60
6.	Phenyl Acetaldehyde	25
7.	Phenyl Ethyl Alcohol	30
8.	Terpineol	150
9.	Ethyl Alcohol 95%	250
10.	Distilled Water	250
		1000

NARCISSUS, SYNTHETIC NO. 2

1.	Benzaldehyde (pure)	25
2.	Benzoic Acid	50
3.	Benzyl Alcohol	300
4.	Cinnamic Alcohol	200
5.	Eugenol	50
6.	Ethyl Alcohol 95%	375
		1000

NARCISSUS, SYNTHETIC NO. 3

1.	Aldehyde C-14 (10% sol'n.)	50
2.	Benzyl Acetate	200
3.	Indole (10% sol'n.)	50
4.	Linalool	200
5.	Phenyl Propyl Acetate	250
6.	Phenyl Propyl Alcohol	250
		1000

NARCISSUS, SYNTHETIC NO. 4

1.	Alcohol C-10	1
2.	Benzyl Acetate	12
3.	Benzyl Alcohol	12
4.	δ-3-Carene	2
5.	Cinnamyl Alcohol	6
6.	Cineol	30
7.	*p*-Cymol	15
8.	Geraniol	2
9.	Indole (10% sol'n.)	16
10.	Limonene	15
11.	Linalool	16
12.	Methyl Anthranilate	17
13.	Methyl Benzoate	3
14.	Methyl Cinnamate	9
15.	Methyl Phenyl Acetate	2
16.	Nerol	1
17.	α-Pinene	8
18.	β-Pinene	2
19.	Sabinene	20
20.	β-Sitosterol	1
21.	α-Terpineol	95
22.	Terpinolene	13
23.	Ethyl Alcohol 95%	702
		1000

NEROLI, IMITATION NO. 1

1.	Bergamot, Oil	80
2.	Citronellol	80

* Formulas which appear in this book

3.	Geraniol	80
4.	Geranyl Acetate	80
5.	Hydroxycitronellal	40
6.	α-Ionone	100
7.	Lemon, Oil (terpeneless)	10
8.	Linalool	200
9.	Linalyl Acetate	80
10.	Methyl Anthranilate	60
11.	Methyl Naphthyl Ketone	60
12.	Nerol	30
13.	Orange, Oil (terpeneless)	10
14.	Petitgrain, Oil (terpeneless)	80
15.	Vanillin (10% sol'n.)	10
		1000

NEROLI, IMITATION NO. 2

1.	Citronellol	200
2.	Geraniol	200
3.	Linalool	80
4.	Linalyl Acetate	50
5.	Methyl Anthranilate	20
6.	Petitgrain, Oil (10% sol'n.)	300
7.	Phenyl Ethyl Alcohol	50
8.	Terpineol	100
		1000

NEROLI, IMITATION NO. 3

1.	Acetate C-8	30
2.	Alcohol C-9	30
3.	Alcohol C-12	30
4.	Aldehyde C-9	15
5.	Aldehyde C-12	15
6.	Bergamot, Oil	10
7.	Citronellol	10
8.	Geraniol	10
9.	Hydroxycitronellal	4
10.	Ionone	1
11.	Lemon, Oil	1
12.	Linalool	20
13.	Linalyl Acetate	10
14.	Methyl Anthranilate	6
15.	Methyl Naphthyl Ketone	6
16.	Nerol	15
17.	Petitgrain, Oil	10
18.	Orange, Oil	1
19.	Vanillin	1
20.	Ethyl Alcohol 95%	388
21.	Distilled Water	387
		1000

NEROLI, IMITATION NO. 4 (FOR SOAP)

1.	Alcohol C-12 (lauric)	30
2.	Amyl Cinnamic Aldehyde	25
3.	Indole (10% sol'n.)	10
4.	Linalool	225
5.	Linalyl Acetate	60
6.	Methyl Anthranilate	30
7.	Nerol	120
8.	Nonyl Acetate	100
9.	Petitgrain, Oil	325
10.	Phenyl Acetic Acid	25
11.	Terpineol	50
		1000

NEROLIN

(β-naphthyl methyl ether or β-naphthyl ethyl ether)

(a) Yara Yara

1.	Methyl Alcohol	60
2.	β-Naphthol	36
3.	Zinc Chloride	4

(b) Bromelia

1.	Ethyl Alcohol	60
2.	β-Naphthol	36
3.	Sulfuric Acid	4

Heat in autoclave at 150 C.
Uses: (a) Perfumes, soaps

NEUTROLEUM, DEODORIZING PERFUME

1.	Ambergris	10
2.	Benzylidene Acetone	100
3.	Butyric Acid	10
4.	Caryophylene	50
5.	Cedar Leaf, Oil	50
6.	Cinnamic Aldehyde	10
7.	Cinnamon Leaf, Oil	50

8.	Clove Leaf, Oil	50
9.	Clove Terpenes, Oil	50
10.	Isovaleric Acid	10
11.	Mercaptan	10
12.	Orange, Oil	50
13.	Pimento Leaf, Oil	50
14.	Propylene Glycol	100
15.	Rosemary, Oil	200
16.	Sage, Oil	200
		1000

NEW MOWN HAY (FOIN COUPÉ), IMITATION NO. 1

1.	Bergamot, Oil	300
2.	Coumarin	300
3.	Lavender, Oil	400
		1000

NEW MOWN HAY (FOIN COUPÉ), IMITATION NO. 2

1.	Acetophenone	55
2.	Benzophenone	15
3.	Benzyl Acetate	55
4.	Bergamot, Oil	55
5.	Clary Sage, Oil	55
6.	Coumarin	100
7.	Geranium, Oil	100
8.	Lavender, Oil	225
9.	Linalool	225
10.	Musk Xylene	40
11.	Oakmoss, Resinoid	15
12.	Patchouli, Oil	40
13.	Sandalwood, Oil	20
		1000

NEW MOWN HAY (FOIN COUPÉ), IMITATION NO. 3

1.	Anisic Aldehyde	23
2.	Anisyl Alcohol	22
3.	Benzyl Benzoate	100
4.	Bergamot, Oil	150
5.	Cananga, Oil	25
6.	Cassia, Absolute	25
7.	Citral	5
8.	Coumarin	20
9.	Geranium, Oil	30
10.	Hydroxycitronellal	100
11.	α-Ionone	5
12.	Isobutyl Salicylate	5
13.	Jasmine, Oil	25
14.	Lavender, Oil	150
15.	Lemon, Oil	20
16.	Linalool	150
17.	Methyl Acetophenone	15
18.	Orange, Oil	25
19.	Orange Flower, Oil	25
20.	Rhodinol	30
21.	Rose, Oil	25
22.	Vanillin	15
23.	Vetiver, Oil	10
		1000

OPOPONAX, IMITATION NO. 1

1.	Bergamot (terpeneless)	300
2.	Heliotropin	70
3.	Ionone	50
4.	Linalyl Acetate	50
5.	Musk Ambrette	60
6.	Opoponax, Resinoid	150
7.	Peru, Resinoid	80
8.	Santalol	80
9.	Vanilla, Resinoid	100
10.	Vetiverol	60
		1000

OPOPONAX, IMITATION NO. 2

1.	Bergamot, Oil	360
2.	Castoreum, Oil	50
3.	Musk Ambrette	150
4.	Neroli, Oil	40
5.	Patchouli, Oil	100
6.	Santalol	100
7.	Vetiverol	100
8.	Vanillin (10% sol'n.)	100
		1000

OPOPONAX, IMITATION NO. 3

1.	Bergamot, Oil	300
2.	Citral	5
3.	Geraniol	150
4.	Jasmine, Oil	35
5.	Musk Ambrette	75
6.	Opoponax, Resinoid	50
7.	Rhodinol	150
8.	Rose, Oil	15
9.	Vanillin	5
10.	Violet, Oil	15
11.	Ethyl Alcohol 95%	100
12.	Distilled Water	100
		1000

OPOPONAX, IMITATION NO. 4 (FOR SOAP)

1.	Amber, Resinoid	50
2.	Benzoin, Resinoid	50
3.	Benzoyl Acetone	60
4.	Bergamot, Oil	200
5.	Labdanum, Resinoid	55
6.	Musk Ambrette	85
7.	Opoponax, Resinoid	60
8.	Rhodinyl Acetate	55
9.	Sandalwood, Oil	150
10.	Sweet Orange, Oil	150
11.	Vanillin	85
		1000

ORANGE BLOSSOM, BOUQUET (FOR SOAP)

1.	Benzyl Acetate	100
2.	Bois De Rose, Oil	175
3.	Bromostyrol	25
4.	Clove, Oil	40
5.	Geranium Palmarosa, Oil	150
6.	Hydroxycinnamic Aldehyde	25
7.	Linalyl Acetate	75
8.	Methyl Anthranilate	50
9.	Methyl Naphthyl Ketone	50
10.	Musk Ambrette	40
11.	Petitgrain, Oil	150
12.	Phenyl Ethyl Alcohol	50
13.	Terpineol	70
		1000

ORANGE FLOWER, IMITATION NO. 1

1.	Aldehyde C-12 (lauric)	30
2.	Cinnamic Alcohol	30
3.	Geraniol	15
4.	Indole (10% sol'n.)	20
5.	Isoeugenol	10
6.	Jasmine, Oil	50
7.	Linalool	100
8.	Linalyl Acetate	30
9.	Methyl Anthranilate	40
10.	Methyl Benzoate	10
11.	Methyl Cinnamate	5
12.	Methyl Naphthyl Ketone	20
13.	Musk Ketone	50
14.	Nerol	50
15.	Orange, Sweet, Oil	40
16.	Petitgrain, Oil	280
17.	Phenyl Acetaldehyde Dimethyl Acetal	10
18.	Phenyl Ethyl Alcohol	200
19.	Sandalwood, Oil	10
		1000

ORANGE FLOWER, IMITATION NO. 2

1.	Acetophenone	5
2.	Bergamot, Oil	10
3.	Geraniol	20
4.	Hydroxycitronellal	50
5.	Linalool	160
6.	Linalyl Acetate	160
7.	Methyl Anthranilate	50
8.	Methyl Ionone	5
9.	Nutmeg	8
10.	Orange, Sweet, Oil	10
11.	Petitgrain	160
12.	Phenyl Acetaldehyde Dimethyl Acetal	2
13.	Phenyl Ethyl Alcohol	350
14.	Sandalwood, Oil	5
15.	Terpineol	5
		1000

ORANGE FLOWER, IMITATION NO. 3

1.	Aldehyde C-8	6
2.	Aldehyde C-10	8
3.	Benzyl Acetate	70
4.	Geranyl Formate	6
5.	Hydroxycitronellal	40
6.	Linalool	200
7.	Methyl Anthranilate	130
8.	Nerol	120
9.	Orange Flowers, Absolute	20
10.	Petitgrain	180
11.	Phenyl Ethyl Alcohol	220
		1000

ORANGE FLOWER, SYNTHETIC NO. 4

1.	Alcohol C-8	20
2.	Alcohol C-9	20
3.	Alcohol C-10	20
4.	Alcohol C-12	18
5.	Aldehyde C-8	18
6.	Aldehyde C-10	20
7.	Aldehyde C-12 (lauric)	20
8.	Aldehyde C-16	10
9.	Cimene	6
10.	Citronellol	20
11.	Citronellyl Acetate	10
12.	Eugenol	3
13.	Farnesol	1
14.	Geraniol	40
15.	Geranyl Acetate	16
16.	Jasmone	1
17.	Limonene	14
18.	Linalool	150
19.	Linalyl Acetate	50
20.	Methyl Anthranilate	150
21.	Nerol	40
22.	Nerolidol	40
23.	Neryl Acetate	40
24.	Phenyl Acetic Acid	1
25.	Phenyl Ethyl Alcohol	250
26.	α-Pinene	1
27.	β-Pinene	1
28.	α-Terpineol	20
		1000

ORCHID, IMITATION

1.	Aldehyde C-9	10
2.	Aldehyde C-11 (undecylenic)	10
3.	Aldehyde C-12, MNA	10
4.	Amyl Benzoate	53
5.	Amyl Salicylate (10% sol'n.)	250
6.	Anisic Aldehyde	54
7.	Ethyl Benzoate	53
8.	Geranium, Oil	50
9.	Isoeugenol	20
10.	Jasmine, Absolute	10
11.	Lavender, Oil	10
12.	Linalool	200
13.	Nerolin	20
14.	Terpineol	200
15.	Ylang Ylang, Oil	50
		1000

ORRIS ROOT, EXTRACT (NATURAL)

1.	Orris Root, Florentine	10	kg
2.	Ethyl Alcohol 95%	10	1

Let stand for 3 days. Express, and to the residue add:

3.	Ethyl Alcohol 95%	20	1
4.	Distilled Water	20	1

Let stand for one week, stirring for 1 h every day. Add:

5.	Distilled Water	20	1
6.	Amyl Acetate	25	ml
7.	Ethyl Acetate	120	ml
8.	Ethyl Oenanthate	45	ml

Distill altogether.
Yield: 60 liters

ORRIS ROOT, FLORENTINE

1.	Citral	25
2.	Cedrol	50
3.	Heliotropin	15
4.	α-Ionone	100
5.	Methylionone (10% sol'n.)	250
6.	Myristic Acid	200
7.	Methyl Myristate	25

8.	Orris, Concrete	25
9.	Orris, Resinoid	100
10.	Stearic Acid	100
11.	Terpineol	75
12.	Vetiverol	25
13.	Vanillin (10% sol'n.)	10
		1000

ORRIS ROOT, SYNTHETIC

1.	Benzyl Alcohol	50
2.	Cineol	10
3.	Ethyl Acetate	250
4.	Ethyl Oenanthate	190
5.	Ethyl Pelargonate	62
6.	Ionone	10
7.	Isoamyl Acetate	420
8.	Linalool	8
		1000

PATCHOULI, IMITATION NO. 1 (FOR SOAP)

1.	Benzyl Acetate	75
2.	Civet, Tincture	75
3.	Clove, Oil	50
4.	Coumarin	75
5.	Geranium, Oil	300
6.	Musk Ambrette	75
7.	Patchouli, Oil	150
8.	Sandalwood, Oil	100
9.	Vetiver, Oil	100
		1000

PATCHOULI, IMITATION NO. 2 (FOR TOILET POWDER)

1.	Aldehyde C-14 (pure)	10
2.	Amber, Tincture	20
3.	Anisaldehyde	50
4.	Benzoin, Resinoid	225
5.	Coumarin	20
6.	Ethyl Cinnamate	55
7.	Heliotropin	75
8.	Jasmine, Oil	75
9.	Linalyl Acetate	135
10.	Orris Root, Extract (Natural)*	225
11.	Patchouli, Oil	55
12.	Rose, Oil	55
		1000

* Formulas which appear in this book

PINE, BOUQUET (FOR SOAP)

1.	Aldehyde C-12 (lauric)	2
2.	Benzaldehyde (pure)	50
3.	Bornyl Acetate	180
4.	Cedarwood, Oil	180
5.	Clove, Oil	65
6.	Diphenyl Methane	50
7.	Geranium, Oil	180
8.	Lemon, Oil	180
9.	Methyl Anthranilate	65
10.	Musk Xylene	48
		1000

PINE, IMITATION NO. 1

1.	α-Phellandrene	200
2.	Pine, Oil	200
3.	Terpineol	200
4.	Terpinolene	200
5.	Ethyl Alcohol 95%	200
		1000

PINE, IMITATION NO. 2

1.	Pine, Oil	200
2.	Sassafras, Oil	40
3.	Terpineol	600
4.	Turpentine	160
		1000

PINE NEEDLE

1.	Pine Needles, Oil	300
2.	Ethyl Alcohol 95%	700
		1000

PINE NEEDLE, SIBERIAN, IMITATION NO. 1

1.	Citral	50
2.	α-Ionone, White	10
3.	Isobornyl Acetate	800
4.	Limonene	100
5.	α-Pinene	10
6.	Rosemary, Oil	20
7.	Spruce, Oil	10
		1000

PINE NEEDLE, SIBERIAN, IMITATION NO. 2

1.	Aldehyde C-12	10
2.	Bois De Rose	10
3.	Diethylene Glycol Monoethyl Ether	80
4.	Geraniol	10
5.	Isobornyl Acetate	80
6.	Musk Ambrette	20
7.	Pine Needle, Siberian, Oil	100
8.	Spruce, Oil	160
9.	Tolu Balsam, Oil (10% sol'n.)	20
10.	Vanillin (10% sol'n.)	10
11.	Ethyl Alcohol 95%	500
		1000

PINE NEEDLE, SIBERIAN, IMITATION NO. 3

1.	Citral (10% sol'n.)	250
2.	α-Ionone	50
3.	Isobornyl Acetate	200
4.	Limonene	100
5.	Pinene	100
6.	Rosemary, Oil	200
7.	Spruce, Oil	100
		1000

ROSE, BULGARIAN TYPE

1.	Alcohol C-8	5
2.	Alcohol C-10	5
3.	Citronellol	23
4.	Citronellyl Acetate	5
5.	Citronellyl Formate	5
6.	Decyl Aldehyde	5
7.	Geraniol	25
8.	Geranium Bourbon	2
9.	Hydroxycitronellal	1
10.	α-Ionone	5
11.	Lemon, Oil (terpeneless)	5
12.	Musk Ambrette	5
13.	Nerol	1
14.	Nonyl Aldehyde	5
15.	Patchouli, Oil	5
16.	Phenyl Ethyl Alcohol	13
17.	Phenyl Ethyl Butyrate	1
18.	Rhodinol	8
19.	Rhodinyl Butyrate	1
20.	Ylang Ylang, Oil	1
21.	Ethyl Alcohol 95%	437
22.	Distilled Water	437
		1000

ROSE, FOR CREAM

1.	Citronellal	180
2.	Geraniol (10% sol'n.)	500
3.	Geranyl Acetate	20
4.	Linalool	60
5.	Phenyl Ethyl Alcohol (10% sol'n.)	170
6.	Rose, Oil (10% sol'n.)	70
		1000

ROSE, FOR FACE POWDER NO. 1

1.	Ambrettolide	50
2.	Benzyl Isoeugenol	20
3.	Citronellol	100
4.	Ethyl Cinnamate	5
5.	Eugenol	10
6.	Geraniol (10% sol'n.)	330
7.	Geranyl Acetate	30
8.	Linalool	80
9.	Linalyl Acetate	20
10.	α-Ionone	43
11.	Jasmine, Oil	40
12.	Methyl Ionone	30
13.	Methyl Nonyl Acetaldehyde	50

14.	Musk Ketone	5
15.	Patchouli, Oil	20
16.	Phenyl Ethyl Alcohol (10% sol'n.)	120
17.	Sandalwood, Oil	30
18.	Vanillin (10% sol'n.)	7
19.	Vetivert, Oil	10
		1000

ROSE, FOR FACE POWDER NO. 2

1.	Anisic Aldehyde	50
2.	Civet	2
3.	Ionone	18
4.	Jasmine, Oil (10% sol'n.)	540
5.	Isoeugenol	60
6.	Neroli, Oil	50
7.	Orris, Oil	10
8.	Phenyl Acetaldehyde	10
9.	Rose, Otto, Oil (10% sol'n.)	60
10.	Sandalwood, Oil	60
11.	Ylang Ylang, Oil	140
		1000

ROSE, IMITATION NO. 1

1.	Citronellol	180
2.	Geraniol	490
3.	Geranyl Acetate	20
4.	Linalool	70
5.	Phenyl Ethyl Alcohol	170
6.	Rose, Oil	70
		1000

ROSE, IMITATION NO. 2

1.	Aldehyde C-8	10
2.	Citral	10
3.	Citronellol	100
4.	Geraniol	800
5.	Linalool	20
6.	Phenyl Ethyl Alcohol	10
7.	Rose, Oil	50
		1000

ROSE, IMITATION NO. 3

1.	Alcohol C-8	5
2.	Alcohol C-10	5
3.	Aldehyde C-9	5
4.	Aldehyde C-10	5
5.	Citronellol	50
6.	Citronellyl Acetate	5
7.	Citronellyl Formate	5
8.	Geraniol	50
9.	Hydroxycitronellal	20
10.	Ionone	5
11.	Lemon, Oil	5
12.	Nerol	10
13.	Patchouli, Oil	5
14.	Phenyl Ethyl Alcohol	25
15.	Phenyl Ethyl Butyrate	10
16.	Rhodinol	15
17.	Rhodinyl Butyrate	10
18.	Rosacetol	5
19.	Ylang Ylang, Oil	10
20.	Ethyl Alcohol 95%	750
		1000

ROSE, IMITATION NO. 4

1.	Aldehyde C-9	20
2.	Citronellol	250
3.	Geraniol	250
4.	Guaiacwood, Oil	5
5.	Methyl Ionone	40
6.	Nerol	50
7.	Phenyl Acetaldehyde (10% sol'n.)	20
8.	Phenyl Acetic Acid (10% sol'n.)	40
9.	Phenyl Ethyl Alcohol	325
		1000

ROSE, IMITATION NO. 5 (FOR COSMETIC CREAM)

1.	Dimethyl Octanol	75
2.	Geranium Palmarosa, Oil	275
3.	Geranyl Acetate	150
4.	Guaiacwood, Oil	75
5.	α-Ionone	30
6.	Musk Xylene	35
7.	Patchouli, Oil	35
8.	Phenyl Ethyl Alcohol	275
9.	Rose, Oil	50
		1000

ROSE, IMITATION NO. 6 (FOR SOAP)

1.	Bois De Rose	250
2.	Civet, Absolute (10% sol'n.)	25
3.	Geraniol	150
4.	Geranium Palmarosa, Oil	150
5.	Musk Xylene	25
6.	Patchouli, Oil	25
7.	Phenyl Ethyl Alcohol	350
8.	Styrax, Resinoid	25
		1000

ROSE, IMITATION NO. 7

1.	Cinnamic Alcohol	200
2.	Ionone	225
3.	Jasmine, Oil	75
4.	Phenyl Ethyl Alcohol	175
5.	Rhodinol	175
6.	Rhodinyl Acetate	150
		1000

ROSE, IMITATION NO. 8

1.	Aldehyde C-11	25
2.	Cinnamic Alcohol	20
3.	Citronellol	150
4.	Eugenol	3
5.	Geranium Palmarosa, Oil	300
6.	Guaiacwood, Oil	75
7.	α-Ionone	100
8.	Phenyl Acetic Acid	25
9.	Phenyl Acetic Aldehyde	2
10.	Phenyl Ethyl Alcohol	150
11.	Rhodinol	150
		1000

ROSE, IMITATION NO. 9 (FOR PERFUME)

1.	Geranium Palmarosa, Oil	50
2.	Jasmine, Oil	200
3.	Rose, Oil	300
4.	Ylang Ylang, Oil	50
5.	Ethyl Alcohol 95%	200
6.	Distilled Water	200
		1000

ROSE, IMITATION NO. 10

1.	Alcohol C-8	5
2.	Alcohol C-10	5
3.	Citronellol	50
4.	Citronellyl Acetate	5
5.	Citronellyl Formate	5
6.	Decyl Aldehyde	5
7.	Geraniol	50
8.	Hydroxycitronellal	20
9.	Lemon, Oil (terpeneless)	2
10.	Nerol, Oil	10
11.	Nonyl Aldehyde	5
12.	Patchouli, Oil	10
13.	Phenyl Ethyl Alcohol (10% sol'n.)	250
14.	Phenyl Ethyl Butyrate	14
15.	Rhodinol	150
16.	Ylang Ylang, Oil	10
17.	Ethyl Alcohol 95%	404
		1000

ROSE, IMITATION NO. 11

1.	Geraniol Extra	40
2.	Geranium Rose, Oil	5
3.	Orange, Bitter, Oil	25
4.	Orange, Sweet, Oil	25
5.	Phenyl Ethyl Alcohol	180
6.	Rhodinol	30
7.	Rose Bulgarian, Oil (10% sol'n.)	5
8.	Ethyl Alcohol 95%	690
		1000

ROSE, IMITATION NO. 12

1.	Citral	1
2.	Geraniol	100
3.	Geranium Rose, Oil	3
4.	Orange, Sweet Oil	25
5.	Rhodinol	25
6.	Rose, Turkish, Oil (10% sol'n.)	5
7.	Ethyl Alcohol 95%	841
		1000

ROSE, IMITATION, NO. 13

1.	Geranium Bourbon	100
2.	Rose, Imitation No. 1*	250

* Formulas which appear in this book

3.	Rose, Imitation No. 2*	250
4.	Rose, Imitation No. 3*	250
5.	Undecylenic Acid	150
		1000

ROSE, IMITATION NO. 14

1.	Geranium Bourbon	100
2.	Undecenal (10% sol'n.)	450
3.	Undecylenic Acid (10% sol'n.)	450
		1000

ROSE, IMITATION NO. 15

1.	Geranium Bourbon	50
2.	Geranium Palmarosa	50
3.	Undecanal (10% sol'n.)	450
4.	Undecylenic Acid (10% sol'n.)	450
		1000

ROSE, IMITATION NO. 16

1.	Rose Macedone, Oil (10% sol'n.)	500
2.	Rose, Imitation No. 6*	500
		1000

ROSE, IMITATION NO. 17

1.	Rose Macedone, Oil (10% sol'n.)	500
2.	Rose, Imitation No. 7*	500
		1000

ROSE, IMITATION NO. 18

1.	Alcohol C-12	10
2.	Citronellol	60
3.	Cedar	30
4.	Geraniol	50
5.	Geranium Palmarosa	100
6.	Guaiacwood	50
7.	Phenyl Ethyl Alcohol (10% sol'n.)	350
8.	Rose Bulgarian, Oil (10% sol'n.)	350
		1000

* Formulas which appear in this book

ROSE, IMITATION NO. 19

1.	Alcohol C-12	10
2.	Citronellol	60
3.	Cedarwood, Oil	30
4.	Geraniol	50
5.	Geranium Palmarosa	100
6.	Guaiacwood	50
7.	Phenyl Ethyl Alcohol (10% sol'n.)	350
8.	Rose Turkish, Oil (10% sol'n.)	350
		1000

ROSE, IMITATION NO. 20

1.	Alcohol C-12	10
2.	Citronellol	60
3.	Cedarwood, Oil	30
4.	Geraniol	50
5.	Geranium Palmarosa	100
6.	Guaiacwood	50
7.	Phenyl Ethyl Alcohol (10% sol'n.)	350
8.	Rose May, Oil (10% sol'n.)	350
		1000

ROSE MACEDONE

1.	Rose Macedone, Oil (10% sol'n.)	500
2.	Undecylenic Acid (10% sol'n.)	500
		1000

ROSE, MOSS

1.	Benzoin, Tincture (10% sol'n.)	200
2.	Cinnamic Alcohol	150
3.	Geranium, Oil	100
4.	Musk Ketone	50
5.	Patchouli, Oil	100
6.	Phenyl Ethyl Alchol (10% sol'n.)	200
7.	Rhodinol, Oil	200
		1000

ROSE, OIL, SYNTHETIC

1.	Citronellol (10% sol'n.)	250
2.	Geraniol (10% sol'n.)	500
3.	Geranium, Oil	30
4.	Geranyl Butyrate	20

5.	Phenyl Ethyl Alcohol	100
6.	Terpineol	100
		1000

ROSE, ORIENTAL

1.	Heliotropin	100
2.	Isoeugenol (10% sol'n.)	250
3.	Labdanum, Resinoid	50
5.	Musk Ambrette	200
6.	Styrax, Tincture	200
7.	Vanillin (10% sol'n.)	100
8.	Vetivert	100
		1000

ROSE OTTO

1.	Geranium Bourbon	50
2.	Geranium Palmarosa	50
3.	Undecylenic Acid (10% sol'n.)	900
		1000

ROSE, SYNTHETIC NO. 1 (GENERAL BASE FOR ROSE ODOR)

1.	Acetate C-8	10
2.	Acetate C-12	10
3.	Alcohol C-8	10
4.	Alcohol C-9	10
5.	Alcohol C-10	10
6.	Alcohol C-12	10
7.	Aldehyde C-9	10
8.	Aldehyde C-10	10
9.	Aldehyde C-11	10
10.	Aldehyde C-16	10
11.	Benzyl Acetate	100
12.	Benzyl Formate	100
13.	Benzyl Propionate	100
14.	Citronellol	100
15.	Geraniol	200
16.	Phenyl Ethyl Alcohol	100
17.	Rhodinol	100
18.	Rosacetol	100
		1000

* Formulas which appear in this book

ROSE, SYNTHETIC NO. 2

1.	Aldehyde C-9	100
2.	Aldehyde C-10	100
3.	Aldehyde C-11	100
4.	Aldehyde C-12	100
5.	Jasmine, Oil	10
6.	Violet, Oil	10
7.	Ethyl Alcohol 95%	300
8.	Distilled Water	280
		1000

ROSE, SYNTHETIC NO. 3

1.	Glycerin	390
2.	Rose, Oil	10
3.	Stearin	300
4.	Ethyl Alcohol 95%	150
5.	Distilled Water	150
		1000

ROSE, SYNTHETIC NO. 4 (MILK-LIKE COMPOUND)

1.	Corn, Oil	165
2.	Rose, Imitation No. 1*	165
3.	Soap	165
4.	Spermaceti	165
5.	Wax	165
6.	Ethyl Alcohol 95%	175
		1000

ROSE, WHITE

1.	Aldehyde C-9 (10% sol'n.)	100
2.	Aldehyde C-10 (10% sol'n.)	100
3.	Aldehyde C-11 (10% sol'n.)	100
4.	Aldehyde C-12 (10% sol'n.)	100
5.	Benzyl Isoeugenol	50
6.	Phenyl Ethyl Alcohol (10% sol'n.)	450
7.	Phenyl Ethyl Propionate	100
		1000

SANDALWOOD "SANTAL," (FOR SOAP)

1.	Benzyl Acetate	70
2.	Cedarwood, Oil	225

3.	Coumarin	55
4.	Geranium, Oil	75
5.	Ionone	70
6.	Mace (or Nutmeg), Oil	25
7.	Musk Xylene	55
8.	Orris, Oleoresin	75
9.	Patchouli, Oil	50
10.	Petitgrain, Oil	25
11.	Sandalwood, Oil	225
12.	Vetiver, Oil	50
		1000

SASSAFRAS, FOR SOAP NO. 1

1.	Camphene	50
2.	Phellandrene	150
3.	Pine, Oil	50
4.	Sassafras, Oil	750
		1000

SASSAFRAS, FOR SOAP NO. 2

1.	Camphene	100
2.	Ocotea Cymbarum	200
3.	Phellandrene	150
4.	Pine, Oil	50
5.	Sassafras, Oil	500
		1000

SEBACIC ACID, STABILIZER FOR PERFUME

1.	Propylene Glycol	750
2.	Sebacic Acid	250
		1000

SOAP, PERFUME NO. 1

1.	Amyl Acetate	10
2.	Benzyl Benzoate	50
3.	Butyl Acetate	10
4.	Citral	50
5.	Ethyl Acetate	10
6.	Ethyl Formate	10
7.	Jasmine, Oil	30
8.	Orris, Oil	10
9.	Rose, Concrete	10
10.	Triacetin	800
11.	Vanillin	10
		1000

SOAP, PERFUME NO. 2

1.	Amyl Acetate	20
2.	Butyl Acetate	20
3.	Citral	80
4.	Ethyl Acetate	20
5.	Ethyl Formate	20
6.	α-Ionone	20
7.	Jasmine, Oil	30
8.	Orris, Oil	30
9.	Rose, Concrete	10
10.	Triacetin	700
11.	Ylang Ylang, Oil	50
		1000

SOAP, PERFUME NO. 3

1.	Aldehyde C-20	250
2.	Soap, Perfume No. 1*	500
3.	Soap, Perfume No. 2*	250
		1000

SOAP, PERFUME NO. 4

1.	Amyl Acetate	25
2.	Butyl Acetate	25
3.	Citral	25
4.	Ethyl Acetate	25
5.	Ethyl Formate	25
6.	Ylang Ylang, Oil	875
		1000

SOAP, PERFUME NO. 5

1.	Apricot Kernel, Oil	250
2.	Pine, Oil	250
3.	Propylene Glycol	500
		1000

* Formulas which appear in this book

SWEET PEA, BLOSSOM

1.	Benzylidene Acetone	1
2.	Hyacinth, Oil	100
3.	Methyl Acetophenone	1
4.	Neroli, Oil	200
5.	Ethyl Alcohol 95%	349
6.	Distilled Water	349
		1000

SYRINGA, IMITATION NO. 1

1.	Lemon, Oil	250
2.	Lime, Oil	250
3.	Terpineol, Extra	500
		1000

SYRINGA, IMITATION NO. 2

1.	Acetophenone	150
2.	Amyl Cinnamic Aldehyde	200
3.	Anisyl Formate	150
4.	Hydroxycitronellal	150
5.	Isobutyl Anthranilate	50
6.	Isobutyl Benzoate	50
7.	Linalool	200
8.	Methyl Ionone	50
		1000

TOBACCO FOR SNUFF

1.	Bergamot, Oil	100
2.	Cascarilla, Oil	400
3.	Cinnamon Leaf, Oil	100
4.	Geranium, Oil	100
5.	Lavender, Oil	100
6.	Nutmeg, Oil	100
7.	Vanilla Beans, Tincture	100
		1000

TOBACCO PERFUMES, GENERAL BASIC MATERIAL NO. 1

1.	Cassia, Absolute	20
2.	Heliotropin	70
3.	Jasmine, Oil	50
4.	Labdanum, Absolute	20
5.	Methyl Ionone	60
6.	Musk Ketone	40
7.	Neroli, Oil	30
8.	Rose, Oil	40
9.	Tuberose, Absolute	10
10.	Vanillin	10
11.	Vetiverol, Oil	60
12.	Ethyl Alcohol 95%	590
		1000

TOBACCO PERFUMES, GENERAL BASIC MATERIAL NO. 2

1.	Bergamot, Oil	110
2.	Birch Tar, Oil	5
3.	Castoreum, Resinoid	2
4.	Clary Sage, Oil	80
5.	Dimethyl Hydroquinone	80
6.	Isopropyl Quinoline	70
7.	Jasmine, Oil	14
8.	Methyl Ionone	40
9.	Methyl Nonyl Acetaldehyde	2
10.	Methyl Phenyl Acetate	15
11.	Musk Ambrette	30
12.	Musk Ketone	80
13.	Neroli, Oil	14
14.	Orris, Oil	10
15.	Phenyl Acetic Acid	15
16.	Rose, Oil	35
17.	Sandalwood, Oil	42
18.	Tetrahydrofurfuryl Acetate	1
19.	Tobacco, Absolute	30
20.	Vanillin	25
21.	Ethyl Alcohol 95%	300
		1000

TOBACCO, STRONG ODOR

1.	Birch Tar, Oil	100
2.	Hydroquinone Dimethyl Ether	100
3.	Immortelle	200
4.	Labdanum, Oil	200
5.	Olibanum, Oil	200
6.	Phenyl Propyl Alcohol	200
		1000

TREFLÉ (CLOVER, TREFOIL) (FOR SOAP)

1.	Amyl Salicylate	400
2.	Anisaldehyde	50
3.	Benzylidene Acetone	25
4.	Benzyl Salicylate	25
5.	Bergamot, Oil	50
6.	Cananga, Oil	225
7.	Clary Sage, Oil	5
8.	Coumarin	45
9.	α-Ionone	25
10.	Lavender, Oil	25
11.	Linalyl Acetate	50
12.	Oakmoss, Resinoid	25
13.	Rose, Oil	35
14.	Vanillin	15
		1000

TUBEROSE, IMITATION (FOR SOAP)

1.	Aldehyde C-18	25
2.	Benzyl Acetate	70
3.	Benzyl Salicylate	70
4.	Hydroxycitronellal	150
5.	Linalool	100
6.	Linalyl Benzoate	175
7.	Methyl Anthranilate	150
8.	Methyl Benzoate	70
9.	Methyl Heptyne Carbonate	15
10.	Methyl Salicylate	70
11.	Tolu Balsam	25
12.	Tuberose	25
13.	Vanillin	5
14.	Ylang Ylang, Oil	50
		1000

TUBEROSE, SYNTHETIC

1.	Alcohol C-10	8
2.	Alcohol C-12	12
3.	Aldehyde C-9	3
4.	Aldehyde C-10	8
5.	Aldehyde C-11	3
6.	Aldehyde C-12	12
7.	Aldehyde C-18	4
8.	Amyl Cinnamic Aldehyde	10
9.	Anisyl Formate	10
10.	Benzyl Alcohol	150
11.	Benzyl Benzoate	150
12.	Benzyl Propionate	150
13.	Butyl Phenyl Acetate	150
14.	Hydroxycitronellal	150
15.	Methyl Anthranilate	10
16.	Methyl Heptyne Carbonate	10
17.	Methyl Nonyl Acetaldehyde	5
18.	Methyl Salicylate	5
19.	Phenyl Propyl Alcohol	150
		1000

UNY COLOGNE, PERFUME BASE

1.	Bergamot, Oil	200
2.	Citral	100
3.	Citronella, Formosa	150
4.	Lavender, Oil	100
5.	Musk Xylol	20
6.	Nerolin	60
7.	Petitgrain, Oil	100
8.	Rosemary, Oil	150
9.	Spike, Oil	120
		1000

VAPOROUS PERFUME, IMITATION NO. 1

1.	Cedarleaf, Oil	10
2.	Eucalyptol, Oil	350
3.	Isobornyl Acetate, Crystals	20
4.	Menthol	500
5.	Menthone, Oil	120
		1000

VAPOROUS PERFUME, IMITATION NO. 2

1.	Eucalyptol, Oil	170
2.	Isoborneol, Crystals	50
3.	Menthol	500
4.	Menthone, Oil	250
5.	Peppermint, Oil	30
		1000

VAPOROUS PERFUME, IMITATION NO. 3

1.	Camphor, Oil	250
2.	Menthone, Oil	250
3.	Vaporous Perfume, Imitation No. 1*	250
4.	Vaporous Perfume, Imitation No. 2*	250
		1000

VIOLET, FOR FACE POWDER

1.	Bergamot	100
2.	α–Ionone (10% sol'n.)	350
3.	Jasmine, Oil	100
4.	Methyl Ionone	50
5.	Musk Ketone	50
6.	Orange, Flower	50
7.	Orris Concrete (10% sol'n.)	200
8.	Vetiver	50
9.	Ylang Ylang	50
		1000

VIOLET, IMITATION NO. 1

1.	Aldehyde C-11	2
2.	Aldehyde C-12	5
3.	Aldehyde C-14	2
4.	Aldehyde C-18	2
5.	Citral	10
6.	Ethyl Myristate	5
7.	Ionone	10
8.	Methyl Heptyne Carbonate	10
9.	Orris Root, Oil	15
10.	Ylang Ylang, Oil	10
11.	Ethyl Alcohol 95%	465
12.	Distilled Water	464
		1000

VIOLET, IMITATION NO. 2

1.	Aldehyde C-18	20
2.	Bergamot, Oil	20
3.	α-Ionone	2
4.	Methyl Heptyne Carbonate	2
5.	Neroli, Oil	2
6.	Orris, Root	130
7.	Rhodinol	10
8.	Vanilla Beans, Oil	10
9.	Ethyl Alcohol 95%	402
10.	Distilled Water	402
		1000

* Formulas which appear in this book

VIOLET, IMITATION NO. 3

1.	Aldehyde C-12 (lauric)	20
2.	Bergamot, Oil	50
3.	Eugenol	25
4.	Heliotropin	25
5.	Hydroxycitronellal	25
6.	α-Ionone	85
7.	β-Ionone	75
8.	Methyl Heptyne Carbonate	15
9.	Methyl Ionone	75
10.	Musk Ambrette	5
11.	Rose, Oil	25
12.	Sandalwood, Oil	10
13.	Vanillin	10
14.	Ylang Ylang	25
15.	Ethyl Alcohol 95%	265
16.	Distilled Water	265
		1000

VIOLET, IMITATION NO. 4 (FOR SOAP)

1.	Cassie, Oil	75
2.	Ethyl Myristate	75
3.	Guaiacwood, Oil	75
4.	α-Ionone	250
5.	Methyl Heptyne Carbonate	50
6.	Orris Root, Concrete	350
7.	Sandalwood, Oil	50
8.	Violet Leaves, Concrete	75
		1000

VIOLET, IMITATION NO. 5 (FOR SOAP)

1.	Anisaldehyde	10
2.	Bergamot, Oil	50
3.	Cassie, Absolute	15
4.	Heliotropin	60
5.	Ionone	250
6.	Methyl Heptyne Carbonate	15

7.	Methyl Ionone	250
8.	Orris Root, Oil	250
9.	Violet Leaf, Absolute	100
		1000

VIOLET, IMITATION NO. 6

1.	Bergamot, Oil	50
2.	Eugenol	20
3.	Heliotropin	40
4.	Hydroxycitronellal	30
5.	α-Ionone (10% sol'n.)	335
6.	β-Ionone (10% sol'n.)	335
7.	Lauric Aldehyde	20
8.	Methyl Ionone	100
9.	Rose, Oil (10% sol'n.)	30
10.	Ylang Ylang, Oil	40
		1000

VIOLET LEAF

1.	Alcohol C-12 (10% sol'n.)	100
2.	Aldehyde C-10 (10% sol'n.)	100
3.	Aldehyde C-12 (10% sol'n.)	100
4.	α-Ionone	100
5.	Methyl Heptyne Carbonate	10
6.	Orris Concrete (10% sol'n.)	100
7.	Phenyl Ethyl Alcohol	100
8.	Ethyl Alcohol 95%	390
		1000

VIOLET, SYNTHETIC

1.	Alcohol C-10	10
2.	Alcohol C-12	50
3.	Aldehyde C-10	5
4.	Aldehyde C-12	15
5.	Cassia, Oil	25
6.	Jasmine, Oil	25
7.	Methyl Heptyne Carbonate	20
8.	Ionone	100
9.	Irone	100
10.	Orris Root, Absolute	50
11.	Ethyl Alcohol 95%	300
12.	Distilled Water	300
		1000

WALLFLOWER

1.	Alcohol C-9	75
2.	Aldehyde C-9	25
3.	Anisaldehyde	25
4.	Heliotropin	25
5.	Hydroxycitronellal	100
6.	Isoeugenol	15
7.	Methyl-*p*-Cresol	200
8.	Methyl Ionone	25
9.	Methyl-β-Naphthyl Ketone	10
10.	Ethyl Alcohol 95%	250
11.	Distilled Water	250
		1000

WINTERGREEN, IMITATION (FOR SOAP)

1.	Cinnamon Bark, Oil	50
2.	Clove, Oil	100
3.	Methyl Salicylate	200
4.	Peppermint, Oil	350
5.	Rhodinol	150
6.	Spearmint, Oil	150
		1000

Stir. Filter.

YLANG YLANG, IMITATION NO. 1

1.	Benzyl Alcohol	250
2.	Benzyl Benzoate	250
3.	Heliotropine	100
4.	α-Ionone, White	20
5.	Vanillin	100
6.	Ylang Ylang, Oil	30
7.	Ethyl Alcohol 95%	125
8.	Distilled Water	125
		1000

YLANG YLANG, IMITATION NO. 2

1.	Benzyl Alcohol	180
2.	Cassia, Oil	30
3.	Citral	50
4.	Ethyl Enanthate	50
5.	Heliotropin	20

6.	Orris, Oil	70
7.	Ylang Ylang, Oil (10% sol'n.)	600
		1000

YLANG YLANG, IMITATION NO. 3

1.	Cananga, Oil (10% sol'n.)	250
2.	α-Ionone	100
3.	Orris, Concrete	150
4.	Ylang Ylang, A	500
		1000

YLANG YLANG, IMITATION NO. 4

1.	Benzyl Alcohol (10% sol'n.)	250
2.	Benzyl Benzoate (10% sol'n.)	250
3.	Heliotropin (10% sol'n.)	100
4.	α-Ionone	20
5.	Phenyl Ethyl Alcohol (10% sol'n.)	250
6.	Vanillin (10% sol'n.)	100
7.	Ylang Ylang, Oil	30
		1000

YLANG YLANG, IMITATION NO. 5

1.	Anisic Aldehyde	100
2.	Benzyl Acetate	20
3.	Benzyl Benzoate	100
4.	Cananga, Oil	10
5.	Cinnamic Acid	10
6.	Citral	10
7.	*p*-Cresol Methyl Ether	10
8.	*p*-Cresyl Acetate	10
9.	*p*-Cresyl Phenyl Acetate	20
10.	Ethyl Benzoate	100
11.	Eugenol	10
12.	Geraniol	100
13.	Geranyl Phenyl Acetate	10
14.	Iraldeine, Balsam	10
15.	Methyl Benzoate	100
16.	Methyl Eugenol	10
17.	Methyl Phenyl Acetate	10
18.	Opoponax, Oil	10
19.	Phenyl Acetic Acid	20
20.	Phenyl Ethyl Alcohol	100
21.	Phenyl Ethyl Cinnamate	20
22.	Terpineol	100
23.	Terpinyl Acetate	100
24.	Vetivert	10
		1000

YLANG YLANG, SYNTHETIC NO. 1

1.	Alcohol C-9	25
2.	Aldehyde C-9	20
3.	Benzyl Acetate	50
4.	Benzyl Alcohol	50
5.	Benzyl Benzoate	50
6.	Cadinene, Oil	50
7.	Eugenol	10
8.	Geraniol	250
9.	Geranyl Benzoate	250
10.	Isoeugenol	20
11.	Linalool	50
12.	Methyl Anthranilate	20
13.	Methyl Benzoate	150
14.	Methyl Salicylate	5
		1000

YLANG YLANG, SYNTHETIC NO. 2

1.	Aldehyde C-18	25
2.	Benzyl Acetate	25
3.	Geraniol	250
4.	Geranyl Benzoate	250
5.	Linalool	100
6.	Linalyl Acetate	50
7.	Methyl Benzoate	250
8.	Methyl Eugenol	25
9.	Terpineol	25
		1000

Chapter XI:
FORMULARY OF FLAVORS

NOTES:

A. The esters of amyl, benzyl, butyl, methyl, and propyl alcohols with acetic, anthranilate, butyric, capric, formic, propionic, and valeric acids are employed to simulate the fruit flavors. For example, a peach flavor is enhanced by Aldehyde C-14, a strawberry flavor by Aldehyde C-16, and a pineapple flavor by ethyl butyrate. All the formulas of these flavors are made with these esters.

B. The proportion used for making essences is 2 or 3 volumes (2 or 3 cc per liter of solvent) for each completed formula.

C. All formulas are alphabetically listed, including their ingredients. The ethyl alcohol 95% and distilled water are always listed last in each formula.

D. Ingredients denoted by an asterisk (*) are formulas which may be found in this book.

GENERAL METHOD FOR THE EXTRACTION OF NATURAL FLAVORS FROM FRESH OR DRY FRUITS

1.	Fruits (fresh, ripe or dry, not rancid) (well crushed, rasped, or ground)	10 kg
2.	Ethyl Alcohol 95%	10 l
3.	Distilled Water	10 l

Let stand for several days (either 10, 8, or 3, depending on the maximum flavor and odor development, which can also be obtained by fermentation with the addition of sugar in double amount, before the addition of alcohol and distilled water). Stir for 1 h daily. Separate the juice. To the residue add:

4.	Ethyl Alcohol 95%	10 l
5.	Distilled Water	10 l

Let stand for another 3 days. Add:

6.	Amyl Valerianate	5 ml

for fresh fruits or

Ethyl Oenanthate	25 ml
Amyl Formate	45 ml

for dry fruits.

Distill altogether. Filter.

Yield: Proportionate to the amount of fruits and doubled ethyl alcohol 95% and distilled water.

"NEUTRAL" ESTERS MIXTURE BASE

1.	Ethyl Acetate	420
2.	Ethyl Formate	250
3.	Isoamyl Acetate	250
4.	Isoamyl Butyrate	80
		1000

Note: This is a general base. It can be used with the simple addition of one or more components for a specific flavor. For example, by increasing the isoamyl acetate in this base, the characteristic "banana" flavor is obtained.

ABBEY, BENEDICTINE TYPE

1.	Angelica, Oil (terpeneless)	2
2.	Camomile, German, Oil (terpeneless)	8
3.	Celery, Oil (terpeneless)	4
4.	Cinnamon, Ceylon, Oil (terpeneless)	8
5.	Mace, Oil (terpeneless)	4
6.	Cognac, Oil	200
7.	Maraschino	350
8.	Orange, Bitter, Oil (terpeneless)	6
9.	Orange, Sweet, Oil (terpeneless)	4
10.	Peppermint, Oil (terpeneless)	14
11.	Ethyl Alcohol 95%	400
		1000

Note: Abbey is the name of a monastery or convent.

ABSINTHE

1.	Absinthe, Oil (10% sol'n.)	50
2.	Anise, Oil	5
3.	Fennel, Oil	2
4.	Lemon, Oil	5
5.	Peppermint, Oil	50
6.	Sugar	238
7.	Ethyl Alcohol 95%	325
8.	Distilled Water	325
		1000

Dissolve sugar in the water; stir together; filter.

Note: Absinthe is not allowed as an alcoholic beverage in the U.S.A.

ADVOCAAT (ADVOKAAT)

1.	Clove, Oil	1
2.	Cloves	2
3.	Cognac	65
4.	Coriander, Oil	1
5.	Mace, Oil	5
6.	Maraschino, Essence	35
7.	Neroli, Oil	1
8.	Nutmeg, Oil	5
9.	Rum, Jamaica	25
10.	Saffron	10
11.	Sassafras, Wood	25
12.	Vanilla, Oil	25
13.	Vanillin (100%)	10
14.	Ethyl Alcohol 95%	395
15.	Distilled Water	395
		1000

Macerate for 10 days, warm. Press the liquid off. Filter through paper. Add:

1.	Yellow Color Sol'n.	2
2.	Ethyl Alcohol 95%	100

Note: Advocaat is a sweet, thick, yellow Dutch liqueur. This essence is a Dutch specialty. It has a peculiar taste, similar to egg yolk. It is also suitable for soft chocolate cream at 1–2 cc/1000 cc.

ALLSPICE, OIL

1.	Caraway, Seeds Oil	100
2.	Celery, Seeds Oil	100
3.	Cinnamon, Seeds Oil	300
4.	Cloves, Seeds Oil	300
5.	Coriander, Seeds Oil	100
6.	Nutmeg, Seeds Oil	100
		1000

ALMOND, BITTER

A variety of the common almond (*Prunus amygdalus amara*) having bitter kernels that yield a highly poisonous oil. It is used for flavoring only when the prussic acid in it has been totally removed.

ALMOND, BITTER ESSENCE (NATURAL)

1.	Almond, Bitter, Oil (pure)	160
2.	Benzaldehyde (pure)	5
3.	Benzyl Alcohol	15
4.	Ethyl Alcohol 95%	410
5.	Distilled Water	410
		1000

ALMOND, BITTER (FOR SOAP)

1.	Benzaldehyde	300
2.	Caraway, Oil	25
3.	Cedarwood, Oil	25
4.	Citronella, Oil	50
5.	Geranium Palmarosa, Oil	150
6.	Phenyl Ethyl Alcohol	150
7.	Terpineol	300
		1000

ALMOND, BITTER IMITATION

1.	Benzaldehyde (pure)	10
2.	Geraniol	70
3.	Petitgrain, Paraguay	50
4.	Phenyl Ethyl Alcohol	80
5.	Ethyl Alcohol 95%	790
		1000

ALMOND, BITTER NO. 1

1.	Benzaldehyde (pure, 10% sol'n.)	450
2.	Benzyl Alcohol (10% sol'n.)	544
3.	Bromelia	1
4.	Vanillin	5
		1000

ALMOND, BITTER NO. 2

1.	Benzaldehyde (pure, 10% sol'n.)	100
2.	Ethyl Acetate (10% sol'n.)	450
3.	Ethyl Benzoate	50
4.	Ethyl Formate (10% sol'n.)	250
5.	Isoamyl Acetate	150
		1000

ALMOND, BITTER NO. 3

1.	Almond, Bitter, Oil (cyanide-free)	200
2.	Benzaldehyde (pure, 10% sol'n.)	50
3.	Benzyl Alcohol	100
4.	Ethyl Alcohol 95%	325
5.	Distilled Water	325
		1000

ALMOND, BITTER NO. 4

1.	Almond, Bitter, Oil (cyanide-free)	500
2.	Benzaldehyde (pure, 10% sol'n.)	150
3.	Benzyl Alcohol (10% sol'n.)	343
4.	Neroli, Oil	2
5.	Vanillin	5
		1000

ALMOND, BITTER NO. 5

1.	Benzaldehyde (pure, 10% sol'n.)	150
2.	Benzyl Alcohol (10% sol'n.)	844
3.	Bromelia	1
4.	Vanillin	5
		1000

ALMOND, BITTER NO. 6

1.	Benzaldehyde (pure, 10% sol'n.)	100
2.	Ethyl Acetate (10% sol'n.)	450
3.	Ethyl Benzoate	50
4.	Ethyl Formate (10% sol'n.)	250
5.	Isoamyl Acetate	150
		1000

ALMOND, BITTER NO. 7

1.	Almond, Bitter No. 1*	750
2.	Almond, Bitter No. 2*	250
		1000

ALMOND, BITTER, SYNTHETIC NO. 1

1.	Benzaldehyde (pure)	10
2.	Ethyl Alcohol 95%	350
3.	Distilled Water	640
		1000

ALMOND, BITTER, SYNTHETIC NO. 2

1.	Benzaldehyde (pure)	5
2.	Benzyl Alcohol	60
3.	Ethyl Benzoate	5
4.	Ethyl Formate	5
5.	Vanillin	5
6.	Ethyl Alcohol 95%	460
7.	Distilled Water	460
		1000

ALMOND, BITTER, SYNTHETIC NO. 3

1.	Benzaldehyde (pure)	12
2.	Benzyl Alcohol	42
3.	Ethyl Acetate	22
4.	Ethyl Benzoate	2
5.	Ethyl Formate	12
6.	Hydrocinnamic Aldehyde	1
7.	Isoamyl Acetate	7
8.	β-Naphthyl Ethyl Ether	2
9.	Rhodinyl Propionate	2
10.	Vanillin	5
11.	Ethyl Alcohol 95%	447
12.	Distilled Water	446
		1000

* Formulas which appear in this book

ALMOND, BITTER SYNTHETIC NO. 4

1.	Anisette, Essence	100
2.	Cognac (liquor at 60%)	50
3.	Curacao, Essence	150
4.	Maraschino, Essence	50
5.	Orange Flowers (collected early morning)	195
6.	Vanillin	5
7.	Ethyl Alcohol 95%	150
8.	Distilled Water	300
		1000

Macerate for 8 days. Agitate with stirrer 1 h daily. Filter.

ALMOND, IMITATION

1.	Benzaldehyde (pure, 10% sol'n.)	9
2.	Isoamyl Isovalerate	10
3.	Malic Acid	1
4.	Ethyl Alcohol 95%	980
		1000

ALMOND, MILK (ORZATA)

1.	Almond, Bitter Essence (Natural)* (pure)	40
2.	Benzoin	10
3.	Sugar	200
4.	Distilled Water	750
		1000

Note: Barley, basis. Barley is a widely cultivated cereal grass (*Hordeum*, Family *Graminaceae*). The grain of this plant is used as food and in making beer, ale, and whiskey.

ALMOND, PEACH

1.	Maraschino, Essence	25
2.	Orange Flowers, Imitation No. 1*	25
3.	Peach, Extract (Natural)*	38
4.	Rose, Imitation No. 1*	25
5.	γ-Undelactone (Aldehyde C-14)	2
6.	Vanillin	3
7.	Ethyl Alcohol 95%	460
8.	Distilled Water	422
		1000

Note: Essences of kernel of maraschino "wild cherry," free of cyanuric acid.

ANGELIC, TINCTURE

1.	Angelic Root (pulverized)	400
2.	Ethyl Alcohol 95%	500
3.	Distilled Water	100
		1000

ANGOSTURA, BITTER

1.	Angostura, Bark (pulverized)	110
2.	Cardamom, Seeds (pulverized)	3
3.	Cinnamon, Bark (pulverized)	40
4.	Clove, Flowers (dry and pulverized)	30
5.	Galangal, Root (pulverized)	7
6.	Gentian, Root (pulverized)	7
7.	Ginger, Root (pulverized)	2
8.	Lemon, Peels (pulverized)	20
9.	Orange (bitter), Peels (pulverized)	40
10.	St. John's Bread (pulverized)	2
11.	Sugar (pulverized)	345
12.	Sweet Flag, Root (pulverized)	7
13.	Tonka Beans, Seeds (pulverized)	40
14.	Ethyl Alcohol 95%	174
15.	Distilled Water	173
		1000

Pulverize #1–13. Macerate with sugar and alcohol (#11, 14) for 10 days, stirring every day for 1 h. Filter. To the residue add double amount of ethyl alcohol 95% and distilled water. Let stand for another 3 days, stirring every day for 1 h. Filter. To the residue add double amount of ethyl alcohol 95% and distilled water. Let stand for another 3 days, stirring every day for 1 h. Put altogether and distill.

Yield: 2 liters

ANISE BASE

1.	Anise Seeds, Oil	820
2.	Cardamom, Oil	20
3.	Cinnamon, Oil	20
4.	Clove, Oil	40
5.	Coriander, Oil	80
6.	Lemon, Oil	20
		1000

ANISEED

1.	Almond, Bitter, Oil (cyanide-free)	2
2.	Angelica, Oil (terpeneless)	2
3.	Anise, Oil (terpeneless)	25
4.	Badiane (Star Anise), Oil	10
5.	Coriander, Oil	6
6.	Fennel, Oil	15
7.	Rose, Bulgarian, Oil (10% sol'n.)	6
8.	Ethyl Alcohol 95%	934
		1000

ANISETTE, OIL NO. 1

1.	Anise, Oil	770
2.	Cardamom, Oil	5
3.	Coriander, Oil	20
4.	Fennel (sweet), Oil	200
5.	Lemon, Oil	5
		1000

Note: Mix well and let stand for 24 h or more. Use 15 cl of this oil to make 1 part of anisette extract.

ANISETTE, OIL NO. 2

1.	Amber, Oil	2
2.	Anise, Seeds Oil	55
3.	Coriander, Oil	3
4.	Fennel (sweet), Oil	6
5.	Orris Root, Oil	9
6.	Sugar	450
7.	Ethyl Alcohol 95%	240
8.	Distilled Water	235
		1000

APPLE, BASE

1.	Apples (freshly sliced)	450
2.	Ethyl Alcohol 95%	550
		1000

Let macerate for 6 days. Then add:

3.	Distilled Water	1250

Distill 1125 cc. Use the distillate to macerate:

4.	Apple (sliced)	450

After 3 days add:

5.	Amyl Valerate	20
6.	Ethyl Butyrate	5
7.	Ethyl Valerate	5
8.	Isobutyl Valerate	100
9.	Distilled Water	200

Distill to obtain a final yield of 1000 cc.

APPLE, ESSENCE (NATURAL) NO. 1

1.	Apples (freshly sliced and chopped)	10 kg
2.	Ethyl Alcohol 95%	20 l

Macerate for 3 days

3.	Distilled Water	10 g

Macerate for another 3 days

4.	Distilled Water	10 g
5.	Amyl Valerate	5 cl

Distill.

APPLE, ESSENCE (NATURAL) NO. 2

1.	Apples (freshly sliced and chopped)	1000
2.	Salt	150

Macerate for 10 days.

3.	Ethyl Alcohol 95%	250
4.	Wine, White	1000

Macerate for another 8 days. Distill, over 1000 cml.

Note: Employ 5–10 cml per liter.

APPLE, ESSENCE (NATURAL) NO. 3

1.	Apple, Essence No. 1 (Natural)*	500
2.	Ethyl Acetate	3
3.	Ethyl Malonate	3
4.	Isobutyl Valerianate	1
5.	Ethyl Alcohol 95%	247
6.	Distilled Water	246
		1000

Distill.

Note: Employ $^1/_2$ cml per liter.

APPLE, ESSENCE (NATURAL) NO. 4

1.	Apple, Concentrated Juice	240
2.	Apple, Essence No. 1 (Natural)*	80
3.	Apple, Essence No. 2 (Natural)*	350
4.	Ethyl Alcohol 95%	165
5.	Propylene Glycol	165
		1000

Distill.

APPLE, ESSENCE (NATURAL) NO. 5

1.	Apples or Apple Peels (dried)	10
2.	Ethyl Alcohol 95%	30

Macerate for 3 days.

3.	Distilled Water	30

Distill.

4. Amyl Valerianate, in small amount to achieve the best odor and flavor.

APPLE, IMITATION NO. 1

1.	Amyl Acetate	34
2.	Amyl Valerate	30
3.	Apple, Base*	200

* Formulas which appear in this book

4.	Benzaldehyde (pure)	1
5.	Clove, Oil	4
6.	Cognac, Oil	1
7.	Ethyl Acetate	65
8.	Ethyl Butyrate	20
9.	Ethyl Pelargonate	15
10.	Ethyl Valerate	45
11.	Isobutyl Valerate	60
12.	Lemon, Oil (terpeneless)	1
13.	Orange, Bitter, Oil (terpeneless)	1
14.	Orange, Sweet, Oil (terpeneless)	3
15.	Ethyl Alcohol 95%	520
		1000

APPLE, IMITATION NO. 2

1.	Amyl Valerianate	125
2.	Ethyl Acetate	85
3.	Ethyl Butyrate	45
4.	Ethyl Malonate	20
5.	Ethyl Nitrate	85
6.	Isobutyl Valerianate	100
7.	Ethyl Alcohol 95%	540
		1000

APPLE, IMITATION NO. 3

1.	Acetaldehyde	20
2.	*n*-Caprylate	10
3.	Geraniol	10
4.	Geranyl Acetate	10
5.	Geranyl Formate	10
6.	Isoamyl Acetate	100
7.	Isoamyl-*n*-Caproate	50
8.	Isoamyl Formate	100
9.	Ethyl Alcohol 95%	345
10.	Distilled Water	345
		1000

APPLE, IMITATION NO. 4

1.	Amyl Acetate	75
2.	Amyl Valerianate	60
3.	Benzaldehyde (pure)	1
4.	Citronellyl Valerate	5
5.	Clove, Oil	10
6.	Ethyl Acetate	140
7.	Ethyl Butyrate	50
8.	Ethyl Malonate	35
9.	Ethyl Valerianate	75
10.	Geranyl Butyrate	5
11.	Isoamyl Valerate	35
12.	Ethyl Alcohol 95%	255
13.	Distilled Water	254
		1000

APPLE, SYNTHETIC NO. 1

1.	Amyl Acetate	13
2.	Amyl Valerianate	26
3.	Benzaldehyde (pure)	2
4.	Ethyl Acetate	13
5.	Ethyl Butyrate	13
6.	Ethyl Valerianate	13
7.	Ethyl Alcohol 95%	460
8.	Propylene Glycol	460
		1000

APPLE, SYNTHETIC NO. 2

1.	Aldehyde C-14	2
2.	Amyl Valerianate	10
3.	Chloroform	1
4.	Ethyl Acetate	1
5.	Ethyl Nitrate	1
6.	Glycerin (neutral)	40
7.	Tartaric Acid	1
8.	Ethyl Alcohol 95%	472
9.	Distilled Water	472
		1000

APPLE, SYNTHETIC NO. 3

1.	Acetaldehyde	1
2.	Amyl Valerianate	10
3.	Chloroform	1
4.	Ethyl Acetate	10
5.	Ethyl Benzoate	10
6.	Ethyl Butyrate	10
7.	Ethyl Nitrate	10
8.	Ethyl Oenanthate	1
9.	Glycerin (neutral)	472
10.	Tartaric Acid	1
11.	Vanillin	2
12.	Ethyl Alcohol 95%	236
13.	Distilled Water	236
		1000

APPLE, SYNTHETIC NO. 4

1.	Amyl Acetate	4
2.	Amyl Valerianate	5
3.	Benzaldehyde (pure)	1
4.	Clove, Oil	1
5.	Ethyl Acetate	3
6.	Ethyl Oenanthate	1
7.	Ethyl Valerianate	5
8.	Ethyl Alcohol 95%	490
9.	Distilled Water	490
		1000

APPLE, SYNTHETIC NO. 5

1.	Apple, Synthetic No. 1*	30
2.	Ethyl Butyrate	5
3.	Isobutyl Valerianate	5
4.	Methyl Ethyl Phenyl Glycidate	5
5.	Ethyl Alcohol 95%	475
6.	Distilled Water	480
		1000

APPLE, SYNTHETIC NO. 6

1.	Acetaldehyde	1
2.	Amyl Valerianate	6
3.	Ethyl Acetate	4
4.	Ethyl Nitrate	4
5.	Ethyl Alcohol 95%	492
6.	Distilled Water	493
		1000

APPLE, SYNTHETIC NO. 7

1.	Acetaldehyde	2
2.	Benzaldehyde	1
3.	*n*-Caprylate	1
4.	Citronellyl Valerianate	22
5.	Ethyl Acetate	3
6.	Ethyl Butyrate	11
7.	Ethyl Isovalerianate	30
8.	Ethyl Malonate	10
9.	Ethyl Oenanthate	16
10.	Eugenol	4
11.	Geranyl Acetate	28
12.	Geranyl Butyrate	26
13.	Isoamyl Acetate	9
14.	Isoamyl Caproate	6
15.	Isoamyl Oenanthate	1
16.	Isoamyl Valerianate	50
17.	Isobutyl Valerianate	10
18.	Malonic Acid	10
19.	Ethyl Alcohol 95%	380
20.	Distilled Water	380
		1000

* Formulas which appear in this book

APPLE, SYNTHETIC NO. 8

1.	Aldehyde C-14	2
2.	Amyl Butyrate	10
3.	Chloroform	1
4.	Ethyl Acetate	1
5.	Ethyl Nitrate	1
6.	Glycerin (neutral)	328
7.	Tartaric Acid	1
8.	Ethyl Alcohol 95%	328
9.	Distilled Water	328
		1000

APPLE, SYNTHETIC NO. 9

1.	Amyl Butyrate	4
2.	Chloroform	3
3.	Ethyl Butyrate	30
4.	Ethyl Salicylate	3
5.	Ethyl Valerianate	15
6.	Glycerin (neutral)	315
7.	Ethyl Alcohol 95%	315
8.	Distilled Water	315
		1000

APPLE, SYNTHETIC NO. 10

1.	Acetaldehyde	2
2.	Amyl Acetate	10
3.	Amyl Valerianate	10
4.	Chloroform	10
5.	Ethyl Acetate	10
6.	Ethyl Nitrate	10
7.	Ethyl Alcohol 95%	474
8.	Distilled Water	474
		1000

APPLE, SYNTHETIC NO. 11

1.	Aldehyde C-14 (pure)	1
2.	Amyl Valerianate	8
3.	Chloroform	2
4.	Ethyl Acetate	2
5.	Ethyl Nitrate	1
6.	Glycerin (neutral)	328
7.	Ethyl Alcohol 95%	330
8.	Distilled Water	328
		1000

APPLE, SYNTHETIC NO. 12

1.	Acetaldehyde	12
2.	Amyl Valerianate	12
3.	Chloroform	12
4.	Ethyl Acetate	12
5.	Ethyl Nitrate	12
6.	Ethyl Alcohol 95%	470
7.	Distilled Water	470
		1000

APPLE, SYNTHETIC NO. 13

1.	Amyl Valerianate	12
2.	Ethyl Acetate	8
3.	Ethyl Butyrate	4
4.	Ethyl Malonate	2
5.	Ethyl Nitrate	8
6.	Isobutyl Valerianate	10
7.	Ethyl Alcohol 95%	478
8.	Distilled Water	478
		1000
9.	Magnesium Oxide	2

Distill, over 1250 cl
Add:

10.	Apple, Essence (Natural) No. 1*	500
11.	Apple, Essence (Natural) No. 2*	500

Filter
Note: Employ 3 cl per liter

* Formulas which appear in this book

APPLE, SYNTHETIC NO. 14

1.	Acetaldehyde	1
2.	Isoamyl Acetate	13
3.	Isoamyl-*n*-Caproate	5
4.	Isoamyl-*n*-Caprylate	2
5.	Isoamyl Valerianate	21
6.	Ethyl Alcohol 95%	479
7.	Distilled Water	479
		1000

APRICOT, ESSENCE (NATURAL) NO. 1

1.	Apricots (chopped, without seeds)	10 kg
2.	Ethyl Alcohol 95%	20 l

Macerate for 3 days

3.	Distilled Water	10 l

Macerate for another 3 days

4.	Distilled Water	10 cl
5.	Ethyl Valerianate	5 cml

Distill

APRICOT, ESSENCE (NATURAL) NO. 2

1.	Apricot, Essence (Natural) No. 1*	500
2.	Benzyl Cinnamate	1
3.	Ethyl Cinnamate	1
4.	γ-Lactone Undecylenic Acid (Persicol)	5
5.	Nonyl Aldehyde (Apricolin)	5
6.	Tannic Acid	1
7.	Vanilla, Oil	2
8.	Vanillin	1
9.	Ethyl Alcohol 95%	242
10.	Distilled Water	242
		1000

APRICOT, IMITATION NO. 1

1.	Almond, Bitter, Oil (cyanide-free)	8
2.	Amyl Butyrate	150

3.	Amyl Propionate	10
4.	Benzaldehyde (pure, 10% sol'n.)	4
5.	Ethyl Butyrate	100
6.	Ethyl Valerate	50
7.	Methyl Salicylate	25
8.	Phenyl Methyl Acetate	25
9.	Phenyl Methyl Formate	25
10.	γ-Undelactone	3
11.	Ethyl Alcohol 95%	600
		1000

APRICOT, IMITATION NO. 2

1.	Almond, Bitter, Oil (cyanide-free)	6
2.	Amyl Butyrate	75
3.	Amyl Propionate	5
4.	Apricot, Base	25
5.	Methyl Heptyne Carbonate	25
6.	Methyl Phenyl Acetate	25
7.	Methyl Phenyl Formate	35
8.	Peach, Base	25
9.	γ-Undelactone	5
10.	Ethyl Alcohol 95%	774
		1000

APRICOT, IMITATION NO. 3

1.	Almond, Bitter, Oil (cyanide-free)	5
2.	Amyl Butyrate	150
3.	Amyl Valerate	25
4.	Benzaldehyde (pure, 10% sol'n.)	5
5.	Ethyl Butyrate	125
6.	Ethyl Valerate	50
7.	Methyl Salicylate	25
8.	Phenyl Methyl Acetate	50
9.	Phenyl Methyl Formate	35
10.	γ-Undelactone	4
11.	Ethyl Alcohol 95%	526
		1000

APRICOT, IMITATION NO. 4

1.	Anethole	5
2.	Amyl Acetate	50
3.	Amyl Alcohol	5
4.	Amyl Butyrate	75
5.	Butyl Butyrate	100
6.	Ethyl Acetate	50
7.	Ethyl Butyrate	75
8.	Ethyl Valerate	55
9.	Eugenol	3
10.	Jasmine, Oil (10% sol'n.)	10
11.	Petitgrain, Oil	10
12.	Phenyl Methyl Carbinyl Acetate	50
13.	Vanillin	12
14.	Ethyl Alcohol 95%	250
15.	Distilled Water	250
		1000

APRICOT, IMITATION NO. 5

1.	Amyl Alcohol	15
2.	Benzaldehyde (pure, 10% sol'n.)	70
3.	Benzyl Acetate	70
4.	Cinnamon, Ceylon, Oil	12
5.	Clove, Oil	6
6.	Cognac, Oil	15
7.	Coriander, Oil	2
8.	Ethyl Acetate	110
9.	Ethyl Butyrate	200
10.	Ethyl Formate	5
11.	Ethyl Pelargonate	25
12.	Ethyl Valerate	40
13.	Geraniol	12
14.	Orange, Sweet, Oil	30
15.	Rose, Oil	3
16.	Vanillin (10% sol'n.)	35
17.	Ethyl Alcohol 95%	350
		1000

APRICOT, SYNTHETIC NO. 1

1.	Amyl Butyrate	1
2.	Chloroform	1
3.	Ethyl Butyrate	10
4.	Ethyl Oenanthate	1
5.	Ethyl Salicylate	2
6.	Ethyl Valerianate	5
7.	Glycerin (neutral)	4
8.	Tartaric Acid	1
9.	Ethyl Alcohol 95%	488
10.	Distilled Water	487
		1000

APRICOT, SYNTHETIC NO. 2

1.	Amyl Acetate	1
2.	Amyl Alcohol	5
3.	Amyl Butyrate	2
4.	Benzyl Acetate	1
5.	Benzyl Propionate	1
6.	Butyl Butyrate	1
7.	Chloroform	2
8.	Ethyl Acetate	5
9.	Ethyl Butyrate	4
10.	Ethyl Oenanthate	2
11.	Ethyl Salicylate	2
12.	Ethyl Valerianate	10
13.	Eugenol	1
14.	Glycerin (neutral)	36
15.	Tartaric Acid	1
16.	Vanillin	1
17.	Ethyl Alcohol 95%	463
18.	Distilled Water	462
		1000

APRICOT, SYNTHETIC NO. 3

1.	Aldehyde C-16	5
2.	Amyl Butyrate	2
3.	Chloroform	1
4.	Ethyl Oenanthate	1
5.	Ethyl Salicylate	2
6.	Ethyl Valerianate	4
7.	Glycerin (neutral)	327
8.	Phenyl Ethyl Acetate	4
9.	Ethyl Alcohol 95%	327
10.	Distilled Water	327
		1000

APRICOT, SYNTHETIC NO. 4

1.	Aldehyde C-16	1
2.	Anethole	1
3.	Apricot, Essence (Natural) No. 1*	20
4.	Benzaldehyde (pure)	3
5.	Benzyl Acetate	2
6.	Butyl Butyrate	2
7.	Ethyl Acetate	5
8.	Ethyl Butyrate	15
9.	Ethyl Formate	4
10.	Ethyl Isovalerianate	8
11.	Ethyl Oenanthate	1
12.	Ethyl Salicylate	1
13.	Eugenol	1
14.	Glycerin (neutral)	300
15.	Isoamyl Acetate	6
16.	Isoamyl Alcohol	2
17.	Isoamyl Butyrate	22
18.	Isoamyl Isovalerianate	2
19.	Isoamyl Propionate	1
20.	Linalool	1
21.	Methyl Heptyne Carbonate	1
22.	Vanillin	1
23.	Ethyl Alcohol 95%	300
24.	Distilled Water	300
		1000

APRICOT, SYNTHETIC NO. 5

1.	Aldehyde C-14	25
2.	Amyl Acetate	16
3.	Amyl Butyrate	16
4.	Amyl Valerianate	16
5.	Benzaldehyde	4
6.	Cinnamic Aldehyde	1
7.	Ethyl Caprylate	18
8.	Ethyl Valerianate	18
9.	Geraniol	1
10.	Neroli, Oil	4
11.	Vanillin	16
12.	Ethyl Alcohol 95%	433
13.	Distilled Water	432
		1000

AUBEPINE (HAWTHORN)

1.	Alcohol C-9	2
2.	Aldehyde C-9	1
3.	Aldehyde C-10	2
4.	Anisic Aldehyde	75
5.	Citral	20
6.	Ethyl Alcohol 95%	450
7.	Distilled Water	450
		1000

AVOCADO

1.	Cloves	3
2.	Cognac	125

* Formulas which appear in this book

3.	Coriander	1
4.	Maraschino	75
5.	Neroli, Oil	1
6.	Nutmeg	15
7.	Rum, Jamaica	50
8.	Saffron	25
9.	Vanilla Beans	20
10.	Ethyl Alcohol 95%	343
11.	Distilled Water	342
		1000

Macerate for 10 days. Press. Filter. Add certified yellow color (2 g), triacetin 100 cc.

BANANA, ESSENCE (NATURAL) NO. 1

1.	Bananas, Peeled (not over-ripened, only the pulp is used)	20 kg
2.	Ethyl Alcohol 95%	20 l

Macerate for 3 days. Express, at least 20 l. To the residue add:

3.	Distilled Water	2 cl
4.	Amyl Butyrate	6 ml
5.	Coriander Oil	12 ml

Macerate for another 3 days. Distill altogether.

Yield: 15 liters

BANANA, ESSENCE (NATURAL) NO. 2

1.	Bananas, Peeled	10 kg
2.	Ethyl Alcohol 95%	10 l

Press after 1 week. Add:

3.	Wine, Brand	2 l
4.	Vanillin	15 g
5.	Ethyl Butyrate	3 ml

BANANA, IMITATION NO. 1

1.	Amyl Acetate	20
2.	Amyl Butyrate	30
3.	Benzyl Benzoate	20
4.	Chamomile, Oil	3
5.	Cinnamon, Oil	2
6.	Ethyl Butyrate	3
7.	Eugenol	3
8.	Lemon, Oil	30
9.	Mandarin, Oil	10
10.	Orange, Sweet, Oil	20
11.	Petitgrain, Oil	7
12.	Vanillin	10
13.	Ethyl Alcohol 95%	421
14.	Distilled Water	421
		1000

BANANA, IMITATION NO. 2

1.	Banana, Essence (Natural) No. 1*	125
2.	Banana, Essence (Natural) No. 2*	375
3.	Amyl Acetate	75
4.	α-Ionone	1
5.	Vanillin	4
6.	Ethyl Alcohol 95%	210
7.	Distilled Water	210
		1000

BANANA, IMITATION NO. 3

1.	Amyl Acetate	40
2.	Benzyl Propionate	21
3.	Butyl Butyrate	45
4.	Ethyl Butyrate	40
5.	Lemon, Oil	25
6.	Orange, Sweet, Oil	21
7.	Propyl Acetate	47
8.	Vanillin	1
9.	Ethyl Alcohol 95%	380
10.	Distilled Water	380
		1000

BANANA, IMITATION NO. 4

1.	Acetaldehyde	2
2.	Amyl Alcohol	5

* Formulas which appear in this book

3.	Benzyl Propionate	10
4.	Chloroform	1
5.	Clove, Oil	1
6.	Glycerin (neutral)	5
7.	Petitgrain, Oil	1
8.	Vanillin	1
9.	Ethyl Alcohol 95%	487
10.	Distilled Water	487
		1000

BANANA, IMITATION NO. 5

1.	Capraldehyde	1
2.	Benzyl Benzoate	12
3.	Cinnamic Aldehyde	1
4.	Ethyl Acetate	12
5.	Ethyl Butyrate	20
6.	Ethyl Sebacate	10
7.	Eugenol	1
8.	Glycerin (neutral)	289
9.	Isoamyl Acetate	37
10.	Isoamyl Butyrate	20
11.	Lemon, Oil	1
12.	δ-Limonene	8
13.	Linalool	6
14.	Methyl Anthranilate	1
15.	Vanillin	3
16.	Ethyl Alcohol 95%	289
16.	Distilled Water	289
		1000

BANANA, SYNTHETIC NO. 1

1.	Amyl Acetate	30
2.	Ethyl Butyrate	30
3.	Ethyl Alcohol 95%	470
4.	Distilled Water	470
		1000

BANANA, SYNTHETIC NO. 2

1.	Amyl Acetate	40
2.	Amyl Butyrate	8
3.	Benzyl Acetate	40
4.	Ethyl Butyrate	8
5.	Vanillin	4
6.	Ethyl Alcohol 95%	450
7.	Distilled Water	450
		1000

BANANA, SYNTHETIC NO. 3

1.	Amyl Acetate	90
2.	Amyl Butyrate	12
3.	Benzyl Acetate	20
4.	Ethyl Butyrate	7
5.	Ethyl Alcohol 95%	436
6.	Distilled Water	435
		1000

BANANA, SYNTHETIC NO. 4

1.	Amyl Acetate	10
2.	Amyl Butyrate	20
3.	Benzyl Acetate	20
4.	Benzyl Propionate	20
5.	Ethyl Butyrate	18
6.	Vanillin	2
7.	Glycerin (neutral)	20
8.	Ethyl Alcohol 95%	445
9.	Distilled Water	445
		1000

BANANA, SYNTHETIC NO. 5

1.	Amyl Acetate	20
2.	Amyl Butyrate	10
3.	Benzyl Acetate	20
4.	Benzyl Phenyl Acetate	2
5.	Ethyl Butyrate	5
6.	Glycerin (neutral)	10
7.	Vanillin, Tincture 1/10%	50
8.	Ethyl Alcohol 95%	442
9.	Distilled Water	441
		1000

BARBECUE

1.	Bay, Leaves	25
2.	Capsicum, Oleoresin	150
3.	Cloves	175
4.	Coriander	50
5.	Garlic, Extract	50

6.	Ginger, Oleoresin	100
7.	Marjoram, Sweet	125
8.	Onion, Extract	50
9.	Pepper, Black	100
10.	Pimenta, Leaves	150
11.	Thyme, White	25
		1000

BARBECUE SAUCE, "HUNT" TYPE

1.	Carrots, Dehydrated	20
2.	Celery, Dehydrated	15
3.	Corn Syrup	60
4.	Flavors, Natural: Basil, Laurel Leaves, Oregano, Parsley, Rosemary, Sage (Oils), 1 ml each	6
5.	Onions, Dehydrated	25
6.	Pectin	5
7.	Pepper, Green Bell, Dehydrated	15
8.	Salt	1
9.	Spices: Cinnamon, Clove, Nutmeg, Paprika, Pepper (Oils) 1 ml each	5
10.	Sugar	20
11.	Tomatoes, Dehydrated	300
12.	Tomatoes, Sauce	350
13.	Vinegar, Distilled	3
14.	Distilled Water	175
		1000

Note: The amount of each ingredient can be increased or decreased in accordance with individual taste.

BARBERRY, ESSENCE (NATURAL)

1.	Barberries, Juice (express from fully ripe berries)	7 1

Macerate the residue for 3 days with:

2.	Ethyl Alcohol 95%	3 1

Mix the residue of the maceration with the juice. Add:

3.	Ethyl Butyrate	12 ml

Distill altogether. Redistill for rectification. Yield: 5 liters

BENEDICTINE NO. 1

Liquor made originally by Benedictine monks.

1.	Absinthe, Oil	250
2.	Angelica, Oil	80
3.	Cardamom, Oil	40
4.	Cinnamon, Oil	20
5.	Coriander, Oil	40
6.	Lemon, Oil	270
7.	Nutmeg, Oil	20
8.	Orange, Oil	90
9.	Peppermint, Oil	170
10.	Thyme, Oil	20
		1000

BENEDICTINE NO. 2

1.	Angelica, Oil	80
2.	Cardamom, Oil	40
3.	Cinnamon, Oil	20
4.	Coriander, Oil	40
5.	Lemon, Oil	270
6.	Nutmeg, Oil	20
7.	Orange, Oil	90
8.	Peppermint, Oil	170
9.	Thyme, Oil	20
10.	Ethyl Alcohol 95%	250
		1000

BERGAMOT, FLAVOR

1.	Bergamot, Oil	100
2.	Lemon, Oil	150
3.	Orange, Oil	50
4.	Ethyl Alcohol 95%	350
5.	Distilled Water	350
		1000

BILBERRY, ESSENCE (NATURAL) NO. 1

1.	Bilberries, Black (crushed)	20 kg
2.	Sugar	20 kg

Let ferment for several days, until the flavor is developed. Express the juice. Macerate the residue for 3 days with:

3.	Amyl Butyrate	4 ml
4.	Coriander, Oil	2 ml
5.	Ethyl Acetate	12 ml
6.	Fennel, Sweet, Oil	2 ml
7.	Ethyl Alcohol 95%	15 l
8.	Distilled Water	15 l

Distill altogether. Redistill for rectification.
Yield: 20 liters

BILBERRY, ESSENCE (NATURAL) NO. 2, RED

1.	Bilberries, Black (crushed)	20 kg
2.	Sugar	20 kg

Let ferment for several days, until the flavor is developed. Express the juice. Macerate the residue for 3 days with:

3.	Ethyl Alcohol 95%	15 l
4.	Distilled Water	15 l
5.	Rose, Oil	1 ml
6.	Ethyl Benzoate	30 ml
7.	Methyl Salicylate	4 ml

Distill altogether. Redistill for rectification.
Yield: 20 liters

BILBERRY, ESSENCE (NATURAL) NO. 3 SCANDINAVIAN TYPE

1.	Bilberries, Juice	485
2.	Amyl Butyrate	5
3.	Benzoic Acid	2
4.	Coriander, Oil	2
5.	Ethyl Acetate	5
6.	Fennel, Sweet, Oil	1
7.	Ethyl Alcohol 95%	500
		1000

Macerate for 2 days. Distill.
Note: Employ 3 ml per liter

BILBERRY, IMITATION NO. 1

1.	Bilberries (crushed)	250
2.	Bilberries, Juice (distilled)	250
3.	Amyl Butyrate	20
4.	Benzoic Acid	1
5.	Coriander	2
6.	Ethyl Acetate	20
7.	Fennel, Oil	2
8.	Ethyl Alcohol 95%	250
9.	Distilled Water	205
		1000

Macerate for 2 days. Distill slowly over 800 cc.

BILBERRY, IMITATION NO. 2

1.	Amyl Acetate	22
2.	Amyl Butyrate	14
3.	Benzyl Acetate	4
4.	Bilberry, Imitation No. 1*	50
5.	Coriander, Oil	1
6.	Ethyl Acetate	38
7.	Ethyl Benzoate	30
8.	Ethyl Valerate	16
9.	Fennel, Oil	2
10.	Methyl Salicylate	1
11.	Petitgrain, Oil	1
12.	Vanillin	3
13.	Ethyl Alcohol 95%	409
14.	Distilled Water	409
		1000

BILBERRY, IMITATION NO. 3

1.	Bilberry, Imitation No. 1*	600
2.	Bilberry, Imitation No. 2*	200
3.	Ethyl Alcohol 95%	200
		1000

* Formulas which appear in this book

BITTER NO. 1, "UNICUM"

1.	Absinthe	1
2.	Angelica, Root	30
3.	Angostura, Bark	75
4.	Calamus, Root	60
5.	Centaury, Root	75
6.	Cinchona (Red), Bark	30
7.	Cinnamon, Bark	35
8.	Gentian, Root	60
9.	Ginger, Root	60
10.	Honey	64
11.	Lemon Balm, Balsam	35
12.	Lemon, Peels	26
13.	Orange, Peels	35
14.	Rhubarb, Roots and Stalks	30
15.	Spearmint, Leaves	30
16.	Sugar	80
17.	Ethyl Alcohol 95%	137
18.	Distilled Water	137
		1000

Macerate the whole pulverized material for 7 days. Express and filter.

BITTER NO. 2, "SPANISH"

1.	Angelica, Oil	3
2.	Angelica, Root	66
3.	Calamus, Oil	5
4.	Calamus, Root	100
5.	Cascarilla, Bark	33
6.	Chamomile, Flowers	33
7.	Chamomile, Oil	5
8.	Clove, Flowers	33
9.	Clove, Oil	3
10.	Coriander, Fruits	33
11.	Galangal, Root	66
12.	Gentian, Bark	66
13.	Juniper, Oil	5
14.	Marjoram	33
15.	Orange, Bitter, Peels	100
16.	Orange, Bitter, Oil	5
17.	Peppermint	33
18.	Pimento, Berry	33
19.	Wormwood, Leaves and Tops	33
20.	Ethyl Alcohol 95%	156
21.	Distilled Water	156
		1000

* Formulas which appear in this book

BITTER NO. 3, "STOMACH"

1.	Aloe, Roots	8
2.	Angelica, Root	8
3.	Calamus, Root	8
4.	Clove, Flowers	8
5.	Gentian, Root	15
6.	Lemon, Peels	15
7.	Licorice, Root	70
8.	Orange, Bitter, Peels	35
9.	Rhubarb, Root	35
10.	Star Anise, Root	49
11.	St. John's Bread (Carob)	70
12.	Wormwood, Leaves and Tops	15
13.	Ethyl Alcohol 95%	332
14.	Distilled Water	332
		1000

BLACKBERRY, ESSENCE (NATURAL)

1.	Blackberries (ripe, crushed)	20 kg
2.	Sugar	20 kg

Let ferment for several days, until the flavor is strongly developed. Express the juice. Macerate the residue for 3 days with:

3.	Ethyl Alcohol 95%	15 1
4.	Distilled Water	15 1
5.	Methyl Salicylate	6 ml

Distill. Redistill.
Yield: 20 liters

BLACKBERRY, IMITATION NO. 1

1.	Apricot, Imitation No. 1*	260
2.	Cherry, Imitation No. 1*	180
3.	Cinnamon, Ceylon, Oil	8
4.	Peach, Imitation No. 1*	60
5.	Pineapple, Imitation No. 1*	40
6.	Raspberry, Imitation No. 1*	140
7.	Ethyl Alcohol 95%	312
		1000

BLACKBERRY, IMITATION NO. 2

1.	Ethyl Acetate	100
2.	Ethyl Butyrate	40
3.	Ethyl Formate	20
4.	Ethyl Pelargonate	30
5.	Isoamyl Butyrate	15
6.	γ-Nonyl Lactone	1
7.	Ethyl Alcohol 95%	794
		1000

BLACKBERRY, IMITATION NO. 3

1.	Amyl Butyrate	6
2.	Benzaldehyde (pure, 10% sol'n.)	4
3.	Benzyl Acetate	100
4.	Ethyl Formate	170
5.	Ethyl Oenanthate	60
6.	Isoamyl Acetate	125
7.	Isoamyl Butyrate	130
8.	Isoamyl Isovalerate	5
9.	Ethyl Alcohol 95%	400
		1000

BLACKBERRY, SYNTHETIC

1.	Amyl Methyl Ketone	1
2.	Benzaldehyde (pure)	4
3.	Benzyl Acetate	10
4.	Ethyl Formate	7
5.	Ethyl Oenanthate	6
6.	Isoamyl Acetate	22
7.	Isoamyl Butyrate	43
8.	Isoamyl Isovalerianate	5
9.	Methyl Salicylate	5
10.	Ethyl Alcohol 95%	449
11.	Distilled Water	448
		1000

BLACK CHERRY

1.	Benzoic Acid (1% sol'n.)	80
2.	Ethyl Acetate (10% sol'n.)	400
3.	Ethyl Benzoate	200
4.	Isoamyl Butyrate	200
5.	Isoamyl Isovalerate	120
		1000

BLACK CURRANT

1.	Acetaldehyde	40
2.	Amyl Acetate	60
3.	Amyl Butyrate	250
4.	Anisaldehyde	15
5.	Buchu, Oil	15
6.	Cinnamon, Oil	20
7.	Ethyl Acetate	160
8.	Ethyl Benzoate	30
9.	Ethyl Heptanoate	20
10.	Ethyl Pelargonate	50
11.	Geraniol	5
12.	Isobutyl Acetate (10% sol'n.)	250
13.	Lemon, Oil (terpeneless)	30
14.	Nerol, Oil	5
15.	Orris, Oil	40
16.	Vanillin	10
		1000

BLACK CURRANT, SYNTHETIC

1.	Acetaldehyde	4
2.	Anisaldehyde	1
3.	Amyl Acetate	5
4.	Amyl Butyrate	25
5.	Cinnamon, Oil	1
6.	Ethyl Acetate	16
7.	Ethyl Benzoate	3
8.	Ethyl Oenanthate	2
9.	Ethyl Pelargonate	5
10.	Geraniol	1
11.	Isobutyl Acetate	25
12.	Neroli, Oil	1
13.	Lemon, Oil	3
14.	Orris, Oil	4
15.	Vanillin	3
16.	Ethyl Alcohol 95%	451
17.	Distilled Water	450
		1000

BLACK PEPPER, IMITATION NO. 1

1.	Borneol	60
2.	Guaiacwood	340

3.	Pepper, Black, Oil	340
4.	Phellandrene (10% sol'n.)	260
		1000

BLACK PEPPER, IMITATION NO. 2

1.	Black Pepper, Oil	350
2.	Borneol	100
3.	Guaiacwood	50
4.	Pepper, Black, Oil	350
5.	Phellandrene	200
		1000

BLUEBERRY, ESSENCE (NATURAL)

1.	Blueberries (ripe, crushed)	20 kg
2.	Sugar	20 kg

Let ferment for several days, until the flavor is strongly developed. Express the juice. Macerate the residue for 3 days with:

3.	Ethyl Alcohol 95%	15 l
4.	Distilled Water	15 l
5.	Isopropyl Hexanoate	1 l
6.	Methyl Ionone	1 l
7.	Rhodinyl Butyrate	1 l

Distill. Redistill.
Yield: 20 liters

BRANDY (COGNAC) NO. 1

1.	Acetic Acid	60 ml
2.	Acetic Ether	60 ml
3.	Kino, Tincture	75 ml
4.	Raisins, Bruised	3 kg
5.	Syrup (simple)	1 kg

Add burnt sugar for color. Let stand 12 days. Filter.

Yield: 20 gal pure, 50% proof spirit

BRANDY (COGNAC) NO. 2

1.	Acetaldehyde	3
2.	Amyl Isobutyrate	3
3.	Benzaldehyde (pure)	1
4.	Cinnamon, Oil	1
5.	Cinnamyl Butyrate	1
6.	Cinnamyl Propionate	1
7.	Cognac, Oil	12
8.	Ethyl Acetate	55
9.	Ethyl Butyrate	2
10.	Fusel, Oil	5
11.	Heliotropine	1
12.	Methyl Eugenol	2
13.	Neroli, Oil	12
14.	Pelargonic Ether	3
15.	Vanillin	6
16.	Ethyl Alcohol 95%	892
		1000

BREAD, FRESH ROASTED FLAVOR

1.	Bread, Fresh Roasted (ground)	2
2.	Propylene Glycol	1
3.	Distilled Water	1

Filter.

BUTTER, FLAVOR, IMITATION NO. 1

1.	Butyl Acetate	60
2.	Butyl Butyrate	20
3.	Diacetyl (10% sol'n.)	350
4.	Ethyl Butyrate	40
5.	Ethyl Alcohol 95%	530
		1000

BUTTER, FLAVOR, IMITATION NO. 2

1.	Butyl Acetate	55
2.	Butyl Butyrate	25
3.	Diacetyl (10% sol'n.)	310
4.	Ethyl Butyrate	35
5.	Ethyl Pelargonate	25
6.	Ethyl Alcohol 95%	550
		1000

BUTTER, FLAVOR, IMITATION NO. 3

1.	Butyl Acetate	15
2.	Butyl Butyrate	5
3.	Diacetyl	170
4.	Ethyl Butyrate	10
5.	Ethyl Alcohol 95%	800
		1000

BUTTER, FLAVOR, IMITATION NO. 4

1.	Butyl Acetate	140
2.	Butyl Butyrate	70
3.	Diacetyl	155
4.	Ethyl Butyrate	70
5.	Ethyl Pelargonate	70
6.	Ethyl Alcohol 95%	495
		1000

BUTTER, FLAVOR, IMITATION NO. 5

1.	Butyl Acetate (10% sol'n.)	250
2.	Butyl Butyrate (10% sol'n.)	250
3.	Diacetyl	200
4.	Ethyl Butyrate	200
5.	Ethyl Pelargonate	100
		1000

BUTTER, FLAVOR, IMITATION NO. 6

1.	Amyl Butyrate	80
2.	Amyl Isobutyrate	130
3.	Butyl Butyrate	65
4.	Ethyl Isobutyrate	155
5.	Ethyl Myristate	55
6.	Ethyl Alcohol 95%	515
		1000

* Formulas which appear in this book

BUTTER, FLAVOR, SYNTHETIC

1.	Amyl Butyrate	7
2.	Butyl Acetate	11
3.	Butyl Butyrate	1
4.	Butyric Acid	12
5.	Diacetyl	43
6.	Ethyl Butyrate	22
7.	Ethyl Myristate	4
8.	Ethyl Pelargonate	1
9.	Triacetin	8
10.	Vanillin	1
11.	Ethyl Alcohol 95%	445
12.	Distilled Water	445
		1000

BUTTER, RUM

1.	Butter, Flavor, Imitation No. 1*	50
2.	Butter, Flavor, Imitation No. 2*	50
3.	Honey	50
4.	Rum, Essence	845
5.	Vanillin	5
		1000

BUTTERSCOTCH, IMITATION NO. 1

1.	Butyl Acetate	120
2.	Butyl Butyrate (10% sol'n.)	570
3.	Cognac, Oil	230
4.	Ethyl Pelargonate	80
		1000

BUTTERSCOTCH, IMITATION NO. 2

1.	Almond, Oil (pure)	75
2.	Amyl Butyrate	35
3.	Butyl Acetate	73
4.	Butyric Acid	100
5.	Butyl Butyrate (10% sol'n.)	250
6.	Butyl Ethyl Ether	35
7.	Ethyl Heptanoate	92
8.	Ethyl Pelargonate	180
9.	Geranium, Oil	40
10.	Lemon, Oil	40
11.	Methyl Salicylate	5

12.	Orange, Oil	20
13.	Pelargonic Aldehyde	20
14.	Vanillin (10% sol'n.)	35
		1000

BUTTERSCOTCH, IMITATION NO. 3

1.	Butyl Acetate	2
2.	Butyl Butyrate	25
3.	Butyric Acid	17
4.	Capraldehyde	1
5.	Cinnamic Aldehyde	1
6.	Ethyl Butyrate	13
7.	Ethyl Oenanthate	9
8.	Ethyl Pelargonate	19
9.	Isoamyl Acetate	11
10.	Isobutyl-α-Toluate	1
11.	Ethyl Alcohol 95%	451
12.	Distilled Water	450
		1000

BUTTERSCOTCH, IMITATION NO. 4

1.	Almond, Oil	18
2.	Amyl Butyrate	5
3.	Butyl Butyrate	5
4.	Butyric Acid	15
5.	Ethyl Butyrate	6
6.	Ethyl Oenanthate	4
7.	Ethyl Pelargonate	4
8.	Geranium, Oil	5
9.	Lemon, Oil	10
10.	Methyl Salicylate	1
11.	Orange, Oil	5
12.	Vanillin	8
13.	Ethyl Alcohol 95%	457
14.	Distilled Water	457
		1000

BUTTERSCOTCH, IMITATION NO. 5

1.	Amyl Acetate	12
2.	Cinnamon, Oil	2
3.	Butyl Butyrate	13
4.	Butyric Acid	3
5.	Ethyl Butyrate	15
6.	Ethyl Cinnamate	7
7.	Ethyl Oenanthate	15
8.	Ethyl Pelargonate	10
9.	Homoquinoline	2
10.	Honey	6
11.	Ethyl Alcohol 95%	458
12.	Distilled Water	457
		1000

* Formulas which appear in this book

BUTTERSCOTCH, IMITATION NO. 6

1.	Butyl Acetate	80
2.	Butyl Butyrate (10% sol'n.)	420
3.	Ethyl Oenanthate	170
4.	Ethyl Pelargonate (10% sol'n.)	330
		1000

CACAO, EXTRACT (NATURAL) NO. 1, COLORLESS

1.	Cacao Beans, Roasted and Ground	10 kg
2.	Ethyl Alcohol 95%	20 l

Macerate for one week. Add:

3.	Distilled Water	3 cl
4.	Cinnamon, Oil	3 ml
5.	Vanillin	20 g

Distill.
Yield: 20 liters

CACAO, EXTRACT (NATURAL) NO. 2, BROWN

1.	Cacao Beans, Roasted and Ground	10 kg
2.	Ethyl Alcohol 95%	20 l

Macerate for one week. Add

3.	Distilled Water	3 cl
4.	Cinnamon, Oil	3 ml
5.	Vanillin	20 g

Filter.
Yield: 20 liters

CACAO, IMITATION

1.	Benzyl Alcohol	70
2.	Cinnamaldehyde	20
3.	Ethyl Acetate (10% sol'n.)	250
4.	Ethyl Oenanthate	80
5.	Eugenol	20
6.	Isoamyl Acetate (10% sol'n.)	250
7.	Isoamyl Butyrate	175
8.	Theobroma, Oil	100
9.	Vanillin (10% sol'n.)	35
		1000

CACAO, SYNTHETIC

1.	Amyl-α-Toluate	1
2.	Benzyl Alcohol	7
3.	Cinnamic Aldehyde	2
4.	Ethyl Acetate	35
5.	Ethyl Oenanthate	8
6.	Eugenol	2
7.	Eugenol Isoamyl Ether	1
8.	Isoamyl Acetate	25
9.	Isoamyl Butyrate	16
10.	Vanillin	3
11.	Ethyl Alcohol 95%	450
12.	Distilled Water	450
		1000

CAKE, FLAVOR NO. 1

1.	Ethyl Vanillin	15
2.	Fenugreek, Tincture	10
3.	Rum Ether	5
4.	Vanilla, Tincture	40
5.	Ethyl Alcohol 95%	465
6.	Distilled Water	465
		1000

CAKE, FLAVOR NO. 2

1.	Rum Ether	5
2.	Vanilla, Tincture	65
3.	Ethyl Alcohol 95%	465
4.	Distilled Water	465
		1000

CAPER, EXTRACT (NATURAL)

1. Capers 2 kg

Cut up small and remove the juice. Macerate with:

2. Alcohol 95% 4 l

for 3 days. Express. To the residue add:

3. Ethyl Alcohol 95% 4 l

Macerate for another 3 days. Distill altogether.

Yield: 10 liters

CAPSICUM, EXTRACT(NATURAL)

1. Capsicum 2 kg

Cut up small and remove the juice (if fresh), or if dry macerate with:

2. Ethyl Alcohol 95% 4 l

for 3 days. Express. To the residue add:

3. Ethyl Alcohol 95% 4 l

Macerate for another 3 days. Distill altogether.

Yield: 10 liters

CARAMEL, FLAVOR NO. 1

1.	Almond, Oil	48
2.	Heliotropin	1
3.	Musk Ambrette	1
4.	Vanillin	15
5.	Ethyl Alcohol 95%	468
6.	Distilled Water	467
		1000

CARAMEL, FLAVOR NO. 2

1.	Almond, Oil (pure)	480
2.	Heliotropin	10
3.	Musk	10
4.	Vanillin (10% sol'n.)	500
		1000

CARAWAY, IMITATION NO. 1

1.	Benzyl Benzoate	200
2.	Orange, Oil	600
3.	Terpineol	200
		1000

CARAWAY, IMITATION NO. 2

1.	Caraway, Imitation No. 1*	320
2.	Caraway, Oil	320
3.	Dill Weed (*Anethum graveolens*)	320
4.	Guaiacwood, Oil	40
		1000

CARAWAY, IMITATION NO. 3

1.	Carvone	200
2.	Limonene (10% sol'n.)	700
3.	Phellandrene	100
		1000

CARAWAY, IMITATION NO. 4

1.	Caraway, Imitation No. 2*	800
2.	Caraway, Oil	200
		1000

CARAWAY, IMITATION NO. 5

1.	Caraway, Imitation No. 3*	800
2.	Dill Weed, Oil	200
		1000

CARDAMOM, IMITATION NO. 1

1.	Cineol	200
2.	Limonene	200
3.	Terpineol (10% sol'n.)	300
4.	Terpinyl Acetate (10% sol'n.)	300
		1000

* Formulas which appear in this book

CARDAMOM, IMITATION NO. 2

1.	Cardamom, Imitation No. 1*	800
2.	Cardamom, Oil	200
		1000

CARNATION, FLAVOR

1.	Cinnamon, Oil	5
2.	Eugenol	50
3.	Heliotropin	50
4.	Hydroxycitronellal	20
5.	Ionone	10
6.	Isoeugenol (10% sol'n.)	350
7.	Methyl Isoeugenol	50
8.	Musk	1
9.	Neroli, Oil	50
10.	Pimento, Oil	50
11.	Rose, Oil	30
12.	Sage, Clary, Oil	20
13.	Vanillin	4
14.	Ylang Ylang, Oil	20
15.	Ethyl Alcohol 95%	290
		1000

CARROT, EXTRACT (NATURAL)

1. Carrot 2 kg

Scrape and express to remove the juice. Macerate with:

2. Alcohol 95% 4 l

for 3 days. Express. To the residue add:

3. Ethyl Alcohol 95% 4 l

Macerate for another 3 days. Distill altogether.

Yield: 10 liters

CASCARILLA, TINCTURE

1.	Cascarilla, Bark (ground)	282
2.	Ethyl Alcohol 95%	178
3.	Distilled Water	540
		1000

CASHEW, EXTRACT (NATURAL)

1.	Cashew, Rasped Kernels	10	kg
2.	Ethyl Alcohol 95%	30	l

Macerate for 10 days, stirring often. Collect all liquid. Add to the residue:

3.	Distilled Water	20	l
4.	Amyl Formate	12	ml
5.	Ethyl Oenanthate	12	ml

Distill altogether.
Yield: 50 liters

CASSIA, IMITATION NO. 1

1.	Cinnamic Aldehyde (10% sol'n.)	958
2.	Clove, Oil	30
3.	Heptaldehyde	2
4.	Menthone	1
5.	α-Methylcinnamic Aldehyde	6
6.	Salicylic Aldehyde	3
		1000

CASSIA, IMITATION NO. 2

1.	Cassia, Imitation No. 1*	200
2.	Cinnamic Aldehyde (10%sol'n.)	800
		1000

CASSIA, IMITATION NO. 3

1.	Cassia, Imitation No. 2*	200
2.	Cedarwood, Oil	100
3.	Cinnamic Aldehyde (10% sol'n.)	700
		1000

CASSIA, IMITATION NO. 4

1.	Cassia, Imitation No. 1*	333
2.	Cassia, Imitation No. 2*	333
3.	Cassia, Imitation No. 3*	334
		1000

* Formulas which appear in this book

CASSIA, IMITATION NO. 5

1.	Cassia, Imitation No. 4*	995
2.	α-Methylcinnamic Aldehyde	5
		1000

CASSIA, IMITATION NO. 6

1.	Cedarwood, Oil	50
2.	Cinnamic Aldehyde (10% sol'n.)	540
3.	Clove, Oil (10% sol'n.)	350
4.	Heptaldehyde	20
5.	Menthone	10
6.	Salicylic Aldehyde (10% sol'n.)	30
		1000

CASSIA, IMITATION NO. 7

1.	Cassia, Imitation No. 5*	790
2.	Cinnamic Aldehyde	30
3.	Propylene Glycol	180
		1000

CASSIA, IMITATION NO. 8

1.	Aldehyde C-10	2
2.	Benzyl Alcohol	40
3.	Cuminic Aldehyde	3
4.	Geraniol	2
5.	Linalool	8
6.	Ionone	2
7.	Irone	5
8.	Methyl Salicylate	35
9.	Terpineol	3
10.	Ethyl Alcohol 95%	450
11.	Distilled Water	450
		1000

CASSIA, IMITATION NO. 9

1.	Acetate C-8	1
2.	Alcohol C-8	2
3.	Alcohol C-11	2
4.	Aldehyde C-9	1
5.	Aldehyde C-10	1
6.	Anisic Aldehyde	5
7.	Benzaldehyde	4
8.	Benzyl Alcohol	45
9.	Isobutyl Salicylate	12

10.	Methyl Acetophenone	4
11.	Methyl Salicylate	23
12.	Ethyl Alcohol 95%	900
		1000

CHAMPAGNE, CEDAR, IMITATION

1.	Amyl Acetate	100
2.	Amyl Valerianate	25
3.	Ethyl Acetate	50
4.	Ethyl Butyrate	100
5.	Ethyl Nitrate	10
6.	Ethyl Valerianate	25
7.	Ginger, Oil	3
8.	Peach, Imitation No. 1*	100
9.	Vanillin	5
10.	Ethyl Alcohol 95%	582
		1000

CHAMPAGNE, FLAVOR

1.	Amyl Acetate	20
2.	Amyl Isobutyrate	4
3.	Cognac, Oil	10
4.	Ethyl Acetate	8
5.	Ethyl Butyrate	40
6.	Lemon, Oil	6
7.	Neroli, Oil	10
8.	Vanillin	2
9.	Ethyl Alcohol 95%	900
		1000

CHARTREUSE

1.	Absinthe, Oil (10% sol'n.)	10
2.	Angelica, Oil	200
3.	Cinnamon, Oil	100
4.	Coriander, Oil	100
5.	Lemon, Oil	60
6.	Neroli, Oil	15
7.	Nutmeg, Oil	100
8.	Orange, Oil	400
9.	Rose, Oil	15
		1000

* Formulas which appear in this book

CHARTREUSE (LIQUEUR) NO. 1

1.	Angelica, Oil	10
2.	Anise, Oil	150
3.	Clove, Oil	150
4.	Hyssop, Oil	150
5.	Lemon, Oil	150
6.	Nutmeg, Oil	150
7.	Peppermint, Oil	20
8.	Ethyl Alcohol 95%	220
		1000

Note: Yellow or green color, sugar, and distilled water may be added according to personal preference.

CHARTREUSE (LIQUEUR) NO. 2

1.	Absinthe, Oil	7
2.	Angelica, Oil	20
3.	Cinnamon, Oil	10
4.	Coriander, Oil	10
5.	Lemon, Oil	4
6.	Nutmeg, Oil	6
7.	Neroli, Oil	2
8.	Orange (Sweet), Oil	40
9.	Rose, Oil	1
10.	Ethyl Alcohol 95%	450
11.	Distilled Water	450
		1000

CHEESE, BLUE, SYNTHETIC NO. 1

1.	Acetoin	1
2.	*n*-Butanol	1
3.	Butanone	1
4.	*n*-Butyric Acid	8
5.	Capric Acid	3
6.	Caproic Acid	21
7.	Caprylic Acid	21
8.	*d*-Decalactone	35
9.	Diacetyl	1
10.	*d*-Dodecalactone	6
11.	Ethyl Acetate	1
12.	Ethyl Butyrate	2
13.	Ethyl Lactate	1
14.	2-Heptanol	3

15.	2-Heptanone	5
16.	*cis*-3-Hexenol	1
17.	2-Nonanone	2
18.	8-Nonen-2-one	23
19.	2-Pentanol	3
20.	2-Pentanone	3
21.	Vegetable Oil	858
		1000

CHEESE, BLUE, SYNTHETIC NO. 2

1.	Acetic Acid	9
2.	Butyric Acid	17
3.	Cinnamic Acid	1
4.	Decanoic Acid	134
5.	5-Decanolide	1
6.	5-Dodecanolide	1
7.	Glycoxylic Acid	71
8.	Heptanoic Acid	12
9.	2-Heptanone	64
10.	Hexanoic Acid	265
11.	Indole	1
12.	Isobutyric Acid	13
13.	Methional	1
14.	3-Methyl Butanoic Acid	3
15.	Nonanoic Acid	5
16.	2-Nonanone	117
17.	Octanoic Acid	90
18.	1-Octen-3-ol	20
19.	2-Oxo-Butanedioic Acid	52
20.	2-Oxo-3-Methyl Pentanoic Acid	18
21.	2-Oxo-4-Methyl Pentanoic Acid	44
22.	2-Oxo-Pentanoic Acid	4
23.	Pentanoic Acid	13
24.	2-Pentanone	10
25.	Pyruvic Acid	21
26.	2-Tridecanone	3
27.	2-Undecanone	10
		1000

CHEESE "ROQUEFORT" TYPE

1.	Ammonium Isovalerianate	20
2.	Butyric Acid	100
3.	Caproic Acid	50
4.	Ethyl Butyrate	200
5.	Isovaleric Acid (pure)	100
6.	Methyl-*n*-Amyl Ketone (free of fusel)	50
7.	Ethyl Alcohol 95%	240
8.	Distilled Water	240
		1000

CHEESE, SYNTHETIC

1.	Caproic Acid	50
2.	Butyl Butyryl Lactate	100
3.	Butyric Acid	100
4.	Ethyl Butyrate	100
5.	Isovaleric Acid (pure)	100
6.	Methyl-*n*-Amyl Ketone (free of fusel)	50
7.	Ethyl Alcohol 95%	250
8.	Propylene Glycol	250
		1000

CHERIMOYA, SYNTHETIC

1.	Aldehyde C-10	5
2.	Aldehyde C-14	5
3.	Allyl Caproate	10
4.	Amyl Acetate	30
5.	Amyl Butyrate	28
6.	Benzyl Acetate	50
7.	Ethyl Butyrate	30
8.	Ethyl Heptylate	20
9.	Ethyl Valerianate	20
10.	Geraniol	100
11.	Isobutyl Butyrate	50
12.	Phenyl Ethyl Alcohol	150
13.	Vanillin	2
14.	Ethyl Alcohol 95%	500
		1000

CHERRY "BLACK", ESSENCE (NATURAL)

1.	Cherries, Black (crushed)	100 kg
2.	Sugar	5 kg

Let ferment for several days. Express the juice. Macerate the residue for another 3 days with:

3.	Ethyl Alcohol 95%	20 1

Express, and add:

4.	Ethyl Benzoate	2 ml
5.	Amyl Formate	3 ml

Distill.
Yield: 20 liters

CHERRY BLOSSOM, NO. 1

1.	Almond, Bitter (cyanide-free)	10
2.	Amyl Acetate	20
3.	Amyl Butyrate	10
4.	Benzaldehyde (pure, 10% sol'n.)	10
5.	Benzyl Alcohol	40
6.	Cinnamon, Leaf	2
7.	Clove, Leaf	2
8.	Lemon, Oil	2
9.	Orange, Oil	2
10.	Vanillin (10% sol'n.)	10
11.	Ethyl Alcohol 95%	446
12.	Distilled Water	446
		1000

CHERRY BLOSSOM NO. 2

1.	Amyl Acetate	100
2.	Amyl Butyrate	50
3.	Benzaldehyde	5
4.	Cherry, Fruit, Juice	160
5.	Cinnamon, Leaf	10
6.	Clove, Leaf	10
7.	Lemon, Oil	100
8.	Neroli, Oil	10
9.	Orange, Oil	100
10.	Vanillin	5
11.	Ethyl Alcohol 95%	225
12.	Distilled Water	225
		1000

CHERRY BRANDY, NO. 1

1.	Almond, Bitter, Oil (cyanide-free)	10
2.	Cherry, Juice	500
3.	Cognac, Oil	50
4.	Ethyl Methylphenylglycidate	32
5.	Neroli, Oil	6
6.	Pineapple, Juice	50
7.	Raspberry, Juice	250
8.	Rum, Essence	100
9.	Vanillin	2
		1000

Distill over 900 cc.

CHERRY BRANDY, NO. 2

1.	Almond, Bitter, Oil (cyanide-free)	8
2.	Cherry, Juice	250
3.	Cognac, Oil	26
4.	Ethyl Methylphenylglycidate	26
5.	Neroli, Oil	2
6.	Pineapple, Juice	50
7.	Raspberry, Juice	250
8.	Rum, Essence	100
9.	Vanillin	2
10.	Ethyl Alcohol 95%	286
		1000

Distill over 900 cc.

CHERRY BRANDY, SYNTHETIC

1.	Amyl Methyl Ketone	1
2.	Benzaldehyde (pure)	4
3.	Benzyl Alcohol	50
4.	Benzoic Acid	1
5.	Benzyl Benzoate	8
6.	Cinnamic Aldehyde	1
7.	Ethyl Oenanthate	25
8.	Ethyl Pelargonate	5
9.	Eugenol	1
10.	Isoamyl Alcohol	1
11.	Isoamyl Caprate	1
12.	Linalool	1
13.	Nerolin	1
14.	Vanillin	1
15.	Ethyl Alcohol 95%	450
16.	Distilled Water	449
		1000

CHERRY, IMITATION NO. 1

1.	Almond, Bitter, Oil (cyanide-free)	20
2.	Amyl Formate	10
3.	Cherry, Juice	260
4.	Ethyl Benzoate	10
5.	Ethyl Alcohol 95%	350
6.	Distilled Water	350
		1000

Distill over 900 cc.

CHERRY, IMITATION NO. 2

1.	Almond, Bitter, Oil (cyanide-free)	15
2.	Amyl Acetate	15
3.	Amyl Alcohol	10
4.	Amyl Formate	60
5.	Benzyl Benzoate	7
6.	Cherry, Juice	150
7.	Cinnamon, Ceylon, Oil	2
8.	Clove, Oil	3
9.	Cognac, Oil	3
10.	Ethyl Acetate	150
11.	Ethyl Pelargonate	15
12.	Raspberry, Juice	150
13.	Ethyl Alcohol 95%	210
14.	Distilled Water	210
		1000

Distill over 900 cc.

CHERRY, IMITATION NO. 3

1.	Almond, Bitter, Oil (cyanide-free)	15
2.	Amyl Acetate	15
3.	Amyl Alcohol	10
4.	Amyl Formate	60
5.	Benzyl Acetate	150
6.	Benzyl Benzoate	7
7.	Cherry, Juice	150
8.	Cinnamon, Ceylon, Oil	2
9.	Clove, Oil	3
10.	Cognac, Oil	3
11.	Ethyl Acetate	150
12.	Raspberry, Juice	150
13.	Vanillin	5
14.	Ethyl Alcohol 95%	140
15.	Distilled Water	140
		1000

Distill over 900 cc.

CHERRY, IMITATION NO. 4

1.	Almond, Bitter, Oil (cyanide-free)	10
2.	Amyl Acetate	2
3.	Amyl Butyrate	8
4.	Cinnamon, Ceylon, Oil	2
5.	Clove, Oil	2
6.	Lemon, Oil	2
7.	Orange, Sweet, Oil	14
8.	Ethyl Alcohol 95%	960
		1000

CHERRY, IMITATION NO. 5

1.	Benzaldehyde (pure, 10% sol'n.)	60
2.	Benzyl Benzoate	25
3.	Cinnamaldehyde	5
4.	Ethyl Acetate (10% sol'n.)	380
5.	Ethyl Oenanthate	100
6.	Ethyl Pelargonate	15
7.	Eugenol	20
8.	Isoamyl Alcohol	70
9.	Isoamyl Formate (10% sol'n.)	300
10.	Vanillin (10% sol'n.)	25
		1000

CHERRY, IMITATION NO. 6

1.	Benzaldehyde (pure, 10% sol'n.)	45
2.	Citral	5
3.	Ethyl Acetate (10% sol'n.)	600
4.	Ethyl Oenanthate	50
5.	Isoamyl Butyrate	100
6.	Isoamyl Formate	200
		1000

CHERRY, IMITATION NO. 7

1.	Benzaldehyde (pure, 10% sol'n.)	100
2.	Benzyl Benzoate	50
3.	Ethyl Acetate (10% sol'n.)	500

4.	Ethyl Benzoate (10% sol'n.)	250
5.	Ethyl Pelargonate	25
6.	Isoamyl Alcohol	50
7.	Vanillin (10% sol'n.)	25
		1000

CHERRY, IMITATION NO. 8

1.	Benzaldehyde (pure, 10% sol'n.)	49
2.	Benzyl Benzoate	90
3.	Bromelia	1
4.	Cinnamaldehyde	20
5.	Ethyl Acetate (10% sol'n.)	540
6.	Ethyl Oenanthate	180
7.	Ethyl Pelargonate	35
8.	Eugenol	60
9.	Isoamyl Alcohol	15
10.	Vanillin	10
		1000

CHERRY, IMITATION NO. 9

1.	Benzaldehyde (pure, 10% sol'n.)	100
2.	Benzoic Acid (1% sol'n.)	100
3.	Ethyl Acetate (10% sol'n.)	400
4.	Isoamyl Formate (10% sol'n.)	400
		1000

CHERRY, IMITATION NO. 10

1.	Benzoic Acid (1% sol'n.)	75
2.	Ethyl Acetate (10% sol'n.)	425
3.	Ethyl Pelargonate	75
4.	Isoamyl Formate (10% sol'n.)	425
		1000

CHERRY, IMITATION NO. 11

1.	Capraldehyde	5
2.	Cinnamaldehyde	55
3.	Citral	10
4.	Ethyl Acetate (10% sol'n.)	450
5.	Eugenol	60
6.	Isoamyl Butyrate	100
7.	Isoamyl Formate (10% sol'n.)	320
		1000

CHERRY, IMITATION NO. 12

1.	Benzaldehyde (pure, 10% sol'n.)	40
2.	Benzoic Acid (1% sol'n.)	80
3.	Ethyl Acetate (10% sol'n.)	400
4.	Ethyl Oenanthate	80
5.	Isoamyl Formate (10% sol'n.)	400
		1000

CHERRY, IMITATION NO. 13

1.	Benzaldehyde (pure, 10% sol'n.)	80
2.	Benzyl Alcohol	55
3.	Cinnamic Aldehyde	30
4.	Ethyl Anthranilate	30
5.	Ethyl Caprate	40
6.	Ethyl Caproate	20
7.	Ethyl Phenyl Acetate	190
8.	Geraniol	60
9.	Geranyl Butyrate	20
10.	Heliotropin	50
11.	Isoamyl Acetate	120
12.	Isobutyl Acetate	120
13.	Methyl Acetate	110
14.	Terpinyl Acetate	5
15.	Vanillin (10% sol'n.)	70
		1000

CHERRY, IMITATION NO. 14

1.	Amyl Acetate (10% sol'n.)	300
2.	Benzaldehyde (pure, 10% sol'n.)	30
3.	Benzyl Benzoate	100
4.	Cinnamaldehyde	20
5.	Ethyl Acetate	200
6.	Ethyl Oenanthate	200
7.	Ethyl Pelargonate	90
8.	Eugenol	15
9.	Isoamyl Alcohol	15
10.	Isoamyl Butyrate	15
11.	Vanillin (10% sol'n.)	15
		1000

CHERRY, IMITATION NO. 15

1.	Almond, Bitter, Oil (cyanide-free)	100
2.	Amyl Acetate	150
3.	Amyl Butyrate	80

4.	Cinnamon, Ceylon, Oil	20
5.	Clove, Oil	20
6.	Lemon, Oil	20
7.	Orange, Sweet, Oil	10
8.	Ethyl Alcohol 95%	600
		1000

CHERRY, IMITATION NO. 16

1.	Almond, Bitter, Oil (pure)	50
2.	Amyl Formate	5
3.	Cherry, "Black," Essence (Natural)*	500
4.	Ethyl Benzoate	5
5.	Ethyl Alcohol 95%	440
		1000

CHERRY, IMITATION NO. 17

1.	Aldehyde C-20	2
2.	Almond, Bitter, Oil (pure)	15
3.	Amyl Acetate	15
4.	Amyl Alcohol	10
5.	Amyl Formate	6
6.	Benzyl Benzoate	7
7.	Cherry "Black" Essence (Natural)*	175
8.	Cherry "Red" Essence (Natural) "Agriot"*	175
9.	Cinnamon, Oil	2
10.	Clove, Oil	5
11.	Cognac, Oil	3
12.	Ethyl Acetate	15
13.	Ethyl Heptoate	15
14.	Lauri Cerasi, Oil (pure)	10
15.	Vanillin	3
16.	Ethyl Alcohol 95%	542
		1000

CHERRY "RED" ESSENCE (NATURAL) "AGRIOT"

1.	Cherries, Red "Agriot" (crushed)	5 kg
2.	Sugar	5 kg

Let ferment for several days. Express the juice. Macerate the residue for another 3 days with:

3.	Ethyl Alcohol 95%	20 l

Express and add:

4.	Amyl Formate	4 ml
5.	Cognac, Oil	4 ml
6.	Ethyl Benzoate	2 ml

Distill.
Yield: 20 liters

CHERRY, SYNTHETIC NO. 1

1.	Ethyl Acetate	50
2.	Ethyl Benzoate	50
3.	Ethyl Oenanthate	10
4.	Glycerin (neutral)	30
5.	Succinic Acid	10
6.	Tartaric Acid	1
7.	Ethyl Alcohol 95%	849
		1000

CHERRY, SYNTHETIC NO. 2

1.	Almond, Bitter, Oil (pure)	30
2.	Amyl Acetate	15
3.	Chloroform	75
4.	Ethyl Acetate	225
5.	Ethyl Benzoate	225
6.	Ethyl Alcohol 95%	430
		1000

CHERRY, SYNTHETIC NO. 3

1.	Aldehyde C-16	10
2.	Benzoic Acid	10
3.	Ethyl Acetate	50
4.	Ethyl Benzoate	50
5.	Ethyl Oenanthate	10
6.	Glycerin (neutral)	30
7.	Ethyl Alcohol 95%	840
		1000

* Formulas which appear in this book

CHERRY, SYNTHETIC NO. 4

1.	Aldehyde C-16	15
2.	Benzoic Acid	10
3.	Ethyl Acetate	45
4.	Ethyl Benzoate	50
5.	Ethyl Oenanthate	10
6.	Glycerin (neutral)	30
7.	Alcohol 95%	840
		1000

CHERRY, SYNTHETIC NO. 5

1.	Amyl Formate	10
2.	Benzaldehyde (pure)	1
3.	Benzoic Acid	1
4.	Clove, Oil	1
5.	Ethyl Acetate	30
6.	Ethyl Benzoate	15
7.	Ethyl Cinnamate	1
8.	Ethyl Oenanthate	8
9.	Ethyl Pelargonate	2
10.	Glycerin (neutral)	9
11.	Ethyl Alcohol 95%	922
		1000

CHERRY, SYNTHETIC NO. 6

1.	Aldehyde C-16	3
2.	Almond, Bitter, Oil (pure)	2
3.	Amyl Acetate	20
4.	Amyl Benzoate	10
5.	Amyl Formate	2
6.	Benzaldehyde (pure)	15
7.	Benzyl Formate	2
8.	Benzyl Propionate	2
9.	Cassia, Oil	2
10.	Cinnamon, Oil	1
11.	Clove, Oil	4
12.	Ethyl Acetate	8
13.	Ethyl Benzoate	1
14.	Ethyl Oenanthate	5
15.	Lemon, Oil	2
16.	Orange, Sweet, Oil	1
17.	Phenyl Ethyl Cinnamate	5
18.	Phenyl Ethyl Phenyl Acetate	4
19.	Vanilla, Oil	1
20.	Vanillin	1
21.	Ethyl Alcohol 95%	909
		1000

CHERRY, SYNTHETIC NO. 7

1.	Aldehyde C-16	2
2.	Almond, Bitter, Oil (pure)	50
3.	Amyl Formate	5
4.	Anisaldehyde	1
5.	Ethyl Acetate	25
6.	Ethyl Benzoate	25
7.	Vanillin	1
8.	Ethyl Alcohol 95%	891
		1000

CHERRY, SYNTHETIC NO. 8

1.	Benzaldehyde (pure)	2
2.	Benzoic Acid	1
3.	Benzyl Benzoate	1
4.	Capraldehyde	1
5.	Cinnamic Aldehyde	1
6.	Citral	1
7.	Ethyl Acetate	4
8.	Ethyl Benzoate	25
9.	Ethyl Oenanthate	3
10.	Ethyl Pelargonate	3
11.	Eugenol	1
12.	Isoamyl Alcohol	1
13.	Isoamyl Butyrate	4
14.	Isoamyl Formate	5
15.	Vanillin	1
16.	Ethyl Alcohol 95%	473
17.	Distilled Water	473
		1000

CHERRY, SYNTHETIC NO. 9

1.	Amyl Methyl Ketone	1
2.	Benzoic Acid	1
3.	Ethyl Acetate	43
4.	Ethyl Benzoate	22
5.	Isoamyl Butyrate	17
6.	Isoamyl Valerianate	6
7.	Ethyl Alcohol 95%	455
8.	Distilled Water	455
		1000

CHERRY "WILD," AGRIOT, SYNTHETIC

1.	Benzaldehyde (pure)	20
2.	Benzoic Acid	2
3.	Ethyl Acetate	10
4.	Ethyl Benzoate	5
5.	Ethyl Oenanthate	5
6.	Tartaric Acid	3
7.	Ethyl Alcohol 95%	955
		1000

CHERVIL, ESSENCE (NATURAL)

1. Chervil 2 kg

Cut up small and add:

2. Ethyl Alcohol 95% 4 l

Macerate for 3 days. Express the juice. To the residue add:

3. Ethyl Alcohol 95% 4 l

Macerate for another 3 days. Distill altogether.
Yield: 10 liters

CHOCOLATE, ESSENCE (FOR PRALINE LIQUEUR)

1.	Cacao (Brown)	498
2.	Cardamom, Tincture	125
3.	Clove, Tincture	125
4.	Cinnamon, Tincture	250
5.	Vanillin	2
		1000

CHOCOLATE, FLAVOR (NATURAL)

1.	Amyl Phenyl Acetate	117
2.	Benzyl Butyrate	12
3.	Cocoa	500
4.	Propylene Glycol	300
5.	Vanillin	60
6.	Veratraldehyde	11
		1000

CHOCOLATE, FLAVOR, SYNTHETIC

1.	Aldehyde C-18	12
2.	Amyl Phenyl Acetate	400
3.	*n*-Butyl Phenyl Ethyl Acetal	50
4.	Propylene Gycol	487
5.	Vanillin	40
6.	Veratraldehyde	11
		1000

CHOCOLATE, HARDENER

1.	Albumin (Eggs) (10% sol'n.)	100
2.	Arabic Gum (10% sol'n.)	100
3.	Flour (10% sol'n.)	100
4.	Gelatin (10% sol'n.)	100
5.	Gluten (10% sol'n.)	100
6.	Pectin (Apple, Lemon, Orange) (10% sol'n.)	300
7.	Malt, Dry	100
8.	Starch, Gum (Dextrin)	100
		1000

CHYPRE, BASE FOR BOUQUET

(Aroma of wine and liquor)

1.	Alcohol C-8	2
2.	Alcohol C-9	1
3.	Alcohol C-10	2
4.	Aldehyde C-8	2
5.	Aldehyde C-9	1
6.	Aldehyde C-10	1
7.	Aldehyde C-12	1
8.	Aldehyde C-16	2
9.	Amber, Tincture	200
10.	Musk Ambrette, Tincture	200
11.	Rose, Oil	2
12.	Tonka Beans, Tincture	200
13.	Vanilla, Tincture	200
14.	Ethyl Alcohol 95%	186
		1000

CINNAMON, IMITATION

1.	Aldehyde C-9	2
2.	Benzaldehyde (pure)	1
3.	Caryophyllene	5
4.	Cinnamic Aldehyde	20
5.	Cuminic Aldehyde	2
6.	Eugenol	5
7.	Isoeugenol	5
8.	Linalool	20
9.	Methyl Amyl Ketone	1
10.	Methyl Isoeugenol	1
11.	Phellandrene	2
12.	Phenyl Propyl Aldehyde	1
13.	Ethyl Alcohol 95%	468
14.	Distilled Water	467
		1000

CITRUS FRUITS, EXTRACT FROM PEELS

1.	Citrus Fruit, Peels from fresh lemon, lime, orange, or tangerine	10	kg
2.	Ethyl Alcohol 95%	20	l

Macerate for 3 days. Express. To the residue add:

3.	Distilled Water	20	l

Distill to separate the terpenes. Redistill altogether with the first expressed juice.
Yield: 30 liters

CLOVE

1.	Clove, Oil	750
2.	Caryophyllene	32
3.	Eugenol	174
4.	Eugenyl Acetate	24
5.	Methyl Eugenol	20
		1000

COCA, FLAVOR

1.	Coca, Tincture	300
2.	Lemon, Oil	40
3.	Orange (Bitter), Oil	15
4.	Tonka Beans, Tincture	50
5.	Vanilla, Tincture	100
6.	Ethyl Alcohol 95%	495
		1000

COCOA, ESSENCE (NATURAL)

1.	Cacao Beans (roasted and powdered	300	g
2.	Vanilla, Beans	4	
3.	Ethyl Alcohol 95%	1500	ml

Macerate for 3 days.

4.	Distilled Water	200	ml

Distill.

COFFEE, EXTRACT (NATURAL) NO. 1, BROWN

1.	Coffee (freshly roasted)	5	kg
2.	Arrack (pure)	3	l
3.	Distilled Water	9	l

Macerate for 1 day. Percolate.

4.	Ethyl Alcohol 95%	2	l
5.	Distilled Water	2	l

Percolate.
Yield: 15 liters
Note: The residue of the percolate can be added as a menstruum to further preparation.

COFFEE, EXTRACT (NATURAL) NO. 2, COLORLESS

1.	Coffee (freshly roasted)	10	kg
2.	Ethyl Alcohol 95%	4	l
3.	Distilled Water	10	l

Macerate for 1 day.

4.	Vanillin	10	g

Distill slowly.
Yield: 10 liters

COFFEE, EXTRACT (NATURAL) NO. 3, BROWN

1.	Coffee, Brown (freshly roasted)	5	kg
2.	Ethyl Alcohol 95%	5	l
3.	Distilled Water	5	l

Let stand 1 day. Percolate 10 l. Add:

4.	Arrack (pure)	1500	ml
5.	Cinnamon, Tincture	150	ml
6.	Mace, Tincture	150	ml
7.	Wine, Brandy (pure)	1000	ml

COFFEE, EXTRACT (NATURAL) NO. 4, COLORLESS

1.	Coffee, Extract (Natural) No. 1, Brown*	5	l
2.	Ethyl Alcohol 95%	3	l
3.	Distilled Water	3	l

Distill.
Yield: 5 liters

COFFEE, IMITATION NO. 1

1.	Benzyl Acetate	60
2.	Bromelia	1
3.	Citral	10
4.	Ethyl Acetate (10% sol'n.)	360
5.	Ethyl Oenanthate	4
6.	Ethyl Formate	180
7.	Ethyl Pelargonate	85
8.	Isoamyl Acetate (10% sol'n.)	280
9.	Vanillin (10% sol'n.)	20
		1000

COFFEE, IMITATION NO. 2

1.	Benzyl Benzoate	130
2.	Bromelia	1
3.	Citral	10
4.	Ethyl Acetate (10% sol'n.)	340
5.	Ethyl Oenanthate	9
6.	Ethyl Formate (10% sol'n.)	340
7.	Ethyl Pelargonate	170
		1000

* Formulas which appear in this book

COFFEE, IMITATION NO. 3

1.	Benzyl Benzoate	60
2.	Bromelia	1
3.	Citral	5
4.	Ethyl Acetate (10% sol'n.)	320
5.	Ethyl Oenanthate	9
6.	Ethyl Formate	200
7.	Ethyl Pelargonate	100
8.	Isoamyl Acetate (10% sol'n.)	300
9.	Vanillin (10% sol'n.)	5
		1000

COFFEE, SYNTHETIC

1.	Benzyl Acetate	13
2.	Benzyl Benzoate	14
3.	Citral	2
4.	Diacetyl	1
5.	Ethyl Acetate	4
6.	Ethyl Formate	6
7.	Ethyl Oenanthate	2
8.	Ethyl Pelargonate	11
9.	Isoamyl Acetate	9
10.	Nerolin	1
11.	Propyl Oenanthate	1
12.	Vanillin	2
13.	Ethyl Alcohol 95%	467
14.	Distilled Water	467
		1000

COGNAC, BASE, SYNTHETIC

1.	Cognac, Oil	10
2.	Ethyl Caprate	10
3.	Ethyl Caproate	10
4.	Ethyl Caprylate	10
5.	Ethyl Oenanthate	10
6.	Ethyl Alcohol 95%	475
7.	Distilled Water	475
		1000

COGNAC, IMITATION NO. 1

1.	Almond Shales (broken)	83
2.	Cognac, White, Oil	22
3.	Ethyl Oenanthate	2
4.	Licorice (sticky)	2

5.	Orris Root (granulated)	16
6.	Peach, Kernels (broken)	37
7.	Plums (dried)	66
8.	Raisins, Blue (dried)	66
9.	Ethyl Alcohol 95%	353
10.	Distilled Water	353
		1000

Macerate for 24 h. Filter.

COGNAC, IMITATION NO. 2

1.	Benzaldehyde (pure)	1
2.	Amyl Acetate	10
3.	Amyl Butyrate	20
4.	Cognac, White, Oil	7
5.	Ethyl Acetate	11
6.	Ethyl Oenanthate	4
7.	Ethyl Pelargonate	20
8.	Neroli, Oil	1
9.	Petitgrain	10
10.	Vanillin	1
11.	Ethyl Alcohol 95%	458
12.	Distilled Water	457
		1000

COGNAC, IMITATION NO. 3

1.	Aldehyde C-20	30
2.	Amyl Butyrate	120
3.	Cardamom, Oil	60
4.	Ethyl Acetate	60
5.	Ethyl Oenanthate	40
6.	Ethyl Pelargonate	50
7.	Mace, Oil	120
8.	Methyl Salicylate	20
9.	Ethyl Alcohol 95%	250
10.	Distilled Water	250
		1000

COGNAC, IMITATION NO. 4

1.	Acetaldehyde	30
2.	Almond, Oil (pure)	5
3.	Amyl Isobutyrate	30
4.	Cinnamon, Oil	5
5.	Cinnamyl Butyrate	10
6.	Cinnamyl Propionate	10
7.	Cognac, Oil	125
8.	Ethyl Acetate (10% sol'n.)	500
9.	Ethyl Butyrate	20
10.	Fusel, Oil	50
11.	Heliotropin	5
12.	Methyl Eugenol	20
13.	Nerol, Oil	100
14.	Pelargonic Aldehyde	30
15.	Vanillin (10% sol'n.)	60
		1000

COGNAC, IMITATION NO. 5

1.	Aldehyde C-20 (10% sol'n.)	60
2.	Amyl Butyrate	180
3.	Cardamom, Oil	80
4.	Ethyl Acetate	90
5.	Ethyl Oenanthate (10% sol'n.)	500
6.	Ethyl Pelargonate	60
7.	Methyl Salicylate (10% sol'n.)	30
		1000

COGNAC, IMITATION NO. 5

1.	Almond, Barks (broken)	250
2.	Cognac, Oil	15
3.	Orris, Root (granulated)	5
4.	Licorice, Stick	5
5.	Peach, Kernels (broken)	100
6.	Plums (dried)	200
7.	Raisin (dried)	200
8.	Sassafras, Wood	225
		1000

Macerate for 24 h. Pour off the juice and filter.

COGNAC, IMITATION NO. 6

1.	Almond, Barks (broken)	24
2.	Cognac, Oil	2
3.	Licorice, Stick	1
4.	Orris, Root (granulated)	1
5.	Peach, Kernels (broken)	10
6.	Plums (dried)	20
7.	Raisin (dried)	20
8.	Sassafras, Wood	2

9.	Ethyl Alcohol 95%	460
10.	Distilled Water	460
		1000

Macerate for 24 h. Pour off the juice and filter.

COGNAC, IMITATION NO. 7

1.	Ethyl Caprate	10
2.	Ethyl Caproate	10
3.	Ethyl Caprylate	10
4.	Ethyl Oenanthate	10
5.	Ethyl Alcohol 95%	960
		1000

COLA, IMITATION NO. 1 (SYRUP)

1.	Bergamot, Oil	25
2.	Cola Nuts, Tincture	400
3.	Orange, Bitter, Oil	275
4.	Orange, Sweet, Oil	100
5.	Tonka Beans, Tincture	100
6.	Vanilla Beans, Tincture	100
		1000

COLA, IMITATION NO. 2 (SYRUP)

1.	Acetic Acid, Glacial 99%	14
2.	Caffeine (powder)	55
3.	Cinnamon, Oil	2
4.	Citric Acid	28
5.	Clove, Oil	1
6.	Cola Tincture	22
7.	Glycerin (neutral)	110
8.	Lemon, Oil	8
9.	Lime, Oil	7
10.	Neroli, Oil	1
11.	Nutmeg, Oil	2
12.	Orange, Oil	7
13.	Patchouli, Oil	22
14.	Vanillin	1
15.	Ethyl Alcohol 95%	360
16.	Distilled Water	360
		1000

Dissolve caffeine in 722 g boiling water. Add 28 g citric acid. Add phosphoric acid syrup. Add glacial acetic acid. Add cola tincture. Dissolve vanillin and all the essential oils. Blend all with stirring. Let stand for 48 h, stirring four times, every 12 h. Let stand for another 48 h without any agitation. Separate the resins at the bottom. Separate the terpenes at the surface. Separate the clear middle portion, siphoning with a rubber tube. Filter all cloudy parts of the bottom with filter paper. Place the oily upper portion in a narrow, small container and siphon off the clear portion. Add to the other clear portion and shake well.

Use 35 ml of this extract and 15 ml of liquid caramel to make a finished syrup. Prepare a simple syrup by mixing 3 kg of sugar, 700 ml of distilled water, and 50 ml of this syrup to make a gallon of imitation cola syrup. Concentration: 30 ml/gal.

COLA, TINCTURE

1.	Cola Nuts (roasted)	10	kg
2.	Ethyl Alcohol 95%	5	l
3.	Distilled Water	5	l

Macerate for 1 week. Filter.
Yield: 10 liters

CORIANDER, IMITATION NO. 1

1.	Camphene	140
2.	Guaiacwood, Oil	20
3.	Limonene	100
4.	Linalool	450
5.	Pinene	150
6.	Terpineol	140
		1000

CORIANDER, IMITATION NO. 2

1.	Coriander, Imitation No. 1*	800
2.	Coriander, Oil	200
		1000

* Formulas which appear in this book

CRANBERRY

1.	Benzyl Acetate	30
2.	Ethyl Acetate (10% sol'n.)	360
3.	Ethyl Benzoate	90
4.	Ethyl Isovalerate	185
5.	Isoamyl Acetate	130
6.	Isoamyl Butyrate	170
7.	Linalool	10
8.	Methyl Salicylate	5
9.	Vanillin (10% sol'n.)	20
		1000

CRANBERRY, SYNTHETIC

1.	Benzyl Acetate	3
2.	Ethyl Acetate	36
3.	Ethyl Benzoate	9
4.	Ethyl isovalerianate	18
5.	Isoamyl Acetate	13
6.	Isoamyl Butyrate	17
7.	Linalool	1
8.	Methyl Salicylate	1
9.	Vanillin	2
10.	Ethyl Alcohol 95%	450
11.	Distilled Water	450
		1000

CREAM PASTE

1.	Corn Syrup	4	l
2.	Gelatin	60	g
3.	Sugar (fine)	10	kg

CRYSTAL BEVERAGES

1.	Any Flavor, from Ethyl Alcohol Extraction	50	ml
2.	Ascorbic Acid	20	g
3.	Citric Acid	70	g
4.	Dextrose	200	g
5.	Sodium Citrate	10	g
6.	Sugar	650	g

Preservative:
Sodium benzoate or
Sodium benzoate 10% (90% distilled water, 10% sodium benzoate) 0.1%

Uses: 100 g of crystals in 1 l distilled water

CUCUMBER, EXTRACT (NATURAL)

1.	Acetate C-8	1
2.	Citral	1
3.	Cucumber, Juice	97
4.	Methyl Heptyne Carbonate	1
5.	Ethyl Alcohol 95%	450
6.	Distilled Water	450
		1000

Express. Filter.

CUCUMBER "MILK" (FOR COSMETICS)

1.	Cucumber, Juice	150
2.	Olive Oil	150
3.	Soap (White)	150
4.	Spermaceti (sperm whale)	150
5.	Wax (Beeswax or Lanolin)	150
6.	Ethyl Alcohol 95%	250
		1000

CULINARY, EXTRACT (NATURAL)

1. Allspice
2. Anise
3. Asparagus
4. Calamus
5. Caper
6. Capsicum
7. Caraway
8. Cardamom
9. Carrot
10. Champignon
11. Chervil
12. Chives
13. Cinnamon
14. Clove
15. Coriander
16. Cumin
17. Curcuma
18. Dill
19. Fennel
20. Garlic
21. Ginger

22. Horseradish
23. Juniper Berries
24. Laurel Leaves
25. Leek
26. Mace
27. Marjoram
28. Morel
29. Mushroom
30. Mustard
31. Nutmeg
32. Onion
33. Parsley
34. Pepper
35. Pimenta
36. Saffron
37. Sage
38. Savory
39. Shallot
40. Tarragon
41. Thyme
42. Truffle

For each listed product, separately dry and cut in very small pieces. Roast slowly and gently stir until each reaches a brownish color. To the weight of each add 50% ethyl alcohol 95% and 50% distilled water. Let stand for 1 week, stirring every day for 1 h. Filter. Reuse the residue for another three times adding 50% ethyl alcohol 95% and 50% distilled water each time. Combine the extract and filter.

CURAÇAO, IMITATION NO. 1, LIQUOR BASE

1.	Almond, Bitter, Oil (cyanide-free)	2
2.	Anise, Oil	1
3.	Cardamom, Oil	1
4.	Cinnamon, Oil	1
5.	Curaçao, Oil	830
6.	Lemon, Oil	5
7.	Mace, Oil	2
8.	Neroli, Oil	2
9.	Orange, Bitter, Oil	156
		1000

25 cc of formula dissolved in ethyl alcohol 95% is sufficient for 100 l of liquor.

* Formulas which appear in this book

CURAÇAO, IMITATION NO. 2, LIQUOR BASE

1.	Curaçao, Imitation No. 1*	50
2.	Curaçao, Oil	900
3.	Orange, Bitter, Oil	50
		1000

25 cc of formula dissolved in ethyl alcohol 95% is sufficient for 100 l of liquor.

CURAÇAO, IMITATION NO. 3, LIQUOR BASE

1.	Almond, Bitter, Oil (cyanide-free)	4
2.	Badian, Oil (terpeneless)	2
3.	Cinnamon, Oil (terpeneless)	2
4.	Curaçao, Oil (terpeneless)	500
5.	Lemon, Oil (terpeneless)	15
6.	Mace, Oil (terpeneless)	2
7.	Neroli, Oil	5
8.	Orange, Bitter, Oil (terpeneless)	150
9.	Ethyl Alcohol 95%	320
		1000

25 cc of formula dissolved in ethyl alcohol 95% is sufficient for 100 l of liquor.

CURAÇAO, IMITATION NO. 4, LIQUOR BASE

1.	Curaçao, Imitation No. 1*	333
2.	Curaçao, Imitation No. 2*	333
3.	Curaçao, Imitation No. 3*	334
		1000

25 cc of formula dissolved in ethyl alcohol 95% is sufficient for 100 l of liquor.

CURAÇAO, IMITATION NO. 5, LIQUOR BASE

1.	Cinnamon, Oil	350
2.	Coriander, Oil	100
3.	Ginger, Oil	150
4.	Lemon, Oil (terpeneless)	148
5.	Neroli, Oil	1

6.	Orange, Oil (terpeneless)	250
7.	Rose, Oil	1
		1000

25 cc of formula dissolved in ethyl alcohol 95% is sufficient for 100 l of liquor.

CURAÇAO, IMITATION NO. 6

1.	Cinnamon	320
2.	Coriander, Oil	80
3.	Ginger, Oil	120
4.	Lemon, Oil	140
5.	Neroli, Oil	1
6.	Orange, Oil	338
7.	Rose, Oil	1
		1000

CURRANT, EXTRACT (NATURAL) NO. 1

1.	Currant (Black), Berries	50 kg
2.	Currant (Red), Berries	50 kg
3.	Sugar	10 kg

Ferment for 1 week or more, until flavor is totally developed. Add:

4.	Ethyl Alcohol 95%	50 l

Distill.
Yield: 60 liters

CURRANT, EXTRACT (NATURAL) NO. 2

1.	Currant (Black), Berries	50 kg
2.	Currant (Red), Berries	50 kg
3.	Sugar	10 kg

Ferment for 1 week or more, until flavor is totally developed. Express. To the residue add:

4.	Currant, Extract (Natural) No. 1*	50 l

Let macerate for another week. Add:

5.	Anisaldehyde	12 ml
6.	Ethyl Acetate	22 ml
7.	Ethyl Benzoate	24 ml
8.	Ethyl Pelargonate	12 ml

Distill altogether.
Yield: 60 liters

CURRANT, IMITATION NO. 1

1.	Black Currant, Fresh Leaves	75
2.	Black Currant	500
3.	Ethyl Alcohol 95%	425
		1000

Macerate, moderately warm, for 6 days. Shake often. Distill. Add:

4.	Distilled Water	875

Distill over 1000 cc. Redistill for above 750 cc.

CURRANT, IMITATION NO. 2

1.	Bilberry, Imitation No. 1*	175
2.	Currant, Imitation No. 1*	300
3.	Ethyl Methylphenylglycidate	22
4.	Pineapple, Imitation No. 1*	15
5.	Raspberry, Imitation No. 1*	60
6.	Raspberry, Imitation No. 2*	12
7.	Ethyl Alcohol 95%	208
8.	Distilled Water	208
		1000

CURRANT, IMITATION NO. 3

1.	Currant, Imitation No. 1*	500
2.	Currant, Imitation No. 2*	500
		1000

CURRANT, IMITATION NO. 4

1.	Currant, Imitation No. 3*	250
2.	Raspberry, Imitation No. 3*	250
3.	Ethyl Alcohol 95%	250
4.	Distilled Water	250
		1000

* Formulas which appear in this book

CURRANT, IMITATION NO. 5

1.	Amyl Butyrate	9
2.	Benzyl Acetate	1
3.	Cinnamon, Ceylon, Oil	2
4.	Ethyl Acetate	5
5.	Isobutyl Acetate	7
6.	Lemon, Oil	5
7.	Orange, Sweet, Oil	5
8.	Orris, Liquid	2
9.	Petitgrain, Oil	2
10.	Rose, Oil	1
11.	Vanillin	1
12.	Ethyl Alcohol 95%	480
13.	Distilled Water	480
		1000

CURRANT, IMITATION NO. 6

1.	Aldehyde C-8	1
2.	Aldehyde C-16	1
3.	Benzyl Acetate	4
4.	Benzyl Phenyl Acetate	1
5.	Clove, Tincture	5
6.	Currant, Extract (Natural) No. 2*	463
7.	Ethyl Benzoate	10
8.	Ethyl Butyrate	20
9.	Ethyl Oenanthate	10
10.	Orange, Oil	5
11.	Orris Root, Tincture	2
12.	Petitgrain, Oil	1
13.	Vanilla Beans, Tincture	5
14.	Ethyl Alcohol 95%	472
		1000

CURRANT, SYNTHETIC NO. 1

1.	Ethyl Acetate (10% sol'n.)	275
2.	Ethyl Benzoate	60
3.	Ethyl Butyrate	60
4.	Ethyl Formate	60
5.	Ethyl Oenanthate	60
6.	Ethyl Sebacate	60
7.	Isoamyl Acetate	60
8.	Isoamyl Butyrate	60
9.	Methyl Salicylate (10% sol'n.)	60
10.	Tartaric Acid (10% sol'n.)	245
		1000

* Formulas which appear in this book

CURRANT, SYNTHETIC NO. 2

1.	Ethyl Acetate (10% sol'n.)	930
2.	Ethyl Benzoate	25
3.	Isoamyl Acetate	10
4.	Propyl Acetate	10
5.	Propyl Propionate	25
		1000

CURRANT, SYNTHETIC NO. 3

1.	Ethyl Isovalerate (10% sol'n.)	500
2.	Ethyl Myristate	5
3.	Ethyl Phenyl Acetate	5
4.	Linalool	60
5.	Methyl Cinnamate (10% sol'n.)	400
6.	Methyl Heptenone	10
7.	Vanillin (10% sol'n.)	20
		1000

CURRANT, SYNTHETIC NO. 4

1.	Aldehyde C-16	1
2.	Benzoic Acid	1
3.	Cyclohexyl Butyrate	10
4.	Cyclohexyl Isovalerianate	18
5.	Ethyl Acetate	10
6.	Ethyl Benzoate	30
7.	Ethyl Butyrate	2
8.	Ethyl Formate	2
9.	Ethyl Myristate	1
10.	Ethyl Oenanthate	4
11.	Ethyl Sebacate	1
12.	Isoamyl Acetate	2
13.	Isoamyl Butyrate	1
14.	Linalool	2
15.	Methyl Cinnamate	8
16.	Methyl Heptenone	1
17.	Methyl Salicylate	1
18.	Propyl Acetate	1
19.	Propyl Propionate	1

20.	Succinic Acid	1
21.	Tartaric Acid	1
22.	Vanillin	1
23.	Ethyl Alcohol 95%	450
24.	Distilled Water	450
		1000

CURRANT, SYNTHETIC NO. 5

1.	Benzoic Acid (1% sol'n.)	70
2.	Ethyl Acetate (10% sol'n.)	350
3.	Ethyl Benzoate	140
4.	Ethyl Oenanthate	70
5.	Succinic Acid (10% sol'n.)	70
6.	Tartaric Acid (10% sol'n.)	300
		1000

CURRANT, SYNTHETIC NO. 6

1.	Ethyl Acetate (10% sol'n.)	350
2.	Ethyl Benzoate	70
3.	Ethyl Butyrate	70
4.	Ethyl Formate	70
5.	Ethyl Oenanthate	70
6.	Isoamyl Acetate	70
7.	Tartaric Acid (10% sol'n.)	300
		1000

DATE, EXTRACT (NATURAL)

1. Dates (dried and chopped) 10 kg
2. Alcohol 95% 20 l

Macerate for 3 days. Add:

3. Distilled Water 20 l

Distill. To the residue add:

4. Ethyl Alcohol 95% 20 l

Macerate for another 3 days. Add:

5. Ethyl Acetate 60 ml

Distill altogether.
Yield: 60 liters

DATE, IMITATION NO. 1

1.	Amyl Acetate	75
2.	Amyl Butyrate	2
3.	Amyl Valerianate	150
4.	Cinnamon, Oil	3
5.	Ethyl Acetate	75
6.	Ethyl Benzoate	150
7.	Eugenol	2
8.	Honey, Imitation No. 1*	20
9.	Nerolin	5
10.	Peach, Imitation No. 1*	6
11.	Ethyl Alcohol 95%	256
12.	Distilled Water	256
		1000

DATE, IMITATION NO. 2

1.	Bromelia	15
2.	Cinnamaldehyde	10
3.	Ethyl Acetate (10% sol'n.)	350
4.	Ethyl Butyrate	150
5.	Eugenol	5
6.	Isoamyl Acetate (10% sol'n.)	250
7.	Isoamyl Butyrate	50
8.	Isoamyl Isovalerate	150
9.	Isobutyl Acetate	5
10.	γ-Undecalactone (10% sol'n.)	15
		1000

DATE, SYNTHETIC

1.	Aldehyde C-14	2
2.	Cinnamaldehyde	2
3.	Ethyl Acetate	30
4.	Ethyl Benzoate	3
5.	Ethyl Butyrate	6
6.	Eugenol	1
7.	Isoamyl Acetate	25
8.	Isoamyl Butyrate	15
9.	Isoamyl Isovalerianate	15
10.	Nerolin	1
11.	Ethyl Alcohol 95%	450
12.	Distilled Water	450
		1000

* Formulas which appear in this book

FERNET "BRANCA" ESSENCE

1.	Angelic, Root	110
2.	Calamus, Root	135
3.	Calisaya, Bark	70
4.	Cardamom, Seeds	15
5.	Curaçao, Peels	70
6.	Gentian, Root	210
7.	Iva, Herb	55
8.	Lemon, Peels	40
9.	Orange, Bitter, Peels	160
10.	Wormwood, Herb	135
		1000

Powder each ingredient and then roast to a brownish color. Macerate altogether for 1 week with:

11.	Ethyl Alcohol 95%	1000
12.	Distilled Water	1000

Filter, and to the residue add:

13.	Ethyl Alcohol 95%	1000
14.	Distilled Water	1000

Macerate again for another week. Filter. Distill altogether.
Yield: 4 liters
Concentration: 60 ml/gal

FIG, ESSENCE (NATURAL)

1.	Figs, Chopped	10 kg
2.	Alcohol 95%	20 kg

Macerate for 3 days. Add:

3.	Distilled Water	20 kg

Express. To the residue add:

4.	Ethyl Alcohol 95%	20 kg

Macerate for another 3 days. Add:

5.	Ethyl Acetate	60 ml

Distill altogether.
Yield: 60 liters

FISH, ODOR (NATURAL)

1.	Fish, Fresh and Chopped	1 kg
2.	Propylene Glycol	2 l
3.	Distilled Water	1 l
4.	Ethyl Alcohol 95%	2 l

Express and filter.

FONDANT—ORGEAT—PRALINE

Fondant—A soft creamy compound of sugar, water, and flavorings, used as a basis for candies or icing.

Orgeat—From the French word "orge" meaning "barley;" a sweet almond-flavored, nonalcoholic syrup used as a cocktail ingredient or food flavoring.

Praline—Generally a confection of nut kernels, especially almonds roasted in boiling sugar until brown and crispy; a patty of creamy-brown sugar and pecan meats.

1.	Benzaldehyde (pure)	2
2.	Cherry Laurel, Water (pure)	50
3.	Condensed Milk	825
4.	Fruit Essence (any type)	100
5.	Rose, Water	15
6.	Vanillin	2
7.	Ethyl Alcohol 95%	6
		1000

Note: Minimal amount of alcohol in fondants.

FORTIFIED EXTRACTS FROM VEGETABLES

1.	Any vegetable (crushed in small pieces)	10 kg
2.	Ethyl Alcohol 95%	20 l
3.	Distilled Water	20 l

Macerate for 1 week. Express. To the 40 l of expressed juice add:

4.	Anise, Oil	5 ml
5.	Calamus, Oil	5 ml

6.	Cardamom, Oil	5 ml
7.	Ginger, Oil	5 ml
8.	Juniper Berries, Oil	5 ml
9.	Mace, Oil	5 ml
10.	Nutmeg, Oil	5 ml
11.	Pepper (Black or White), Oil	5 ml

Stir and filter.

FRUIT EXTRACT, NATURAL FLAVOR

Base:

1.	Ethyl Alcohol 95%	70
2.	Glycerin (neutral)	5
3.	Distilled Water	25

1.	Fresh Fruit Juice (any single)	4 l
2.	Base	4 l
3.	Ethyl Alcohol 95%	2 l

Stir. Filter.
Yield: 10 liters

FRUIT SODA

1.	Champagne Cedar, Essence	125
2.	Cherry, Imitation No. 1*	175
3.	Grenadine, Imitation No. 1*	175
4.	Pineapple, Imitation No. 1*	175
5.	Raspberry, Imitation No. 1*	175
6.	Strawberry, Imitation No. 1*	175
		1000

FUNGI EXTRACT (NATURAL)

1.	Dried Fungi (Champignons, Morels, Mushrooms, or Truffles, single type)	1
2.	Ethyl Alcohol 95%	1
3.	Distilled Water	1

Macerate for 1 week. Separate the liquid without pressure. To the residue add:

4.	Distilled Water	1

Let stand for another day. Express. Blend the two liquids and filter.
Yield: 3 liters

* Formulas which appear in this book

GARLIC, EXTRACT (NATURAL)

Use garlic, well peeled and finely cut. Press well. Discard the juice (no value).

1.	Garlic	1 kg
2.	Ethyl Alcohol 95%	4 l

Let stand for 3 days. Express. To the residue add:

3.	Ethyl Alcohol 95%	2 l
4.	Distilled Water	2 l

Let stand for another 3 days. Express. Put the liquid together. Add:

5.	Mustard Oil	16 ml

Filter.
Yield: 8 liters

GIN, IMITATION

1.	Angelic Root, Oil	8
2.	Anise, Oil	4
3.	Coriander, Oil	12
4.	Juniper, Oil	930
5.	Lemon, Oil	30
6.	Orange, Oil	16
		1000

GINGER, ESSENCE (NATURAL)

1.	Cinnamon, Oil	60
2.	Clove, Oil	40
3.	Ginger, Oil	850
4.	Lemon, Oil	50
		1000

GINGER, EXTRACT (NATURAL), "GINGERINE"

1.	Ginger Roots (unpeeled)	10 kg

(Previously washed in 12 l of water and 1 kg

of sodium bicarbonate. Discard dirty water after 1 day; wash the roots again 3 times.)

2.	Ethyl Alcohol 95%	10 1

Let stand for 3 days. Percolate. Add to the residue (roots)

3.	Ethyl Alcohol 95%	4 1
4.	Distilled Water	4 1

Let stand for another 3 days. Percolate. Put together the two percolates. Distill.

Yield: 18 liters

GINGER, IMITATION NO. 1

1.	Amyl Butyrate	250
2.	Cardamom, Oil	12
3.	Clove, Oil	10
4.	Ethyl Acetate	350
5.	Ethyl Oenanthate	150
6.	Galanga, Oil	16
7.	Ginger, Oil	200
8.	Petitgrain, Oil	12
		1000

GINGER, IMITATION NO. 2

1.	Ginger, Oil	700
2.	Lemon, Oil	25
3.	Orange, Oil	50
4.	Pineapple, Imitation No. 1*	225
		1000

GINGER, IMITATION NO. 3

1.	Cinnamon, Oil	60
2.	Clove, Oil	40
3.	Ginger, Oil	850
4.	Lemon, Oil (terpeneless)	50
		1000

GINGER, IMITATION NO. 4

1.	Camphene	50
2.	Ginger, Imitation No. 1*	300
3.	Methylheptenone	100
4.	Phellandrene	200
5.	Pinene, Imitation No. 1*	100
6.	Terpineol	250
		1000

* Formulas which appear in this book

GINGER, IMITATION NO. 5

1.	Ginger, Imitation No. 1*	400
2.	Ginger, Imitation No. 2*	400
3.	Ginger, Oil	200
		1000

GINGERGRASS (PALMAROSA)

1.	Clove, Oil (10% sol'n.)	500
2.	Geraniol	300
3.	Geranium, Palmarosa	200
		1000

GIROFLÉ (CLOVE), TINCTURE

1.	Eugenol	90
2.	Ethyl Alcohol 95%	910
		1000

GLACE CAKE MIX

(Candied for fruit cakes and desserts, encrusted or coated with sugar, or baked with sugar or syrup until translucent)

1. Drained Fruits
    1. Cherries, Crushed
    2. Grapefruits, Peels
    3. Lemon, Peels
    4. Orange, Peels
    5. Pineapples, Pulp (cut) (Ananas)
    6. Any Other Fruits
2. Syrup
    1. Corn Syrup
    2. Sugar Syrup
3. Preservatives
    1. Citric Acid (1% sol'n.)
    2. Sodium Benzoate (1% sol'n.)
    3. Sulfur Dioxide (trace)
4. Synthetic Flavor
5. Color FD&C Yellow No. 5

GOOSEBERRY, EXTRACT (NATURAL)

1.	Gooseberries, Red or Yellow (not green)	10	kg

Express the juice (7 kg). To the residue (3 kg) add:

2.	Ethyl Alcohol 95%	3	l

Macerate for 3 days. Express. Mix all juice and add:

3.	Amyl Acetate	25	ml
4.	Ethyl Acetate	25	ml
5.	Ethyl Butyrate	45	ml

Filter.
Yield: 10 liters

GOOSEBERRY, IMITATION NO. 1

1.	Aldehyde C-14	10
2.	Ethyl Acetate	50
3.	Ethyl Benzoate	10
4.	Ethyl Oenanthate	10
5.	Gooseberry, Extract (Natural)*	425
6.	Orange, Oil	70
7.	Ethyl Alcohol 95%	425
		1000

GOOSEBERRY, IMITATION NO. 2

1.	Anethole	10
2.	Ethyl Acetate (10% sol'n.)	340
3.	Ethyl Benzoate	50
4.	Ethyl Butyrate (10% sol'n.)	275
5.	Isoamyl Acetate (10% sol'n.)	275
6.	Phenyl Ethyl Alcohol	1
7.	Safrole	10
8.	Vanillin	39
		1000

* Formulas which appear in this book

GOOSEBERRY, IMITATION NO. 3

1.	Amyl Acetate	15
2.	Buchu, Leaves Extract	50
3.	Currant, Juice	28
4.	Ethyl Acetate	13
5.	Ethyl Benzoate	17
6.	Ethyl Butyrate	50
7.	Fennel, Oil	4
8.	Orris, Juice	3
9.	Raspberry, Juice	300
10.	Rose, Oil (10% sol'n.)	6
11.	Safrole, Oil	10
12.	Vanillin	2
13.	Ethyl Alcohol 95%	502
		1000

GOOSEBERRY, IMITATION NO. 4

1.	Anethole	4
2.	Bromelia	1
3.	Ethyl Acetate (10% sol'n.)	400
4.	Ethyl Benzoate	30
5.	Ethyl Butyrate (10% sol'n.)	270
6.	Isoamyl Acetate (10% sol'n.)	265
7.	Vanillin (10% sol'n.)	30
		1000

GOOSEBERRY, IMITATION NO. 5

1.	Anethole	13
2.	Ethyl Acetate (10% sol'n.)	350
3.	Ethyl Butyrate (10% sol'n.)	275
4.	Isoamyl Acetate (10% sol'n.)	275
5.	Isoamyl Butyrate	50
6.	Phenyl Ethyl Alcohol	1
7.	Safrole	6
8.	Vanillin (10% sol'n.)	30
		1000

GOOSEBERRY, SYNTHETIC NO. 1

1.	Acetaldehyde	1
2.	Aldehyde C-16	10
3.	Ethyl Acetate	10

4.	Ethyl Benzoate	10
5.	Ethyl Oenanthate	10
6.	Ethyl Alcohol 95%	480
7.	Distilled Water	479
		1000

GOOSEBERRY, SYNTHETIC NO. 2

1.	Anethole	2
2.	Anisaldehyde	1
3.	Ethyl Acetate	20
4.	Ethyl Benzoate	20
5.	Ethyl Butyrate	40
6.	Ethyl Oenanthate	2
7.	Isoamyl Acetate	4
8.	Isoamyl Butyrate	2
9.	Nerolin	1
10.	Phenyl Ethyl Alcohol	1
11.	Ethyl Alcohol 95%	447
12.	Distilled Water	460
		1000

GOOSEBERRY, SYNTHETIC NO. 3

1.	Benzoic Acid (1% sol'n.)	100
2.	Ethyl Acetate (10% sol'n.)	500
3.	Ethyl Benzoate	100
4.	Ethyl Oenanthate	100
5.	Succinic Acid (10% sol'n.)	100
6.	Tartaric Acid (10% sol'n.)	100
		1000

GOOSEBERRY, SYNTHETIC NO. 4

1.	Benzoic Acid (1% sol'n.)	50
2.	Ethyl Acetate (10% sol'n.)	250
3.	Ethyl Aldehyde	50
4.	Ethyl Benzoate	50
5.	Ethyl Pelargonate	50
6.	Glycerol	350
7.	Succinic Acid (10% sol'n.)	50
8.	Tartaric Acid (10% sol'n.)	150
		1000

GRAPE, EXTRACT (NATURAL) NO. 1

1.	Raisin, Seedless (unbleached)	2 kg
2.	Distilled Water	1 l

Let stand for 24 h and sieve expressing all juice. Add to the residue:

3.	Ethyl Alcohol 95%	1 l

Let stand for another 24 h and sieve expressing all juice. Add to the residue:

4.	Distilled Water	1 l

Let stand for another 24 h and sieve expressing all juice. Distill altogether.

Yield: 3 liters

GRAPE, EXTRACT (NATURAL) NO. 2

1.	Raisins	10 kg
2.	Sweet Clear Wine (hot)	10 l

Let stand for 3 days. Express. To the residue add:

3.	Ethyl Alcohol 95%	8 l
4.	Sweet Clear Wine	2 l

Let stand for another 3 days. Express and add:

5.	Cognac	13 ml
6.	Ethyl Oenanthate	10 ml
7.	Mace, Oil	12 ml

Distill altogether the expressed juice.

Yield: 20 liters

Note: This type of grape extract is called "wine flavor" for fondants. Fondants are sweet, creamy sugar paste, eaten as a candy or employed for filling other candies.

GRAPE, IMITATION NO. 1

1.	Grape, Extract (Natural) No. 1*	250
2.	Grape, Extract (Natural) No. 2*	250
3.	Ethyl Alcohol 95%	250
4.	Distilled Water	250
		1000

* Formulas which appear in this book

GRAPE, IMITATION NO. 2

1.	Amyl Butyrate	6
2.	Cardamom, Oil	3
3.	Cognac, Oil	238
4.	Ethyl Acetate	25
5.	Ethyl Oenanthate	125
6.	Ethyl Pelargonate	175
7.	Mace, Oil	6
8.	Methyl Anthranilate	62
9.	Ethyl Alcohol 95%	180
10.	Distilled Water	180
		1000

GRAPE, SYNTHETIC NO. 1

1.	Aldehyde C-14 (pure)	20
2.	Chloroform (pure)	20
3.	Ethyl Oenanthate	120
4.	Glycerin (neutral)	180
5.	Lees (dregs)**	10
6.	Methyl Anthranilate	10
7.	Ethyl Alcohol 95%	320
8.	Distilled Water	320
		1000

GRAPE, SYNTHETIC NO. 2

1.	Aldehyde C-14 (pure)	20
2.	Chloroform (pure)	20
3.	Ethyl Formate	10
4.	Ethyl Oenanthate	120
5.	Glycerin (neutral)	130
6.	Ethyl Alcohol 95%	350
7.	Distilled Water	350
		1000

GRAPE, SYNTHETIC NO. 3

1.	Butyl Anthranilate	24
2.	Cinnamyl Anthranilate	29
3.	Cinnamyl Formate	4
4.	Cinnamyl Propionate	18
5.	Diethyl Anthranilate	255
6.	Dimethyl Anthranilate	113
7.	Ethyl Butyrate	44
8.	Ethyl Cinnamate	18
9.	Ethyl Formate	35
10.	Ethyl Lactate	141
11.	Ethyl Oenanthate	37
12.	Nerolin	1
13.	Propyl Cinnamate	18
14.	Ethyl Alcohol 95%	263
		1000

GRAPE, SYNTHETIC NO. 4

1.	Cardamom, Oil	11
2.	Ethyl Acetate	11
3.	Ethyl Anthranilate	12
4.	Ethyl Butyrate	2
5.	Ethyl Cinnamate	4
6.	Ethyl Formate	1
7.	Ethyl Oenanthate	32
8.	Ethyl Pelargonate	1
9.	Isoamyl Acetate	1
10.	Isoamyl Butyrate	3
11.	Isoamyl Oenanthate	1
12.	Isoamyl Valerianate	4
13.	Mace, Oil	1
14.	Methyl Anthranilate	12
15.	Propyl Cinnamate	4
16.	Ethyl Alcohol 95%	450
17.	Distilled Water	450
		1000

GRAPE, SYNTHETIC NO. 5

1.	Ethyl Anthranilate (10% sol'n.)	450
2.	Ethyl Formate	100
3.	Ethyl Oenanthate (10% sol'n.)	450
		1000

GRAPE, SYNTHETIC NO. 6

1.	Ethyl Anthranilate	150
2.	Ethyl Butyrate	40
3.	Ethyl Cinnamate (10% sol'n.)	220
4.	Ethyl Oenanthate (10% sol'n.)	370
5.	Propyl Acetate (10% sol'n.)	220
		1000

** The settling of liquor during fermentation and aging

GRAPE, SYNTHETIC NO. 7

1.	Cardamom, Oil	5
2.	Ethyl Acetate (10% sol'n.)	550
3.	Ethyl Oenanthate (10% sol'n.)	310
4.	Ethyl Pelargonate	30
5.	Isoamyl Butyrate	90
6.	Isoamyl Isovalerate	3
7.	Mace, Oil	10
8.	Methyl Salicylate	2
		1000

GRAPE, SYNTHETIC NO. 8

1.	Ethyl Butyrate	30
2.	Ethyl Oenanthate (10% sol'n.)	220
3.	Isoamyl Acetate	30
4.	Isoamyl Isovalerate	95
5.	Methyl Anthranilate (10% sol'n.)	625
		1000

GRAPE, SYNTHETIC NO. 9

1.	Ethyl Formate	200
2.	Ethyl Oenanthate (10% sol'n.)	400
3.	Ethyl Salicylate (10% sol'n.)	10
4.	Succinic Acid (10% sol'n.)	190
5.	Tartaric Acid (10% sol'n.)	200
		1000

GRAPEFRUIT, SYNTHETIC

1.	Citral	5
2.	Ethyl Butyrate	10
3.	Linalool	20
4.	Limonene	40
5.	Ethyl Alcohol 95%	463
6.	Distilled Water	462
		1000

GREEN GAGE, EXTRACT (NATURAL)

1. Green Gages (Blue) (crushed in small pieces) 5
2. Sugar

Let ferment for a few days. Express the juice. To the residue add:

3. Ethyl Alcohol 95% 15 1

Let macerate for another 3 days. Add:

4. Amyl Valerianate 12 ml

Distill altogether.
Yield: 20 liters

Note: Gage refers to any of the rather small, rounded, greenish or greenish-yellow cultivated plums. The name "gage" is from the English botanist Sir William Gage, 1724–1820.

GREEN GAGE, IMITATION

1.	Amyl Alcohol	5
2.	Amyl Butyrate	30
3.	Benzaldehyde (pure)	30
4.	Cinnamon, Oil	4
5.	Clove, Oil	2
6.	Cognac, Oil	5
7.	Ethyl Acetate	20
8.	Ethyl Butyrate	35
9.	Ethyl Oenanthate	60
10.	Ethyl Pelargonate	20
11.	Geranium, Oil	3
12.	Orange (Sweet), Oil	15
13.	Rose, Oil	1
14.	Vanillin	6
15.	Ethyl Alcohol 95%	382
16.	Distilled Water	382
		1000

GRENADINE

See Pomegranate

GUAVA, EXTRACT (NATURAL)

1. Guava Fruits, Crushed 10 kg
2. Sugar 5 kg

Let ferment for 1 week. Express all juice. To the residue add:

3. Ethyl Alcohol 95% 10 1

Let stand for 1 week. Express, and to the

residue add:

4.	Distilled Water	10 l

Let stand for another 3 days. Add:

5.	Vanilla Beans, Oil	2 ml

Distill altogether.
Yield: 20 liters

HAM, BAKED "GLAZE"

1.	Pineapple (Ananas) Extract (Natural)*	260
2.	Clove, Tincture	100
3.	Guar, Gum	5
4.	Sodium Benzoate	1
5.	Sorbic Acid	1
6.	Strawberry, Extract (Natural)*	260
7.	Sugar	300
8.	Vinegar	3
9.	Distilled Water	70
		1000

HAZELNUT, EXTRACT (NATURAL)

1.	Hazelnut Kernels (crushed near powder, fresh with good taste, not rancid)	10 kg
2.	Ethyl Alcohol 95%	30 l

Macerate for 10 days, stirring each day for 1 h. Collect, without pressure, the extract (20 l). To the residue add:

3.	Distilled Water	20 l

Let stand for another 3 days.

4.	Amyl Formate	50 ml
5.	Ethyl Oenanthate	25 ml

Distill altogether.
Yield: 40 liters

* Formulas which appear in this book

HERBAL CREAM (CELERY OR ANY OTHER HERB)

1.	Celery, Oil	10
2.	Sugar	250
3.	Ethyl Alcohol 95%	495
4.	Distilled Water	245
		1000

HONEY, IMITATION NO. 1

1.	Ethyl Phenyl Acetate	1
2.	Farnesol, Oil	2
3.	Fennel, Oil	16
4.	Honey, Oil	480
5.	Rose, Oil	1
6.	Ethyl Alcohol 95%	500
		1000

HONEY, IMITATION NO. 2

1.	Cognac, Oil	10
2.	Honey, Imitation No. 1*	490
3.	Ethyl Alcohol 95%	500
		1000

HONEY, IMITATION NO. 3

1.	Ethyl Pelargonate	50
2.	Farnesol, Oil	5
3.	Honey, Imitation No. 1*	200
4.	Honey, Imitation No. 2*	250
5.	Phenyl Isobutyrate	100
6.	Ethyl Alcohol 95%	395
		1000

HONEY, IMITATION NO. 4

1.	Ethyl Pelargonate	10
2.	Farnesol, Oil	2
3.	Honey, Oil	400
4.	Phenyl Isobutyrate	50
5.	Ethyl Alcohol 95%	538
		1000

HONEY, IMITATION NO. 5

1.	Ethyl Pelargonate	50
2.	Honey, Imitation No. 2*	500
3.	Honey, Oil	400
4.	Phenyl Ethyl Isobutyrate	50
		1000

HONEY, IMITATION NO. 6

1.	Celery, Oil	7
2.	Geranium, Oil	7
3.	Methyl Acetophenone	15
4.	Methyl Phenyl Acetate	240
5.	Phenyl Acetic Acid	240
6.	Propylene Glycol	371
7.	Vanillin	120
		1000

HONEY, IMITATION NO. 7

1.	Ethyl Acetate	21
2.	Ethyl Isovalerianate	63
3.	Ethyl Pelargonate	20
4.	Linalool	27
5.	Methyl Anthranilate	10
6.	Neroli, Oil	4
7.	Phenyl Ethyl Acetate	15
8.	Phenyl Ethyl Alcohol	10
9.	Propylene Glycol	820
10.	Rhodinyl Phenyl Acetate	10
		1000

HONEY, SYNTHETIC NO. 1

1.	Amyl Acetate	50
2.	Amyl Valerianate	200
3.	Ethyl Acetate	100
4.	Ethyl Oenanthate	175
5.	Propylene Glycol	300
6.	Rhodinyl Phenyl Acetate	175
		1000

* Formulas which appear in this book

HONEY, SYNTHETIC NO. 2 (FOR PERFUMES)

1.	Dimethyl Hydroquinone	110
2.	Geraniol	110
3.	Phenyl Acetic Acid	110
4.	Phenyl Acetic Aldehyde	110
5.	Phenyl Ethyl Acetate	110
6.	Phenyl Ethyl Alcohol	120
7.	Hydroxycitronellal	110
8.	Linalool	110
9.	Quinoline	110
		1000

HONEY, SYNTHETIC NO. 3 (FOR PERFUMES)

1.	Aldehyde C-14 (1% sol'n.)	60
2.	Benzoic Acid	20
3.	Cinnamic Alcohol	50
4.	Dimethyl Hydroquinone	80
5.	Ethyl Naphtholate	10
6.	Ethyl Phenyl Acetate	90
7.	Geraniol	90
8.	Hydroxycitronellal	80
9.	Indole (1% sol'n.)	30
10.	Isopropyl Quinoline (10% sol'n.)	20
11.	Methyl Cinnamate	30
12.	Methyl Naphtholate	10
13.	β–Methyl Naphthyl Acetone	40
14.	Methyl Phenyl Acetate	90
15.	Musk Ketone	30
16.	Musk Xylene (10% sol'n.)	50
17.	Phenoxy Ethanol	10
18.	Phenyl Acetic Acid	10
19.	Phenyl Ethyl Alcohol	30
20.	Phenyl Ethyl Isobutyrate	40
21.	Phenyl Ethyl Phenyl Acetate	70
22.	Skatole (1/1000 sol'n.)	30
23.	Trichloromethyl Phenyl Carbinyl Acetate	30
		1000

HONEY, SYNTHETIC NO. 4

1.	Amyl Acetate (10% sol'n.)	570
2.	Ethyl Acetate	160
3.	Ethyl Isovalerate (10% sol'n.)	225
4.	Ethyl Pelargonate	25
5.	Isobutyl-α-Toluate	20
		1000

HONEY, SYNTHETIC NO. 5

1.	Ethyl Acetate (10% sol'n.)	700
2.	Ethyl Butyrate	30
3.	Ethyl Isovalerate	200
4.	Ethyl Pelargonate	15
5.	Phenyl Ethyl Acetate	55
		1000

HOP, EXTRACT (NATURAL)

1.	Hop, Flowers (freshly dried)	1 kg
2.	Ethyl Alcohol 95%	5 l
3.	Distilled Water	5 l

Macerate for 1 week. Express all extract.
Yield: 9 liters

HOP, IMITATION

1.	Amyl Acetate	20
2.	Amyl Butyrate	20
3.	Cinnamon, Oil	2
4.	Clove, Oil	8
5.	Ethyl Acetate	20
6.	Ethyl Oenanthate	20
7.	Ethyl Pelargonate	20
8.	Hop, Extract (Natural)*	500
9.	Orange, Sweet, Oil	10
10.	Petitgrain, Oil	10
11.	Ethyl Alcohol 95%	185
12.	Distilled Water	185
		1000

HOP, SYNTHETIC NO. 1

1.	Anisaldehyde	1
2.	Butyric Acid	14
3.	Capraldehyde	2
4.	Cinnamic Aldehyde	1
5.	Ethyl Acetate	16
6.	Ethyl Oenanthate	12
7.	Ethyl Pelargonate	22
8.	Ethyl Isovalerianate	45
9.	Eugenol	2
10.	Heliotropin	1
11.	Isoamyl Acetate	29
12.	Isoamyl Butyrate	29
13.	Limonene	1
14.	Phenyl Ethyl Alcohol	1
15.	Ethyl Alcohol 95%	412
16.	Distilled Water	412
		1000

* Formulas which appear in this book

HOP, SYNTHETIC NO. 2

1.	Butyric Acid	5
2.	Capraldehyde	20
3.	Cinnamaldehyde	4
4.	Ethyl Acetate (10% sol'n.)	500
5.	Ethyl Oenanthate	120
6.	Ethyl Pelargonate	45
7.	Eugenol	12
8.	Isoamyl Acetate	150
9.	Isoamyl Butyrate	130
10.	Limonene	14
		1000

HOP, SYNTHETIC NO. 3

1.	Anethole	12
2.	Butyric Acid	20
3.	Ethyl Acetate (10% sol'n.)	400
4.	Ethyl Isovalerate	160
5.	Eugenol	10
6.	Heliotropin	13
7.	Isoamyl Acetate	200
8.	Isoamyl Butyrate	160
9.	Phenyl Ethyl Alcohol	25
		1000

HUCKLEBERRY, SYNTHETIC NO. 1

1.	Anethole	10
2.	Ethyl Acetate (10% sol'n.)	357
3.	Ethyl Benzoate (10% sol'n.)	300
4.	Isoamyl Acetate	200
5.	Isoamyl Butyrate	130
6.	Linalool	3
		1000

HUCKLEBERRY, SYNTHETIC NO. 2

1.	Anethole	1
2.	Ethyl Acetate	35
3.	Ethyl Benzoate	30
4.	Isoamyl Acetate	20
5.	Isoamyl Butyrate	13
6.	Linalool	1
7.	Ethyl Alcohol 95%	450
8.	Distilled Water	450
		1000

JUICES, GENERAL

1.	Juice Concentrate (from any fruit)	1 l
2.	Distilled Water	1 l
3.	Potassium Sorbate (preservative, 20% sol'n.)	1 g

KERNEL (NUT), GENERAL

See Nuts, Kernels (General Method of Flavor Extraction).

KETCHUP (CATSUP), MUSHROOM FLAVOR

1.	Acetic Acid	1 kg
2.	Cardamom, Seeds (ground)	1 kg
3.	Cloves (ground)	1 kg
4.	Ginger, Root (ground)	1 kg
5.	Mushrooms (well crushed)	6 kg
6.	Pepper, Black (ground)	1 l
7.	Pimienta (ground)	1 kg
8.	Salt (20% sol'n.)	1 l
9.	Ethyl Alcohol 95%	10 l
10.	Distilled Water	10 l

Macerate for 10 days, stirring for 1 h every day. Express, and to the residue add:

11.	Ethyl Alcohol 95%	10 l
12.	Distilled Water	10 l

Let stand for another 3 days. Boil gently for 1 h. Cool and express. Put all juices together and filter.

Yield: 40 liters.

KETCHUP (CATSUP), SPICE

1.	Cassia, Oil	10
2.	Celery, Seeds, Oil	5
3.	Clove, Oil	50
4.	Mace, Oil	10
5.	Mustard, Oil	5
6.	Nutmeg, Oil	10
7.	Pimenta, Oil	10
8.	Ethyl Alcohol 95%	900
		1000

KETCHUP (CATSUP), TOMATO FLAVOR

1.	Basil, Oil	1 ml
2.	Cinnamon, Oil	1 ml
3.	Clary Sage, Oil	1 ml
4.	Clove, Oil	1 ml
5.	Corn Syrup	3 l
6.	Laurel Leaves, Oil	1 ml
7.	Mace, Oil	1 ml
8.	Marjoram, Oil	1 ml
9.	Nutmeg, Oil	1 ml
10.	Onion, Extract (Natural)*	500 ml
11.	Oregano, Oil	1 ml
12.	Paprika, Oil	1 ml
13.	Parsley, Oil	1 ml
14.	Pepper, Oil	1 ml
15.	Tomato, Juice (from ripe crushed tomatoes)	1 ml
16.	Vinegar	1 ml
17.	Ethyl Alcohol 95%	5 ml
18.	Distilled Water	5 ml

Macerate altogether for 10 days. Express and separate the residue. To the residue add:

19.	Ethyl Alcohol 95%	5 l
20.	Distilled Water	5 l

Let stand for another 3 days. Express and put the juices together. Filter.

Yield: 20 liters

* Formulas which appear in this book

KUMMEL

1.	Badian (Star Anise), Oil (terpeneless)	3
2.	Chamomile, German, Oil	5
3.	Carvi (Caraway), Oil (terpeneless)	25
4.	Cognac, Oil	175
5.	Coriander, Oil (terpeneless)	10
6.	Ethyl Propionate	10
7.	Maraschino, Imitation No. 1*	100
8.	Ethyl Alcohol 95%	672
		1000

LAVENDER, FLAVOR

1.	Bergamot, Oil	150
2.	Clove, Oil	7
3.	Lavender, Oil (10% sol'n.)	600
4.	Neroli, Oil	3
5.	Patchouli	3
6.	Rose, Oil	10
7.	Ethyl Alcohol 95%	227
		1000

LEMON, EXTRACT (NATURAL)

1.	Lemon, Peels (fresh)	10	kg
2.	Ethyl Alcohol 95%	10	l
3.	Distilled Water	10	l

Macerate for 3 days. Express. To the residue add:

4.	Ethyl Alcohol 95%	10	l
5.	Distilled Water	10	l

Let stand for another 3 days. Distill to separate the terpenes and the residue. Mix the juice and the distillate. Redistill altogether. Filter.

Yield: 40 liters

LEMON, IMITATION NO. 1

1.	Citral	13
2.	Ethyl Acetate	6
3.	Ethyl Butyrate	3
4.	Isoamyl Acetate	8
5.	Isoamyl Butyrate	9
6.	Lemon, Oil	44
7.	Orange, Oil	3
8.	Tartaric Acid (10% sol'n.)	10
9.	Ethyl Alcohol 95%	452
10.	Distilled Water	452
		1000

LEMON, IMITATION NO. 2

1.	Aldehyde C-8	20
2.	Chloroform (pure)	10
3.	Citral	10
4.	Citronellal	1
5.	Ethyl Acetate	100
6.	Ethyl Nitrate	10
7.	Glycerin (neutral)	50
8.	Linalyl Acetate	50
9.	Methyl Anthranilate	25
10.	Lemon, Oil	50
11.	Rhodinyl Acetate	10
12.	Tartaric Acid (10% sol'n.)	10
13.	Ethyl Alcohol 95%	327
14.	Distilled Water	327
		1000

LEMON, IMITATION NO. 3

1.	Aldehyde C-8	5
2.	Aldehyde C-10	20
3.	Ethyl Acetate	50
4.	Ethyl Nitrate	10
5.	Glycerin (neutral)	50
6.	Lemon, Extract (Natural)*	500
7.	Tartaric Acid (10% sol'n.)	10
8.	Ethyl Alcohol 95%	178
9.	Distilled Water	177
		1000

LEMON, IMITATION NO. 4

1.	Amyl Acetate	15
2.	Amyl Butyrate	35
3.	Citral	5
4.	Ethyl Acetate	30
5.	Lemon, Oil (terpeneless)	457
6.	Ethyl Alcohol 95%	458
		1000

* Formulas which appear in this book

LEMON, IMITATION NO. 5

1.	Lemon, Imitation No. 1*	550
2.	Lemon, Oil	140
3.	Lime, Oil	10
4.	Ethyl Alcohol 95%	300
		1000

LEMON, IMITATION NO. 6

1.	Citral	50
2.	Lemon, Imitation No. 2*	300
3.	Lemon, Oil (terpeneless)	50
4.	Lime, Oil (terpeneless)	25
5.	Orange, Sweet, Oil	10
6.	Ethyl Alcohol 95%	565
		1000

LEMON, IMITATION NO. 7

1.	Citral	25
2.	Lemon, Imitation No. 3*	325
3.	Ethyl Alcohol 95%	650
		1000

LEMON, IMITATION NO. 8

1.	Lemon, Oil	500
2.	Lemon, Oil (terpeneless)	50
3.	Lime, Oil	25
4.	Ethyl Alcohol 95%	425
		1000

LEMON, IMITATION NO. 9

1.	Ethyl Acetate (10% sol'n.)	720
2.	Lemon, Oil	140
3.	Tartaric Acid (10% sol'n.)	140
		1000

LEMON, IMITATION NO. 10

1.	Ethyl Acetate	70
2.	Isoamyl Acetate	100
3.	Isoamyl Butyrate (10% sol'n.)	280
4.	Lemon, Oil (10% sol'n.)	400
5.	Orange, Oil	150
		1000

* Formulas which appear in this book

LEMON, IMITATION NO. 11

1.	Ethyl Acetate	200
2.	Ethyl Butyrate	170
3.	Isoamyl Acetate (10% sol'n.)	340
4.	Isoamyl Butyrate	170
5.	Lemon, Oil	60
6.	Tartaric Acid (10% sol'n.)	60
		1000

LEMON, IMITATION NO. 12

1.	Citral	18
2.	Lemon, Oil (terpeneless)	8
3.	Ethyl Alcohol 95%	974
		1000

LEMON, IMITATION NO. 13

1.	Citral (10% sol'n.)	680
2.	Lemon, Oil (terpeneless, 10% sol'n.)	320
		1000

LEMON, IMITATION NO. 14

1.	Ethyl Acetate (10% sol'n.)	320
2.	Lemon, Oil (10% sol'n.)	320
3.	Succinic Acid (10% sol'n.)	40
4.	Tartaric Acid (10% sol'n.)	320
		1000

LEMON, IMITATION NO. 15

1.	Citral (10% sol'n.)	500
2.	Geraniol	50
3.	Lemon, Oil	100
4.	Linalool	150
5.	Methylheptenone	20
6.	Terpineol	180
		1000

LEMON, IMITATION NO. 16

1.	Citral	40
2.	Lemon, Imitation No. 1*	800
3.	Limonene	160
		1000

LEMON, POWDERED (CONCENTRATE)

1.	Color, Certified	1
2.	Lemon, Oil	250
3.	Malic Acid (powdered)	249
4.	Sugar (granulated)	500
		1000

LEMON, SYNTHETIC NO. 1

1.	Acetaldehyde	2
2.	Amyl Valerianate	20
3.	Chloroform	1
4.	Citric Acid	10
5.	Ethyl Acetate	30
6.	Glycerin (neutral)	15
7.	Tartaric Acid	1
8.	Ethyl Alcohol 95%	461
9.	Distilled Water	460
		1000

LEMON, SYNTHETIC NO. 2

1.	Aldehyde C-9 (10% sol'n.)	2
2.	Citral	40
3.	Geraniol	25
4.	Geranyl Acetate	2
5.	Linalyl Acetate	25
6.	Linalool	25
7.	Terpineol	35
8.	Ethyl Alcohol 95%	423
9.	Distilled Water	423
		1000

LEMON, SYNTHETIC NO. 3

1.	Amyl Butyrate	10
2.	Citral	25
3.	Chloroform	10
4.	Ethyl Acetate	20
5.	Ethyl Nitrate	10
6.	Glycerin (neutral)	50
7.	Ethyl Alcohol 95%	438
8.	Distilled Water	437
		1000

LICORICE, ROOT, EXTRACT (NATURAL)

1.	Licorice, Root (well ground)	5 kg
2.	Distilled Water	20 l

Let stand for 3 days, stirring for 1 h each day. Percolate. To the residue add:

3.	Distilled Water	10 l
4.	Ethyl Alcohol 95%	10 l

Let stand for another 3 days. Heat to the boiling point. Cool and filter. Evaporate to a viscid point. Add while stirring:

5.	Sodium Benzoate (10% sol'n.)	1 ml

Note: The desired coloration, as well as the amount of essence, could be increased or decreased.

LIME, EXTRACT (NATURAL)

1.	Lime, Peels (fresh)	10 kg
2.	Ethyl Alcohol 95%	10 l
3.	Distilled Water	10 l

Let stand for 3 days. Express off all juice (20 l). To the residue add:

4.	Ethyl Alcohol 95%	10 l
5.	Distilled Water	10 l

Let stand for another 3 days. Distill altogether, separating all terpenes. Filter.

Yield: 40 liters

* Formulas which appear in this book

LIME, IMITATION

1.	Ethyl Acetate	25
2.	Isoamyl Acetate	15
3.	Isoamyl Butyrate	12
4.	Lemon, Oil	30
5.	Lime, Oil	30
6.	Menthol	1
7.	Ethyl Alcohol 95%	444
8.	Distilled Water	443
		1000

LIME, SYNTHETIC NO. 1

1.	Benzoin	10
2.	Benzyl Acetate	30
3.	Geraniol	30
4.	Linalool	30
5.	Methyl Anthranilate	30
6.	Musk Ketone	10
7.	Peru Balsam	10
8.	Ethyl Alcohol 95%	425
9.	Distilled Water	425
		1000

LIME, SYNTHETIC NO. 2

1.	Lime, Oil (terpeneless)	500
2.	Orange, Sweet, Oil (terpeneless)	100
3.	Ethyl Alcohol 95%	400
		1000

LIME, SYNTHETIC NO. 3

1.	Lemon, Oil (terpeneless)	150
2.	Lime, Imitation No. 1*	175
3.	Lime, Oil (terpeneless)	175
4.	Ethyl Alcohol 95%	500
		1000

LIME, SYNTHETIC NO. 4

1.	Isoamyl Acetate	100
2.	Isoamyl Butyrate	95
3.	Lemon, Oil (10% sol'n.)	400
4.	Lime, Oil (10% sol'n.)	400
5.	Menthol	5
		1000

* Formulas which appear in this book

LIME, SYNTHETIC NO. 5

1.	Ethyl Acetate (10% sol'n.)	250
2.	Isoamyl Acetate	200
3.	Isoamyl Butyrate	145
4.	Lemon, Oil	200
5.	Lime, Oil	200
6.	Menthol	5
		1000

MALT, EXTRACT (NATURAL)

1.	Malt (slightly dried and well crushed)	10	kg
2.	Cardamom, Seeds	300	g
3.	Distilled Water	24	l

Heat at 60 C and let stand for 2 h at this temperature. Cool and add:

4.	Ethyl Alcohol 95%	5	l
5.	Distilled Water	5	l

Distill slowly. Dissolve into it:

6.	Maltol	2	kg

Filter.
Yield: 25 liters

MALT, IMITATION NO. 1

1.	Ethyl Acetate	52
2.	Ethyl Formate	25
3.	Ethyl Oenanthate	13
4.	Ginger, Oil	1
5.	Isoamyl Alcohol	2
6.	Linalool	6
7.	Orange, Sweet, Oil	3
8.	Phenyl Ethyl Acetate	1
9.	Ethyl Alcohol 95%	449
10.	Distilled Water	448
		1000

MALT, IMITATION NO. 2

1.	Ethyl Acetate (10% sol'n.)	525
2.	Ethyl Formate (10% sol'n.)	250
3.	Ethyl Oenanthate	100
4.	Ginger, Oil	10
5.	Isoamyl Alcohol	20
6.	Linalool	60
7.	Orange, Sweet, Oil	30
8.	Phenyl Ethyl Acetate	5
		1000

MANDARIN, IMITATION NO. 1

1.	Mandarin, Oil (terpeneless)	500
2.	Orange, Sweet, Oil (terpeneless)	500
		1000

MANDARIN, IMITATION NO. 2

1.	Mandarin, Oil (terpeneless)	150
2.	Mandarin, Imitation No. 1*	100
3.	Orange, Bitter, Oil (terpeneless)	75
4.	Ethyl Alcohol 95%	675
		1000

MANDARIN, IMITATION NO. 3

1.	Mandarin, Imitation No. 2*	500
2.	Orange, Sweet, Oil (terpeneless)	100
3.	Ethyl Alcohol 95%	400
		1000

MANDARIN, IMITATION NO. 4

1.	Mandarin, Imitation No. 1*	250
2.	Mandarin, Imitation No. 2*	250
3.	Mandarin, Imitation No. 3*	250
4.	Mandarin, Oil (terpeneless)	250
		1000

* Formulas which appear in this book

MANDARIN, IMITATION NO. 5

1.	Citral	40
2.	Grapefruit, Oil	20
3.	Lime, Oil	20
4.	Limonene (10% sol'n.)	500
5.	Methyl Anthranilate	20
6.	Orange, Oil	400
		1000

MANDARIN, IMITATION NO. 6

1.	Citral (10% sol'n.)	320
2.	Decyl Aldehyde	10
3.	Limonene	150
4.	Dipentene	100
5.	Linalool	150
6.	Methyl Anthranilate	50
7.	Nonyl Aldehyde	20
8.	Orange, Oil	200
		1000

MANDARIN, IMITATION NO. 7

1.	Aldehyde C-9	5
2.	Aldehyde C-10	5
3.	Citral	20
4.	Grapefruit, Oil	100
5.	Lemon, Oil	100
6.	Lime, Oil	55
7.	Limonene (10% sol'n.)	240
8.	Mandarin, Oil	400
9.	Methyl Anthranilate	20
10.	Orange, Oil	55
		1000

MANDARIN, IMITATION NO. 8

1.	Citral	20
2.	Lime, Oil	10
3.	Limonene	70
4.	Mandarin, Oil	850
5.	Orange, Oil	50
		1000

MANDARIN, IMITATION NO. 9

1.	Aldehyde C-8 (10% sol'n.)	20
2.	Aldehyde C-9	5
3.	Aldehyde C-14 (pure)	20
4.	Amyl Acetate	10
5.	Chloroform	20
6.	Citral	2
7.	Ethyl Benzoate	10
8.	Ethyl Butyrate	20
9.	Ethyl Formate	10
10.	Glycerin (neutral)	50
11.	Linalool	1
12.	Mandarin, Oil	75
13.	Methyl Anthranilate	1
14.	Neroli, Oil	1
15.	Tartaric Acid (10% sol'n.)	10
16.	Ethyl Alcohol 95%	373
17.	Distilled Water	372
		1000

MANDARIN, SYNTHETIC NO. 1

1.	Aldehyde C-9	20
2.	Aldehyde C-10	10
3.	Dipentene	250
4.	Limonene	660
5.	Linalool	10
6.	Methyl Anthranilate	40
7.	Terpineol	10
		1000

MANGO, EXTRACT (NATURAL)

1.	Mango Fruits (ripe, freshly cut, separated from the stone, and crushed)	10 kg
2.	Ethyl Alcohol 95%	10 l
3.	Distilled Water	10 l

Macerate for 3 days. Express. To the residue add:

4.	Ethyl Alcohol 95%	10 l
5.	Distilled Water	10 l

Let stand for another 3 days. Add:

6.	Cinnamon, Oil	1 ml
7.	Clove, Oil	1 ml

Distill altogether.
Yield: 40 liters

MANGO, IMITATION

1.	Aldehyde C-14 (pure)	1
2.	Pineapple (Ananas) Extract (Natural)*	249
3.	Mango, Extract (Natural)*	500
4.	Peach, Extract (Natural)*	250
		1000

MAPLE

1.	Cacao, Extract	15
2.	Coffee, Extract	15
3.	Fenugreek, Extract	120
4.	Glycerin	150
5.	Malta, Syrup	120
6.	Maple, Syrup	150
7.	Vanillin (10% sol'n.)	30
8.	Ethyl Alcohol 95%	200
9.	Distilled Water	200
		1000

MAPLE, FLAVOR

1.	Angelic, Tincture	15
2.	Coffee, Tincture	75
3.	Ethyl Oenanthate	4
4.	Fenugreek, Tincture	371
5.	Peru Balsam	28
6.	Vanillin	45
7.	Ethyl Alcohol 95%	462
		1000

MAPLE, SYRUP

1.	Maple, Flavor	300
2.	Sugar, Dark Brown	600
3.	Distilled Water	100
		1000

* Formulas which appear in this book

MARASCHINO, IMITATION NO. 1

1.	Almond, Bitter, Oil (cyanide-free)	40
2.	Cardamom, Oil	10
3.	Jasmine, Oil	1
4.	Mace, Oil	33
5.	Neroli, Oil	66
6.	Orange, Sweet, Oil	100
7.	Raspberry, Imitation No. 1*	200
8.	Rose, Oil	6
9.	Ethyl Alcohol 95%	544
		1000

MARASCHINO, IMITATION NO. 2

1.	Cardamom, Oil	5
2.	Cinnamon, Ceylon, Oil	30
3.	Clove, Oil (terpeneless)	35
4.	Mace, Oil (terpeneless)	20
5.	Maraschino, Imitation No. 1*	100
7.	Neroli, Oil	20
7.	γ-Nonyl Lactone	10
8.	Orange, Sweet, Oil (terpeneless)	150
9.	Petitgrain, Oil (terpeneless)	35
10.	Rose, Oil	1
11.	Ethyl Alcohol 95%	594
		1000

MARASCHINO, IMITATION NO. 3

1.	Almond, Oil (pure)	300
2.	Cinnamon, Oil	30
3.	Lemon, Oil	350
4.	Neroli, Oil	10
5.	Orange, Oil	300
6.	Rose, Oil	10
		1000

MARASCINO, IMITATION NO. 4

1.	Almond, Oil	350
2.	Cinnamon, Oil	30
3.	Lemon, Oil	300
4.	Neroli, Oil	10
5.	Orange, Oil	300
6.	Rose, Oil	10
		1000

MARSHMALLOW

1.	Marshmallow, Roots	300
2.	Ethyl Alcohol 95%	700

Macerate warm for 3 days. Filter and add:

3.	Malt, Extract	30
4.	Distilled Water (boiling)	30

Let cool and mix with:

5.	Ethyl Formate	235
6.	Peach, Imitation No. 1*	235
7.	Pear, Imitation No. 1*	235
8.	Pineapple, Imitation No. 1*	235

Blend altogether and distill, recovering 1800 cc.

MAYONNAISE

1.	Eggs (whole or just yolk)	200
2.	Lemon, Juice	200
3.	Oil, Edible	380
4.	Pepper	9
5.	Salt	1
6.	Sugar	200
7.	Vinegar	10
		1000

MAYONNAISE, REAL

1.	Basil, Oil	1
2.	Calcium Disodium EDTA	1
3.	Clary Sage, Oil	1
4.	Eggs (whole or just yolk)	200
5.	Garlic (dehydrated)	50
6.	Laurel Leaves, Oil	1
7.	Lemon, Juice	150
8.	Marjoram, Oil	1
9.	Onion (dehydrated)	50
10.	Oregano, Oil	1
11.	Paprika, Oil	1

* Formulas which appear in this book

12.	Parsley, Oil	1
13.	Rosemary, Oil	1
14.	Salt	1
15.	Soybeans, Oil	380
16.	Sugar	150
17.	Vinegar	10
		1000

MAYONNAISE, SPICE

1.	Celery, Oil	100
2.	Lemon, Oil	300
3.	Mustard, Oil	400
4.	Nutmeg, Oil	100
5.	Pepper, Black, Oil	100
		1000

MEAT, FLAVOR

1. Meat

Boil in water until dissolved to the maximum. Freeze to separate from the water. Dissolve in propylene glycol.

MELON, EXTRACT (NATURAL)

1.	Melon (fresh, peeled, and crushed)	100 kg

Remove the seeds with a sieve

2.	Ethyl Alcohol 95%	10 l
3.	Distilled Water	10 l

Macerate the pulp for 3 days. Add:

4.	Ethyl Butyrate	45 ml

Distill.
Yield: 20 liters

MELON, IMITATION NO. 1

1.	Apple, Essence (Natural)	150
2.	Ethyl Pelargonate	50
3.	Lemon, Oil	50
4.	Orange, Oil	50
5.	Pear, Extract (Natural)*	150
6.	Pineapple (Ananas) Extract (Natural)*	150
7.	Raspberry, Extract (Natural)*	250
8.	Ethyl Alcohol 95%	150
		1000

MELON, IMITATION NO. 2

1.	Apple, Extract (Natural)*	150
2.	Ethyl Pelargonate	50
3.	Lemon, Extract (Natural)*	50
4.	Orange, Extract (Natural)*	100
5.	Pear, Extract (Natural)*	50
6.	Pineapple (Ananas), Extract (Natural)*	150
7.	Raspberry, Extract (Natural) No. 1*	250
8.	Vanillin	35
9.	Ethyl Alcohol 95%	165
		1000

MELON, IMITATION NO. 3

1.	Apple, Imitation No. 1*	45
2.	Ethyl Pelargonate	11
3.	Lemon, Oil	12
4.	Orange, Oil	10
5.	Pear, Imitation No. 1*	37
6.	Pineapple, Imitation No. 1*	50
7.	Raspberry, Imitation No. 1*	25
8.	Vanillin	5
9.	Ethyl Alcohol 95%	805
		1000

MELON, SYNTHETIC NO. 1

1.	Citral	10
2.	Ethyl Butyrate (10% sol'n.)	300
3.	Ethyl Formate	100
4.	Ethyl Isovalerate (10% sol'n.)	400
5.	Isoamyl Butyrate	165
6.	Vanillin (10% sol'n.)	25
		1000

* Formulas which appear in this book

MELON, SYNTHETIC NO. 2

1.	Butyric Acid	15
2.	Citral	10
3.	Ethyl Acetate	150
4.	Ethyl Isovalerate	180
5.	Ethyl Pelargonate	40
6.	Isoamyl Acetate	120
7.	Isoamyl Butyrate	180
8.	Isoamyl Isovalerate (10% sol'n.)	280
9.	Vanillin (10% sol'n.)	25
		1000

MELON, SYNTHETIC NO. 3

1.	Ethyl Butyrate	200
2.	Ethyl Formate	50
3.	Ethyl Isovalerate (10% sol'n.)	250
4.	Ethyl Sebacate (10% sol'n.)	500
		1000

MELON, SYNTHETIC NO. 4

1.	Ethyl Butyrate (10% sol'n.)	300
2.	Ethyl Formate	170
3.	Ethyl Isovalerate (10% sol'n.)	300
4.	Ethyl Salicylate	10
5.	Ethyl Sebacate (10% sol'n.)	220
		1000

MELON, SYNTHETIC NO. 5

1.	Aldehyde C-14 (myristic)	10
2.	Aldehyde C-14 (pure)	20
3.	Ethyl Butyrate	40
4.	Ethyl Formate	10
5.	Ethyl Sebacate	100
6.	Ethyl Valerianate	45
7.	Glycerin (neutral)	40
8.	Ethyl Alcohol 95%	370
9.	Distilled Water	365
		1000

MELON, SYNTHETIC NO. 6

1.	Acetaldehyde	3
2.	Chloroform	10
3.	Clove, Oil	10
4.	Glycerin (neutral)	157
5.	Ethyl Acetate	10
6.	Ethyl Butyrate	90
7.	Ethyl Formate	20
8.	Ethyl Sebacate	20
9.	Ethyl Valerianate	70
10.	Ethyl Alcohol 95%	305
11.	Distilled Water	305
		1000

MELON, SYNTHETIC NO. 7

1.	Aldehyde C-14 (pure)	20
2.	Ethyl Butyrate	75
3.	Ethyl Formate	10
4.	Ethyl Sebacate	10
5.	Ethyl Valerianate	50
6.	Glycerin (neutral)	185
7.	Ethyl Alcohol 95%	325
8.	Distilled Water	325
		1000

MELON, SYNTHETIC NO. 8

1.	Butyric Acid	1
2.	Citral	1
3.	Ethyl Acetate	3
4.	Ethyl Butyrate	27
5.	Ethyl Formate	5
6.	Ethyl Isovalerianate	25
7.	Ethyl Pelargonate	1
8.	Ethyl Sebacate	15
9.	Isoamyl Acetate	3
10.	Isoamyl Butyrate	8
11.	Isoamyl Isovalerianate	7
12.	Vanillin	1
13.	Ethyl Alcohol 95%	452
14.	Distilled Water	451
		1000

MENTHA, CREAM

1.	Menthol	5
2.	Menthone	15
3.	Menthyl Acetate	15
4.	Menthyl Isovalerianate	15
5.	Ethyl Alcohol 95%	475
6.	Distilled Water	475
		1000

MILK, CARAMEL

1.	Amyl Butyrate	60
2.	Benzaldehyde (pure)	1
3.	Butyric Acid	4
4.	Cardamom, OIl	5
5.	Cinnamon, Oil	1
6.	Coriander, Oil	12
7.	Ethyl Acetate	40
8.	Ethyl Butyrate	50
9.	Geranium, Oil	8
10.	Honey (natural)	10
11.	Thymol	1
12.	Ethyl Alcohol 95%	404
13.	Distilled Water	404
		1000

MINT

1.	Eucalyptol	50
2.	Menthol	200
3.	Menthyl Acetate	150
4.	Peppermint	500
5.	Phellandrene	50
6.	Terpineol	50
		1000

MIRABELLE

1.	Benzaldehyde (pure, 10% sol'n.)	75
2.	Cinnamaldehyde	15
3.	Citral	15
4.	Decyl Acetate	5
5.	Ethyl Acetate (10% sol'n.)	290
6.	Ethyl Butyrate (10% sol'n.)	220
7.	Ethyl Formate	140
8.	Ethyl Oenanthate	175
9.	Eugenol	30
10.	Isoamyl Alcohol	15
11.	Vanillin (10% sol'n.)	20
		1000

MIRABELLE (PLUM), EXTRACT (NATURAL)

1.	Mirabelles, Yellow (separated from the stones, and well crushed)	100	kg
2.	Sugar	5	kg

Let ferment for 1 week or more until flavor and odor develop. Express the juice, and to the residue add:

3.	Ethyl Alcohol 95%	10	l
4.	Distilled Water	10	l

Let stand for another 3 days. Add:

5.	Amyl Valerate	12	ml

Distill altogether. Redistill to rectify.
Yield: 20 liters

MIRABELLE (PLUM), IMITATION

1.	Amyl Alcohol	65
2.	Benzaldehyde (pure)	5
3.	Cinnamon, Oil	60
4.	Clove, Oil	10
5.	Ethyl Acetate	90
6.	Ethyl Butyrate	150
7.	Ethyl Formate	60
8.	Ethyl Oenanthate	65
9.	Geranium, Oil	10
10.	Lemon, Oil	60
11.	Vanilla Beans, Tincture	65
12.	Ethyl Alcohol 95%	180
13.	Distilled Water	180
		1000

MIRABELLE (PLUM), SYNTHETIC

1.	Benzaldehyde (pure)	1
2.	Cinnamic Aldehyde	3
3.	Citral	2
4.	Ethyl Acetate	22
5.	Ethyl Butyrate	29
6.	Ethyl Formate	14
7.	Ethyl Oenanthate	17
8.	Eugenol	6
9.	Isoamyl Butyrate	1
10.	Linalool	3
11.	Vanillin	2
12.	Ethyl Alcohol 95%	450
13.	Distilled Water	450
		1000

MUGUET, FOR CREAM

1.	Bergamot (terpeneless)	50
2.	Cinnamic Alcohol	50
3.	Citronellol	50
4.	Coriander, Oil	30
5.	Dimethyl Benzyl Carbinol	30
6.	Jasmine, Absolute	10
7.	Linalool, Oil (10% sol'n.)	500
8.	Orange Flower, Absolute	10
9.	Rose, Absolute	20
10.	Terpineol, Extra	50
11.	Trichlorophenylmethyl Carbinyl Acetate (rose crystals)	20
12.	Vanillin (10% sol'n.)	10
13.	Ylang Ylang, Oil	170
		1000

MULBERRY, EXTRACT (NATURAL)

1.	Mulberries, Black or Red (crushed)	1 kg
2.	Sugar	2 kg

Let ferment for 1 week. Express the juice, and to the residue add:

3.	Ethyl Alcohol 95%	10 l
4.	Distilled Water	10 l

Let stand for another 3 days and add:

5.	Distilled Water	20 l
6.	Coriander, Oil	3 ml
7.	Ethyl Acetate	24 ml
8.	Fennel, Oil	5 ml

Distill altogether. Redistill to rectify.
Yield: 40 liters

MULBERRY, IMITATION

1.	Ethyl Acetate	150
2.	Ethyl Butyrate	300
3.	Mulberry, Extract (Natural)*	530
4.	Orris, Tincture	20
		1000

* Formulas which appear in this book

MULBERRY, SYNTHETIC NO. 1

1.	Benzaldehyde (pure)	2
2.	Benzyl Acetate	10
3.	Ethyl Acetate	22
4.	Ethyl Butyrate	27
5.	Ethyl Formate	13
6.	Ethyl Oenanthate	37
7.	Ethyl Pelargonate	61
8.	Isoamyl Acetate	25
9.	Ethyl Alcohol 95%	402
10.	Distilled Water	401
		1000

MULBERRY, SYNTHETIC NO. 2

1.	Benzaldehyde (pure)	1
2.	Benzyl Acetate	23
3.	Ethyl Acetate (10% sol'n.)	280
4.	Ethyl Butyrate (10% sol'n.)	550
5.	Ethyl Formate	70
6.	Ethyl Oenanthate	15
7.	Ethyl Pelargonate	5
8.	Isoamyl Acetate	56
		1000

MULBERRY, SYNTHETIC NO. 3

1.	Benzaldehyde (pure, 10% sol'n.)	4
2.	Benzyl Acetate	100
3.	Ethyl Acetate	170
4.	Ethyl Formate	200
5.	Ethyl Oenanthate	60
6.	Ethyl Pelargonate	15
7.	Isoamyl Acetate (10% sol'n.)	450
8.	Ionone	1
		1000

MUSHROOM, IMITATION NO. 1

1.	Basil, Oil	20
2.	Chamomile, Oil	20
3.	Carrot, Oil	30
4.	Celery, Oil	20
5.	Copaiba, Oil	20
6.	Cotton Seeds, Oil	750

7.	Isobutyl Phenyl Acetate	20
8.	Marjoram, Oil	20
9.	Nonyl Acetate	10
10.	Oregano, Oil	20
11.	Parsley, Oil	30
12.	Sage, Oil	20
13.	Thyme, Oil	20
		1000

MUSHROOM, IMITATION NO. 2

1.	Isobutyl Phenyl Acetate	100
2.	Nonyl Acetate	100
3.	Phenyl Propyl Aldehyde	100
4.	Ethyl Alcohol 95%	350
5.	Distilled Water	350
		1000

NECTARINE

1.	Aldehyde C-14 (pure)	2
2.	Pineapple (Ananas) Extract (Natural)*	500
3.	Lemon, Extract (Natural)*	200
4.	Vanilla Beans, Tincture	298
		1000

NOISETTE

1.	Hazelnuts (roasted and powdered)	10	kg
2.	Sugar	6	kg

Blend and totally pulverize. Add:

3.	Cocoa	200	g
4.	Ethyl Alcohol 95%	5	l
5.	Distilled Water	5	l

Note: The amount of cocoa, alcohol, and distilled water can be either reduced or increased per individual taste preference.

NOUGATINE

1.	Almonds or Peanuts	3	kg
2.	Hazelnuts (chopped)	3	kg
3.	Sugar (melted)	10	kg

Melt the sugar together with other ingredients.

NUTMEG, IMITATION NO. 1

1.	Camphene, Oil	80
2.	Limonene	20
3.	Nutmeg, Oil	640
4.	Pinene	240
5.	Terpineol	20
		1000

NUTMEG, IMITATION NO. 2

1.	Camphene (10% sol'n.)	250
2.	Guaiacwood	50
3.	Limonene (10% sol'n.)	350
4.	Pinene (10% sol'n.)	250
5.	Terpineol	100
		1000

NUTMEG, IMITATION NO. 3

1.	Isoeugenol	50
2.	Nutmeg, Imitation No. 1*	700
3.	Nutmeg, Imitation No. 2*	250
		1000

NUTMEG, IMITATION NO. 4

1.	Camphene (10% sol'n.)	270
2.	Guaiacwood	50
3.	Limonene	100
4.	Pinene (10% sol'n.)	300
5.	Terpineol (10% sol'n.)	280
		1000

NUTMEG, IMITATION NO. 5

1.	Nutmeg, Imitation No. 3*	375
2.	Nutmeg, Imitation No. 4*	375
3.	Nutmeg, Oil	250
		1000

* Formulas which appear in this book

NUTS, FLAVOR FOR PASTRY

1.	Noisette*	200
2.	Vanilla Beans, Tincture	200
3.	Ethyl Alcohol 95%	350
4.	Distilled Water	250
		1000

NUTS, KERNELS (GENERAL METHOD OF FLAVOR EXTRACTION)

(Kernels of fresh nuts of any type such as hazel, walnut, peanuts, macadamia, pistachio, etc., not rancid, well rasped or crushed, almost pulverized)

1.	Nuts	10 kg
2.	Ethyl Alcohol 95%	15 l
3.	Distilled Water	15 l

Macerate for 10 days, stirring for 1 h each day. Collect, without any pressure, 20 l of extract. To the residue add:

4.	Amyl Formate	45 ml
5.	Ethyl Oenanthate	25 ml
6.	Distilled Water	20 l

Distill altogether.
Yield: 40 liters

ONION

1.	Asafetida (10% sol'n. in water)	100
2.	Ethyl Alcohol 95%	900
		1000

Note: This may be modified with traces of allyl sulfide.** If it is cloudy, filter with magnesium carbonate.

ONION, EXTRACT (NATURAL)

(Onions, well peeled and finely cut with its juice totally discarded since it has no value. For every kilogram of residue, add 2 l of ethyl alcohol 95%.)

1.	Onions, Residue	10 kg
2.	Ethyl Alcohol 95%	20 l

Let stand for 3 days. Express. To the residue add:

3.	Ethyl Alcohol 95%	10 l
4.	Distilled Water	10 l

Let stand for another 3 days. Add:

5.	Mustard Oil (1 ml for every kilogram of juice)	40 ml

Put all juices together and filter.
Yield: 40 liters

ONION, IMITATION

1.	Allyl Sulfide**	1 drop
2.	Asafetida	253
3.	Ethyl Alcohol 95%	493
4.	Distilled Water	253

Filter with magnesium carbonate.
Note: Mixed with water it makes a milky emulsion.

ORANGE, EXTRACT (NATURAL)

1.	Orange, Peels (fresh)	10 kg
2.	Ethyl Alcohol 95%	20 l

Macerate for 3 days. Express 20 l of extract. To the residue add:

3.	Distilled Water	20 l

Let stand for another 3 days. Distill to separate the terpenes. Distill the extract altogether and add:

FOR ORANGE BITTER TYPE:

1.	Petitgrain, Oil	500 ml
2.	Orange, Bitter, Oil	500 ml

Distill. Filter.

* Formulas which appear in this book

** Highly toxic by ingestion and inhalation; irritant of the eyes and skin

FOR SWEET ORANGE TYPE:

1.	Cinnamon, Oil	60 ml
2.	Orange, Sweet, Oil	10 1

Distill. Filter.
Yield: 50 liters

ORANGE, IMITATION NO. 1

1.	Capraldehyde	10
2.	Ethyl Acetate	30
3.	Ethyl Benzoate	30
4.	Ethyl Butyrate	100
5.	Ethyl Formate	30
6.	Isoamyl Acetate	160
7.	Isoamyl Butyrate	150
8.	Lemon, Oil	200
9.	Linalool	10
10.	Orange, Oil	260
11.	Pimenta, Oil	10
12.	Tartaric Acid	10
		1000

Note: 25 cc is sufficient for 100 1 of orange liquor.

ORANGE, IMITATION NO. 2

1.	Aldehyde C-8	30
2.	Aldehyde C-14 (pure)	29
3.	Amyl Acetate	10
4.	Chloroform (pure)	20
5.	Ethyl Formate	10
6.	Glycerin (neutral)	50
7.	Linalool	13
8.	Methyl Anthranilate	25
9.	Neroli, Oil	2
10.	Orange, Oil	50
11.	Tartaric Acid	1
12.	Ethyl Alcohol 95%	380
13.	Distilled Water	380
		1000

Note: 25 cc is sufficient for 100 1 of orange liquor.

ORANGE, IMITATION NO. 3

1.	Citral	350
2.	Decyl Aldehyde (10%)	10
3.	D-Limonene	250
4.	Linalool (Ex Bois De Rose)	150
5.	Nonyl Alcohol (10%)	20
6.	Orange, Sweet	100
7.	Terpineol, Extra	120
		1000

Note: 25 cc is sufficient for 100 1 of orange liquor.

ORANGE, IMITATION NO. 4

1.	Ethyl Butyrate	15
2.	Mandarin, Oil (terpeneless)	20
3.	Orange, Bitter, Oil (terpeneless)	300
4.	Orange, Sweet, Oil (terpeneless)	300
5.	Ethyl Alcohol 95%	365
		1000

Note: 25 cc is sufficient for 100 1 of orange liquor.

ORANGE, IMITATION NO. 5

1.	Lemon, Oil (terpeneless)	15
2.	Mandarin, Oil (terpeneless)	12
3.	Orange, Imitation No. 1*	473
4.	Ethyl Alcohol 95%	500
		1000

Note: 25 cc is sufficient for 100 1 of orange liquor.

ORANGE, IMITATION NO. 6

1.	Lemon, Oil (terpeneless)	75
2.	Orange, Imitation No. 2*	250
3.	Orange, Sweet, Oil (terpeneless)	225
4.	Ethyl Alcohol 95%	450
		1000

Note: 25 cc is sufficient for 100 1 of orange liquor.

* Formulas which appear in this book

ORANGE, IMITATION NO. 7

1.	Lemon, Oil (terpeneless)	25
2.	Lemon, Imitation No. 1*	25
3.	Orange, Bitter, Oil (terpeneless)	50
4.	Orange, Imitation No. 3*	175
5.	Orange, Sweet, Oil (terpeneless)	125
6.	Ethyl Alcohol 95%	600
		1000

Note: 25 cc is sufficient for 100 l of orange liquor.

ORANGE, IMITATION NO. 8

1.	Mandarin, Oil	10
2.	Orange, Sweet, Oil (terpeneless)	240
3.	Orange, Imitation No. 4*	250
4.	Ethyl Alcohol 95%	500
		1000

ORANGE, IMITATION NO. 9

1.	Capraldehyde	25
2.	Ethyl Acetate	110
3.	Isoamyl Acetate (10% sol'n.)	420
4.	Isoamyl Butyrate (10% sol'n.)	420
5.	Orange, Oil	25
		1000

ORANGE, IMITATION NO. 10

1.	Ethyl Acetate	60
2.	Isoamyl Acetate	120
3.	Isoamyl Butyrate (10% sol'n.)	350
4.	Lemon, Oil	120
5.	Orange, Oil (10% sol'n.)	350
		1000

ORANGE, IMITATION NO. 11

1.	Ethyl Acetate (10% sol'n.)	250
2.	Ethyl Benzoate	50
3.	Ethyl Butyrate	50
4.	Ethyl Formate	50
5.	Isoamyl Acetate	50
6.	Orange, Oil (10% sol'n.)	500
7.	Tartaric Acid (10% sol'n.)	50
		1000

* Formulas which appear in this book

ORANGE, IMITATION NO. 12

1.	Ethyl Acetate	45
2.	Isoamyl Acetate	120
3.	Isoamyl Butyrate (10% sol'n.)	310
4.	Linalool	60
5.	Orange, Oil (10% sol'n.)	460
6.	Pimenta, Oil	5
		1000

ORANGE, IMITATION NO. 13

1.	Orange, Bitter, Oil (terpeneless)	250
2.	Orange, Imitation No. 5*	250
3.	Ethyl Alcohol 95%	500
		1000

ORANGE, IMITATION NO. 14

1.	Mandarin, Oil	75
2.	Lemon, Oil	75
3.	Orange, Imitation No. 6*	250
4.	Ethyl Alcohol 95%	600
		1000

ORANGE, SYNTHETIC NO. 1

1.	Alcohol C-8	30
2.	Aldehyde C-8	20
3.	Aldehyde C-10	20
4.	Aldehyde C-12, MNA	50
5.	Amyl Acetate	150
6.	Citral	5
7.	Cuminic Aldhyde	25
8.	Ethyl Acetate	10
9.	Ethyl Butyrate	85
10.	Ethyl Formate	20
11.	Isobutyl Anthranilate	25
12.	Linalyl Acetate	50
13.	Rhodinyl Acetate	150
14.	Ethyl Alcohol 95%	180
15.	Distilled Water	180
		1000

ORANGE, SYNTHETIC NO. 2

1.	Acetaldehyde	2
2.	Amyl Acetate	70
3.	Chloroform	20
4.	Citric Acid	10
5.	Ethyl Acetate	20
6.	Ethyl Benzoate	20
7.	Ethyl Butyrate	150
8	Ethyl Formate	20
9.	Ethyl Oenanthate	40
10.	Glycerin (neutral)	200
11.	Tartaric Acid	10
12.	Vanillin	10
13.	Ethyl Alcohol 95%	214
14.	Distilled Water	214
		1000

ORANGE, SYNTHETIC NO. 3

1.	Capraldehyde	20
2.	Ethyl Acetate (10% sol'n.)	500
3.	Ethyl Benzoate	100
4.	Ethyl Butyrate	100
5.	Ethyl Formate	100
6.	Isoamyl Acetate	100
7.	Tartaric Acid (10% sol'n.)	80
		1000

ORANGE, SYNTHETIC NO. 4

1.	Amyl Butyrate	100
2.	Ethyl Acetate	50
3.	Ethyl Aldehyde	20
4.	Ethyl Benzoate	100
5.	Ethyl Butyrate	100
6.	Ethyl Formate	100
7.	Ethyl Salicylate (10% sol'n.)	10
8.	Ethyl Alcohol 95%	520
		1000

OREGANO, TYPE

1.	Bergamot	40
2.	Ethyl Vanillin (10% sol'n.)	120
3.	Jasmine, Absolute (10% sol'n.)	240
4.	Heliotropin (10% sol'n.)	300
5.	Mandarin, Oil	60
6.	Orange, Sweet, Oil	150
7.	Tonka, Resinoid	60
8.	Verbena, Oil	30
		1000

PEACH, EXTRACT (NATURAL)

1.	Peaches (dried, without stones, well crushed)	10 kg
2.	Ethyl Alcohol 95%	10 l
3.	Distilled Water	10 l

Macerate for 3 days. Express all the juice. To the residue add:

4.	Distilled Water	20 l

Let stand for another 3 days. Add:

5.	Amyl Valerate	5 ml
6.	Ethyl Valerate	3 ml

Distill altogether.
Yield: 40 liters

PEACH, IMITATION NO. 1

1.	Peaches (crushed or sliced, with kernels broken)	1000
2.	Ethyl Alcohol 95%	500
3.	Distilled Water	486

Distill and add:

4.	Amyl Valerate	7
5.	Ethyl Valerate	5
6.	Phenyl Ethyl Acetate	1
7.	γ-Undecalactone	1
		2000

Redistill over 1250 cc.

PEACH, IMITATION NO. 2

1.	Peach, Fruit Pulp	500
2.	Ethyl Alcohol 95%	250
3.	Distilled Water	250
		1000

PEACH, IMITATION NO. 3

1.	Acetaldehyde	30
2.	Almond, Oil (pure)	50
3.	Amyl Acetate	120
4.	Amyl Butyrate	100
5.	Anisaldehyde	20
6.	Cardamom, Oil	10
7.	Ethyl Acetate	150
8.	Ethyl Butyrate	50
9.	Ethyl Valerate	20
10.	Eugenol	10
11.	Lemon, Oil	50
12.	Nerol, Oil	10
13.	Orange, Oil	20
14.	γ-Undelactone	10
15.	Vanillin (10% sol'n.)	40
16.	Ethyl Alcohol 95%	310
		1000

Macerate for 3 days. Distill over 1800 cc.

PEACH, IMITATION NO. 4

1.	Amyl Acetate (10% sol'n.)	225
2.	Amyl Butyrate	24
3.	Benzaldehyde (pure, 10% sol'n.)	14
4.	Cardamom, Oil	6
5.	Ethyl Acetate (10% sol'n.)	225
6.	Ethyl Butyrate	115
7.	Isoamyl Butyrolactone	25
8.	Lemon, Oil	24
9.	Orange, Sweet, Oil	12
10.	Peach, Kernel Extract	100
11.	Petitgrain, Oil	3
12.	Pimento, Oil	3
13.	γ-Undecalactone	3
14.	Vanillin	10
15.	Ethyl Alcohol 95%	211
		1000

Add Peach Imitation No. 1* and distill over 1800 cc.

PEACH, IMITATION NO. 5

1.	Almond, Bitter, Oil (cyanide-free)	6
2.	Ethyl Methylphenylglycidate	10
3.	Ethyl Pelargonate	25
4.	γ-Nonyl Lactone	10
5.	Peach, Imitation No. 1*	722
6.	γ-Undecalactone	2
7.	Ethyl Alcohol 95%	225
		1000

PEACH, IMITATION NO. 6

1.	Apricot, Imitation No. 1*	500
2.	Peach, Imitation No. 2*	500
3.	Ethyl Alcohol 95%	500
4.	Distilled Water	500
		2000

Distill over 1800 cc.

PEACH, IMITATION NO. 7

1.	Acetaldehyde	1
2.	Aldehyde C-14 (pure)	1
3.	Almond, Oil	15
4.	Amyl Acetate	12
5.	Amyl Butyrate	10
6.	Anisaldehyde	5
7.	Cardamom, Oil	1
8.	Ethyl Acetate	15
9.	Ethyl Butyrate	15
10.	Ethyl Valerianate	2
11.	Eugenol	1
12.	Lemon, Oil	5
13.	Neroli, Oil	1
14.	Orange, Sweet, Oil	2
15.	Vanillin	4
16.	Ethyl Alcohol 95%	455
17.	Distilled Water	455
		1000

PEACH, IMITATION NO. 8

1.	Aldehyde C-14 (10% sol'n.)	50
2.	Amyl Acetate	130
3.	Amyl Butyrate	10
4.	Amyl Valerate	15
5.	Benzaldehyde (pure, 10% sol'n.)	8
6.	Ethyl Butyrate	15
7.	Ethyl Cinnamate	20
8.	Ethyl Oenanthate	10
9.	Ethyl Vanillin (10% sol'n.)	22

* Formulas which appear in this book

10.	Orange, Sweet, Oil	100
11.	Phenyl Acetic Acide	20
12.	Wine, Residue (green)	10
13.	Ethyl Alcohol 95%	590
		1000

PEACH, IMITATION NO. 9

1.	Almond, Bitter, Oil (cyanide-free)	5
2.	Amyl Acetate	80
3.	Amyl Butyrate	10
4.	Cardamom, Oil	6
5.	Ethyl Acetate	25
6.	Ethyl Butyrate	25
7.	Lemon, Oil	10
8.	Methyl Heptyne Carbonate	10
9.	Methyl Phenyl Acetate	25
10.	Methyl Pelargonate	25
11.	Orange, Sweet, Oil	6
12.	Peach, Imitation No. 1*	100
13.	Peach, Imitation No. 2*	100
14.	Peach, Imitation No. 3*	100
15.	Peach, Imitation No. 4*	100
16.	Peach, Imitation No. 5*	100
17.	Peach, Imitation No. 6*	100
18.	Petitgrain, Oil	4
19.	Phenyl Ethyl Acetate	50
20.	Pimenta, Oil	4
21.	Raspberry, Imitation No. 1*	100
22.	γ-Undelactone	10
23.	Vanillin	5
		1000

PEACH, IMITATION NO. 10

1.	Aldehyde C-14 (10% sol'n.)	100
2.	Apple	30
3.	Cherry	20
4.	Orange, Oil (10% sol'n.)	100
5.	Pine, Siberian, Oil (10% sol'n.)	50
6.	Ethyl Alcohol 95%	350
7.	Distilled Water	350
		1000

PEACH, IMITATION NO. 11

1.	Almond, Bitter, Oil (cyanide-free)	10
2.	Amyl Butyrate	100
3.	Amyl Valerianate	100
4.	Ethyl Formate	25
5.	Peach, Imitation No. 7*	762
6.	γ-Undecalactone	3
		1000

PEACH, IMITATION NO. 12

1.	Benzaldehyde (pure, 10% sol'n.)	40
2.	Ethyl Butyrate	200
3.	Ethyl Isovalerate	140
4.	Isoamyl Acetate (10% sol'n.)	280
5.	Isoamyl Alcohol	20
6.	Isoamyl Butyrate	70
7.	Lemon, Oil	70
8.	Linalool	70
9.	Orange, Sweet, Oil	70
10.	Pimenta, Oil	20
11.	Vanillin (10% sol'n.)	20
		1000

PEACH, SYNTHETIC NO. 1

1.	Aldehyde C-14 (pure)	35
2.	Benzaldehyde (pure)	10
3.	Benzyl Butyrate	140
4.	Ethyl Acetate	25
5.	Ethyl Cinnamate	140
6.	Ethyl Isobutyrate	25
7.	Ethyl Isovalerianate	20
8.	Geranyl Formate	10
9.	Isoamyl Acetate	15
10.	Isoamyl Butyrate	70
11.	Isoamyl Salicylate	10
12.	Vanillin	10
13.	Ethyl Alcohol 95%	245
14.	Distilled Water	245
		1000

PEACH, SYNTHETIC NO. 2

1.	Aldehyde C-14 (pure)	20
2.	Ethyl Acetate	50
3.	Ethyl Butyrate	50

* Formulas which appear in this book

4.	Ethyl Formate	50
5.	Ethyl Oenanthate	50
6.	Ethyl Salicylate	20
7.	Ethyl Valerianate	50
8.	Glycerin (neutral)	50
9.	Sebacic Acid	1
10.	Ethyl Alcohol 95%	330
11.	Distilled Water	329
		1000

PEACH, SYNTHETIC NO. 3

1.	Aldehyde C-14 (pure, 10% sol'n.)	840
2.	Benzaldehyde (pure)	10
3.	Ethyl Isobutyrate	30
4.	Ethyl Isovalerianate	20
5.	Isoamyl Acetate	10
6.	Vanillin	90
		1000

PEACH, SYNTHETIC NO. 4

1.	Aldehyde C-14	70
2.	Amyl Acetate	45
3.	Amyl Butyrate	250
4.	Amyl Isovalerianate	230
5.	Benzaldehyde (pure)	27
6.	Ethyl Acetate	120
7.	Ethyl Butyrate	90
8.	Ethyl Formate	70
9.	Ethyl Oenanthate	50
10.	Ethyl Salicylate	20
11.	Ethyl Sebacate	20
12.	Vanillin	8
		1000

PEACH, SYNTHETIC NO. 5

1.	Acetaldehyde	4
2.	Amyl Valerianate	10
3.	Ethyl Acetate	10
4.	Ethyl Butyrate	10
5.	Ethyl Formate	10
6.	Ethyl Alcohol 95%	478
7.	Distilled Water	478
		1000

PEACH, SYNTHETIC NO. 6

1.	Ethyl Acetate	140
2.	Ethyl Butyrate (10% sol'n.)	600
3.	Ethyl Cinnamate	140
4.	Geranyl Formate	10
5.	Isoamyl Butyrate	70
6.	Isobutyl Salicylate	20
7.	γ-Undecalactone (10% sol'n.)	20
		1000

PEACH, SYNTHETIC NO. 7

1.	Benzaldehyde (pure, 10% sol'n.)	40
2.	Ethyl Acetate	100
3.	Isoamyl Butyrate (10% sol'n.)	430
4.	Isoamyl Isovalerate (10% sol'n.)	430
		1000

PEACH, SYNTHETIC NO. 8

1.	Benzaldehyde (pure, 10% sol'n.)	40
2.	Ethyl Acetate	190
3.	Isoamyl Butyrate (10% sol'n.)	385
4.	Isoamyl Isovalerate (10% sol'n.)	385
		1000

PEACH, SYNTHETIC NO. 9

1.	Benzaldehyde (pure, 10% sol'n.)	20
2.	Ethyl Acetate (10% sol'n.)	360
3.	Ethyl Butyrate	125
4.	Geranyl Formate	10
5.	Isoamyl Acetate (10% sol'n.)	360
6.	Isoamyl Butyrate	30
7.	Lemon, Oil	30
8.	Linalool	5
9.	Orange, Sweet, Oil	15
10.	Pimenta, Oil	5
11.	γ-Undecalactone (10% sol'n.)	25
12.	Vanillin (10% sol'n.)	15
		1000

PEACH, SYNTHETIC NO. 10

1.	Aldehyde C-14 (pure)	100
2.	Jasmine, Oil	1
3.	Phenyl Ethyl Acetate	4

4.	Ethyl Alcohol 95%	448
5.	Distilled Water	447
		1000

PEACH, SYNTHETIC NO. 11

1.	Benzaldehyde (pure, 10% sol'n.)	30
2.	Ethyl Acetate	50
3.	Ethyl Oenanthate	50
4.	Ethyl Sebacate	125
5.	Isoamyl Butyrate (10% sol'n.)	350
6.	Isoamyl Isovalerate (10% sol'n.)	350
7.	Vanillin (10% sol'n.)	45
		1000

PEACH, SYNTHETIC NO. 12

1.	Ethyl Acetate	150
2.	Ethyl Butyrate (10% sol'n.)	270
3.	Ethyl Isobutyrate	180
4.	Ionone	1
5.	Methyl Heptyne Carbonate	140
6.	Methyl Phenyl Acetate	180
7.	γ-Nonyl Lactone	9
8.	γ-Undecalactone (10% sol'n.)	45
9.	Vanillin (10% sol'n.)	25
		1000

PEAR, EXTRACT (NATURAL)

1.	Pears (sliced and well crushed)	10 kg
2.	Ethyl Alcohol 95%	10 l
3.	Distilled Water	10 l

Macerate for 3 days. Express, and to the residue add:

4.	Distilled Water	20 l

Let stand for another 3 days, and add:

5.	Amyl Acetate	25 ml
6.	Amyl Valerate	5 ml
7.	Bergamot, Oil	5 ml
8.	Coriander, Oil	5 ml

Distill altogether.
Yield: 40 liters

PEAR, IMITATION NO. 1

1.	Pears (crushed or sliced)	500
2.	Ethyl Alcohol 95%	250
3.	Distilled Water	250
		1000

Macerate for 8 days and distill over 800 cc.

PEAR, IMITATION NO. 2

1.	Pears (crushed or sliced)	500
2.	Amyl Acetate	90
3.	Coriander, Oil	4
4.	Ethyl Acetate	7
5.	Ethyl Butyrate	14
6.	Ethyl Nitrate	14
7.	Ginger, Oil	3
8.	Vanillin	5
9.	Ethyl Alcohol 95%	182
10.	Distilled Water	181
		1000

Macerate for 3 days and distill over 800 cc.

PEAR, IMITATION NO. 3

1.	Amyl Acetate	440
2.	Amyl Butyrate	50
3.	Bergamot, Oil	50
4.	Clary Sage, Oil	20
5.	Cognac, Oil	10
6.	Ethyl Acetate	120
7.	Eugenol	10
8.	Geranyl Butyrate	20
9.	Isobutyl Acetate	100
10.	Lemon, Oil	50
11.	Orange, Oil	100
12.	Petitgrain, Oil	10
13.	Vanillin	20
		1000

PEAR, IMITATION NO. 4

1.	Amyl Acetate	150
2.	Amyl Valerate	100

3.	Ethyl Acetate	5
4.	Ethyl Butyrate	150
5.	Ethyl Nitrate	50
6.	Ethyl Valerate	10
7.	Eugenol	3
8.	Ginger, Oil (terpeneless)	3
9.	Lemon, Oil (terpeneless)	3
10.	Petitgrain, Oil	5
11.	Vanillin (10% sol'n.)	10
12.	Ethyl Alcohol 95%	511
		1000

PEAR, IMITATION NO. 5

1.	Amyl Acetate	150
2.	Amyl Butyrate	50
3.	Bergamot, Oil	50
4.	Clary Sage, Oil	20
5.	Cognac, Oil	5
6.	Eugenol	5
7.	Geranyl Butyrate	7
8.	Isobutyl Acetate	100
9.	Lemon, Oil	3
10.	Orange, Oil	10
11.	Petitgrain, Oil	10
12.	Vanillin (10% sol'n.)	20
13.	Ethyl Alcohol 95%	570
		1000

PEAR, IMITATION NO. 6

1.	Ethyl Acetate	210
2.	Eugenol	1
3.	Isoamyl Acetate (10% sol'n.)	700
4.	Linalool	9
5.	Linalyl Acetate	20
6.	Orange, Oil	50
7.	Vanillin (10% sol'n.)	10
		1000

PEAR, IMITATION NO. 7

1.	Ethyl Acetate	160
2.	Eugenol	5
3.	Isoamyl Acetate (10% sol'n.)	600
4.	Linalool	15
5.	Linalyl Acetate	70
6.	Orange, Oil	120
7.	Vanillin (10% sol'n.)	30
		1000

PEAR, IMITATION NO. 8

1.	Amyl Acetate	50
2.	Ethyl Acetate	50
3.	Ethyl Butyrate	50
4.	Ethyl Nitrate	50
5.	Ginger, Oil	5
6.	Vanillin	5
7.	Ethyl Alcohol 95%	790
		1000

PEAR, IMITATION NO. 9

1.	Amyl Acetate (10% sol'n.)	315
2.	Ethyl Acetate	75
3.	Ethyl Butyrate	125
4.	Ethyl Nitrate	50
5.	Ginger, Oil	5
6.	Vanillin	5
7.	Ethyl Alcohol 95%	425
		1000

PEAR, IMITATION NO. 10

1.	Amyl Valerianate	100
2.	Bergamot, Oil	10
3.	Ethyl Valerianate	150
4.	Isobutyl Valerianate	150
5.	Pear, Imitation No. 1*	295
6.	Ethyl Alcohol 95%	295
		1000

PEAR, SYNTHETIC NO. 1

1.	Ethyl Acetate	50
2.	Glycerin (neutral)	190
3.	Sebacic Acid (10% sol'n.)	10
4.	Ethyl Alcohol 95%	375
5.	Distilled Water	375
		1000

* Formulas which appear in this book

PEAR, SYNTHETIC NO. 2

1.	Amyl Acetate	300
2.	Ethyl Nitrate	150
3.	Glycerin (neutral)	300
4.	Ethyl Alcohol 95%	250
		1000

PEAR, SYNTHETIC NO. 3

1.	Amyl Acetate	330
2.	Ethyl Acetate	166
3.	Ethyl Nitrate	166
4.	Ethyl Alcohol 95%	338
		1000

PEAR, SYNTHETIC NO. 4

1.	Amyl Acetate	100
2.	Ethyl Acetate	50
3.	Ethyl Nitrate	50
4.	Glycerin (neutral)	100
5.	Ethyl Alcohol 95%	350
6.	Distilled Water	350
		1000

PEAR, SYNTHETIC NO. 5

1.	Amyl Acetate	310
2.	Amyl Butyrate	10
3.	Ethyl Acetate	160
4.	Glycerin (neutral)	110
5.	Vanillin (10% sol'n.)	10
6.	Ethyl Alcohol 95%	200
7.	Distilled Water	200
		1000

PEAR, SYNTHETIC NO. 6

1.	Amyl Acetate	150
2.	Ethyl Acetate	50
3.	Ethyl Cinnamate	120
4.	Ethyl Nitrate	150
5.	Glycerin (neutral)	350
6.	Isoamyl Butyrate	20
7.	Isoamyl Pelargonate	150
8.	Sebacic Acid (10% sol'n.)	10
		1000

PEAR, SYNTHETIC NO. 7

1.	Ethyl Acetate	160
2.	Ethyl Butyrate	160
3.	Ethyl Isovalerate	100
4.	Ginger, Oil	5
5.	Isoamyl Acetate (10% sol'n.)	500
6.	Isobutyl Isovalerate	60
7.	Linalyl Acetate	5
8.	Vanillin (10% sol'n.)	10
		1000

PEAR, SYNTHETIC NO. 8

1.	Benzoic Acid (1% in ethyl alcohol 95%)	50
2.	Ethyl Acetate (10% sol'n.)	250
3.	Ethyl Benzoate (10% sol'n.)	250
4.	Ethyl Pelargonate	50
5.	Ethyl Alcohol 95%	400
		1000

PEAR, SYNTHETIC NO. 9

1.	Ethyl Acetate (10% sol'n.)	450
2.	Isoamyl Acetate (10% sol'n.)	450
3.	Isoamyl Butyrate	100
		1000

PEAR, SYNTHETIC NO. 10

1.	Ethyl Acetate (10% sol'n.)	300
2.	Isoamyl Acetate (10% sol'n.)	700
		1000

PEAR, SYNTHETIC NO. 11

1.	Ethyl Acetate	140
2.	Ethyl Butyrate (10% sol'n.)	240
3.	Isoamyl Acetate (10% sol'n.)	600
4.	Ginger, Oil	10
5.	Vanillin (10% sol'n.)	10
		1000

PEAR, SYNTHETIC NO. 12

1.	Butyl Acetate	120
2.	Ethyl Cinnamate (10% sol'n.)	525
3.	Geraniol	55
4.	Geranyl Butyrate (10% sol'n.)	220
5.	Isoamyl Formate	55
6.	Propyl Propionate	25
		1000

PEAR, SYNTHETIC NO. 13

1.	Ethyl Acetate	200
2.	Isoamyl Acetate (10% sol'n.)	800
		1000

PEAR, SYNTHETIC NO. 14

1.	Butyl Acetate	13
2.	Ethyl Acetate	17
3.	Ethyl Butyrate	44
4.	Ethyl Cinnamate	58
5.	Ethyl Isovalerianate	11
6.	Eugenol	1
7.	Geraniol	6
8.	Geranyl Butyrate	24
9.	Ginger, Oil	2
10.	Isoamyl Acetate	59
11.	Isoamyl Butyrate	11
12.	Isoamyl Formate	5
13.	Isoamyl Isovalerianate	6
14.	Isobutyl Isovalerianate	6
15.	Linalool	2
16.	Linalyl Acetate	10
17.	Orange, Oil	18
18.	Propyl Propionate	2
19.	Vanillin	6
20.	Ethyl Alcohol 95%	350
21.	Distilled Water	349
		1000

PEA, SWEET, IMITATION NO. 1

1.	Anisic Aldehyde	100
2.	Bergamot, Oil	230
3.	Ethyl Phenyl Acetate	100
4.	Isobutyl Benzoate	100
5.	Musk Ambrette	20
6.	Petitgrain, Oil	100
7.	Phenylacetic Aldehyde	50
8.	Terpineol	300
		1000

PEA, SWEET, IMITATION NO. 2

1.	Benzylidene Acetone	180
2.	Ethyl Phthalate (10% sol'n.)	100
3.	Methyl Heptyne Carbonate	10
4.	Pea, Sweet, Imitation No. 1*	710
		1000

PEA, SWEET, IMITATION NO. 3

1.	Pea, Sweet, Imitation No. 1*	500
2.	Pea, Sweet, Imitation No. 2*	500
		1000

PEA, SWEET, SYNTHETIC NO. 1

1.	Alcohol C-10	2
2.	Aldehyde C-9	4
3.	Aldehyde C-10	2
4.	Bergamot, Oil	180
5.	Cinnamic Alcohol	80
6.	Heliotropin	60
7.	Hydroxycitronellal	60
8.	Ionone	45
9.	Jasmine, Absolute	10
10.	Linalool	120
11.	Methyl Anthranilate	60
12.	Musk Ambrette	40
13.	Neroli, Oil	20
14.	Phenyl Ethyl Alcohol	120
15.	Rhodinol	60
16.	Rose, Oil	60
17.	Terpineol	65
18.	Vanillin	2
19.	Ylang Ylang, Oil	10
		1000

* Formulas which appear in this book

PEA, SWEET, SYNTHETIC NO. 2

1. Benzophenone 75
2. Benzylidene Acetone 200
3. Heliotropin 115
4. Isobutyl Phenyl Acetate 115
5. Musk Ambrette 85
6. Petitgrain, Oil 85
7. Phenyl Acetaldehyde 75
8. Rose, Absolute 80
9. Terpineol 85
10. Violet Leaves, Absolute 85

1000

PEPPERMINT, IMITATION NO. 1

1. Camphor, Oil 130
2. Menthol 700
3. Mint, Sweet (10% sol'n.) 150
4. Terpinyl Acetate 20

1000

PEPPERMINT, IMITATION NO. 2

1. Camphor, Oil 200
2. Menthol 100
3. Peppermint, Imitation No. 1* 700

1000

PEPPERMINT, IMITATION NO. 3

1. Camphor, Oil 100
2. Eucalyptol 80
3. Menthol (10% sol'n.) 370
4. Menthone (10% sol'n.) 250
5. Menthyl Acetate 80
6. Phellandrene 120

1000

* Formulas which appear in this book

PEPPERMINT, IMITATION NO. 4

1. Anethole 10
2. Lemon, Oil 5
3. Peppermint, Oil (10% sol'n.) 485
4. Peppermint, Imitation No. 1* 125
5. Peppermint, Imitation No. 2* 125
6. Peppermint, Imitation No. 3* 125
7. Peppermint, Oil 125

1000

PEPPERMINT, IMITATION NO. 5

1. Anethole 20
2. Lemon, Oil 10
3. Menthol 250
4. Menthone 175
5. Menthyl Acetate 60
6. Menthyl Isovalerianate 15
7. Peppermint, Oil 270
8. Ethyl Alcohol 95% 200

1000

PEPPERMINT, IMITATION NO. 6

1. Menthol (10% sol'n.) 300
2. Menthone 200
3. Menthyl Acetate 50
4. Peppermint 50
5. Ethyl Alcohol 95% 400

1000

"PERSICOT," (PEACH KERNEL IMITATION)

1. Aldehyde C-16 15
2. Benzaldehyde (pure) 15
3. Laurel Leaves, Oil (pure) 1
4. Parsely, Oil 10
5. Ethyl Alcohol 95% 480
6. Distilled Water 479

1000

PICKLE SPICE SALTS

1.	Capsicum, Oil	140
2.	Celery, Oil	88
3.	Dill, Oil	88
4.	Mustard, Oil	44
5.	Pepper, Oil	70
6.	Pimenta, Oil	39
7.	Table Salt (refined sodium chloride)	45
8.	Tarragon, Oil	26
9.	Ethyl Alcohol 95%	230
10.	Distilled Water	230
		1000

PINEAPPLE (ANANAS) EXTRACT (NATURAL) NO. 1

PEELED PINEAPPLE:

1.	Pineapple (Ananas) (fresh, peeled, and ground)	10 kg
2.	Ethyl Alcohol 95%	10 1

Let macerate for 3 days. Express, and to the residue add:

3.	Ethyl Alcohol 95%	10 1

Let stand for another 3 days. Add:

4.	Vanillin	15 g

Distill.
Yield: 20 liters

PINEAPPLE PEELS:

1.	Pineapple Peels (well ground)	10 kg
2.	Ethyl Alcohol 95%	10 1

Let stand for three days. Express, and to the residue add:

3.	Ethyl Alcohol 95%	10 1

Let stand for another three days. Add:

4.	Amyl Butyrate	12 ml

Distill.
Yield: 20 liters

Put together the two distillates (from the peeled pineapple and the peels of pineapple). Redistill.

Yield: 40 liters

PINEAPPLE, (ANANAS) EXTRACT (NATURAL) NO. 2

1.	Pineapple (grated)	500
2.	Ethyl Alcohol 95%	250
3.	Distilled Water	250
		1000

Macerate for 5 days. Distill over 800 cc. Add:

4.	Pineapple (grated)	500
5.	Ethyl Butyrate	3

Macerate for 5 days. Distill over 1200 cc.

PINEAPPLE (ANANAS), IMITATION NO. 1

1.	Acetaldehyde	1
2.	Amyl Acetate	16
3.	Amyl Butyrate	3
4.	Chloroform	3
5.	Citric Acid	1
6.	Ethyl Acetate	2
7.	Ethyl Butyrate	8
8.	Ethyl Pelargonate	1
9.	Glycerin (neutral)	313
10.	Lime, Oil	9
11.	Orange, Oil	10
12.	Vanillin	1
13.	Ethyl Alcohol 95%	316
14.	Distilled Water	316
		1000

PINEAPPLE (ANANAS), IMITATION NO. 2

1.	Amyl Acetate	4
2.	Amyl Butyrate	4
3.	Butyl Acetate	7

4.	Butyraldehyde	2
5.	Butyric Acid	1
6.	Ethyl Acetate	2
7.	Ethyl Butyrate	2
8.	Ethyl Pelargonate	1
9.	Ethyl Sebacate	4
10.	Isoamyl Acetate	6
11.	Isoamyl Isovalerianate	11
12.	Lemon, Oil	1
13.	Orange, Oil	1
14.	Vanillin	1
15.	Ethyl Alcohol 95%	477
16.	Distilled Water	476
		1000

PINEAPPLE (ANANAS), IMITATION NO. 3

1.	Amyl Acetate	5
2.	Amyl Butyrate	50
3.	Amyl Isobutyrate	50
4.	Ethyl Butyrate	25
5.	Ethyl Pelargonate	2
6.	Ethyl Valerianate	3
7.	α-Ionone	1
8.	Isoethyl Acetate	10
9.	Lemon, Oil	2
10.	Orange, Oil	1
11.	Vanillin	1
12.	Ethyl Alcohol 95%	425
13.	Distilled Water	425
		1000

PINEAPPLE (ANANAS), IMITATION NO. 4

1.	Amyl Acetate	10
2.	Amyl Butyrate	25
3.	Ethyl Acetate	30
4.	Ethyl Butyrate	35
5.	Ethyl Vanillin	20
6.	Lemon, Oil (terpeneless)	2
7.	Orange, Oil (terpeneless)	1
8.	Ethyl Alcohol 95%	877
		1000

PINEAPPLE (ANANAS), IMITATION NO. 5

1.	Butyric Acid	2
2.	Ethyl Acetate	64
3.	Ethyl Butyrate	170
4.	Ethyl Pelargonate	120
5.	Ethyl Sebacate	60
6.	Isoamyl Acetate (10% sol'n.)	320
7.	Isoamyl Butyrate (10% sol'n.)	260
8.	Lemon, Oil	2
9.	Vanillin	2
		1000

PINEAPPLE (ANANAS), IMITATION NO. 6

1.	Orris, Roots (granulated)	50
2.	Pineapple (grated)	450
3.	Ethyl Alcohol 95%	250
4.	Distilled Water	250
		1000

Macerate, cool, for 20 days. Shake often. Press and filter. Distill over 800 cc.

PINEAPPLE (ANANAS), IMITATION NO. 7

1.	Bornyl Acetate	150
2.	Butyl Butyrate	150
3.	Ethyl Butyrate	150
4.	Ethyl Isoamyl Butyrate	10
5.	Ethyl Propionate	200
6.	Pineapple, Imitation No. 1*	340
		1000

PINEAPPLE (ANANAS), IMITATION NO. 8

1.	Pineapple, Imitation No. 2*	250
2.	Pineapple, Imitation No. 3*	250
3.	Wine, White	250
4.	Ethyl Alcohol 95%	250
		1000

* Formulas which appear in this book

PINEAPPLE (ANANAS), IMITATION NO. 9

1.	Pineapple (Ananas), Extract (Natural) No 1*	500
2.	Pineapple (Ananas), Extract (Natural) No. 2*	500
		1000

PINEAPPLE (ANANAS), IMITATION NO. 10

1.	Butyric Acid	2
2.	Ethyl Acetate	64
3.	Ethyl Butyrate	170
4.	Ethyl Pelargonate	120
5.	Ethyl Sebacate	60
6.	Isoamyl Acetate (10% sol'n.)	320
7.	Isoamyl Butyrate (10% sol'n.)	260
8.	Lemon, Oil	2
9.	Vanillin	2
		1000

PINEAPPLE (ANANAS), SYNTHETIC NO. 1

1.	Aldehyde C-14	10
2.	Amyl Acetate	10
3.	Amyl Butyrate	90
4.	Chloroform	10
5.	Ethyl Butyrate	50
6.	Glycerin (neutral)	330
7.	Ethyl Alcohol 95%	250
8.	Distilled Water	250
		1000

PINEAPPLE (ANANAS), SYNTHETIC NO. 2

1.	Acetaldehyde	1
2.	Amyl Butyrate	150
3.	Chloroform	9
4.	Ethyl Butyrate	150
5.	Glycerin (neutral)	230
6.	Ethyl Alcohol 95%	230
7.	Distilled Water	230
		1000

* Formulas which appear in this book

PINEAPPLE (ANANAS), SYNTHETIC NO. 3

1.	Amyl Butyrate	5
2.	Chloroform	5
3.	Ethyl Butyrate	2
4.	Glycerin (neutral)	170
5.	Ethyl Alcohol 95%	408
6.	Distilled Wate	410
		1000

PINEAPPLE (ANANAS), SYNTHETIC NO. 4

1.	Aldehyde C-10	4
2.	Allyl Caproate	2
3.	Ethyl Formate	4
4.	Ethyl Hepthylate	4
5.	Ethyl Valerianate	4
6.	Geraniol	20
7.	Isobutyl Butyrate	10
8.	Phenyl Ethyl Alcohol	30
9.	Ethyl Alcohol 95%	461
10.	Distilled Water	461
		1000

PINEAPPLE (ANANAS), SYNTHETIC NO. 5

1.	Ethyl Butyrate	190
2.	Isoamyl Isovalerate	162
3.	Ethyl Alcohol 95%	648
		1000

PINEAPPLE (ANANAS), SYNTHETIC NO. 6

1.	Amyl Butyrate	100
2.	Chloroform	10
3.	Ethyl Aldehyde	100
4.	Ethyl Butyrate (10% sol'n.)	290
5.	Ethyl Alcohol 95%	500
		1000

PINEAPPLE (ANANAS), SYNTHETIC NO. 7

1.	Ethyl Acetate	75
2.	Ethyl Butyrate (10% sol'n.)	550
3.	Ethyl Sebacate	150
4.	Isoamyl Acetate	75
5.	Isoamyl Butyrate	150
		1000

PINEAPPLE (ANANAS), SYNTHETIC NO. 8

1.	Ethyl Butyrate	190
2.	Isoamyl Isovalerate (10% sol'n.)	810
		1000

PINEAPPLE (ANANAS), SYNTHETIC NO. 9

1.	Ethyl Butyrate (10% sol'n.)	330
2.	Isoamyl Butyrate (10% sol'n.)	670
		1000

PINEAPPLE (ANANAS), SYNTHETIC NO. 10

1.	Ethyl Butyrate (10% sol'n.)	300
2.	Isoamyl Acetate	85
3.	Isoamyl Butyrate (10% sol'n.)	600
4.	Lemon, Oil	5
5.	Orange, Oil	10
		1000

PINEAPPLE (ANANAS), SYNTHETIC NO. 11

1.	Ethyl Acetate	50
2.	Ethyl Butyrate (10% sol'n.)	820
3.	Ethyl Sebacate	130
		1000

PISTACHIO NUT, EXTRACT (NATURAL)

1.	Pistachio Nuts (rasped and totally ground)	10	kg
2.	Ethyl Alcohol 95%	15	l
3.	Distilled Water	15	l

Macerate for 10 days, stirring for 1 h each day. Collect, without any pressure, 20 l of extract. To the residue add:

4.	Distilled Water	20	l

Let stand for another 3 days. Add:

5.	Amyl Formate	5	ml
6.	Ethyl Oenanthate	25	ml

Distill altogether.
Yield: 30 liters

PISTACHIO NUT, IMITATION NO. 1

1.	Almond Extract (Natural)	200
2.	Neroli, Oil	1
3.	Vanilla Beans, Tincture	400
4.	Ethyl Alcohol 95%	200
5.	Distilled Water	199
		1000

PISTACHIO NUT, IMITATION NO. 2

1.	Almond, Bitter, Oil (pure)	30
2.	Calamus, Oil	30
3.	Cinnamon, Oil	2
4.	Cloves, Oil	60
5.	Magnesium Carbonate	6
6.	Nutmeg, Oil	2
7.	Orange, Oil	10
8.	Ethyl Alcohol 95%	550
9.	Distilled Water	310
		1000

PISTACHIO NUT, IMITATION NO. 3

1.	Aldehyde C-14 (pure)	2
2.	Benzaldehyde (pure)	12
3.	Benzyl Benzoate	12
4.	Butyric Acid	1
5.	Ethyl Acetate	17
6.	Ethyl Butyrate	33
7.	Ethyl Oenanthate	5
8.	Heliotropin	1
9.	Isoamyl Acetate	10
10.	Mandarin, Oil	1
11.	Nutmeg, Oil	2
12.	Orange, Sweet, Oil	12
13.	Pimento, Oil	2
14.	Ethyl Alcohol 95%	445
15.	Distilled Water	445
		1000

PISTACHIO NUT, IMITATION NO. 4

1.	Peach, Imitation No. 1*	199
2.	Peach, Imitation No. 2*	199
3.	Peach, Imitation No. 3*	199
4.	Peach, Imitation No. 4*	199
5.	Raspberry, Imitation No. 1*	199
6.	γ-Undelactone	5
		1000

PISTACHIO NUT, IMITATION NO. 5

1.	Almond, Oil	100
2.	Almond, Bitter, Oil (cyanide-free)	30
3.	Calamus, Oil	30
4.	Cinnamon, Oil	2
5.	Clove, Oil	60
6.	Nerol, Oil	2
7.	Nutmeg, Oil	4
8.	Orange, Oil	6
9.	Vanilla, Oil	20
10.	Ethyl Alcohol 95%	373
11.	Distilled Water	373
		1000

* Formulas which appear in this book

PISTACHIO NUT, IMITATION NO. 6

1.	Almond, Bitter, Oil (cyanide-free)	20
2.	Calamus, Oil	30
3.	Cassia, Oil	20
4.	Clove	20
5.	Nerol, Oil	1
6.	Nutmeg, Oil	1
7.	Orange, Oil	4
8.	Vanilla, Oil	4
9.	Ethyl Alcohol 95%	450
10.	Distilled Water	450
		1000

PISTACHIO NUT, IMITATION NO. 7

1.	Benzaldehyde (pure, 10% sol'n.)	80
2.	Benzyl Benzoate	15
3.	Butyric Acid	10
4.	Ethyl Acetate (10% sol'n.)	350
5.	Ethyl Butyrate	180
6.	Ethyl Oenanthate	100
7.	Heliotropin	30
8.	Isoamyl Acetate	80
9.	Mandarin, Oil	15
10.	Nutmeg, Oil	40
11.	Orange, Sweet, Oil	40
12.	Pimenta, Oil	40
13.	γ-Undelactone	20
		1000

PISTACHIO NUT, IMITATION NO. 8

1.	Benzaldehyde (pure, 10% sol'n.)	70
2.	Ethyl Acetate (10% sol'n.)	310
3.	Ethyl Butyrate	170
4.	Isoamyl Acetate	150
5.	Orange, Sweet, Oil (10% sol'n.)	300
		1000

PLUM, EXTRACT (NATURAL)

1.	Plums, Fruits (without stones)	10	kg
2.	Ethyl Alcohol 95%	10	l
3.	Distilled Water	10	l

Macerate for 3 days. Express and to the residue add:

4.	Distilled Water	20	l

Let stand for another 3 days and add:

5.	Amyl Valerianate	5	ml

Distill altogether.
Yield: 40 liters

PLUM, IMITATION NO. 1

1.	Aldehyde C-14 (pure)	4
2.	Benzaldehyde (pure)	8
3.	Benzyl Acetate	15
4.	Cinnamic Aldehyde	2
5.	Cineol	1
6.	Citral	6
7.	Ethyl Acetate	10
8.	Ethyl Benzoate	3
9.	Ethyl Butyrate	26
10.	Ethyl Caprate	5
11.	Ethyl Formate	6
12.	Ethyl Heptyne Carbonate	7
13.	Ethyl Oenanthate	5
14.	Ethyl Pelargonate	13
15.	Eugenol	7
16.	Geraniol	1
17.	Ionone	1
18.	Isoamyl Acetate	3
19.	Isoamyl Alcohol	17
20.	Isoamyl Butyrate	19
21.	Isoamyl Formate	6
22.	Linalool	2
23.	Methyl Anthranilate	2
24.	Nerolin	1
25.	Orange, Oil	6
26.	Phenyl Ethyl Alcohol	1
27.	Vanillin	2
28.	Ethyl Alcohol 95%	411
29.	Distilled Water	410
		1000

PLUM, IMITATION NO. 2

1.	Aldehyde C-14 (pure)	50
2.	Ethyl Acetate	20
3.	Ethyl Butyrate	50
4.	Ethyl Formate	10
5.	Parsley, Oil	30
6.	Glycerin (neutral)	280
7.	Ethyl Alcohol 95%	280
8.	Distilled Water	280
		1000

PLUM, IMITATION NO. 3

1.	Benzaldehyde (pure, 10% sol'n.)	45
2.	Benzyl Acetate	60
3.	Bromelia	1
4.	Cinnamaldehyde	5
5.	Ethyl Acetate (10% sol'n.)	280
6.	Ethyl Butyrate	190
7.	Ethyl Caprate	5
8.	Ethyl Formate	80
9.	Ethyl Oenanthate	80
10.	Ethyl Pelargonate	30
11.	Eugenol	2
12.	Geraniol	2
13.	Isoamyl Alcohol	5
14.	Isoamyl Butyrate	190
15.	Orange, Oil	15
16.	Vanillin (10% sol'n.)	10
		1000

PLUM, IMITATION NO. 4

1.	Benzaldehyde (pure, 10% sol'n.)	40
2.	Benzyl Acetate	20
3.	Cinnamaldehyde	5
4.	Ethyl Acetate	150
5.	Ethyl Butyrate	180
6.	Ethyl Caprate	5
7.	Ethyl Oenanthate	150
8.	Ethyl Pelargonate	50
9.	Eugenol	20
10.	Geraniol	2
11.	Isoamyl Alcohol	20
12.	Isoamyl Butyrate (10% sol'n.)	300
13.	Orange, Oil	20
14.	Phenyl Ethyl Alcohol	30
15.	Vanillin (10% sol'n.)	8
		1000

PLUM, IMITATION NO. 5

1.	Benzaldehyde (pure, 10% sol'n.)	45
2.	Benzyl Acetate	60
3.	Cinnamaldehyde	10
4.	Ethyl Acetate (10% sol'n.)	271
5.	Ethyl Butyrate	170
6.	Ethyl Caprate	9
7.	Ethyl Oenanthate	100
8.	Ethyl Pelargonate	25
9.	Eugenol	5
10.	Geraniol	5
11.	Isoamyl Alcohol	15
12.	Isoamyl Butyrate (10% sol'n.)	240
13.	Orange, Oil	20
14.	Phenyl Ethyl Alcohol	10
15.	Vanillin (10% sol'n.)	15
		1000

PLUM, IMITATION NO. 6

1.	Almond, Bitter, Oil (cyanide-free)	10
2.	Amyl Alcohol	15
3.	Amyl Butyrate	75
4.	Amyl Formate	50
5.	Clove, Oil	10
6.	Coriander, Oil	10
7.	Ethyl Acetate	100
8.	Ethyl Butyrate	40
9.	Ethyl Formate	20
10.	Ethyl Methylphenylglycidate	5
11.	Lemon, Oil	25
12.	Mandarin, Oil	25
13.	γ-Nonyl Lactone	10
14.	Pineapple, Imitation No.1*	50
15.	Raspberry, Imitation No. 1*	100
16.	Ethyl Alcohol 95%	455
		1000

PLUM, SYNTHETIC NO. 1

1.	Benzaldehyde (pure, 10% sol'n.)	20
2.	Ethyl Acetate	140
3.	Ethyl Butyrate	160
4.	Ethyl Formate	80
5.	Ethyl Alcohol 95%	600
		1000

* Formulas which appear in this book

PLUM, SYNTHETIC NO. 2

1.	Benzaldehyde (pure, 10% sol'n.)	90
2.	Citral	5
3.	Ethyl Acetate	90
4.	Ethyl Formate	180
5.	Eugenol	15
6.	Isoamyl Alcohol	40
7.	Isoamyl Butyrate (10% sol'n.)	270
8.	Isoamyl Formate (10% sol'n.)	270
9.	Linalool	20
10.	Methyl Anthranilate	20
		1000

PLUM, SYNTHETIC NO. 3

1.	Ethyl Acetate (10% sol'n.)	350
2.	Ethyl Butyrate (10% sol'n.)	350
3.	Ethyl Caprylate	60
4.	Eugenol	2
5.	Ionone	1
6.	Isoamyl Butyrate	200
7.	γ-Nonyl Lactone	17
8.	Vanillin (10% sol'n.)	20
		1000

PLUM, SYNTHETIC NO. 4

1.	Benzaldehyde (pure, 10% sol'n.)	40
2.	Cineol	5
3.	Cinnamaldehyde	10
4.	Ethyl Acetate (10% sol'n.)	400
5.	Ethyl Benzoate (10% sol'n.)	280
6.	Ethyl Oenanthate	140
7.	Eugenol	10
8.	Isoamyl Acetate	30
9.	Isoamyl Alcohol	50
10.	Isoamyl Butyrate	30
11.	Vanillin	5
		1000

PLUM, SYNTHETIC NO. 5

1.	Benzaldehyde (pure, 10% sol'n.)	60
2.	Cinnamaldehyde	5
3.	Ethyl Acetate	140
4.	Ethyl Formate	200
5.	Eugenol	5
6.	Isoamyl Alcohol	8

7.	Isoamyl Butyrate (10% sol'n.)	300
8.	Isoamyl Formate (10% sol'n.)	250
9.	Methyl Anthranilate	1
10.	Phenyl Ethyl Alcohol (10% sol'n.)	31
		1000

PLUM, SYNTHETIC NO. 6

1.	Acetaldehyde	2
2.	Aldehyde C-14 (pure)	50
3.	Ethyl Acetate	20
4.	Ethyl Butyrate	50
5.	Ethyl Formate	10
6.	Ethyl Nitrate	10
7.	Ethyl Oenanthate	10
8.	Ethyl Salicylate	8
9.	Glycerin (neutral)	280
10.	Ethyl Alcohol 95%	280
11.	Distilled Water	280
		1000

POMEGRANATE (GRENADINE), IMITATION NO.1

1.	Lemon, Imitation No. 1*	245
2.	Orange, Imitation No. 1*	245
3.	Pineapple, Imitation No. 1*	245
4.	Raspberry, Imitation No. 1*	245
5.	Vanillin	20
		1000

POMEGRANATE (GRENADINE), IMITATION NO. 2

1.	Pineapple, Imitation No. 2*	250
2.	Pomegranate (Grenadine), Imitation No. 1*	750
		1000

* Formulas which appear in this book

POMEGRANATE (GRENADINE), IMITATION NO. 3

1.	Pineapple, Imitation No. 3*	150
2.	Pomegranate (Grenadine), Imitation No. 2*	850
		1000

POMEGRANATE (GRENADINE), IMITATION NO. 4

1.	Benzyl Benzoate	100
2.	Bromelia	12
3.	Cinnamaldehyde	8
4.	Ethyl Acetate (10% sol'n.)	450
5.	Eugenol	5
6.	Isoamyl Acetate	200
7.	Isoamyl Isovalerate	180
8.	Isobutyl Propionate	5
9.	Limonene	20
10.	γ-Undelactone	20
		1000

POMEGRANATE (GRENADINE), IMITATION NO. 5

1.	Benzaldehyde (pure, 10% sol'n.)	80
2.	Benzyl Benzoate	160
3.	Cinnamaldehyde	10
4.	Ethyl Acetate (10% sol'n.)	300
5.	Eugenol	10
6.	Isoamyl Acetate	160
7.	Isoamyl Isovalerate (10% sol'n.)	240
8.	Limonene	20
9.	γ-Undelactone	20
		1000

POMEGRANATE (GRENADINE), IMITATION NO. 6

1.	Ethyl Acetate (10% sol'n.)	250
2.	Ethyl Benzoate (10% sol'n.)	250
3.	Ethyl Butyrate	200
4.	Ethyl Salicylate	10
5.	Isoamyl Acetate	200
6.	Isoamyl Butyrate	80
7.	Vanillin (10% sol'n.)	10
		1000

POMEGRANATE (GRENADINE), IMITATION NO. 7

1.	Pineapple (Ananas), Extract (Natural)*	170
2.	Lemon, Oil	100
3.	Raspberry, Extract (Natural) No. 1*	325
4.	Orange, Oil	105
5.	Orris Root, Tincture	150
6.	Vanilla Beans, Tincture	150
		1000

POMEGRANATE (GRENADINE), IMITATION NO. 8

1.	Amyl Acetate	10
2.	Amyl Valerianate	10
3.	Benzyl Benzoate	4
4.	Cinnamon, Oil	6
5.	Clove, Oil	4
6.	Ethyl Acetate	10
7.	Honey, Natural	30
8.	Nerolin	2
9.	Peach, Extract (Natural)*	220
10.	Petitgrain, Oil	4
11.	Ethyl Alcohol 95%	355
12.	Distilled Water	345
		1000

POMEGRANATE (GRENADINE), SYNTHETIC

1.	Aldehyde C-14 (pure)	1
2.	Benzaldehyde	1
3.	Benzyl Benzoate	8
4.	Cinnamic Aldehyde	1
5.	Ethyl Acetate	11
6.	Ethyl Benzoate	8
7.	Ethyl Butyrate	4
8.	Eugenol	1
9.	Isoamyl Acetate	17
10.	Isoamyl Butyrate	4
11.	Isoamyl Valerianate	15
12.	Isobutyl-α-Toluate	1
13.	Limonene	1
14.	Nerolin	1
15.	Vanillin	1
16.	Ethyl Alcohol 95%	470
17.	Distilled Water	455
		1000

* Formulas which appear in this book

POTATO, FLAVOR

1. Potatoes (peeled)
2. Propylene Glycol

Add propylene glycol to potatoes. Boil at 187 F for 15 min. Drain by pressing (gravity) or by centrifuge.

Note: This procedure could be applied to other natural products.

POUND CAKE, FLAVOR

1.	Almond, Bitter, Oil (pure)	175
2.	Cardamom, Oil	120
3.	Cinnamon, Oil	120
4.	Clove, Oil	120
5.	Lemon, Oil	200
6.	Nutmeg, Oil	120
7.	Vanillin	145
		1000

POWDERED FLAVORS

1.	Color, Certified	1
2.	Essence (Any Extract or Synthetic)	247
3.	Malic Acid	2
4.	Sugar (granulated)	750
		1000

Note: The amount of certified color could be increased or decreased to suit. The amount of sugar could be reduced adding arabic gum (*Acacia senegal*). The amount of essence could be reduced or increased.

PRALINE** FLAVOR (CRYSTALS)

1.	Almond (blanched)	10 kg
2.	Hazelnuts	10 kg
3.	Sugar	18 kg

Roast the almonds and hazelnuts at 143–149 C. Dissolve the sugar with the minimum amount possible of distilled water. Heat altogether at 158 C. Pour all on a water-cooled table. Pulverize.

PROTEINIC BASIC FLAVOR

1. Raw Material
2. Propylene Glycol
3. Ethyl Alcohol 95%

Use raw material from any plant or animal substance. Separate off solids. Boil in water until dissolved to the maximum. Freeze. Separate water. Dissolve in proPylene glycol. Add alcohol to 10% the entire amount.

PRUNELLE, EXTRACT (NATURAL)

1.	Prunelles (chopped)	10 kg
2.	Ethyl Alcohol 95%	10 l
3.	Distilled Water	10 l

Let macerate for 3 days. Express. To the residue add:

4.	Distilled Water	20 l

Let stand for another 3 days. Add:

5.	Amyl Valerianate	5 ml

Distill altogether.
Yield: 40 liters

QUINCE, EXTRACT (NATURAL)

1.	Quinces (well ripe, crushed)	100 kg
2.	Ethyl Alcohol 95%	20 l

Macerate for 3 days. Express. To the residue add:

3.	Ethyl Alcohol 95%	10 l
4.	Distilled Water	10 l

Let stand for another 3 days. Add:

5.	Amyl Acetate	24 ml
6.	Ethyl Pelargonate	24 ml
7.	Ethyl Valerianate	12 ml

Distill altogether.
Yield: 40 liters

QUINCE, IMITATION

1.	Benzaldehyde (pure)	15
2.	Ethyl Butyrate	40
3.	Ethyl Isobutyrate	310
4.	Ethyl Oenanthate	8
5.	Ethyl Pelargonate	60
6.	Eugenol	15
7.	Isoamyl Acetate	310
8.	Isoamyl Isovalerianate	180
9.	Linalyl Acetate	2
10.	Orange, Sweet, Oil	60
		1000

QUINCE, SYNTHETIC NO. 1

1.	Amyl Acetate	5
2.	Ethyl Butyrate	150
3.	Ethyl Oenanthate	1
4.	Ethyl Pelargonate	50
5.	Ethyl Alcohol 95%	397
6.	Distilled Water	397
		1000

QUINCE, SYNTHETIC NO. 2

1.	Alcohol C-11 (undecylenic)†	100
2.	Amyl Valerianate	2
3.	Ethyl Acetate	20
4.	Ethyl Caprate	35

** Confection of nut kernels (almond, hazel, pecan, etc.) roasted in boiling sugar until brown colored.

† Alcohol C-11 (undecylenic) is obtained by heating undecylenic acid (from destructive distillation of castor oil) with alcohol in presence of sulfuric acid (as a catalyst), washing it with alkaline water (sodium bicarbonate), and distilling. It has the quince fruit aroma.

5.	Ethyl Formate	5
6.	Ethyl Pelargonate	15
7.	Glycerin (neutral)	411
8.	Ethyl Alcohol 95%	412
		1000

QUINCE, SYNTHETIC NO. 3

1.	Benzaldehyde (pure, 10% sol'n.)	15
2.	Ethyl Butyrate	60
3.	Ethyl Isobutyrate (10% sol'n.)	310
4.	Ethyl Oenanthate	8
5.	Eugenol	15
6.	Isoamyl Acetate (10% sol'n.)	370
7.	Isoamyl Isovalerate	180
8.	Linalyl Acetate	2
9.	Orange, Sweet, Oil	40
		1000

RAISIN, SYNTHETIC

1.	Aldehyde C-14 (pure)	20
2.	Chloroform (pure)	10
3.	Ethyl Formate	20
4.	Ethyl Oenanthate	92
5.	Glycerin (neutral)	140
6.	Methyl Anthranilate	10
7.	Succinic Acid	3
8.	Tartaric Acid	5
9.	Ethyl Alcohol 95%	700
		1000

RASPBERRY, EXTRACT (NATURAL) NO. 1

1.	Raspberries	100 kg
2.	Sugar	5 kg

Let ferment fror 1 week or more, until the flavor is well developed. Add:

3.	Ethyl Alcohol 95%	24 1

Let stand for another week. Express and to the residue add:

4.	Ethyl Alcohol 95%	12 1
5.	Distilled Water	12 1

Let stand for another 3 days. Add:

6.	Anisaldehyde	12 ml
7.	Cognac, Oil	8 ml
8.	Ethyl Acetate	24 ml
9.	Ethyl Benzoate	24 ml
10.	Ethyl Pelargonate	12 ml
11.	Vanillin	12 g

Distill altogether. Redistill for rectification.
Yield: 50 liters

RASPBERRY, EXTRACT (NATURAL) NO. 2

1.	Raspberry, Juice (fresh)	40 1
2.	Ethyl Alcohol 95%	4 1

Distill.
Yield: 8 liters

RASPBERRY, EXTRACT (NATURAL) NO. 3

1.	Raspberry, Extract (Natural) No. 1*	10 1
2.	Raspberry, Extract (Natural) No. 2*	10 1
3.	Sugar Syrup (60%)	40 1
4.	Ethyl Alcohol 95%	20 1
5.	Distilled Water	20 1

Filter.
Yield: 100 liters

RASPBERRY, IMITATION NO. 1

1.	Acetaldehyde	2
2.	Aldehyde C-20	1
3.	Amyl Acetate	5
4.	Amyl Butyrate	25
5.	Amyl Isobutyrate	25
6.	Cinnamon, Oil	1
7.	Clove, Oil	3
8.	Ethyl Acetate	5
9.	Ethyl Butyrate	15
10.	Ethyl Formate	5

* Formulas which appear in this book

11.	Ethyl Isobutyrate	15
12.	Ethyl Salicylate	1
13.	α-Ionone	2
14.	Isobutyl Acetate	15
15.	Lemon, Oil	2
16.	Neroli, Oil	2
17.	Orris, Oil	2
18.	Vanillin	5
19.	Ethyl Alcohol 95%	435
20.	Distilled Water	434
		1000

RASPBERRY, IMITATION NO. 2

1.	Aldehyde C-16	10
2.	Amyl Acetate	10
3.	Benzoic Acid	1
4.	Ethyl Acetate	50
5.	Ethyl Benzoate	10
6.	Ethyl Butyrate	10
7.	Ethyl Formate	10
8.	Ethyl Nitrate	10
9.	Ethyl Oenanthate	10
10.	Ethyl Salicylate	10
11.	Glycerin (neutral)	106
12.	Orange, Oil	62
13.	Sebacic Acid	1
14.	Ethyl Alcohol 95%	350
15.	Distilled Water	350
		1000

RASPBERRY, IMITATION NO. 3

1.	Aldehyde C-20	30
2.	Amyl Acetate	60
3.	Benzyl Butyrate	12
4.	Benzyl Formate	10
5.	Benzyl Propionate	10
6.	Butyl Acetate	60
7.	Ethyl Acetate	60
8.	Isobutyl Acetate	20
9.	Isocinnamic Acetate	40
10.	Orris, Oil	12
11.	Phenyl Ethyl Butyrate	80
12.	Vanillin	6
13.	Ethyl Alcohol 95%	300
14.	Distilled Water	300
		1000

RASPBERRY, IMITATION NO. 4

1.	Orris, Roots (granulated)	100
2.	Amyl Acetate	175
3.	Amyl Butyrate	25
4.	Ethyl Acetate	80
5.	Ethyl Butyrate	150
6.	Ethyl Nitrate	25
7.	Ethyl Oenanthate	15
8.	Isobutyl Formate	5
9.	Orange, Oil	20
10.	Raspberry, Juice	400
11.	Vanillin	5
		1000

Macerate for 1 day and distill over 800 cc.

RASPBERRY, IMITATION NO. 5

1.	Almond, Bitter, Oil (cyanide-free)	8
2.	Benzyl Acetate	100
3.	Cinnamon, Ceylon, Oil	15
4.	Civette, Tincture (3%)	1
5.	Clove, Oil	15
6.	Neroli, Oil	4
7.	Orris, Root, Extract (10%)	5
8.	Phenyl Ethyl Alcohol	75
9.	Peru Balsam	15
10.	Propyl Acetate	30
11.	Raspberry, Imitation No. 1*	346
12.	Rose, Oil	7
13.	Tolu, Extract (10%)	15
14.	Vanillin (10% sol'n.)	18
15.	Ethyl Alcohol 95%	346
		1000

RASPBERRY, IMITATION NO. 6

1.	Aldehyde C-12	10
2.	γ-Nonyl Lactone	20

* Formulas which appear in this book

3.	Raspberry, Imitation No. 1*	485
4.	Ethyl Alcohol 95%	485
		1000

RASPBERRY, IMITATION NO. 7

1.	Aldehyde C-20	10
2.	γ-Nonyl Lactone	10
3.	Raspberry, Imitation No. 2*	490
4.	Ethyl Alcohol 95%	490
		1000

RASPBERRY, IMITATION NO. 8

1.	Almond, Bitter, Oil (cyanide-free)	3
2.	Benzyl Acetate	40
3.	Cinnamon, Ceylon, Oil	5
4.	Civette, Tincture (10%)	1
5.	Clove, Oil	5
6.	Neroli, Oil	2
7.	Orris, Extract (10%)	1
8.	Phenyl Ethyl Alcohol	50
9.	Peru, Balsam, Oil	10
10.	Propyl Acetate	10
11.	Raspberry, Imitation No. 3*	432
12.	Rose, Oil	3
13.	Vanillin	5
14.	Ethyl Alcohol 95%	433
		1000

RASPBERRY, IMITATION NO. 9

1.	γ-Nonyl Lactone	10
2.	Raspberry, Imitation No. 1*	165
3.	Raspberry, Imitation No. 2*	165
4.	Raspberry, Imitation No. 3*	165
5.	Raspberry, Imitation No. 4*	165
6.	Raspberry, Imitation No. 5*	165
7.	Ethyl Alcohol 95%	165
		1000

* Formulas which appear in this book

RASPBERRY, IMITATION NO. 10

1.	Acetaldehyde	50
2.	Aldehyde C-20	3
3.	Amyl Acetate	50
4.	Amyl Butyrate	150
5.	Amyl Isobutyrate	150
6.	Cinnamon, Ceylon, Oil	15
7.	Clove, Oil	15
8.	Ethyl Acetate	50
9.	Ethyl Butyrate	150
10.	Ethyl Formate	50
11.	Ethyl Isobutyrate	100
12.	α-Ionone	15
13.	Isobutyl Acetate	150
14.	Lemon, Oil (terpeneless)	12
15.	Methyl Salicylate	5
16.	Neroli, Oil	15
17.	Orris, Oil	15
18.	Vanillin	5
		1000

RASPBERRY, SYNTHETIC NO. 1

1.	Aldehyde C-20	40
2.	Amyl Acetate	10
3.	Amyl Valerianate	10
4.	Ethyl Acetate	5
5.	Ethyl Benzoate	10
6.	Ethyl Formate	10
7.	Ethyl Nitrate	10
8.	Glycerin (neutral)	100
9.	Tartaric Acid	5
10.	Ethyl Alcohol 95%	400
11.	Distilled Water	400
		1000

RASPBERRY, SYNTHETIC NO. 2

1.	Acetaldehyde	2
2.	Aldehyde C-20	30
3.	Amyl Acetate	10
4.	Amyl Butyrate	20
5.	Amyl Valerianate	20
6.	Ethyl Acetate	10
7.	Ethyl Benzoate	10
8.	Ethyl Butyrate	20

9.	Ethyl Formate	10
10.	Ethyl Nitrate	10
11.	Ethyl Oenanthate	20
12.	Ethyl Salicylate	1
13.	Ethyl Sebacate	4
14.	Ethyl Succinate	1
15.	Ethyl Valerianate	10
16.	Glycerin (neutral)	120
17.	Succinic Acid	1
18.	Tartaric Acid	1
19.	Ethyl Alcohol 95%	350
20.	Distilled Water	350
		1000

RASPBERRY, SYNTHETIC NO. 3

1.	Aldehyde C-20	15
2.	Amyl Acetate	10
3.	Amyl Butyrate	5
4.	Amyl Valerianate	25
5.	Ethyl Acetate	15
6.	Ethyl Benzoate	10
7.	Ethyl Formate	10
8.	Ethyl Nitrate	10
9.	Glycerin (neutral)	293
10.	Tartaric Acid	5
11.	Vanillin	2
12.	Ethyl Alcohol 95%	300
13.	Distilled Water	300
		1000

RASPBERRY, SYNTHETIC NO. 4

1.	Amyl Acetate	45
2.	Amyl Butyrate	220
3.	Ethyl Acetate	45
4.	Ethyl Formate	45
5.	Ethyl Pelargonate	45
6.	Glycerin (neutral)	160
7.	Ethyl Alcohol 95%	220
8.	Distilled Water	220
		1000

RASPBERRY, SYNTHETIC NO. 5

1.	Benzyl Acetate	1
2.	Benzyl Benzoate	35
3.	Ethyl Acetate	200
4.	Ethyl Formate	20
5.	Eugenol	5
6.	Geraniol	2
7.	Ionone	2
8.	Isoamyl Acetate	200
9.	Isobutyl Acetate	400
10.	Linalool	120
11.	Nerolin	10
12.	Vanillin	5
		1000

RASPBERRY, SYNTHETIC NO. 6

1.	Aldehyde C-18	4
2.	Amyl Butyrate	140
3.	Benzaldehyde (pure)	2
4.	Benzyl Acetate	68
5.	Benzyl Benzoate	12
6.	Butyl-β-Naphthyl Ether	36
7.	Cinnamic Aldehyde	8
8.	Ethyl Acetate	44
9.	Ethyl Benzoate	62
10.	Ethyl Butyrate	146
11.	Ethyl Cinnamate	10
12.	Ethyl Formate	54
13.	Ethyl Oenanthate	60
14.	Ethyl Salicylate	36
15.	Ethyl Sebacate	36
16.	Eugenol	10
17.	Geraniol	4
18.	Ionone	8
19.	Isoamyl Acetate	24
20.	Isoamyl Butyrate	74
21.	Isoamyl Isovalerianate	10
22.	Isobutyl Acetate	18
23.	Isobutyl Formate	8
24.	Linalool	4
25.	Nerolin	4
26.	Phenyl Ethyl Alcohol	90
27.	Propyl Acetate	14
28.	Succinic Acid	2
29.	Tartaric Acid	4
30.	Vanillin	8
		1000

RASPBERRY, SYNTHETIC NO. 7

1.	Ethyl Acetate	50
2.	Ethyl Benzoate	3
3.	Ethyl Butyrate	5
4.	Ethyl Formate	3
5.	Ethyl Heptanoate	3
6.	Ethyl Nitrate	10
7.	Ethyl Salicylate	5
8.	Ethyl Sebacate	10
9.	γ-Nonyl Lactone	10
10.	Raspberry, Synthetic No. 1*	260
11.	Raspberry, Synthetic No. 2*	100
12.	Ethyl Alcohol 95%	541
		1000

RASPBERRY, SYNTHETIC NO. 8

1.	Ethyl Benzoate	120
2.	Ethyl Butyrate	120
3.	Isoamyl Acetate	25
4.	Isoamyl Formate	20
5.	Ionone	10
6.	Vanillin	5
7.	Ethyl Alcohol 95%	700
		1000

RASPBERRY, SYNTHETIC NO. 9

1.	Ethyl Acetate (10% sol'n.)	550
2.	Ethyl Benzoate	110
3.	Ethyl Butyrate	110
4.	Ionone	10
5.	Isoamyl Acetate	110
6.	Isoamyl Butyrate	110
		1000

RASPBERRY, SYNTHETIC NO. 10

1.	Benzaldehyde (pure, 10% sol'n.)	20
2.	Benzyl Acetate (10% sol'n.)	350
3.	Bromelia	2
4.	Cinnamaldehyde	40
5.	Ethyl Acetate (10% sol'n.)	350
6.	Eugenol	40
7.	Geraniol	20
8.	Ionone	10
9.	Isoamyl Acetate	20
10.	Phenyl Ethyl Acetate (10% sol'n.)	50
11.	Propyl Acetate	80
12.	Vanillin (10% sol'n.)	18
		1000

RASPBERRY, SYNTHETIC NO. 11

1.	Benzyl Acetate	1
2.	Benzyl Benzoate	50
3.	Cinnamaldehyde	5
4.	Ethyl Acetate	200
5.	Ethyl Formate	60
6.	Eugenol	15
7.	Geraniol	1
8.	Ionone	3
9.	Isoamyl Acetate (10% sol'n.)	250
10.	Isobutyl Acetate (10% sol'n.)	380
11.	Linalool	15
12.	Vanillin (10% sol'n.)	20
		1000

RASPBERRY, SYNTHETIC NO. 12

1.	Benzyl Acetate	2
2.	Benzyl Benzoate	20
3.	Bromelia	15
4.	Ethyl Acetate	200
5.	Ethyl Formate	35
6.	Eugenol	6
7.	Geraniol	1
8.	Ionone	1
9.	Isoamyl Acetate (10% sol'n.)	275
10.	Isobutyl Acetate (10% sol'n.)	425
11.	Linalool	10
12.	Vanillin (10% sol'n.)	10
		1000

* Formulas which appear in this book

RASPBERRY, SYNTHETIC NO. 13

1.	Ethyl Acetate	120
2.	Ethyl Oenanthate	180
3.	Isoamyl Acetate (10% sol'n.)	300
4.	Isobutyl Acetate (10% sol'n.)	240
5.	Isobutyl Formate	45
6.	Linalool	10
7.	β-Naphthyl Ethyl Ether (10% sol'n.)	80
8.	γ-Nonyl Lactone (10% sol'n.)	25
		1000

RATAFIA

Ratafias are liqueurs made with extract from fresh fruits macerated with alcohol and synthetic flavor.

Liqueurs are flavored with fruit kernels and bitter almonds.

Sweet biscuits are made with almond paste.

Note: Liqueur is a sweet alcoholic beverage flavored with fruits or aromatics.

Liquor is a distilled, rather than fermented, alcoholic beverage.

RHODIUM

1.	Bois De Rose, Oil	200
2.	Geranium Bourbon, Oil	200
3.	Rhodium, Oil	200
4.	Triacetin	400
		1000

ROOT BEER, IMITATION

1.	Amyl Butyrate	45
2.	Anise, Oil	2
3.	Cassia, Oil	90
4.	Clove, Oil	10
5.	Ethyl Salicylate	110
6.	Lemon, Oil	90
7.	Nutmeg, Oil	5
8.	Vanilla Beans, Oil	113
9.	Ethyl Alcohol 95%	535
		1000

ROSE, FLAVOR

1.	Citral	1
2.	Geraniol	100
3.	Geranium Rose (10% sol'n.)	250
4.	Orange, Sweet	47
5.	Rhodinol	150
6.	Rose, Turkish, Oil	2
7.	Ethyl Alcohol 95%	450
		1000

ROSE, LIQUOR

1.	Cardamom, Oil	35
2.	Cedar, Oil	15
3.	Cinnamon, Oil	20
4.	Clove, Oil	15
5.	Iris, Florentine	15
6.	Lemon, Oil	50
7.	Melissa, Oil	25
8.	Mint, Oil	15
9.	Nutmeg, Oil	25
10.	Orange Flower, Oil	135
11.	Orange, Oil	100
12.	Rose, Oil	25
13.	Rosemary, Oil	25
14.	Storax	3
15.	Vanilla	25
16.	Ethyl Alcohol 95%	236
17.	Distilled Water	236
		1000

ROSEMARY, CHILI

1.	Rosemary, Leaves	30	kg
2.	Vinegar, Natural	240	l

Let stand for 1 week. Sieve, and add:

3.	Vinegar, Natural	1600	l

Let stand several months. Filter.

RUM, ETHER FLAVOR

1.	Acetic Acid	3
2.	Ethyl Alcohol 95%	624
3.	Manganese Dioxide	5
4.	Pyroligneous Acid (tar-free)	150
5.	Charcoal	3

Distill slowly with low flame under cap. Add:

6.	Peru Balsam, Oil	210
7.	Charcoal	5
		1000

Redistill. Filter.

RUM, IMITATION NO. 1

1.	Angelic, Root, Extract	25
2.	Catechu, Extract	25
3.	Cinnamon, Ceylon, Oil	30
4.	Ethyl Acetate	110
5.	Ethyl Butyrate	120
6.	Ethyl Formate	50
7.	Neroli, Oil	5
8.	Vanilla, Oil (10% sol'n.)	35
9.	Ethyl Alcohol 95%	600
		1000

RUM, IMITATION NO. 2

1.	Ethyl Formate	100
2.	Ethyl Nitrate	150
3.	Rum, Imitation No. 1*	745
4.	Vanillin	5
		1000

RUM, IMITATION NO. 3

1.	Birch Tar, Oil (10% sol'n.)	50
2.	Ethyl Acetate	50
3.	Rum, Imitation No. 2*	450
4.	Ethyl Alcohol 95%	450
		1000

RUM, IMITATION NO. 4

1.	Rum, Imitation No. 2*	488
2.	Rum, Imitation No. 3*	487
3.	Saffron, Extract	25
		1000

* Formulas which appear in this book

RUM, IMITATION NO. 5

1.	Rum, Imitation No. 4*	500
2.	Sugar, Syrup (32 Bé)	500
		1000

RUM "JAMAICA," NO. 1

1.	Acetic Acid (10% sol'n.)	30 ml
2.	Butyric Acid (2% sol'n.)	1 ml
3.	Kino, Tincture	45 ml
4.	Ethyl Alcohol 95%	10 1
5.	Distilled Water	10 1

Color with burnt sugar (caramel). Let stand 5 days, stirring for 1 h every day. Filter.

RUM "JAMAICA," NO. 2

1.	Amyl Acetate	100
2.	Amyl Butyrate	100
3.	Amyl Formate	100
4.	Birch Tar (rectified)	20
5.	Clove, Oil	35
6.	Ethyl Acetate	28
7.	Ethyl Butyrate	58
8.	Ethyl Formate	56
9.	Ethyl Oenanthate	58
10.	Ethyl Propionate	72
11.	Peru Balsam, Oil	50
12.	Styrax, Resinoid	68
13.	Vanillin	133
14.	Ethyl Alcohol 95%	122
		1000

RUM, OIL

1.	Birch Tar, Oil	3
2.	Ethyl Acetate	42
3.	Ethyl Butyrate	14
4.	Ethyl Formate	12
5.	Lemon, Oil	4
6.	Peru Balsam, Oil	75
7.	Vanillin	15
8.	Ethyl Alcohol 95%	418
9.	Distilled Water	417
		1000

RUM, SYNTHETIC NO. 1

1.	Amyl Butyrate	100
2.	Amyl Isobutyrate	100
3.	Caramel	249
4.	Ethyl Formate	100
5.	Furfural	1
6.	Isobutyl Acetate	100
7.	Isobutyl Butyrate	100
8.	Ethyl Alcohol 95%	250
		1000

RUM, SYNTHETIC NO. 2

1.	Acetic Acid (10% sol'n.)	80
2.	Amyl Butyrate	60
3.	Butyric Acid	28
4.	Ethyl Acetate	86
5.	Ethyl Butyrate	118
6.	Heliotropin	38
7.	Rum Ether	62
8.	Vanillin	28
9.	Ethyl Alcohol 95%	500
		1000

RUM, SYNTHETIC NO. 3

1.	Amyl Acetate	10
2.	Angelica, Oil (terpeneless)	1
3.	Birch Tar, Oil (10% sol'n.)	1
4.	Cinnamon, Ceylon, Oil (terpeneless)	1
5.	Ethyl Acetate	10
6.	Ethyl Butyrate	100
7.	Ethyl Formate	200
8.	Ethyl Nitrate	100
9.	Neroli, Oil	1
10.	Rum, Synthetic No. 1*	571
11.	Vanillin	5
		1000

SAINT JOHN'S BREAD (CAROB), TINCTURE

1.	St. John's Bread (Carob) (roasted and powdered)	457
2.	Ethyl Alcohol 95%	355
3.	Distilled Water	188
		1000

* Formulas which appear in this book

SARSAPARILLA, IMITATION NO. 1

1.	Anise	200
2.	Caraway	50
3.	Cinnamon	50
4.	Fennel	50
5.	Sassafras	25
6.	Wintergreen	50
7.	Ethyl Alcohol 95%	288
8.	Distilled Water	287
		1000

SARSAPARILLA, IMITATION NO. 2

1.	Anise, Oil	4
2.	Fennel, Oil	2
3.	Sweet Birch, Oil	35
4.	Wintergreen, Oil	92
5.	Ethyl Alcohol 95%	434
6.	Distilled Water	433
		1000

SASSAFRAS, IMITATION NO. 1

1.	Benzyl Benzoate (10% sol'n.)	300
2.	Limonene	60
3.	Sassafras, Oil	100
4.	Ocotea Cymbarum, Oil (10% sol'n.)	540
		1000

SASSAFRAS, IMITATION NO. 2

1.	Benzyl Benzoate (10% sol'n.)	300
2.	Limonene	30
3.	Sassafras, Oil	120
4.	Ocotea Cymbarum, Oil (10% sol'n.)	550
		1000

SASSAFRAS, IMITATION NO. 3

1.	Benzyl Benzoate (10% sol'n.)	280
2.	Citral	10
3.	Fenchone	110
4.	Lemongrass	70
5.	Limonene (10% sol'n.)	250
6.	Pine, Oil	110
7.	Terpineol	170
		1000

SASSAFRAS, IMITATION NO. 4

1.	Camphene	50
2.	Phellandrene	150
3.	Pinene	50
4.	Sassafras, Imitation No. 1*	250
5.	Sassafras, Imitation No. 2*	250
6.	Sassafras, Oil	250
		1000

SASSAFRAS, SYNTHETIC NO. 1

1.	Camphene	100
2.	Maple, Lactone	1
3.	Musk	10
4.	Ocotea Cymbarum	200
5.	Phellandrene	150
6.	Pine, Oil	50
7.	Sassafras, Oil	489
		1000

SASSAFRAS, SYNTHETIC NO. 2

1.	Citral	10
2.	Benzyl Benzoate	280
3.	Fenchone, Oil	110
4.	Lemongrass	70
5.	Limonene	250
6.	Pine, Oil	110
7.	Terpineol	170
		1000

* Formulas which appear in this book

SAUCE FLAVORS

Note: Sauces can be made with either fruits or vegetables, e.g., apple, date, mango or onion, garlic, etc. These formulas can be applied to any type of fruit or vegetable.

SAUCE, FLAVOR BASE

1.	Any Fruit or Vegetable	25	kg
2.	Distilled Water	35	l
3.	Sugar Syrup	55	l
4.	Vinegar, Natural	35	l

Let macerate for 10 days and then add:

5.	Acetic Acid (10% sol'n.)	5	l
6.	Caramel (10% sol'n.)	2	l
7.	Cinnamon (ground)	187	g
8.	Cloves (ground)	120	g
9.	Paprika (ground)	200	g
10.	Pepper (ground)	120	g
11.	Pimienta (ground)	200	g
12.	Tragacanth, Gum	16	g

Let macerate for another 10 days. Sieve and percolate.

SAUCE, SOY FLAVOR

1.	Soy Beans (roasted, powdered, @ 250 F)	2	kg
2.	Propylene Glycol	1	l
3.	Ethyl Alcohol 95%	5	l
4.	Distilled Water	1	l

SAVORY, OIL NO. 1

1.	Cinnamic Aldehyde	400
2.	Geraniol	10
3.	Ocotea Cymbarum	100
4.	Propylene Glycol	480
5.	Vetiver, Oil	10
		1000

SAVORY, OIL NO. 2

1.	Cassia, Oil	750
2.	Ocotea Cymbarum	150
3.	Vetiver, Oil	100
		1000

SCOTCH, SMOKE TYPE TASTE

1.	Barley, Malted (dried on peat fuel instead of coal)	250
2.	Rye or Oats (unmalted and with no smoke taste)	250
3.	Ethyl Alcohol 95%	250
4.	Distilled Water	250
		1000

SMOKE, FLAVOR

1. Hardwoods (Hickory or Maple) Burning

Introduce smoke to a liquid:

2.	Glycerin (neutral), or Propylene Glycol, or Triethylene Glycol, or Tween	
3.	Ethyl Alcohol 95%	25% of total amount

SMOKE, FLAVOR FOR FISH (SEASONING)

1.	Cassia, Oil	40
2.	Capsicum, Oil	30
3.	Clove, Oil	80
4.	Ginger, Oil	10
5.	Pimenta Berries, Oil	140
6.	Propylene Glycol	210
7.	Tween 80	490
		1000

SMOKE, FLAVOR FOR MEAT

1.	Cade, Oil (rectified)	687
2.	Capsicum, Oleoresin	187
3.	Pepper, Black, Oil	126
		1000

SPEARMINT-WINTERGREEN-PEPPERMINT NO. 1

1.	Benzyl Alcohol	200
2.	Camphora	50
3.	Eucalyptol	170
4.	Menthol	120
5.	Menthone	60
6.	Menthyl Acetate	40
7.	Phellandrene (10% sol'n.)	360
		1000

SPEARMINT-WINTERGREEN-PEPPERMINT NO. 2

1.	Benzyl Alcohol	200
2.	Methyl Salicylate (10% sol'n.)	25
3.	Phellandrene (10% sol'n.)	375
4.	Spearmint-Wintergreen-Peppermint No. 1*	400
		1000

SPICE, IMITATION NO. 1

1.	Calamus, Oil	150
2.	Capsicum, Oil	150
3.	Cardamom, Oil	150
4.	Cassia, Oil	25
5.	Cinnamon, Oil	40
6.	Clove, Oil	60
7.	Coriander, Oil	30
8.	Nutmeg, Oil	80
9.	Pepper, Oil	150
10.	Pimento, Oil	15
11.	Tarragon, Oil	150
		1000

SPICE, IMITATION NO. 2

1.	Cassia, Oil (10% sol'n.)	250
2.	Cinnamon, Oil (10% sol'n.)	400
3.	Clove, Oil	60
4.	Coriander, Oil	30
5.	Nutmeg, Oil	80
6.	Orange, Oil	30
7.	Pimento, Oil	150
		1000

* Formulas which appear in this book

STRAWBERRY, EXTRACT (NATURAL) NO. 1

1.	Strawberries (freshly harvested)	100	kg

Express and to the residue add:

2.	Ethyl Alcohol 95%	30	l

Let stand for 3 days. Distill altogether. Add:

3.	Allspice, Oil	10	ml
4.	Cognac, Oil	5	ml
5.	Ethyl Acetate	8	ml
6.	Ethyl Salicylate	8	ml

Redistill to rectify.
Yield: 50 liters

STRAWBERRY, EXTRACT (NATURAL) NO. 2

1.	Strawberry Fruits	500
2.	Ethyl Alcohol 95%	250
3.	Distilled Water	250
		1000

Macerate for 5 days and distill over 750 cc.

STRAWBERRY, IMITATION NO. 1

1.	Aldehyde C-16	210
2.	Almond, Bitter (pure)	2
3.	Amyl Butyrate	25
4.	Amyl Formate	4
5.	Amyl Valerianate	3
6.	Benzyl Acetate	5
7.	Benzyl Valerianate	3
8.	Cinnamon, Oil	2
9.	Cognac, Oil	5
10.	Ethyl Acetate	15
11.	Ethyl Butyrate	35
12.	Ethyl Cinnamate	206
13.	Ethyl Formate	4
14.	Ethyl Phenyl Glycidate	206
15.	Eugenol	2
16.	Isoamyl Butyrate	25
17.	Isoethyl Butyrate	35
18.	Neroli, Oil	2
19.	Methyl Cinnamate	206
20.	Orange, Oil	1
21.	Orris, Oil	2
22.	Vanillin	2
		1000

STRAWBERRY, IMITATION NO. 2

1.	Acetaldehyde	2
2.	Acetic Acid	2
3.	Aldehyde C-9	5
4.	Aldehyde C-10	5
5.	Aldehyde C-14 (pure)	16
6.	Aldehyde C-16	25
7.	Almond, Bitter, Oil (pure)	1
8.	Amyl Acetate	20
9.	Amyl Butyrate	30
10.	Amyl Formate	9
11.	Amyl Valerianate	6
12.	Anethole	5
13.	Anisaldehyde	10
14.	Benzyl Acetate	8
15.	Benzyl Butyrate	6
16.	Benzyl Propionate	30
17.	Butyric Acid	1
18.	Cinnamon, Oil	2
19.	Cinnamyl Butyrate	4
20.	Citral	4
21.	Citronellol	2
22.	Citronellyl Acetate	2
23.	Citronellyl Formate	1
24.	Ethyl Acetate	15
25.	Ethyl Cinnamate	20
26.	Ethyl Formate	10
27.	Ethyl Oenanthate	1
28.	Ethyl Phenyl Glycidate	25
29.	Ethyl Salicylate	10
30.	Eugenol	2
31.	Geraniol	30
32.	Glycerin (neutral)	235
33.	Hexyl Cinnamic Aldehyde	20
34.	β-Ionone	20
35.	Isoethyl Butyrate	26
36.	Isojasmone	2
37.	Isovaleric Acid	2

38.	Lactic Acid	2
39.	Methyl Anthranilate	10
40.	Methyl Cinnamate	20
41.	Methyl Heptyne Carbonate	20
42.	Neroli, Oil	3
43.	Orange, Oil	1
44.	Orris, Oil	2
45.	Phenyl Ethyl Acetate	10
46.	Phenyl Ethyl Alcohol	20
47.	Phenyl Ethyl Butyrate	20
48.	Phenyl Ethyl Propionate	30
49.	Rhodinol	1
50.	Rhodinyl Butyrate	2
51.	Vanillin	10
52.	Ethyl Alcohol 95%	235
		1000

STRAWBERRY, IMITATION NO. 3

1.	Aldehyde C-16	50
2.	Aldehyde C-20	50
3.	Ethyl Phenyl Glycidate	50
4.	Strawberry, Extract (Natural) No. 1*	500
5.	Ethyl Alcohol 95%	175
6.	Distilled Water	175
		1000

STRAWBERRY, IMITATION NO. 4

1.	Ethyl Methylphenylglycidate	15
2.	β-Naphthyl Ethyl Ether	5
3.	Pineapple, Imitation No. 1*	150
4.	Raspberry, Imitation No. 1*	330
5.	Strawberry, Imitation No. 1*	500
		1000

STRAWBERRY, IMITATION NO. 5

1.	Ethyl Methylphenylglycidate	25
2.	β-Naphthyl Ethyl Ether	15
3.	Strawberry, Imitation No. 2*	480
4.	Ethyl Alcohol 95%	480
		1000

* Formulas which appear in this book

STRAWBERRY, IMITATION NO. 6

1.	Ethyl Methylphenylglycidate	25
2.	Pineapple, Imitation No. 2*	325
3.	Raspberry, Imitation No. 2*	325
4.	Strawberry, Imitation No. 3*	325
		1000

STRAWBERRY, IMITATION NO. 7

1.	Ethyl Methylphenylglycidate	10
2.	Pineapple, Imitation No. 3*	248
3.	Pineapple, Imitation No. 4*	248
4.	Raspberry, Imitation No. 3*	248
5.	Strawberry, Imitation No. 4*	246
		1000

STRAWBERRY, IMITATION NO. 8

1.	Ethyl Methylphenylglycidate	3
2.	β-Naphthyl Ethyl Ether	2
3.	Pineapple, Imitation No. 4*	335
4.	Raspberry, Imitation No. 4*	330
5.	Strawberry, Imitation No. 5*	330
		1000

STRAWBERRY, IMITATION NO. 9

1.	Ethyl Methylphenylglycidate	2
2.	β-Naphthyl Ethyl Ether	3
3.	Pineapple, Imitation No. 5*	100
4.	Pineapple, Imitation No. 6*	50
5	Raspberry, Imitation No. 5*	95
5.	Strawberry, Imitation No. 6*	750
		1000

STRAWBERRY, IMITATION NO. 10

1.	Amyl Acetate	30
2.	Amyl Butyrate	10
3.	Amyl Formate	10
4.	Amyl Valerianate	20

5.	Ethyl Acetate	15
6.	Ethyl Methylphenylglycidate	10
7.	Orris, Roots, Extract	50
8.	Strawberry, Imitation No. 7*	100
9.	Ethyl Alcohol 95%	755
		1000

STRAWBERRY, IMITATION NO. 11

1.	β-Naphthyl Ethyl Ether	50
2.	Strawberry, Imitation No. 8*	300
3.	Ethyl Alcohol 95%	650
		1000

STRAWBERRY, SYNTHETIC NO. 1

1.	Almond, Oil (pure)	20
2.	Amyl Butyrate	100
3.	Amyl Formate	50
4.	Amyl Valerate	3
5.	Benzyl Acetate	100
6.	Benzyl Valerate	3
7.	Cinnamon, Oil	15
8.	Cognac, Oil	20
9.	Ethyl Acetate	100
10.	Ethyl Butyrate	150
11.	Ethyl Cinnamate	2
12.	Ethyl Formate	50
13.	Eugenol	20
14.	Isoamyl Butyrate	100
15.	Isoethyl Butyrate	150
16.	Methyl Ethylphenylglycidate	2
17.	Neroli, Oil	20
18.	Orange, Oil (terpeneless)	50
19.	Orris, Oil	15
20.	Vanillin (10% sol'n.)	30
		1000

STRAWBERRY, SYNTHETIC NO. 2

1.	Amyl Acetate	30
2.	Amyl Butyrate	10
3.	Amyl Formate	10
4.	Amyl Valerianate	20
5.	Ethyl Acetate	15
6.	Ethyl Methylphenylglycidate	10
7.	Orris, Root, Oil	50
8.	Strawberry, Imitation No. 9*	428
9.	Ethyl Alcohol 95%	427
		1000

* Formulas which appear in this book

STRAWBERRY, SYNTHETIC NO. 3

1.	Aldehyde C-16	15
2.	Amyl Acetate	240
3.	Amyl Butyrate	120
4.	Ethyl Acetate	300
5.	Ethyl Benzoate	10
6.	Ethyl Butyrate	45
7.	Ethyl Formate	45
8.	Ethyl Nitrate	10
9.	Ethyl Salicylate	10
10.	Vanillin	5
11.	Glycerin (neutral)	200
		1000

STRAWBERRY, SYNTHETIC NO. 4

1.	Acetic Acid, Glacial	10
2.	Aldehyde C-14	4
3.	Aldehyde C-16	22
4.	Anethole	1
5.	Benzyl Acetate	20
6.	Ethyl Salicylate	3
7.	β-Ionone	3
8.	Methyl Anthranilate	20
9.	Methyl Cinnamate	5
10.	Methyl Heptyne Carbonate	2
11.	Vanillin	10
12.	Propylene Glycol	450
13.	Ethyl Alcohol 95%	450
		1000

STRAWBERRY, SYNTHETIC NO. 5

1.	Acetic Acid	3
2.	Aldehyde C-16	35
3.	Amyl Formate	42

4.	Benzyl Butyrate	8
5.	Benzyl Propionate	15
6.	Butyric Acid	2
7.	Cinnamyl Butyrate	2
8.	Ethyl Acetate	95
9.	Ethyl Butyrate	15
10.	Ethyl Cinnamate	30
11.	Isopropyl Butyrate	43
12.	Isovaleric Acid	5
13.	Methyl Heptyne Carbonate	5
14.	Phenyl Butyl Ketone	4
15.	Phenyl Ethyl Butyrate	21
16.	Phenyl Ethyl Formate	5
17.	Phenyl Ethyl Propionate	15
18.	Vanillin	5
19.	Ethyl Alcohol 95%	325
20.	Distilled Water	325
		1000

STRAWBERRY, SYNTHETIC NO. 6

1.	Amyl Butyrate	200
2.	Amyl Formate	48
3.	Benzyl Acetate	200
4.	Ethyl Acetate	200
5.	Ethyl Benzoate	85
6.	Ethyl Butyrate	135
7.	Ethyl Phenyl Glycidate	20
8.	Ethyl Salicylate	6
9.	Nerolin	2
10.	Vanillin	4
11.	Ethyl Alcohol 95%	100
		1000

STRAWBERRY, SYNTHETIC NO. 7

1.	Aldehyde C-14 (pure)	18
2.	Aldehyde C-16	12
3.	Benzaldehyde (pure)	3
4.	Benzyl Acetate	45
5.	Benzyl Benzoate	11
6.	Cinnamic Aldehyde	2
7.	Ethyl Acetate	17
8.	Ethyl Benzoate	15
9.	Ethyl Butyrate	24
10.	Ethyl Cinnamate	40
11.	Ethyl Formate	5
12.	Ethyl Pelargonate	20
13.	Ethyl Phenyl Glycidate	20
14.	Ethyl Salicylate	3
15.	Geraniol	10
16.	Isoamyl Acetate	11
17.	Isoamyl Butyrate	40
18.	Isoamyl Formate	25
19.	Isoamyl Isovalerianate	18
20.	Isobutyl Isovalerianate	1
21.	Nerolin	5
22.	Vanillin	5
23.	Ethyl Alcohol 95%	325
24.	Distilled Water	325
		1000

STRAWBERRY, SYNTHETIC NO. 8

1.	Amyl Acetate	90
2.	Amyl Butyrate	60
3.	Ethyl Acetate	150
4.	Ethyl Butyrate	150
5.	Ethyl Formate	30
6.	Ethyl Nitrate	30
7.	Ethyl Salicylate	30
8.	Glycerin (neutral)	60
9.	Ethyl Alcohol 95%	400
		1000

STRAWBERRY, SYNTHETIC NO. 9

1.	Aldehyde C-16	20
2.	Amyl Acetate	30
3.	Amyl Butyrate	20
4.	Ethyl Acetate	50
5.	Ethyl Butyrate	50
6.	Ethyl Formate	10
7.	Ethyl Nitrate	10
8.	Ethyl Salicylate	10
9.	Ethyl Alcohol 95%	400
10.	Distilled Water	400
		1000

STRAWBERRY, SYNTHETIC NO. 10 "GENERAL BASE"

1.	Aldehyde C-16	300
2.	Ethyl Phenyl Glycidate	200
3.	Methyl Cinnamate	200
4.	Methyl Heptyne Carbonate	5
5.	Nerolin	20
6.	Ethyl Alcohol 95%	138
7.	Distilled Water	137
		1000

STRAWBERRY, SYNTHETIC NO. 11

1.	Alcohol C-7	50
2.	Aldehyde C-14	25
3.	Aldehyde C-16	25
4.	Cinnamyl Isobutyrate	25
5.	Cinnamyl Isovalerate	35
6.	Ethyl Lactate	10
7.	Ethyl Valerate	25
8.	Propylene Glycol	400
9.	Vanillin	5
10.	Ethyl Alcohol 95%	400
		1000

STRAWBERRY, SYNTHETIC NO. 12

1.	Aldehyde C-16 (10% sol'n.)	20
2.	Ethyl Butyrate	200
3.	Ethyl Pelargonate	75
4.	Ethyl Phenyl Glycidate (10% sol'n.)	250
5.	Glycerol	125
6.	Methyl Anthranilate	10
7.	Methyl Cinnamate	10
8.	Vanillin (10% sol'n.)	10
9.	Ethyl Alcohol 95%	300
		1000

STRAWBERRY, SYNTHETIC NO. 13

1.	Aldehyde C-16 (10% sol'n.)	20
2.	Borneol	5
3.	Bornyl Acetate	5
4.	Ethyl Butyrate	100
5.	Ethyl Caproate	25
6.	Ethyl Phenyl Glycidate	200
7.	Ionone	10
8.	Methyl Cinnamate	50
9.	Vanillin (10% sol'n.)	10
10.	Ethyl Alcohol 95%	575
		1000

SYRUP, BASE FOR FLAVOR (PANCAKE)

1.	Caramel**	
2.	Citric Acid (10% sol'n.)	1
3.	Corn Sweetener (syrup)	300
4.	Flavor, Natural (10% sol'n.)†	10
5.	Flavor, Synthetic (10% sol'n.)†	5
6.	Potassium Sorbate (10% sol'n.)	1
7.	Sodium Benzoate (10% sol'n.)	1
8.	Distilled Water	70

SYRUP, SIMPLE, BASE FOR FLAVOR

1.	Sugar	3000	g
2.	Distilled Water	700	ml

TAMARIND, EXTRACT (NATURAL)

1.	Tamarind, Fruit Pulp	10	kg
2.	Ethyl Alcohol 95%	10	l
3.	Distilled Water	10	l

Let stand for 10 days, stirring for 1 h each day. Collect the juice, without any pressure. Add to the residue:

4.	Ethyl Alcohol 95%	10	l
5.	Distilled Water	10	l

** Quantity depending on desired color
† Flavor depending on individual preference

Let stand for 10 days, stirring for 1 h each day. Collect the juice, without any pressure. Add to the residue:

6.	Ethyl Alcohol 95%	10 l
7.	Distilled Water	10 l

Let stand for 10 days, stirring for 1 h each day. Put altogether and distill.
Yield: 60 liters

Note: The pulp of the tamarind fruit is the most useful for beverages. The pulp is about 75% of the fruit, with 30–40% sugar and 9–15% tartaric acid. The tartaric acid is useful for effervescent beverages.

Sugar can be added according to personal taste to make the beverage sweeter or more pleasant.

In large quantities, the beverage has a slightly purgative action.

The leaves of tamarind must not be used due to their acidic content.

The seeds of tamaraind, if pounded and boiled, form adhesives.

TANGERINE, EXTRACT (NATURAL)

1.	Tangerine, Peels (fresh, well ground)	10 kg
2.	Ethyl Alcohol 95%	20 l

Let stand for 3 days. Express and to the residue add:

3.	Distilled Water	20 l

Let stand for another 3 days and add:

4.	Orange, Sweet, Oil	6 l
5.	Tangerine, Oil	4 l
6.	Thyme, Oil	3 ml

Distill altogether.
Yield: 50 liters

TANGERINE, IMITATION NO. 1

1.	Ethyl Acetate	150
2.	Isoamyl Acetate	100
3.	Isoamyl Butyrate	350
4.	Orange, Bitter, Oil	100
5.	Tangerine, Oil	200
6.	Lemon, Oil	100
		1000

TANGERINE, IMITATION NO. 2

1.	Ethyl Acetate	150
2.	Ethyl Butyrate (10% sol'n.)	350
3.	Isoamyl Acetate	100
4.	Lemon, Oil	100
5.	Orange, Bitter, Oil	100
6.	Tangerine, Oil	200
		1000

TARRAGON

1.	Tarragon	30 kg

Blend with:

2.	Vinegar, Natural	240 l

Let stand for 1 week. Sieve and add:

3.	Vinegar, Natural	1600 l

Filter.

TEA, IMITATION NO. 1

1.	Benzyl Acetate	50
2.	Ethyl Acetate	400
3.	Ethyl Formate	100
4.	Ethyl Oenanthate	10
5.	Ethyl Pelargonate	60
6.	Isoamyl Butyrate	200
7.	Lemon, Oil	10
8.	Nerolin	2
9.	Phenyl Ethyl Alcohol	158
10.	Vanillin	10
		1000

TEA, IMITATION NO. 2

1.	Benzyl Acetate	50
2.	Bromelia	2
3.	Ethyl Acetate (10% sol'n.)	420
4.	Ethyl Formate	140
5.	Ethyl Oenanthate	7
6.	Ethyl Pelargonate	60
7.	Isoamyl Butyrate (10% sol'n.)	280
8.	Lemon, Oil	10
9.	Phenyl Ethyl Alcohol	1
10.	Vanillin (10% sol'n.)	30
		1000

TEA, NATURAL NO. 1

1.	Tea, Leaves (dry)	3 kg
2.	Ethyl Alcohol 95%	10 l
3.	Distilled Water	10 l

Let stand for 3 days. Filter.

TEA, NATURAL NO. 2

1.	Rose, Flower Petals	1 kg
2.	Tea, Leaves (dry)	2 kg
3.	Ethyl Alcohol 95%	10 l

Let stand for 1 day and then add:

4.	Water, Boiling	8 l

Let cool and express. Add:

5.	Pineapple (Ananas) Extract (Natural) No. 1*	1 l
6.	Lemon, Oil	24 ml
7.	Orange Flowers, Oil	8 ml

Filter.
Yield: 10 liters

TEA, NATURAL NO. 3

1.	Pineapple (Ananas), Extract (Natural) No. 1*	1500 ml
2.	Arrack	1 kg
3.	Lemon, Oil	150 ml
4.	Orange Flowers, Oil	15 ml
5.	Rose Petals (dry)	150 g
6.	Tea, Ceylon (black)	3 kg
7.	Ethyl Alcohol 95%	2 l
8.	Distilled Water	2 l

Let stand for 3 days. Percolate and then add:

9.	Distilled Water	q.s. 20 l

Concentration: 60 ml/gal

TOBACCO FORMULAS FOR IMPROVING FLAVOR AND ODOR

Family: Solanaceae
Genus: Nicotiana

SPECIES OF NATURAL TOBACCO

1. *N. acuminata*, Northern Syria
2. *N. latakia*, Turkey, Syria
3. *N. multivalis*
4. *N. nepansa*, Havana
5. *N. persica*, Iran, Shiraz
6. *N. quadrivalis*
7. *N. rustica*, southern Europe, Turkey
8. *N. tabacum*, South America

These formulas can be used to improve the natural flavor and odor of tobacco, for cigarettes, cigars, chewing tobacco, snuff tobacco, pipe tobacco, etc.

TOBACCO, CHEWING, FLAVOR NO. 1

1.	Cascarilla, Oil	50
2.	Cassia, Oil	50
3.	Clove, Oil	50
4.	Heliotropin	20
5.	Nutmeg, Oil	80
6.	Orange, Sweet, Oil	150
7.	Rhodinyl Valerianate	50
8.	Rose, Oil	30
9.	Tonka Beans, Tincture	500
10.	Vanillin	20
		1000

* Formulas which appear in this book

TOBACCO, CHEWING, FLAVOR NO. 2

1.	Anise Seeds, Oil	150
2.	Caraway, Oil	150
3.	Cascarilla, Oil	100
4.	Clove, Oil	150
5.	Nutmeg, Oil	100
6.	Valerian, Oil	200
7.	Vanilla Beans, Tincture	150
		1000

TOBACCO, CIGARETTE, FLAVOR NO. 1

1.	Bergamot, Oil	40
2.	Clove, Oil	10
3.	Cascarilla, Oil	100
4.	Geranium, Oil	400
5.	Isobutyl Valerianate	50
6.	Lavender, Oil	80
7.	Menthol	40
8.	Orange, Sweet, Oil	100
9.	Orris, Tincture	100
10.	Rose Otto, Oil	20
11.	Tonka Beans, Oil	60
		1000

TOBACCO, CIGARETTE, FLAVOR NO. 2

1.	Bergamot, Oil	30
2.	Cassia, Oil	5
3.	Clove, Oil	15
4.	Geranium, Oil	50
5.	Lemon, Oil	30
6.	Orange, Sweet, Oil	70
7.	Orris, Tincture	500
8.	Phenyl Ethyl Valerianate	20
9.	Tonka Beans, Tincture	30
10.	Vanilla, Tincture	250
		1000

* Formulas which appear in this book

TOBACCO, CIGARETTE, FLAVOR NO. 3

1.	Angelica Roots, Oil	8
2.	Cardamom, Oil	2
3.	Coriander Seeds, Oil	125
4.	Mace, Oil	15
5.	Tonka Beans, Oil	125
6.	Ethyl Alcohol 95%	363
7.	Distilled Water	362
		1000

TOBACCO FLAVOR, GENERAL

1.	Bergamot, Oil	50
2.	Clary Sage, Oil	10
3.	Cascarilla, Oil	50
4.	Castoreum, Resinoid	50
5.	Labdanum, Resinoid	50
6.	Licorice, Extract	200
7.	Methyl Ionone	50
8.	Phenyl Acetic Acid	100
9.	Rum, Ether Flavor*	350
10.	Sandalwood or Cedarwood, Oil	50
11.	γ-Valerolactone	20
12.	Vetiver, Oil	20
		1000

TOBACCO FLAVOR NO. 1

1.	Cascarilla, Oil	20
2.	Cinnamon Leaf, Oil	30
3.	Cognac, Oil	70
4.	Rose Otto, Oil	5
5.	Sandalwood, Oil	25
6.	Vanilla Beans, Tincture	100
7.	Ethyl Alcohol 95%	750
		1000

TOBACCO FLAVOR NO. 2

1.	Cedar, Oil	350
2.	Mastic (*Pistacia lentiscus*), Resinoid	60
3.	Methyl Eugenol	340
4.	Storax, Resinoid	250
		1000

TOBACCO FLAVOR NO. 3

1.	Cascarilla, Oil	300
2.	Cedar, Oil	250
3.	Clove, Oil	350
4.	Vanillin	100
		1000

TOBACCO FLAVOR NO. 4

1.	Amyl Valerianate	25
2.	Cascarilla, Oil	13
3.	Castor, Tincture	48
4.	Butyric Acid	36
5.	Ethyl Butyrate	135
6.	Ethyl Valerianate	13
7.	Geranium, Oil	25
8.	Lavender, Oil	15
9.	Peru Balsam	36
10.	Rum, Ether Flavor*	140
11.	Sandalwood, Oil	32
12.	St. John's Bread, Tincture	96
13.	Valerian, Oil	7
14.	Vanillin	25
15.	Ethyl Alcohol 95%	177
16.	Distilled Water	177
		1000

TOBACCO FLAVOR NO. 5

1.	Butyl Butyrate	275
2.	Cardamom, Oil	50
3.	Cinnamon, Oil	150
4.	Clove, Oil	125
5.	Ginger, Oil	250
6.	Isoeugenol	125
7.	Vanillin	25
		1000

TOBACCO FLAVOR NO. 6

1.	Bergamot, Oil	175
2.	Clove, Oil	50
3.	Cinnamon, Oil	50
4.	Ethyl Valerianate	50
5.	Geranium, Oil	175
6.	Lemon, Oil	175
7.	Methyl Ionone	50
8.	Orange, Oil	50
9.	Tonka Beans, Resinoid	175
10.	Vanillin	50
		1000

TOBACCO FLAVOR NO. 7

1.	Bergamot, Oil	40
2.	Cascarilla, Oil	40
3.	Clove, Oil	40
4.	Ethyl Valerianate	40
5.	Geranium, Oil	180
6.	Lavender, Oil	180
7.	Methyl Ionone	40
8.	Orange, Oil	180
9.	Rose, Oil	40
10.	Tonka Beans, Resinoid	180
11.	Vanillin	40
		1000

TOBACCO FLAVOR NO. 8

1.	Geranium, Oil	9
2.	Jasmine, Absolute	2
3.	Lavender, Oil	8
4.	Methyl Phenyl Acetate	1
5.	Orange Blossom, Absolute	5
6.	Orris, Tincture	800
7.	Patchouli, Oil	2
8.	Rose Otto, Oil	5
9.	Tonka, Absolute	5
10.	Tuberose, Absolute	3
11.	Vanilla Beans, Tincture	160
		1000

TOBACCO FLAVOR NO. 9

1.	Honey, Imitation No. 1*	20
2.	Lovage, Oil	20
3.	Peru Balsam	85
4.	Phenyl Ethyl Valerianate	20
5.	Propylene Glycol	238
6.	Rhodinol Acetate	20
7.	Rum, Oil*	245
8.	Rose, Otto, Oil	2
9.	Snakeroot, Oil	20
10.	Styrax	85

* Formulas which appear in this book

11.	Tolu Balsam	85
12.	Valerian, Oil	20
13.	Vanillin	140
		1000

TUTTI FRUTTI

1.	Pineapple (Ananas) Extract (Natural) No. 1*	360
2.	Lemon, Extract (Natural)*	240
3.	Raspberry, Extract (Natural) No. 1*	130
4.	Rum, Ether Flavor*	130
5.	Strawberry, Extract (Natural)*	140
		1000

VALERIAN, ROOT, EXTRACT (NATURAL)

1.	Valerian, Roots (well powdered)	300
2.	Ethyl Alcohol 95%	350
3.	Distilled Water	350
		1000

Macerate and let stand for 8 days. Distill.

VANILLA

1.	Vanilla, Oil	100
2.	Ethyl Alcohol 95%	900
		1000

VANILLA, CONCENTRATED FLAVOR

1.	Caramel Coloring (10% sol'n.)	100
2.	Glycerol	500
3.	Sugar	100
4.	Vanillin (10% sol'n.)	100
5.	Ethyl Alcohol 95%	200
		1000

* Formulas which appear in this book

VANILLA, FLAVOR NO. 1

1.	Caramel Coloring	10
2.	Glycerol	100
3.	Vanillin (10% sol'n.)	20
4.	Ethyl Alcohol 95%	870
		1000

VANILLA, FLAVOR NO. 2

1.	Bourbonal (Ethyl Vanillin) (10% sol'n.)	100
2.	Heliotropin, Piperonal	100
3.	Tonka, Oil	100
4.	Vanilla Beans, Oil	200
5.	Ethyl Alcohol 95%	500
		1000

VANILLA, FLAVOR NO. 3

1.	Vanilla, Beans Bourbonal	20
2.	Vanillin (10% sol'n.)	83
3.	Ethyl Alcohol 95%	897
		1000

VANILLA, IMITATION NO. 1

1.	Cascara Sagrada, Bark	100
2.	Chicory, Seeds	45
3.	Prune Juice	55
4.	Vanillin	30
5.	Ethyl Alcohol 95%	385
6.	Distilled Water	385
		1000

Boil and distill.

VANILLA, IMITATION NO. 2

1.	Furfuryl Alcohol	125
2.	Propylene Glycol	250
3.	Tolu Balsam	25
4.	Vanillin	600
		1000

VANILLA BEANS, EXTRACT (NATURAL) NO. 1

1.	Vanilla Beans (well crushed)	10	kg
2.	Ethyl Alcohol 95%	20	l
3.	Distilled Water	20	l

Macerate for 10 days. Express and to the residue add:

4.	Ethyl Alcohol 95%	20	l
5.	Distilled Water	20	l

Macerate for 10 days. Express and to the residue add:

6.	Ethyl Alcohol 95%	20	l
7.	Distilled Water	20	l

Let stand for another 10 days. Distill altogether.

Yield: 120 liters

VANILLA BEANS, EXTRACT (NATURAL) NO. 2

1.	Sugar	100
2.	Vanilla Beans (cut very fine)	100
3.	Ethyl Alcohol 95%	400
4.	Distilled Water	400
		1000

VANILLA BEANS, IMITATION

1.	Caramel (per desired color)		
2.	Sugar	2	kg
3.	Vanilla Beans, Extract (Natural) No. 1*	6	l
4.	Vanillin	200	g
5.	Ethyl Alcohol 95%	6	l
6.	Distilled Water	6	l

Yield: 20 liters

VANILLA BEANS, TINCTURE NO. 1

1.	Vanilla Beans (finely cut)	10	g
2.	Ethyl Alcohol 95%	990	ml

* Formulas which appear in this book

VANILLA BEANS, TINCTURE NO. 2

1.	Vanilla Beans (finely cut)	10	g
2.	Vanillin	10	g
3.	Ethyl Alcohol 95%	980	ml

VANILLIN, CRYSTAL (PARTIAL)

1.	Anisic Aldehyde	10
2.	Benzyl Benzoate	550
3.	Cinnamic Alcohol	40
4.	Heliotropin	100
5.	Vanillin	200
6.	Ethyl Alcohol 95%	100
		1000

VANILLIN, FLAVORED MIXTURE

1.	Cardamom, Oil	15
2.	Cinnamaldehyde	30
3.	Ethyl Acetate (10% sol'n.)	500
4.	Ethyl Oenanthate	85
5.	Eugenol	40
6.	Isoamyl Acetate (10% sol'n.)	250
7.	Vanillin (10% sol'n.)	80
		1000

VANILLIN NO. 1

1.	Glycerin (neutral)	50	ml
2.	Heliotropin	50	g
3.	Vanillin	450	g
4.	Ethyl Alcohol 95%	250	ml
5.	Distilled Water	200	ml

VANILLIN NO. 2 (ESTER MIXTURE)

1.	Cinnamic Aldehyde	30
2.	Ethyl Acetate	500
3.	Ethyl Oenanthate	85
4.	Eugenol	40
5.	Isoamyl Acetate	250
6.	Vanillin	95
		1000

VANILLIN, SUPER ODOR

1.	Anisic Aldehyde	10
2.	Benzyl Alcohol	200
3.	Benzyl Benzoate	200
4.	Cinnamic Alcohol	20
5.	Heliotropin	50
6.	Vanillin	100
7.	Ethyl Alcohol 95%	210
8.	Distilled Water	210
		1000

VANILLIN, WATER SOLUBLE

1.	Anisic Aldehyde	10
2.	Cinnamic Alcohol	20
3.	Heliotropin	50
4.	Propylene Glycol	300
5.	Vanillin	100
6.	Ethyl Alcohol 95%	260
7.	Distilled Water	260
		1000

VERMOUTH

1.	Agaric, White	8
2.	Aloe	18
3.	Angelica, Roots	13
4.	Anise, Seeds	5
5.	Balm	8
6.	Benzoin	5
7.	Calamus, Roots	16
8.	Chamomile, Flowers	2
9.	Cardamom	2
10.	Centaury	8
11.	Cinchona, Bark (Peruvian or Bolivian)	18
12.	Cinnamon, Ceylon, Quills	13
13.	Cloves	8
14.	Coriander, Seeds	18
15.	Dittany (Origanum leaves of Creta)	38
16.	Elder	18
17.	Elecampane, Roots	13
18.	Galangal, Roots	10
19.	Gentian, Roots	18
20.	Germander	13
21.	Hops, Flowers	13
22.	Hyssop	18
23.	Marjoram	2
24.	Nutmeg	23
25.	Orange, Bitter, Peels	10
26.	Orris, Roots and Powdered Flowers	10
27.	Pimento	3
28.	Quassia, Bitter, Wood	8
29.	Rhubarb, Roots	18
30.	Saffron, Thread	2
31.	Sage, Flowers and Leaves	10
32.	Star Anise, Seeds	5
33.	Sugar	50
34.	Thistle	13
35.	Thyme	18
36.	Vanilla	2
37.	Wine, White	500
38.	Wormwood	20
39.	Wort, Roots	13
40.	Zedoary	10
		1000

Macerate for 20 days in a double amount of ethyl alcohol 95% (2000 cc). Blend every day. Press and filter. Add caramel 2%. Filter.

Use: 1 liter for 100 liters of wine.

VERMOUTH, ITALIAN TYPE NO. 1

1.	Absinthe (Artemisia), Wormwood Oil	1
2.	Angelica, Root	10
3.	Cardamom, Seeds	35
4.	Cardo Benedict, Herb	20
5.	Calamus, Root	20
6.	Centaury	20
7.	Elecampane, Root	20
8.	Gentian, Root	10
9.	Germander	2
10.	Nutmeg	2
11.	Orange, Peels (dried)	1
12.	Ethyl Alcohol 95%	439
13.	Distilled Water	420
		1000

Let macerate for 10 days. Press and filter.
Use: 1 liter for 100 liters of wine.

VERMOUTH, ITALIAN TYPE NO. 2

1.	Absinthe	1	kg
2.	Angelica, Root	240	g
3.	Calamus, Root	1	kg
4.	Cardamom	150	g
5.	Cardo Santo (Blessed Thistle)	1	kg
6.	Centaury	1	kg
7.	Cinnamon, Bark	109	g
8.	Elecampane, Root	1	kg
9.	Gentian, Root	40	g
10.	Germander	1	kg
11.	Nutmeg	60	g
12.	Wine, White Sweet	375	l
13.	Ethyl Alcohol 95%	20	l

Let stand for 8 days. Press. Filter. Bottle.
Concentration: 1 liter for 100 liters of wine.

VINEGAR, SPICED

1.	Chilies, Hot Pepper	22	kg
2.	Cloves	14	kg
3.	Coriander	25	kg
4.	Ginger	15	kg
5.	Mustard Seeds	15	kg
6.	Pepper, Black	14	kg
7.	Pimiento	15	kg
8.	Vinegar, Natural (boiling)	280	gal

Let stand for 1 week for maceration. Sieve and blend with:

9.	Vinegar, Natural	600	gal

Filter.
Yield: 1000 gal

VIOLET, FLAVOR

1.	Bergamot, Oil	50
2.	Eugenol	20
3.	Heliotropin	40
4.	Hydroxycitronellal	30
5.	α-Ionone	200
6.	β-Ionone	150
7.	Lauric Aldehyde	2
8.	Methyl Ionone	100
9.	Musk	10
10.	Rose, Oil	30
11.	Sandalwood	10
12.	Vanillin (10% sol'n.)	20
13.	Ylang Ylang, Oil	40
14.	Ethyl Alcohol 95%	298
		1000

WALNUT, EXTRACT (NATURAL)

1.	Walnut Kernels (fresh without rancid taste, very well rasped or totally pulverized)	10	kg
2.	Ethyl Alcohol 95%	15	l
3.	Distilled Water	15	l

Macerate for 10 days, stirring for 1 h every day. Collect 20 l, without any pressure, and to the residue add:

4.	Distilled Water	20	l

Let stand for another 3 days and then add:

5.	Amyl Formate	45	ml
6.	Ethyl Oenanthate	25	ml

Distill altogether.
Yield: 30 liters

WALNUT, FLAVOR FOR KETCHUP

1.	Acetic Acid	1	ml
2.	Cardamom, Seeds (ground)	1	kg
3.	Cloves (ground)	1	kg
4.	Ginger, Root	1	kg
5.	Pepper, Black (ground)	1	kg
6.	Pimenta (ground)	1	kg
7.	Salt (20% sol'n.)	1	l
8.	Walnut Kernels (fresh, without rancid taste, well pulverized)	6	kg
9.	Ethyl Alcohol 95%	10	l
10.	Distilled Water	10	l

Macerate for 10 days, stirring for 1 h every day. Express and to the residue add:

11.	Ethyl Alcohol 95%	10	1
12.	Distilled Water	10	1

Let stand for another 3 days. Boil gently for 1 h. Cool and express. Put all juices together and filter.

Yield: 40 liters

WALNUT, IMITATION NO. 1

1.	Ethyl Valerianate	77
2.	Maple Flavor*	248
3.	Methyl-*p*-Cresol	38
4.	Valerian Root, Extract (Natural)*	637
		1000

WALNUT, IMITATION NO. 2

1.	Amyl Valerianate	57
2.	Anisaldehyde	23
3.	Benzaldehyde (pure)	21
4.	Butyric Acid	23
5.	Cardamom, Oil	7
6.	Clove, Oil	26
7.	Ethyl Acetate	45
8.	Ethyl Oenanthate	57
9.	Lemon, Oil	115
10.	Mace, Oil	100
11.	Orange, Sweet, Oil	50
12.	Vanillin	21
13.	Ethyl Alcohol 95%	455
		1000

WALNUT, IMITATION NO. 3

1.	Anisaldehyde	9
2.	Benzaldehyde (pure)	28
3.	Butyric Acid	6
4.	Cardamom, Oil	20
5.	Ethyl Acetate	34
6.	Ethyl Oenanthate	23
7.	Eugenol	10
8.	Isoamyl Isovalerianate	24
9.	Lemon, Oil	31
10.	Mace, Oil	45
11.	Nutmeg, Oil	6
12.	Orange, Oil	8
13.	Vanillin	21
14.	Ethyl Alcohol 95%	368
15.	Distilled Water	367
		1000

* Formulas which appear in this book

WALNUT, IMITATION NO. 4

1.	Anisaldehyde	12
2.	Benzaldehyde (pure, 10% sol'n.)	25
3.	Butyric Acid	10
4.	Cardamom, Oil	3
5.	Ethyl Acetate (10% sol'n.)	320
6.	Ethyl Oenanthate	190
7.	Eugenol	15
8.	Isoamyl Isovalerate (10% sol'n.)	220
9.	Lemon, Oil	75
10.	Mace, Oil	75
11.	Orange, Oil	25
12.	Vanillin (10% sol'n.)	30
		1000

WALNUT, IMITATION NO. 5

1.	Anisaldehyde	10
2.	Benzaldehyde (pure, 10% sol'n.)	20
3.	Butyric Acid	3
4.	Cardamom, Oil	2
5.	Ethyl Acetate (10% sol'n.)	300
6.	Ethyl Oenanthate (10% sol'n.)	300
7.	Eugenol	5
8.	Isoamyl Isovalerate (10% sol'n.)	300
9.	Lemon, Oil	10
10.	Nutmeg, Oil	20
11.	Orange, Oil	20
12.	Vanillin (10% sol'n.)	10
		1000

WALNUT, IMITATION NO. 6

1.	Anisaldehyde	5
2.	Benzaldehyde (pure, 10% sol'n.)	40
3.	Butyric Acid	7
4.	Cardamom, Oil	3
5.	Ethyl Acetate (10% sol'n.)	400

6.	Ethyl Oenanthate	200
7.	Eugenol	10
8.	Isoamyl Isovalerate	200
9.	Lemon, Oil	10
10.	Mace, Oil	60
11.	Orange, Oil	40
12.	Vanillin (10% sol'n.)	25
		1000

WINTERGREEN

1.	Ethyl Salicylate (10% sol'n.)	30
2.	Ethyl Alcohol 95%	970
		1000

WINTERGREEN, SYNTHETIC NO. 1

1.	Methyl Salicylate	50
2.	Ethyl Alcohol 95%	750
3.	Distilled Water	200
		1000

Stir. Filter.

WINTERGREEN, SYNTHETIC NO. 2

1.	Methyl Salicylate	30
2.	Ethyl Alcohol 95%	570
3.	Distilled Water	400
		1000

Stir. Filter.

WINTERGREEN, SYNTHETIC NO. 3

1.	Methyl Salicylate (10% sol'n.)	20
2.	Ethyl Alcohol 95%	980
		1000

* Formulas which appear in this book

WOODRUFF, EXTRACT (NATURAL)

1.	Pineapple (Ananas), Extract (Natural) No. 1*	1	l
2.	Grape, Extract (Natural) No. 1*	2	l
3.	Orange Flower, Extract (Natural)*	120	ml
4.	Tonka Beans (ground)	120	g
5.	Wine (Brandy)	1	l
6.	Woodruff Flowering Tops (fresh, crushed, and expressed**)	8	kg
7.	Ethyl Alcohol 95%	4	l

Let stand for 3 days. Express 10 l.

WOODRUFF, IMITATION

1.	Tonka Beans, Tincture (1:5)	1	l
2.	Vanillin	30	g
3.	Ethyl Alcohol 95% (hot)	450	ml
4.	Ethyl Alcohol 95%	4	l
5.	Distilled Water	5	l

Yield: 10 liters

WOODRUFF, SYNTHETIC NO. 1

1.	Benzyl Acetate	75
2.	Ethyl Acetate	240
3.	Ethyl Oenanthate	170
4.	Ethyl Pelargonate	100
5.	Isoamyl Butyrate	280
6.	Vanillin	135
		1000

WOODRUFF, SYNTHETIC NO. 2

1.	Benzyl Acetate	75
2.	Ethyl Acetate (10% sol'n.)	280
3.	Ethyl Oenanthate	170
4.	Ethyl Pelargonate	100
5.	Isoamyl Butyrate (10% sol'n.)	240
6.	Vanillin (10% sol'n.)	135
		1000

** The juice is discarded because of its greasy taste.

WORCESTERSHIRE SAUCE NO. 1

1.	Brandy	7	l
2.	Cherry Essence (Natural)*	5	l
3.	Coriander (ground)	1	kg
4.	Mace (ground)	1	kg
5.	Mushroom (dried and ground)	10	kg
6.	Pepper, Cayenne (pulverized)	1	kg
7.	Pimenta (ground)	1	kg
8.	Sugar	3	kg
9.	Tamarind, Extract (Natural)*	10	l
10.	Vinegar, Natural	70	l
11.	Walnut, Flavor for Ketchup*	10	l

Percolate after 10 days of stirring for 1 h each day. Filter.

Yield: 100 liters

Note: Well chopped garlic or onion may be added (1 kg).

WORCESTERSHIRE SAUCE NO. 2

1.	Cloves (ground)	3	kg
2.	Lemon, Peels (ground)	6	kg
3.	Nutmeg (ground)	3	kg
4.	Pepper, Cayenne (ground)	4	kg
5.	Soy Sauce, Flavor	4	l
6.	Sugar	3	kg
7.	Vinegar, Natural	70	l
8.	Walnut, Flavor for Ketchup*	8	l

Percolate after 10 days of stirring for 1 h each day. Filter.

Yield: 75 liters

Note: Well chopped garlic or onion may be added (1 kg).

---

* Formulas which appear in this book

Chapter XII:
CHEMICAL SPECIFICATIONS FOR PERFUME AND FLAVOR COMPONENTS

NOTE ON SOLVENTS:
An explanation is offered regarding the solvents listed for each ingredient of the formulas:

1. Fixed Oil—A nonvolatile fatty oil from a plant distinguished from the essential oil.
2. Mineral Oil—Any of various oils of mineral origin, especially the distillate from petroleum (petrolatum). Naphtha derives from a crude petroleum used as a solvent and is considered a mineral spirit.
3. Vegetable Oil—Any of the various oils obtained from plants and used industrially and in food products. Major vegetable oils include: linseed, cottonseed, soybean, castor, corn, sesame.
4. Volatile Oil—An oil that volatilizes with a distinctive flavor and odor of the original plant, and which is called an essential oil. It is used for flavor and perfume compositions.
5. Tincture—An alcoholic or aqueous-alcoholic solution of plants or minerals. Tincture is more diluted than fluid extract and less volatile than spirit.

ACETALDEHYDE

SYNONYMS: Acetic aldehyde; Aldehyde; Ethanal; Ethyl aldehyde
CAS NUMBER: 75-07-0
MOLECULAR FORMULA: C_2H_4O
MOLECULAR WEIGHT: 44.05
CHARACTERISTICS: *Form:* Liquid; *Color:* Colorless; *Odor:* Fruity, pungent
PHYSICAL PROPERTIES: *Specific gravity:* 0.783 (18 C); *Refractive index:* 1.3316 (20 C); *Boiling point:* 20.2 C; *Freezing point:* –123.5 C; *Flash point:* –40 F (Open Cup); *Solubility:* Soluble in benzene, gasoline, naphtha, toluene, xylene, turpentine, acetone
DERIVATION: Oxidation of ethylene; vapor-phase oxidation of propane and butane; direct conversion of ethylene

WARNING AND CAUTION: Highly flammable and toxic; dangerous fire and explosion risk

ACETATE C-8

SYNONYMS: Octyl acetate
MOLECULAR FORMULA: $C_{10}H_{20}O_2$
MOLECULAR WEIGHT: 172.27
CHARACTERISTICS: *Form:* Liquid; *Color:* Colorless; *Odor:* Orange, jasmine
PHYSICAL PROPERTIES: *Specific gravity:* 0.865–0.868 (25/25 C); *Refractive index:* 1.4180–1.4210 (20 C); *Flash point:* 185 F (TCC); *Solubility:* Soluble in 4 parts 70% ethyl alcohol 95%
DERIVATION: From oil of green tea and *Heracleum giganteum L.*

ACETATE C-9

SYNONYMS: Nonyl acetate
MOLECULAR FORMULA: $C_{11}H_{22}O_2$
MOLECULAR WEIGHT: 186.30
CHARACTERISTICS: *Form:* Liquid; *Color:* Colorless; *Odor:* Fruity floral, strong
PHYSICAL PROPERTIES: *Specific gravity:* 0.864–0.868 (25/25 C); *Refractive index:* 1.4220–1.4260 (20 C); *Flash point:* > 212 F (TCC)

ACETATE C-10

SYNONYMS: Decyl acetate
MOLECULAR FORMULA: $C_{12}H_{24}O_2$
MOLECULAR WEIGHT: 200.32
CHARACTERISTICS: *Form:* Liquid; *Color:* Colorless; *Odor:* Floral, orange-rose
PHYSICAL PROPERTIES: *Specific gravity:* 0.862–0.866 (25/25 C); *Refractive index:* 1.4250–1.4300 (20 C); *Boiling point:* 187–190 C; *Flash point:* > 212 F (TCC); *Solubility:* Soluble in ethyl alcohol 95% (2 parts 80%), ether, glacial acetic acid, benzene; insoluble in water

ACETATE C-11

SYNONYMS: 10-Undecen-1-yl acetate
MOLECULAR FORMULA: $C_{13}H_{24}O_2$
MOLECULAR WEIGHT: 212.33
CHARACTERISTICS: *Form:* Liquid; *Color:* Colorless; *Odor:* Floral-fatty
PHYSICAL PROPERTIES: *Specific gravity:* 0.876–0.880 (25/25 C); *Refractive index:* 1.4380–1.4420 (20 C); *Flash point:* 212 F (TCC); *Solubility:* Soluble in ethyl alcohol 95% (2 parts 80%)

ACETATE C-12

SYNONYMS: Lauryl acetate; Dodecyl acetate
MOLECULAR FORMULA: $C_{14}H_{28}O_2$
MOLECULAR WEIGHT: 228.37
CHARACTERISTICS: *Form:* Liquid; *Color:* Colorless; *Odor:* Light citrus-rose
PHYSICAL PROPERTIES: *Specific gravity:* 0.860–0.865 (25/25 C); *Refractive index:*

1.4320–1.4360 (20 C); *Flash point:* > 212 F (TCC); *Solubility:* Soluble in ethyl alcohol 95% (4 parts 80%)

ALDEHYDE C-14 PURE

SYNONYMS: 4-Hydroxyundecanoic acid lactone; γ-Undelactone; Peach aldehyde; γ-*n*-Heptylbutyrolactone; Undecanolide-1,4; Persicol; γ-Undecalactone
CAS NUMBER: 710-04-3
MOLECULAR FORMULA: $C_{11}H_{20}O_2$
MOLECULAR WEIGHT: 184.28
CHARACTERISTICS: *Form:* Liquid; *Color:* Slightly yellow to yellowish; *Odor:* Strong peach; *Taste:* Peach
PHYSICAL PROPERTIES: *Specific gravity:* 0.940–0.944 (25/25 C); *Refractive index:* 1.4500–1.4540 (20 C); *Flash point:* 212 F (TCC); *Solubility:* Soluble in ethyl alcohol 95% (5 parts 60%), benzyl alcohol, benzyl benzoate, organic solvents
DERIVATION: From β-ionone and methyl or ethyl chloroacetate

ALDEHYDE C-16 PURE

SYNONYMS: Ethyl α,β-epoxy-β-methylhydrocinnamate; Strawberry aldehyde; Ethyl methylphenylglycidate
MOLECULAR FORMULA: $C_{12}H_{14}O_2$
MOLECULAR WEIGHT: 206.24
CHARACTERISTICS: *Form:* Liquid; *Color:* Colorless to yellowish; *Odor:* Strong strawberry; *Taste:* Strawberry
PHYSICAL PROPERTIES: *Specific gravity:* 1.0887–1.0920 (25/25 C); *Refractive index:* 1.5040–1.5090 (20 C); *Solubility:* Soluble clear in ethyl alcohol 95% (4 parts 70%)
WARNING AND CAUTION: Low toxicity

ALDEHYDE C-18

SYNONYMS: 4-Hydroxynonanoic acid lactone; γ-Nonalactone; Prunolide; γ-*n*-Amylbutyrolactone; Nonanolide-1,4; Coconut aldehyde
MOLECULAR FORMULA: $C_9H_{16}O_2$
MOLECULAR WEIGHT: 156.23
CHARACTERISTICS: *Form:* Liquid; *Color:* Slightly yellow to yellow; *Odor:* Strong coconut-like
PHYSICAL PROPERTIES: *Specific gravity:* 0.958–0.965 (25/25 C); *Refractive index:* 1.4460–1.4500 (20 C); *Flash point:* 212 F (TCC); *Solubility:* Soluble in ethyl alcohol 95% (2 parts 60%)

ALLYL SULFIDE

SYNONYMS: Diallyl sulfide; Thioallyl ether; Garlic oil; 3,3-Thiobis (1-propene)
MOLECULAR FORMULA: $C_6H_{10}S$
MOLECULAR WEIGHT: 114.20
CHARACTERISTICS: *Form:* Liquid; *Color:* Colorless; *Odor:* Garlic
PHYSICAL PROPERTIES: *Specific gravity:* 0.888 (27/4 C); *Refractive index:* 1.4877 (27 C); *Boiling point:* 139 C; *Solubility:* Soluble in alcohol, chloroform, ether,

carbon tetrachloride; insoluble in water
DERIVATION: From allyl bromide and sulfur in solution with sodium
WARNING AND CAUTION: Highly toxic

AMYL ACETATE
SYNONYMS: Amyl acetate ester; Banana oil; Pear oil; Pentyl acetate; Amyl acetic ester
CAS NUMBER: 628-63-7
MOLECULAR FORMULA: $C_7H_{14}O_2$
MOLECULAR WEIGHT: 130.13
CHARACTERISTICS: *Form:* Liquid; *Color:* Colorless; *Odor:* Banana
PHYSICAL PROPERTIES: *Flash point:* 65–95 F (CC); *Solubility:* Soluble in alcohol; slightly soluble in water
DERIVATION: From amyl alcohol with acetic acid and a small amount of sulfuric acid as a catalyst
WARNING AND CAUTION: Flammable; moderately toxic

AMYL ALCOHOL
SYNONYMS: (a) Primary (normal): *n*-Butylcarbinol; *n*-Amyl alcohol; 1-Pentanol; (b) Secondary (iso): 1-Methylbutanol; 2-Pentanol; (c) Tertiary: Amylene hydrate; Dimethylethyl carbinol; 1-Dimethylpropyl alcohol
CAS NUMBER: (a) 71-41-0 (primary); (b) 6032-29-7 (secondary); (c) 75-85-4 (tertiary)
MOLECULAR FORMULA: $C_5H_{12}O$
MOLECULAR WEIGHT: 88.11
CHARACTERISTICS: *Form:* Liquid; *Color:* Colorless; *Odor:* Camphor; *Taste:* Burning
PHYSICAL PROPERTIES: *Specific gravity:* 0.825 (20 C); *Refractive index:* 1.4025 (20 C); *Boiling point:* (a) 137 C (primary); (b) 118 C (secondary); (c) 102 C (tertiary); *Flash point:* 70 F (TOC); *Solubility:* Soluble in alcohol; slightly soluble in water
DERIVATION: Fractional distillation of mixed alcohol from chlorination and alkaline hydrolysis of pentane
WARNING AND CAUTION: Flammable; moderately toxic

AMYL BUTYRATE
SYNONYMS: Butanoic acid pentyl ester; Isoamyl *n*-butyrate; Isoamyl butyric ester
CAS NUMBER: 106-27-4
MOLECULAR FORMULA: $C_9H_{18}O_2$
MOLECULAR WEIGHT: 158.23
CHARACTERISTICS: *Form:* Liquid; *Color:* Colorless; *Odor:* Apricot
PHYSICAL PROPERTIES: *Specific gravity:* 0.8832–0.866 (15 C); *Refractive index:* 1.4110 (20 C); *Boiling point:* 150–180 C; *Freezing point:* –73.2 C; *Solubility:* Soluble in alcohol, ether; slightly soluble in water
DERIVATION: By treating isoamyl alcohol with butyric acid
WARNING AND CAUTION: Combustible; low toxicity

AMYL FORMATE

MOLECULAR FORMULA: $C_6H_{12}O_2$
MOLECULAR WEIGHT: 116.13
CHARACTERISTICS: *Form:* Liquid; *Color:* Colorless; *Odor:* Plum
PHYSICAL PROPERTIES: *Specific gravity:* 0.880–0.885 (25/25 C); *Boiling point:* 123.5 C; *Flash point:* 80 F (TCC); *Solubility:* Soluble in alcohol, oils, hydrocarbons, ketones; slightly soluble in water
WARNING AND CAUTION: Flammable; moderately toxic

AMYL VALERATE

SYNONYMS: Isoamyl valerate; Apple essence; Apple oil; Isoamyl isovalerate; Amyl valerianate; Amyl isovalerate; Isoamyl valerianate
MOLECULAR FORMULA: $C_{10}H_{20}O_2$
MOLECULAR WEIGHT: 172.26
CHARACTERISTICS: *Form:* Liquid; *Color:* Clear, colorless; *Odor:* Apple when diluted with alcohol
PHYSICAL PROPERTIES: *Specific gravity:* 0.8812 (25/25 C); *Refractive index:* 1.413 (19 C); *Boiling point:* 203.7 C; *Solubility:* Soluble in alcohol, ether; slightly soluble in water
DERIVATION: By adding sulfuric acid to a mixture of amyl alcohol and valeric acid further distilling
WARNING AND CAUTION: Combustible; low toxicity

ANETHOLE

SYNONYMS: Isoestragole; *p*-Propenylphenyl methyl ether; 1-Methoxy-4-(1-propenyl) benzene; *p*-Propenyl anisole; Anise camphor
MOLECULAR FORMULA: $C_{10}H_{12}O$
MOLECULAR WEIGHT: 148.20
CHARACTERISTICS: *Form:* Liquid; *Color:* Colorless; *Odor:* Anise
PHYSICAL PROPERTIES: *Specific gravity:* 0.984–0.987 (25/25 C); *Refractive index:* 1.5570–1.5610 (20 C); *Optical rotation:* 0.15°; *Freezing point:* 20 C; *Flash point:* 212 F (TCC); *Solubility:* Soluble in 2 parts of 90% ethyl alcohol
DERIVATION: From aniseed, star anise, fennel oils, from leaves of *Clausena anisata hook, Backhousia anisata,* and *Magnolia salicifolia maxim*

ANISALDEHYDE

SYNONYMS: Anisyl aldehyde; *p*-Methoxybenzaldehyde; 4-Methoxybenzaldehyde; Anisic aldehyde
CAS NUMBER: 123-11-5
MOLECULAR FORMULA: $C_8H_8O_2$
MOLECULAR WEIGHT: 136.14
CHARACTERISTICS: *Form:* Liquid; *Color:* Colorless to yellowish; *Odor:* Hawthorn
PHYSICAL PROPERTIES: *Specific gravity:* 1.119–1.122 (25/25 C); *Refractive index:* 1.572–1.5764 (20 C); *Boiling point:* 245 C; *Freezing point:* 0 C; *Solubility:*

Soluble in 5 parts 50% ethyl alcohol 95%
DERIVATION: From anethole or anisole by oxidation
WARNING AND CAUTION: Combustible

BENZALDEHYDE
SYNONYMS: Benzoic aldehyde; Artificial essential oil of almond
CAS NUMBER: 100-52-7
MOLECULAR FORMULA: C_7H_6O
MOLECULAR WEIGHT: 106.12
CHARACTERISTICS: *Form:* Liquid; *Color:* Colorless; *Odor:* Bitter almond; *Taste:* Burning aromatic
PHYSICAL PROPERTIES: *Specific gravity:* 1.041–1.046 (25/25 C); *Refractive index:* 1.5440–1.5456 (20 C); *Boiling point:* 178 C; *Freezing point:* –56 C; *Flash point:* 145 F (TCC); *Solubility:* Soluble in 3 parts 60% ethyl alcohol 95%
DERIVATION: Occurs in kernels of bitter almond; synthetically made from benzyl chloride and lime, or by oxidation of toluene
WARNING AND CAUTION: Narcotic in high concentration; causes dermatitis by contact

BENZOIC ACID
SYNONYMS: Carboxybenzene; Benzenecarboxylic acid; Dracylic acid; Phenylformic acid
CAS NUMBER: 65-85-0
MOLECULAR FORMULA: $C_7H_6O_2$
MOLECULAR WEIGHT: 122.12
CHARACTERISTICS: *Form:* Scales, needle crystals; *Color:* White; *Odor:* Benzoin or benzaldehyde
PHYSICAL PROPERTIES: *Specific gravity:* 1.2659 (25/25 C); *Boiling point:* 249.2 C; *Freezing point:* 121.25 C
DERIVATION: Occurs naturally in benzoin resin; decarboxylation of phthalic acid by steam in the presence of catalyst; chlorination of toluene to yield benzotrichloride which is hydrolyzed to benzoic acid; oxidation of toluene; from benzoin resin
WARNING AND CAUTION: May cause nausea and gastroenteric disturbance, allergic reactions

BENZYL ACETATE
SYNONYMS: Phenylmethyl acetate; Acetic acid phenylmethyl ester; Acetic acid benzyl ester
MOLECULAR FORMULA: $C_9H_{10}O_2$
MOLECULAR WEIGHT: 150.17
CHARACTERISTICS: *Form:* Liquid; *Color:* White; *Odor:* Floral, pear
PHYSICAL PROPERTIES: *Specific gravity:* 1.059–1.062 (15 C); *Refractive index:* 1.5015–1.5035 (20 C); *Flash point:* 216 F (TCC); *Solubility:* Soluble in alcohol, ether
DERIVATION: From benzyl chloride with sodium acetate in a solvent; by esterification of benzyl alcohol with acetic anhydride or acetic acid triethylamine; naturally

in jasmine and other plants
WARNING AND CAUTION: Moderately toxic; irritant of the skin

BENZYL ALCOHOL
SYNONYMS: α-Hydroxytoluene; Phenyl methanol; Phenyl carbinol; Benzene methanol
CAS NUMBER: 100-51-6
MOLECULAR FORMULA: C_7H_8O
MOLECULAR WEIGHT: 108.13
CHARACTERISTICS: *Form:* Liquid; *Color:* White; *Odor:* Slight; *Taste:* Sharp burning
PHYSICAL PROPERTIES: *Specific gravity:* 1.040–1.050 (25/25 C); *Refractive index:* 1.5385–1.5405; *Boiling point:* 206 C; *Flash point:* 213 F (TCC); *Solubility:* Soluble in alcohol, chloroform, ether, water
DERIVATION: By hydrolysis of benzyl chloride; from benzaldehyde by catalystic reduction or Cannizaro reaction
WARNING AND CAUTION: Combustible; low toxicity

BENZYL BENZOATE
SYNONYMS: Benzoic acid phenyl methyl ester; Benzoic acid benzyl ester; Benzyl benzene carboxylate; Ascabin; Ascabiol; Benylate; Venzonate; Vanzoate
CAS NUMBER: 120-51-4
MOLECULAR FORMULA: $C_{14}H_{12}O_2$
MOLECULAR WEIGHT: 212.24
CHARACTERISTICS: *Form:* Liquid; *Color:* White; *Odor:* Faint aromatic; *Taste:* Sharp burning
PHYSICAL PROPERTIES: *Specific gravity:* 1.116–1.120 (25/25 C); *Refractive index:* 1.568–1.569 (20 C); *Boiling point:* 325 F; *Freezing point:* 18.8 C; *Flash point:* 298 F (TCC); *Solubility:* Soluble in alcohol, chloroform, ether; insoluble in water, glycerin
DERIVATION: Contained in Peru and Tolu balsam; by esterifying benzyl alcohol with benzoic acid, in presence of triethylamine; action of sodium benzylate on benzaldehyde
WARNING AND CAUTION: Combustible; low toxicity

BENZYL FORMATE
SYNONYMS: Formic acid phenylmethyl ester; Formic acid benzyl ester
MOLECULAR FORMULA: $C_8H_8O_2$
MOLECULAR WEIGHT: 136.14
CHARACTERISTICS: *Form:* Liquid; *Odor:* Fruity, spicy
PHYSICAL PROPERTIES: *Specific gravity:* 1.083–1.087 (25/25 C); *Refractive index:* 1.511–1.513 (20 C); *Boiling point:* 203 C; *Solubility:* Soluble in alcohol; insoluble in water
DERIVATION: From formic acid and benzyl alcohol
WARNING AND CAUTION: Combustible

BORNEOL

SYNONYMS: endo-1,7,7-Trimethylbicyclo (2,2,1) heptane-2-ol; endo-2-Bornanol; endo-2-Camphanol; endo-2-Hydrocamphane; Bornyl alcohol; Baros camphor; Sumatra camphor; Dryobalanops camphor; Bhimsaim camphor; Malayan camphor; Camphol; Borneo camphor
CAS NUMBER: 507-70-0
MOLECULAR FORMULA: $C_{10}H_{18}O$
MOLECULAR WEIGHT: 154.24
CHARACTERISTICS: *Form:* Lumps; *Color:* White, translucent; *Odor:* Camphor
PHYSICAL PROPERTIES: *Specific gravity:* 1.011 (25/25 C); *Boiling point:* 212 C; *Freezing point:* 203 C; *Flash point:* 150 F (TCC); *Solubility:* Soluble in alcohol, ether; insoluble in water
DERIVATION: By reduction of camphor; from wood of *Dyrobalanops camphora*, a tree of Sumatra and Borneo (solid crystalline mass deposited in the trunks)
WARNING AND CAUTION: Moderately toxic; flammable

BORNYL ACETATE

SYNONYMS: 1,7,7-Trimethylbicyclo (2,2,1) heptan-2-ol acetate; Borneol acetate; Bornyl acetic ether; Bornyl acetate pure laevo
MOLECULAR FORMULA: $C_{12}H_{20}O_2$
MOLECULAR WEIGHT: 196.28
CHARACTERISTICS: *Form:* Crystals; *Color:* Colorless; *Odor:* Camphoraceous
PHYSICAL PROPERTIES: *Specific gravity:* 0.980–0.984 (25/25 C); *Refractive index:* 1.463–1.465 (20 C); *Solubility:* Soluble in 3 parts 70% ethyl alcohol, ether
DERIVATION: Interaction of borneol and acetic anhydride in presence of formic acid
WARNING AND CAUTION: Moderately toxic; flammable

BROMELIA

See Nerolin

***n*-BUTYL ACETATE**

SYNONYMS: Acetic acid butyl ester
CAS NUMBER: 123-86-4
MOLECULAR FORMULA: $C_6H_{12}O_2$
MOLECULAR WEIGHT: 116.16
CHARACTERISTICS: *Form:* Liquid; *Color:* Colorless; *Odor:* Fruity
PHYSICAL PROPERTIES: *Specific gravity:* 0.8826 (20/20 C); *Refractive index:* 1.3951 (20 C); *Boiling point:* 126.3 C; *Freezing point:* –75 C; *Flash point:* 92 F (TOC); *Solubility:* Soluble in alcohol, ether, hydrocarbons; slightly soluble in water
DERIVATION: Esterification and distillation after contact of butyl alcohol in the presence of a catalyst such as sulfuric acid
WARNING AND CAUTION: Flammable; moderately toxic; skin irritant

***n*-BUTYL BUTYRATE**

SYNONYMS: Butyl butanoate; Butanoic acid butyl ester; Butyric acid butyl ester; *n*-Butyl *n*-butyrate

CAS NUMBER: 109-21-7
MOLECULAR FORMULA: $C_8H_{16}O_2$
MOLECULAR WEIGHT: 144.21
CHARACTERISTICS: *Form:* Liquid
PHYSICAL PROPERTIES: *Specific gravity:* 0.8692 (20/20 C); *Refractive index:* 1.4064 (20 C); *Boiling point:* 165 C; *Freezing point:* –91.5 C; *Flash point:* 128 F (OC); *Solubility:* Soluble in alcohol, ether; insoluble in water
WARNING AND CAUTION: Moderately toxic; irritant and narcotic; flammable

BUTYRIC ACID
SYNONYMS: *n*-Butyric acid; Butanoic acid; Ethylacetic acid; Propylformic acid
CAS NUMBER: 107-92-6
MOLECULAR FORMULA: $C_4H_8O_2$
MOLECULAR WEIGHT: 88.10
CHARACTERISTICS: *Form:* Liquid; *Color:* Colorless; *Odor:* Rancid; *Taste:* Unpleasant
PHYSICAL PROPERTIES: *Specific gravity:* 0.9583 (20/4 C); *Refractive index:* 1.3981 (20 C); *Boiling point:* 163.5 C; *Freezing point:* –5 to –8 C; *Flash point:* 170 F (TCC); *Solubility:* Soluble in alcohol, ether, water
DERIVATION: Occurs as glyceride in animal fats; produced as a by-product in hydrocarbon synthesis, by oxidation of butyraldehyde, and by fermentation of molasses or starch
WARNING AND CAUTION: Combustible; low toxicity

CAPRALDEHYDE
SYNONYMS: *n*-Decanal; Capric aldehyde; *n*-Decyl aldehyde; Aldehyde C-10
MOLECULAR FORMULA: $C_{10}H_{20}O$
MOLECULAR WEIGHT: 156.27
CHARACTERISTICS: *Form:* Liquid; *Color:* Colorless to light yellow; *Odor:* Floral fatty
PHYSICAL PROPERTIES: *Specific gravity:* 0.831-0.838 (15 C); *Refractive index:* 1.427–1.431 (20 C); *Solubility:* Soluble in 80% alcohol, fixed oils, volatile oils, mineral oils; insoluble in water and glycerol
DERIVATION: Lemongrass; citronella; orange; synthetically by oxidation of the alcohol or reduction of the acid
WARNING AND CAUTION: Combustible; low toxicity

CARAMEL, COLORING
CHARACTERISTICS: *Form:* Powder or thick liquid; *Color:* Dark brown; *Odor:* Burnt sugar; *Taste:* Bitter taste
PHYSICAL PROPERTIES: *Specific gravity:* 1.35 (25/25 C); *Solubility:* Soluble in diluted alcohol, water; insoluble in chloroform, ether, organic solvents
DERIVATION: Heating sugar or glucose, adding small quantities of alkali, alkaline carbonate, or trace of mineral acid during the heating; heating sucrose, adding small quantities of sodium carbonate during heating

CHLOROFORM

SYNONYMS: Trichloromethane
CAS NUMBER: 67-66-3
MOLECULAR FORMULA: $CHCl_3$
MOLECULAR WEIGHT: 119.39
CHARACTERISTICS: *Form:* Liquid; *Color:* Colorless; *Odor:* Characteristic; *Taste:* Sweet
PHYSICAL PROPERTIES: *Specific gravity:* 1.485 (20/20 C); *Refractive index:* 1.4476 (20 C); *Boiling point:* 61.2 C; *Freezing point:* –63.5 C; *Solubility:* Soluble in alcohol, ether, benzene, naphtha, fixed volatile oils; slightly soluble in water
DERIVATION: Chlorinated lime with acetone, acetaldehyde, or ethyl alcohol; by-product from chlorination of methane; purification with concentrated sulfuric acid and rectification; from acetone and bleaching powder by addition of sulfuric acid; methane chlorination
WARNING AND CAUTION: Highly toxic; narcotic; prolonged inhalation or ingestion may be fatal

CINEOL

SYNONYMS: Eucalyptol; Cajeputol; Cineole
CAS NUMBER: 470-82-6
MOLECULAR FORMULA: $C_{10}H_{18}O$
MOLECULAR WEIGHT: 154.25
CHARACTERISTICS: *Form:* Liquid; *Color:* Colorless; *Odor:* Camphor, pungent; *Taste:* Spicy
PHYSICAL PROPERTIES: *Specific gravity:* 0.921–0.923 (25/25 C); *Refractive index:* 1.4550–1.4600 (20 C); *Boiling point:* 174–177 C; *Freezing point:* 0 C; *Solubility:* Soluble in alcohol, chloroform, ether, glacial acetic acid, and fixed or volatile oils; slightly soluble in water
DERIVATION: By fractional distillation of eucalyptus oil, followed by freezing
WARNING AND CAUTION: Combustible; moderately toxic

CINNAMIC ALDEHYDE

SYNONYMS: Cinnamaldehyde; 3-Phenylpropenal; Cinnamyl aldehyde
CAS NUMBER: 104-55-2
MOLECULAR FORMULA: C_9H_8O
MOLECULAR WEIGHT: 132.16
CHARACTERISTICS: *Form:* Oil; *Color:* Yellowish; *Odor:* Cinnamon; *Taste:* Sweet
PHYSICAL PROPERTIES: *Specific gravity:* 1.048–1.052 (25/25 C); *Refractive index:* 1.618–1.623 (20 C); *Boiling point:* 248 C; *Freezing point:* –8 C; *Solubility:* Soluble in 5 volumes 60% alcohol; slightly soluble in water
DERIVATION: From Ceylon and Chinese cinnamon oils; by condensation of benzaldehyde and acetaldehyde
WARNING AND CAUTION: Combustible

CITRAL

SYNONYMS: Geranial; Geranialdehyde; 3,7-Dimethyl-2,6-octadienal
CAS NUMBER: 5392-40-5

MOLECULAR FORMULA: $C_{10}H_{16}O$
MOLECULAR WEIGHT: 152.24
CHARACTERISTICS: *Form:* Liquid; *Color:* Pale yellow; *Odor:* Strong lemon
PHYSICAL PROPERTIES: *Specific gravity:* 0.891–0.897 (15 C); *Refractive index:* 1.4860–1.4900 (20 C); *Solubility:* Soluble in alcohol, benzyl benzoate, diethyl phthalate, glycerin, propylene glycol, mineral oils, fixed oils
DERIVATION: Lemongrass oil by fractional distillation; synthetically by oxidation of geraniol, nerol, or linalool by chromic acid
WARNING AND CAUTION: Combustible

CITRONELLAL

SYNONYMS: 3,7-Dimethyl-6-octen-1-al; 3,7-Dimethyloct-6 (or 7)-enal
MOLECULAR FORMULA: $C_{10}H_{18}O$
MOLECULAR WEIGHT: 154.25
CHARACTERISTICS: *Form:* Liquid; *Color:* Colorless to slightly yellow; *Odor:* Strong and intense lemon
PHYSICAL PROPERTIES: *Specific gravity:* 0.848–0.856 (25/25 C); *Refractive index:* 1.4460–1.4520 (20 C); *Optical rotation:* 8–11°; *Boiling point:* 205 C; *Flash point:* 178 F (TCC); *Solubility:* Soluble in 5 parts 70% alcohol, ether; slightly soluble in water
DERIVATION: Found as a main constituent in oils of citronella, lemongrass, and other oils

CITRONELLOL

SYNONYMS: 3,7-Dimethyl-6-octen-1-ol; 2,6-Dimethyl-2-octen-8-ol; Cephrol
CAS NUMBER: 106-22-9
MOLECULAR FORMULA: $C_{10}H_{20}O$
MOLECULAR WEIGHT: 156.27
CHARACTERISTICS: *Form:* Liquid; *Color:* Colorless; *Odor:* Light rosy
PHYSICAL PROPERTIES: *Specific gravity:* 0.852–0.860 (25/25 C); *Refractive index:* 1.4530–1.4600 (20 C); *Optical rotation:* –1.30 to 3°; *Boiling point:* 108.4 C; *Solubility:* Soluble in alcohol, ether; slightly soluble in water
DERIVATION: Constituent of rose, geranium, *Eucalyptus citriodora*, Ceylon and Java citronella oils, verbena, savin, oakmoss, palmarosa

DECYL ACETATE

See Acetate C-10

DIACETYL

SYNONYMS: 2,3-Butanedione; Butanedione; Biacetyl; Dimethyl diketone; Dimethyl glyoxal; 2,3-Diketobutane
CAS NUMBER: 431-03-8
MOLECULAR FORMULA: $C_4H_6O_2$
MOLECULAR WEIGHT: 86.09
CHARACTERISTICS: *Form:* Liquid; *Color:* Yellowish-green; *Odor:* Quinone
PHYSICAL PROPERTIES: *Specific gravity:* 0.990 (15/15 C); *Refractive index:* 1.3933

(18 C); *Boiling point:* 88–91 C; *Freezing point:* –3 to –4 C; *Flash point:* 80 F (TCC); *Solubility:* Soluble in ether, 4 parts water

DERIVATION: Found in bay and other oils and in butter; made from methyl ethyl ketone by converting to the isonitroso compound, then, with HCl, decomposing to diacetyl by hydrolysis and by special fermentation of glucose via methylacetylcarbinol

WARNING AND CAUTION: Flammable

ETHYL ACETATE

SYNONYMS: Acetic ether; Acetic ester; Acetic acide ethyl ester; Vinegar naphtha

CAS NUMBER: 141-78-6

MOLECULAR FORMULA: $C_4H_8O_2$

MOLECULAR WEIGHT: 88.10

CHARACTERISTICS: *Form:* Liquid; *Color:* Colorless; *Odor:* Fragrant

PHYSICAL PROPERTIES: *Specific gravity:* 0.8945 (25/25 C); *Boiling point:* 77 C; *Freezing point:* –83.6 C; *Flash point:* 24 F (TCC); *Solubility:* Soluble in alcohol, chloroform, ether; slightly soluble in water

DERIVATION: By heating acetic acid and ethyl alcohol in presence of sulfuric acid and distilling

WARNING AND CAUTION: Flammable; moderately toxic by inhalation and skin absorption

ETHYL ACETOACETATE

SYNONYMS: Diacetic ester; Acetoacetic ester; 3-Oxobutanoic acid ethyl ester; Acetoacetic acid ethyl ester; Ethyl 3-oxobutanoate

MOLECULAR FORMULA: $C_6H_{10}O_2$

MOLECULAR WEIGHT: 130.14

CHARACTERISTICS: *Form:* Liquid; *Color:* Colorless; *Odor:* Fruity

PHYSICAL PROPERTIES: *Specific gravity:* 1.0250 (20/4 C); *Boiling point:* 180–181 C; *Flash point:* 185 F (TCC); *Solubility:* Soluble in alcohol, water

DERIVATION: Action of metallic sodium on ethyl acetate and distillation

WARNING AND CAUTION: Moderately toxic by ingestion and inhalation; irritant to skin and eyes

ETHYL ALCOHOL

SYNONYMS: Alcohol; Grain alcohol; Ethanol; Spirit of wine; Absolute alcohol; Ethyl hydrate; Spirit

CAS NUMBER: 64-17-5

MOLECULAR FORMULA: C_2H_6O

MOLECULAR WEIGHT: 46.046

CHARACTERISTICS: *Form:* Liquid, volatile; *Color:* Colorless; *Odor:* Ethereal, vinous

PHYSICAL PROPERTIES: *Specific gravity:* 0.816 (15.56 C); *Refractive index:* 1.3651 (15 C); *Boiling point:* 78 C; *Freezing point:* –117.3 to –114 C; *Flash point:* 55 F; *Solubility:* Miscible with chloroform, ether, water, other solvents

WARNING AND CAUTION: Flammable

ETHYL ALDEHYDE

See Acetaldehyde

ETHYL ANTHRANILATE

SYNONYMS: Ethyl *o*-aminobenzoate
CAS NUMBER: 87-25-2
MOLECULAR FORMULA: $C_9H_{11}NO_2$
MOLECULAR WEIGHT: 165.20
CHARACTERISTICS: *Form:* Liquid; *Color:* Slightly yellow to brownish; *Odor:* Fruity
PHYSICAL PROPERTIES: *Specific gravity:* 1.115–1.120 (25/25 C); *Refractive index:* 1.5630–1.5660 (20 C); *Boiling point:* 260 C; *Solubility:* Soluble in alcohol, propylene glycol

ETHYL BENZOATE

SYNONYMS: Benzoic acid ethyl ester
CAS NUMBER: 93-89-0
MOLECULAR FORMULA: $C_9H_{10}O_2$
MOLECULAR WEIGHT: 150.18
CHARACTERISTICS: *Form:* Liquid; *Color:* Colorless; *Odor:* Aromatic, suggestive of wintergreen
PHYSICAL PROPERTIES: *Specific gravity:* 1.043–1.046 (25/25 C); *Refractive index:* 1.5030–1.5060 (20 C); *Boiling point:* 212.9 C; *Freezing point:* –32.7 C; *Flash point:* 190 F (TCC); *Solubility:* Soluble in alcohol, chloroform, ether
DERIVATION: By heating ethyl alcohol and benzoic acid in presence of sulfuric acid

ETHYL BUTYRATE

SYNONYMS: Ethyl butanoate; Butanoic acid ethyl ester; Butyric acid ethyl ester; Ethyl *n*-butyrate
CAS NUMBER: 105-54-4
MOLECULAR FORMULA: $C_6H_{12}O_2$
MOLECULAR WEIGHT: 116.16
CHARACTERISTICS: *Form:* Liquid; *Color:* Colorless; *Odor:* Pineapple
PHYSICAL PROPERTIES: *Specific gravity:* 0.8788 (25/25 C); *Refractive index:* 1.400 (20 C); *Boiling point:* 120.6 C; *Freezing point:* –93.3 C; *Flash point:* 78 F (TCC); *Solubility:* Soluble in alcohol, ether; insoluble in water, glycerin
DERIVATION: From ethyl alcohol and butyric acid heated in presence of sulfuric acid and distillation
WARNING AND CAUTION: Flammable; irritating to eyes; narcotic in high concentration

ETHYL CAPRATE

SYNONYMS: Ethyl decanoate; Decanoic acid ethyl ester
CAS NUMBER: 110-38-3
MOLECULAR FORMULA: $C_{12}H_{24}O_2$
MOLECULAR WEIGHT: 200.31
CHARACTERISTICS: *Form:* Liquid; *Color:* Colorless; *Odor:* Fragrant
PHYSICAL PROPERTIES: *Specific gravity:* 0.862 (25/25 C); *Boiling point:* 243 C;

Solubility: Soluble in alcohol, ether; insoluble in water
DERIVATION: By heating capric acid, absolute alcohol, sulfuric acid, and distilling
WARNING AND CAUTION: Combustible; low toxicity

ETHYL CAPROATE
SYNONYMS: Ethyl hexoate; Ethyl hexanoate; Hexanoic acid ethyl ester
CAS NUMBER: 123-66-0
MOLECULAR FORMULA: $C_8H_{16}O_2$
MOLECULAR WEIGHT: 144.21
CHARACTERISTICS: *Form:* Liquid; *Color:* Colorless; *Odor:* Pleasant
PHYSICAL PROPERTIES: *Specific gravity:* 0.873 (25/25 C); *Boiling point:* 167 C; *Solubility:* Soluble in alcohol, ether; insoluble in water, glycerin
DERIVATION: Heating absolute alcohol and *n*-caproic acid in presence of sulfuric acid, and distilling
WARNING AND CAUTION: Low toxicity, combustible

ETHYL CAPRYLATE
SYNONYMS: Ethyl octoate; Ethyl octanoate; Octanoic acid ethyl ester; Ethyl octylate
CAS NUMBER: 106-32-1
MOLECULAR FORMULA: $C_{10}H_{20}O_2$
MOLECULAR WEIGHT: 172.17
CHARACTERISTICS: *Form:* Liquid; *Color:* Colorless; *Odor:* Pineapple
PHYSICAL PROPERTIES: *Specific gravity:* 0.865–0.869 (25/25 C); *Boiling point:* 207–209 C; *Freezing point:* –48 C; *Solubility:* Soluble in alcohol, ether; insoluble in water, glycerin
DERIVATION: Heating caprylic acid, alcohol, sulfuric acid, and distilling
WARNING AND CAUTION: Combustible; low toxicity

ETHYL CARBONATE
SYNONYMS: Diethyl carbonate; Carbonic acid diethyl ester
CAS NUMBER: 105-58-8
MOLECULAR FORMULA: $C_5H_{10}O_3$
MOLECULAR WEIGHT: 118.30
CHARACTERISTICS: *Form:* Liquid; *Color:* Colorless; *Odor:* Mild
PHYSICAL PROPERTIES: *Specific gravity:* 0.975 (20.4 C); *Boiling point:* 126 C; *Freezing point:* –43 C; *Flash point:* 77 F (OC); *Solubility:* Soluble in alcohol, ketones, esters, aromatic hydrocarbons, aliphatic solvents; insoluble in water
DERIVATION: Reacting chlorine and carbon monoxide to produce phosgene ($COCl_2$); reacting phosgene with ethyl alcohol to make ethyl chlorocarbonate ($ClCO_2C_2H_5$); reacting ethyl chlorocarbonate with anhydrous ethyl alcohol to produce diethyl carbonate
WARNING AND CAUTION: Flammable; moderately toxic; strong irritant

ETHYL CINNAMATE
SYNONYMS: Ethyl phenyl acrylate; Cinnamylic ether
MOLECULAR FORMULA: $C_{11}H_{12}O_2$
MOLECULAR WEIGHT: 176.22

CHARACTERISTICS: *Form:* Liquid; *Color:* Colorless; *Odor:* Sweet, balsamic honey note
PHYSICAL PROPERTIES: *Specific gravity:* 1.045–1.048 (25/25 C); *Refractive index:* 1.5590–1.5610 (20 C); *Boiling point:* 271 C; *Freezing point:* 7 C; *Flash point:* > 212 F; *Solubility:* Soluble in alcohol, ether; insoluble in water
DERIVATION: Heating ethyl alcohol and cinnamic acid in presence of sulfuric acid; found in storax oil and *Kaempferia galanga*
WARNING AND CAUTION: Low toxicity

ETHYL FORMATE
SYNONYMS: Ethyl formic ester
CAS NUMBER: 109-94-4
MOLECULAR FORMULA: $C_3H_6O_2$
MOLECULAR WEIGHT: 74.07
CHARACTERISTICS: *Form:* Unstable; *Color:* Colorless; *Odor:* Pleasant aromatic
PHYSICAL PROPERTIES: *Specific gravity:* 0.9236 (20/20 C); *Refractive index:* 1.35975 (20 C); *Boiling point:* 54.3 C; *Freezing point:* –80.5 C; *Flash point:* –4 F (TCC); *Solubility:* Soluble in alcohol, ether, benzene; slightly soluble in water with gradual decomposition
DERIVATION: Heating ethyl alcohol with formic acid in presence of sulfuric acid
WARNING AND CAUTION: Highly flammable; narcotic; irritating to skin and eyes

ETHYL ISOBUTYRATE
SYNONYMS: Methyl propanoic acid ethyl ester
CAS NUMBER: 97-62-1
MOLECULAR FORMULA: $C_6H_{12}O_2$
MOLECULAR WEIGHT: 116.6
CHARACTERISTICS: *Form:* Liquid, volatile; *Color:* Colorless
PHYSICAL PROPERTIES: *Specific gravity:* 0.870 (25/25 C); *Refractive index:* 1.3903 (20 C); *Boiling point:* 110–111 C; *Freezing point:* –88 C; *Solubility:* Soluble in alcohol, ether; slightly soluble in water
DERIVATION: Heating isobutyric acid and ethyl alcohol and distilling
WARNING AND CAUTION: Moderately toxic

ETHYL ISOVALERATE
SYNONYMS: Ethyl valerate; Ethyl valeriate; Ethyl 2-methyl butyrate; 3-Methylbutanoic acid ethyl ester; Pentanoic acid ethyl ester
CAS NUMBER: 108-64-5
MOLECULAR FORMULA: $C_7H_{14}O_2$
MOLECULAR WEIGHT: 130.18
CHARACTERISTICS: *Form:* Liquid, oily; *Color:* Colorless; *Odor:* Fruity
PHYSICAL PROPERTIES: *Specific gravity:* 0.864 (20/20 C); *Refractive index:* 1.3950–1.3990 (20 C); *Boiling point:* 135 C; *Freezing point:* –99 C; *Solubility:* Soluble in alcohol, ether, benzene; slightly soluble in water
DERIVATION: Heating sodium valerate and ethyl alcohol in presence of sulfuric acid or hydrochloric acid, and distilling
WARNING AND CAUTION: Low toxicity

ETHYL MALONATE

SYNONYMS: Propanechoic acid diethyl ester; Diethyl malonate; Malonic ester
CAS NUMBER: 105-53-3
MOLECULAR FORMULA: $C_7H_{12}O_4$
MOLECULAR WEIGHT: 160.17
CHARACTERISTICS: *Form:* Liquid; *Color:* Colorless; *Odor:* Aromatic, pleasant
PHYSICAL PROPERTIES: *Specific gravity:* 1.055 (25/25 C); *Refractive index:* 1.4143 (20 C); *Boiling point:* 198–199 C; *Freezing point:* –50 C; *Flash point:* 200 F; *Solubility:* Soluble in alcohol, ether; slightly soluble in water
DERIVATION: From chloroacetic acid and sodium cyanide; esterification with ethanol and sulfuric acid
WARNING AND CAUTION: Combustible; low toxicity

ETHYL METHYL PHENYL GLYCIDATE

See Aldehyde C-16 Pure

ETHYL MYRISTATE

SYNONYMS: Ethyl tetradecanoate; Tetradecanoic acid ethyl ester
MOLECULAR FORMULA: $C_{16}H_{32}O_2$
MOLECULAR WEIGHT: 256.44
CHARACTERISTICS: *Form:* Liquid; *Color:* Colorless; *Odor:* Orris, fatty
PHYSICAL PROPERTIES: *Specific gravity:* 0.856–0.860 (25/25 C); *Refractive index:* 1.4340–1.4380 (20 C); *Freezing point:* 4 C; *Flash point:* > 212 F (TCC); *Solubility:* Soluble in 2 parts 90% ethyl alcohol; slightly soluble in ether; insoluble in water
WARNING AND CAUTION: Combustible; low toxicity

ETHYL NITRATE

SYNONYMS: Aether nitricus
CAS NUMBER: 625-58-1
MOLECULAR FORMULA: $C_2H_5NO_3$
MOLECULAR WEIGHT: 91.09
CHARACTERISTICS: *Form:* Liquid; *Color:* Colorless; *Odor:* Pleasant; *Taste:* Sweet
PHYSICAL PROPERTIES: *Specific gravity:* 1.116 (25/25 C); *Boiling point:* 87.6 C; *Freezing point:* –112 C; *Flash point:* 50 F (CC); *Solubility:* Soluble in alcohol, ether; insoluble in water
DERIVATION: Heating alcohol, urea nitrate, and nitric acid, and distilling
WARNING AND CAUTION: Flammable; explodes at 185 F

ETHYL OENANTHATE

SYNONYMS: Ethyl enanthate; Ethyl heptanoate; Ethyl *n*-heptoate; Oenanthic ether; Heptanoic acid ethyl ester; Cognac oil synthetic; Oil of grapes; Aether oenanthicus; Oleum vitis viniferae
MOLECULAR FORMULA: $C_9H_{18}O_2$
MOLECULAR WEIGHT: 158.23
CHARACTERISTICS: *Form:* Liquid; *Color:* Colorless; *Odor:* Fruity

PHYSICAL PROPERTIES: *Specific gravity:* 0.87 (25/25 C); *Boiling point:* 187 C; *Solubility:* Soluble in alcohol, chloroform, ether; insoluble in water
DERIVATION: Heating oenanthic acid and ethyl alcohol in presence of sulfuric acid, and distilling
WARNING AND CAUTION: Low toxicity; combustible

ETHYL PELARGONATE

SYNONYMS: Ethyl nonoate; Wine ether; Nonanoic acid ethyl ester
MOLECULAR FORMULA: $C_{11}H_{22}O_2$
MOLECULAR WEIGHT: 186.29
CHARACTERISTICS: *Form:* Liquid; *Color:* Colorless; *Odor:* Fruity
PHYSICAL PROPERTIES: *Specific gravity:* 0.863–0.865 (25/25 C); *Refractive index:* 1.4210–1.4260 (20 C); *Boiling point:* 220 C; *Freezing point:* –44 C; *Solubility:* Insoluble in water; soluble in alcohol and ether
WARNING AND CAUTION: Low toxicity

ETHYL PHENYL ACETATE

SYNONYMS: Ethyl α-toluate; Benzeneacetic acid ethyl ester; α-Toluic acid ethyl ester
CAS NUMBER: 101-97-3
MOLECULAR FORMULA: $C_{10}H_{12}O$
MOLECULAR WEIGHT: 164.21
CHARACTERISTICS: *Form:* Liquid; *Color:* Colorless; *Odor:* Sweet honey-rose
PHYSICAL PROPERTIES: *Specific gravity:* 1.027–1.032 (25/25 C); *Refractive index:* 1.4960–1.4980 (20 C); *Boiling point:* 276 C; *Flash point:* > 212 F (TCC); *Solubility:* Soluble in 10 parts 60% ethyl alcohol, 3 parts 70% ethyl alcohol

ETHYL PHENYL GLYCIDATE

SYNONYMS: Ethyl β-phenyl glycidate
MOLECULAR FORMULA: $C_{11}H_{12}O_3$
MOLECULAR WEIGHT: 192.13
CHARACTERISTICS: *Form:* Liquid; *Color:* Colorless to slightly yellow; *Odor:* Strong strawberry
PHYSICAL PROPERTIES: *Specific gravity:* 1.120–1.125 (25/25 C); *Refractive index:* 1.5160–1.5210 (20 C); *Flash point:* > 212 F (TCC); *Solubility:* Soluble in 6 parts 70% ethyl alcohol, 1 part 80% ethyl alcohol

ETHYL SALICYLATE

SYNONYMS: Ethyl hydroxybenzoate; Salicylic acid ethyl ester; Salicylic ether; Sal ethyl
CAS NUMBER: 118-61-6
MOLECULAR FORMULA: $C_9H_{10}O_2$
MOLECULAR WEIGHT: 166.18
CHARACTERISTICS: *Form:* Liquid; *Color:* Colorless; *Odor:* Faint methyl salicylate
PHYSICAL PROPERTIES: *Specific gravity:* 1.126–1.129 (25/25 C); *Refractive index:*

1.5210–1.5230 (20 C); *Boiling point:* 231–234 C; *Solubility:* Insoluble in water
WARNING AND CAUTION: Combustible

ETHYL SEBACATE
SYNONYMS: Decanedioic acid diethyl ester; Diethyl sebacate
MOLECULAR FORMULA: $C_{14}H_{26}O_4$
MOLECULAR WEIGHT: 258.35
CHARACTERISTICS: *Form:* Liquid; *Color:* Colorless to yellowish
PHYSICAL PROPERTIES: *Specific gravity:* 0.965 (20 C); *Refractive index:* 1.4369 (20 C); *Boiling point:* 307 C; *Solubility:* Soluble in alcohol, ether, organic solvents

ETHYL VALERATE
See Ethyl isovalerate

ETHYL VANILLIN
SYNONYMS: Bourbonal; 3-Ethoxy-4-hydroxybenzaldehyde; Ethyl protal; Ethovan; Ethyl protocatechuic aldehyde; Vanillal
CAS NUMBER: 121-32-4
MOLECULAR FORMULA: $C_9H_{10}O_3$
MOLECULAR WEIGHT: 166.17
CHARACTERISTICS: *Form:* Crystals; *Color:* White, affected by light; *Odor:* Intense vanillin; *Taste:* Vanilla
PHYSICAL PROPERTIES: *Melting point:* 76.5 C; *Solubility:* Soluble in alcohol, chloroform, ether, glycerol, propylene glycol; slightly soluble in water
WARNING AND CAUTION: Low toxicity; combustible

EUGENOL
SYNONYMS: 4-Allyl-2-methoxyphenol; Eugenic acid; 4-Allylguaiacol; 2-Methoxy-4-(2-propenyl) phenol; Caryophyllic acid
CAS NUMBER: 97-53-0
MOLECULAR FORMULA: $C_{10}H_{12}O_2$
MOLECULAR WEIGHT: 164.21
CHARACTERISTICS: *Form:* Liquid; *Color:* Light yellow; *Odor:* Pungent, spicy cloves, characteristic
PHYSICAL PROPERTIES: *Specific gravity:* 1.064–1.068 (25/25 C); *Refractive index:* 1.5400–1.5420 (20 C); *Boiling point:* 253.5 C; *Freezing point:* –9.2 to –9.1 C; *Flash point:* 230 F (TCC); *Solubility:* Soluble in 2 parts 60% ethyl alcohol
DERIVATION: Found mainly in oil of clove, cinnamon leaf, pimento, and in minor quantity in many other oils such as ylang ylang, cananga, patchouli, rose, violet, hyacinth, tuberose, orange flower, acacia
WARNING AND CAUTION: Low toxicity; combustible

GERANIOL
SYNONYMS: *trans*-3,7-Dimethyl-2,6-octadien-1-ol; (E)-3,7-Dimethyl-2,6-octadien-1-ol; 2,6-Dimethyl-2,6-octadien-8-ol; Lemonol
MOLECULAR FORMULA: $C_{10}H_{18}O$

MOLECULAR WEIGHT: 154.25
CHARACTERISTICS: *Form:* Liquid; *Color:* Colorless; *Odor:* Rosy
PHYSICAL PROPERTIES: *Specific gravity:* 0.870–0.880 (25/25 C); *Refractive index:* 1.4710–1.4760 (20 C); *Optical rotation:* 2°; *Boiling point:* 229–230 C; *Flash point:* 217 F (TCC); *Solubility:* Soluble in 2 parts 70% ethyl alcohol; insoluble in water
DERIVATION: Main constituent of oils of palmarosa, rose geranium, citronella, and in lesser amounts in verbena, lemongrass, rosewood, linaloe, petitgrain, and many other oils

GERANYL ACETATE

SYNONYMS: *trans*-3,7-Dimethyl-2,6-octadienyl acetate; Geraniol acetate
CAS NUMBER: 105-87-3
MOLECULAR FORMULA: $C_{12}H_{20}O_2$
MOLECULAR WEIGHT: 196.29
CHARACTERISTICS: *Form:* Liquid; *Color:* Colorless to slightly yellow; *Odor:* Sweet rose-lavender note
PHYSICAL PROPERTIES: *Specific gravity:* 0.900–0.910 (25/25 C); *Refractive index:* 1.4570–1.4620 (20 C); *Optical rotation:* –2 to 2°; *Boiling point:* 128–129 C; *Flash point:* 228 F (TCC); *Solubility:* Soluble in 2 parts 80% ethyl alcohol
DERIVATION: Found in citronella, lemongrass, palmarosa, geranium, coriander, lavender, neroli, petitgrain, and others, and in greater amounts in *Eucalyptus staigeriana*, *E. macarthurii*, *Dancus carota*; by heating geraniol and sodium acetate with acetic anhydride
WARNING AND CAUTION: Combustible; nontoxic

GERANYL BENZOATE

SYNONYMS: *trans*-3,7-Dimethyl-2,6-octadienyl benzoate
MOLECULAR FORMULA: $C_{17}H_{22}O_2$
MOLECULAR WEIGHT: 258.37
CHARACTERISTICS: *Form:* Liquid; *Color:* Slightly yellow; *Odor:* Sweet, suggestive of ylang ylang
PHYSICAL PROPERTIES: *Specific gravity:* 0.978–0.984 (25/25 C); *Refractive index:* 1.5130–1.5180 (20 C); *Optical rotation:* 1°; *Flash point:* 212 F (TCC); *Solubility:* Soluble in 4 parts 90% ethyl alcohol

GERANYL BUTYRATE

SYNONYMS: Geraniol butyrate; *trans*-3,7-Dimethyl-2,6-octadienyl butyrate
MOLECULAR FORMULA: $C_{14}H_{24}O_2$
MOLECULAR WEIGHT: 224.34
CHARACTERISTICS: *Form:* Liquid; *Color:* Colorless to slightly yellow; *Odor:* Fruity-rosy
PHYSICAL PROPERTIES: *Specific gravity:* 0.891–0.896 (25/25 C); *Refractive index:* 1.4560–1.4620 (20 C); *Optical rotation:* 1°; *Boiling point:* 151 C; *Flash point:* 200 F (TCC); *Solubility:* Soluble in 7 parts 80% ethyl alcohol, 1 part 90% ethyl alcohol, ether; insoluble in water and glycerin

DERIVATION: Occurs in several essential oils
WARNING AND CAUTION: Combustible; nontoxic

GERANYL FORMATE
SYNONYMS: *trans*-3,7-Dimethyl-2,6-octadienyl formate; Geraniol formate
CAS NUMBER: 105-86-2
MOLECULAR FORMULA: $C_{11}H_{18}O_2$
MOLECULAR WEIGHT: 182.26
CHARACTERISTICS: *Form:* Liquid; *Color:* Colorless to slightly yellow; *Odor:* Fresh, light leafy-rose
PHYSICAL PROPERTIES: *Specific gravity:* 0.906–0.914 (25/25 C); *Refractive index:* 1.4580–1.4640 (20 C); *Flash point:* 186 F (TCC); *Solubility:* Soluble in 3 parts 80% ethyl alcohol, ether; insoluble in water and glycerin
DERIVATION: Found in oil of geranium
WARNING AND CAUTION: Combustible; nontoxic

GERANYL PHENYLACETATE
SYNONYMS: *trans*-3,7-Dimethyl-2,6-octadienyl phenylacetate
MOLECULAR FORMULA: $C_{18}H_{24}O_2$
MOLECULAR WEIGHT: 272.39
CHARACTERISTICS: *Form:* Liquid; *Color:* Yellow; *Odor:* Soft honey-rose
PHYSICAL PROPERTIES: *Specific gravity:* 0.971–0.978 (25/25 C); *Refractive index:* 1.5070–1.5110 (20 C); *Optical rotation:* 1°; *Flash point:* 210 F (TCC); *Solubility:* Soluble in 4 parts 90% ethyl alcohol

GERANYL PROPIONATE
SYNONYMS: *trans*-3,7-Dimethyl-2,6-octadienyl propionate; Geraniol propionate
MOLECULAR FORMULA: $C_{13}H_{22}O_2$
MOLECULAR WEIGHT: 210.32
CHARACTERISTICS: *Form:* Liquid; *Color:* Slightly yellow; *Odor:* Fruity-rose
PHYSICAL PROPERTIES: *Specific gravity:* 0.896–0.909 (25/25 C); *Refractive index:* 1.4570–1.4620 (20 C); *Optical rotation:* 1°; *Flash point:* 210 F (TCC); *Solubility:* Soluble in 3 parts 80% ethyl alcohol, most oils; insoluble in glycerol
WARNING AND CAUTION: Combustible; nontoxic

GLYCEROL
SYNONYMS: Glycerin; Glycerinum; 1,2,3-Propanetriol; Propenyl hydrate; Glycerol alcohol; Trihydroxypropane; Trihydric (polyhydric) alcohol
CAS NUMBER: 56-81-5
MOLECULAR FORMULA: $C_3H_8O_3$
MOLECULAR WEIGHT: 92.09
CHARACTERISTICS: *Form:* Liquid, syrup; *Color:* Colorless; *Odor:* Odorless; *Taste:* Sweet, warm
PHYSICAL PROPERTIES: *Specific gravity:* 1.2653 (25/25 C); *Boiling point:* 290 C; *Freezing point:* 17 C (solidifies at lower temperature); *Flash point:* 320 F (TCC); *Solubility:* Soluble in water and alcohol; insoluble in chloroform, ether, benzene,

fixed and volatile oils, organic solvents
DERIVATION: By saponification of fats and oils; from propylene and chlorine with hydrochlorous acid
WARNING AND CAUTION: Combustible; low toxicity

HELIOTROPIN
SYNONYMS: Piperonal; Piperonyl aldehyde; 3,4-(Methylenedioxy) benzaldehyde; 1,3-Benzodioxole-5-carboxaldehyde; Dioxymethyleneprotocatechuic aldehyde; Protocatechuic aldehyde methylene ether
CAS NUMBER: 120-57-0
MOLECULAR FORMULA: $C_8H_6O_3$
MOLECULAR WEIGHT: 150.13
CHARACTERISTICS: *Form:* Crystals; *Color:* White, lustrous; turns red-brown; *Odor:* Sweet heliotrope
PHYSICAL PROPERTIES: *Boiling point:* 263 C; *Freezing point:* 35.5–37 C; *Solubility:* Soluble in alcohol, ether; slightly soluble in water and glycerol
DERIVATION: By oxidation of isosafrole; found in oils of *Vanilla tahitiana*
WARNING AND CAUTION: Combustible; low toxicity

HEXYL ACETATE
CAS NUMBER: 142-92-7
MOLECULAR FORMULA: $C_8H_{16}O_2$
MOLECULAR WEIGHT: 144.2
CHARACTERISTICS: *Form:* Liquid; *Color:* Colorless; *Odor:* Sweet ester
PHYSICAL PROPERTIES: *Specific gravity:* 0.890 (25/25 C); *Boiling point:* 169.2 C; *Solubility:* Soluble in alcohol, ether; insoluble in water
DERIVATION: From primary and secondary hexyl alcohol
WARNING AND CAUTION: Combustible

HEXYL ALCOHOL
SYNONYMS: 1-Hexanol; Amyl carbinol; *n*-Hexyl alcohol; Pentylcarbinol; 1-Hydroxyhexane
CAS NUMBER: 111-27-3
MOLECULAR FORMULA: $C_6H_{14}O$
MOLECULAR WEIGHT: 102.17
CHARACTERISTICS: *Form:* Liquid; *Color:* Colorless
PHYSICAL PROPERTIES: *Specific gravity:* 0.886 (25/25 C); *Refractive index:* 1.469 (25 C); *Boiling point:* 157.2 C; *Freezing point:* –51.6 C; *Flash point:* 149 F (TCC); *Solubility:* Soluble in alcohol, ether; slightly soluble in water
DERIVATION: By reducing ethyl caproate with sodium in absolute alcohol; from olefins by the oxo process
WARNING AND CAUTION: Combustible; low toxicity

HYDROXYCITRONELLAL
SYNONYMS: Citronellal hydrate; 3,7-Dimethyl-7-hydroxyoctanal; Laurine; 7-Hydroxy-3,7-dimethyloctan-1-al

CAS NUMBER: 107-75-5
MOLECULAR FORMULA: $C_{10}H_{20}O_2$
MOLECULAR WEIGHT: 172.27
CHARACTERISTICS: *Form:* Liquid, viscous; *Color:* Colorless or faint yellow; *Odor:* Sweet and intense odor of linden blossom
PHYSICAL PROPERTIES: *Specific gravity:* 0.917–0.921 (25/25 C); *Refractive index:* 1.4470–1.4500 (20 C); *Optical rotation:* 9–10°; *Boiling point:* 94–96 C; *Flash point:* 270 F (TCC); *Solubility:* Soluble in 1 part 50% ethyl alcohol, fixed oils; slightly soluble in water, glycerol, mineral oils
DERIVATION: From citronella or *Eucalyptus citriodora*
WARNING AND CAUTION: Combustible; nontoxic

IONONE

SYNONYMS: α or β-Cyclocitrylidenacetone; Irisone; 4-(2,6,6-Trimethyl-2-cyclohexenyl)-2-buten-2-one; α- or β-Ionone; 4-(2,6,6-Trimethyl-1-cyclohexenyl)-3-buten-2-one
CAS NUMBER: 8013-90-9
MOLECULAR FORMULA: $C_{13}H_{20}O$
MOLECULAR WEIGHT: 193.30
CHARACTERISTICS: *Form:* Liquid; *Color:* Light yellow; *Odor:* Violet
PHYSICAL PROPERTIES: *Specific gravity:* 0.927–0.933 (25/25 C); *Refractive index:* 1.4970–1.5020 (20 C); *Boiling point:* 126–128 C; *Flash point:* > 212 F (TCC); *Solubility:* Soluble in 2–3 parts 70% alcohol, chloroform, ether, mineral oils, propylene glycol, benzene; insoluble in water and glycerin
DERIVATION: Condensing citral with acetone; reaction of acetylene with acetone, followed by hydrogenation, condensation with diketone, and further reaction with acetylene

ISOAMYL ACETATE

CAS NUMBER: 123-92-2
MOLECULAR FORMULA: $C_7H_{14}O_2$
MOLECULAR WEIGHT: 130.18
CHARACTERISTICS: *Form:* Liquid; *Color:* Colorless; *Odor:* Banana, pear
PHYSICAL PROPERTIES: *Specific gravity:* 0.876 (15.4 C); *Refractive index:* 1.400 (20 C); *Boiling point:* 142 C; *Freezing point:* –78.5 C; *Flash point:* 80 F (TCC); *Solubility:* Soluble in alcohol, ether; slightly soluble in water
DERIVATION: Rectification of commercial amyl acetate
WARNING AND CAUTION: Flammable; moderately toxic and irritating

ISOAMYL ALCOHOL

SYNONYMS: 3-Methyl-1-butanol; Isobutyl carbinol
CAS NUMBER: 123-51-3
MOLECULAR FORMULA: $C_5H_{12}O$
MOLECULAR WEIGHT: 88.11
CHARACTERISTICS: *Form:* Liquid; *Color:* Colorless; *Odor:* Disagreeable; *Taste:* Pungent

PHYSICAL PROPERTIES: *Specific gravity:* 0.813 (15.4 C); *Refractive index:* 1.4075 (20 C); *Boiling point:* 132 C; *Freezing point:* –117.2 C; *Flash point:* 109 F (CC); *Solubility:* Soluble in alcohol, ether; slightly soluble in water

DERIVATION: Distillation of fusel oil or the mixed alcohol resulting from chlorination and hydrolysis of pentane (amyl hydride)

WARNING AND CAUTION: Flammable; moderately toxic and irritating

ISOAMYL BUTYRATE

CAS NUMBER: 106-27-4

MOLECULAR FORMULA: $C_9H_{18}O_2$

MOLECULAR WEIGHT: 158.23

CHARACTERISTICS: *Form:* Liquid; *Color:* White; *Odor:* Aromatic, pear

PHYSICAL PROPERTIES: *Specific gravity:* 0.866–0.868 (15.5 C); *Boiling point:* 150–180 C; *Solubility:* Soluble in alcohol, ether; very slightly soluble in water

DERIVATION: By treating isoamyl alcohol with butyric acid and distilling

WARNING AND CAUTION: Combustible; low toxicity

ISOAMYL FORMATE

CAS NUMBER: 110-45-2

MOLECULAR FORMULA: $C_6H_{12}O_2$

MOLECULAR WEIGHT: 116.09

CHARACTERISTICS: *Form:* Liquid; *Color:* Colorless; *Odor:* Fruity

PHYSICAL PROPERTIES: *Specific gravity:* 0.87 (20 C); *Refractive index:* 1.391 (20 C); *Boiling point:* 12.3 C; *Solubility:* Soluble in alcohol, ether; slightly soluble in water

WARNING AND CAUTION: Highly toxic by ingestion and inhalation; strong irritant to tissues

ISOAMYL ISOVALERATE

See Amyl valerate

ISOAMYL PROPIONATE

SYNONYMS: Amyl propionate

MOLECULAR FORMULA: $C_8H_{16}O_2$

MOLECULAR WEIGHT: 144.42

CHARACTERISTICS: *Form:* Liquid; *Color:* Colorless; *Odor:* Apple

PHYSICAL PROPERTIES: *Specific gravity:* 0.869–0.873 (20 C); *Refractive index:* 1.4065 (20 C); *Boiling point:* 160–161 C; *Flash point:* 106 F (TCC); *Solubility:* Soluble in alcohol, ether; insoluble in water

DERIVATION: From amyl alcohol with propionic acid in presence of sulfuric acid as a catalyst, and distilling

WARNING AND CAUTION: Flammable; moderately toxic

ISOAMYL SALICYLATE

SYNONYMS: Amyl salicylate

CAS NUMBER: 87-20-7

MOLECULAR FORMULA: $C_{12}H_{16}O$
MOLECULAR WEIGHT: 208.25
CHARACTERISTICS: *Form:* Liquid; *Color:* Colorless to faint yellow; *Odor:* Pleasant, orchid-like
PHYSICAL PROPERTIES: *Specific gravity:* 1.053–1.059 (15 C); *Refractive index:* 1.5050–1.5080 (20 C); *Optical rotation:* 0–2.30°; *Boiling point:* 280 C; *Solubility:* Soluble in alcohol, ether; insoluble in water and glycerol
DERIVATION: By esterifying salicylic acid with amyl alcohol, and distilling
WARNING AND CAUTION: Combustible; low toxicity

ISOBUTYL ACETATE
CAS NUMBER: 110-19-0
MOLECULAR FORMULA: $C_6H_{12}O$
MOLECULAR WEIGHT: 116.16
CHARACTERISTICS: *Form:* Liquid; *Color:* Colorless; *Odor:* Fruit-like
PHYSICAL PROPERTIES: *Specific gravity:* 0.8685 (15 C); *Refractive index:* 1.392 (20 C); *Boiling point:* 116–117 C; *Freezing point:* –99 C; *Flash point:* 88 F (OC); *Solubility:* Soluble in alcohol, ether, hydrdocarbons; insoluble in water
DERIVATION: Treating isobutyl alcohol with acetic acid in presence of catalysts
WARNING AND CAUTION: Flammable; moderately toxic by ingestion and inhalation

ISOBUTYL ISOBUTYRATE
SYNONYMS: Isobutyl *n*-butyrate
CAS NUMBER: 97-85-8
MOLECULAR FORMULA: $C_8H_{16}O_2$
MOLECULAR WEIGHT: 144.21
CHARACTERISTICS: *Form:* Liquid; *Color:* Colorless; *Odor:* Fruity
PHYSICAL PROPERTIES: *Specific gravity:* 0.853–0.857 (20/20 C); *Refractive index:* 1.3999 (20 C); *Boiling point:* 148.7 C; *Freezing point:* 80.7 C; *Solubility:* Soluble in alcohol, ether; insoluble in water
WARNING AND CAUTION: Combustible; may be toxic

ISOBUTYL FORMATE
SYNONYMS: Tetryl formate
MOLECULAR FORMULA: $C_5H_{10}O_2$
MOLECULAR WEIGHT: 102.13
CHARACTERISTICS: *Form:* Liquid
PHYSICAL PROPERTIES: *Specific gravity:* 0.885 (25/25 C); *Refractive index:* 1.3858 (20 C); *Boiling point:* 98 C; *Freezing point:* –95 C; *Solubility:* Soluble in alcohol, ether; slightly soluble in water

ISOBUTYL ISOVALERATE
SYNONYMS: Isobutyl valerate
MOLECULAR FORMULA: $C_9H_{18}O_2$
MOLECULAR WEIGHT: 158.23

CHARACTERISTICS: *Form:* Liquid; *Color:* Colorless; *Odor:* Ethereal
PHYSICAL PROPERTIES: *Specific gravity:* 0.853 (25/25 C); *Refractive index:* 1.4064 (20 C); *Boiling point:* 170–172 C; *Solubility:* Soluble in alcohol, ether; insoluble in water

ISOBUTYL PROPIONATE
CAS NUMBER: 540-42-1
MOLECULAR FORMULA: $C_7H_{14}O_2$
MOLECULAR WEIGHT: 130.18
CHARACTERISTICS: *Form:* Liquid; *Odor:* Ethereal, agreeable
PHYSICAL PROPERTIES: *Specific gravity:* 0.8600–0.8635 (20/20 C); *Refractive index:* 1.3975 (20 C); *Boiling point:* 138 C; *Freezing point:* –71.4 C; *Solubility:* Soluble in alcohol; insoluble in water

ISOBUTYL SALICYLATE
SYNONYMS: Isobutyl *o*-hydroxybenzoate
CAS NUMBER: 87-19-4
MOLECULAR FORMULA: $C_{11}H_{14}O_3$
MOLECULAR WEIGHT: 194.23
CHARACTERISTICS: *Form:* Liquid; *Color:* Colorless to slightly yellow; *Odor:* Clove-orchid, amyl salicylate
PHYSICAL PROPERTIES: *Specific gravity:* 1.061–1.065 (25/25 C); *Refractive index:* 1.5070–1.5100 (20 C); *Boiling point:* 259 C; *Flash point:* > 212 F (TCC); *Solubility:* Soluble in 9 parts 80% ethyl alcohol, 2 parts 90% ethyl alcohol, mineral oils; insoluble in water and glycerol
WARNING AND CAUTION: Combustible; low toxicity

ISOBUTYL-α-TOLUATE
SYNONYMS: Isobutyl phenyl acetate
MOLECULAR FORMULA: $C_{12}H_{16}O_2$
MOLECULAR WEIGHT: 192.26
CHARACTERISTICS: *Form:* Liquid; *Color:* Colorless; *Odor:* Musk, honey, rose
PHYSICAL PROPERTIES: *Specific gravity:* 0.984–0.986 (25/25 C); *Refractive index:* 1.4860–1.4875 (20 C); *Flash point:* 212 F (TCC); *Solubility:* Soluble in 8 parts 70% ethyl alcohol, 2 parts 80% ethyl alcohol

ISOEUGENOL
SYNONYMS: 2-Methoxy-4-propenylphenol; 4-Hydroxy-3-methoxy-1-propenyl benzene; 4-Propenyl guaiacol; 1-Hydroxy-2-methoxy-4-propenyl benzene
CAS NUMBER: 97-54-1
MOLECULAR FORMULA: $C_{10}H_{12}O_2$
MOLECULAR WEIGHT: 164.20
CHARACTERISTICS: *Form:* Oily; *Color:* Pale yellow; *Odor:* Spicy clove
PHYSICAL PROPERTIES: *Specific gravity:* 1.081–1.084 (25/25 C); *Refractive index:* 1.5739 (19 C); *Boiling point:* 268 C; *Freezing point:* 19 C; *Solubility:* Soluble in alcohol, ether, organic solvents; slightly soluble in water

DERIVATION: Occurs in ylang ylang and other essential oils; from eugenol by isomerization with caustic potash

WARNING AND CAUTION: Combustible; low toxicity

LAURIC ALDEHYDE

SYNONYMS: Lauryl aldehyde; Dodecyl aldehyde; Aldehyde C-12 lauric; Dodecanal; Lauraldehyde; *n*-Dodecylic aldehyde

CAS NUMBER: 112-54-9

MOLECULAR FORMULA: $C_{12}H_{24}O$

MOLECULAR WEIGHT: 184.32

CHARACTERISTICS: *Form:* Crystals, powder, leaflet; *Color:* White or colorless; *Odor:* Bay oil, slight

PHYSICAL PROPERTIES: *Specific gravity:* 0.828–0.836 (25/25 C); *Refractive index:* 1.433–1.440 (20 C); *Boiling point:* 225 C; *Melting point:* 44 C; *Flash point:* 212 F (TCC); *Solubility:* Soluble in 90% alcohol; insoluble in water

DERIVATION: Small constituent in oils of sweet orange, petitgrain, and several species of pinus

WARNING AND CAUTION: Combustible; low toxicity

LIMONENE

SYNONYMS: 1-Methyl-4-(1-methylethenyl) cyclohexene; *p*-Mentha-1,8-diene; Cinene; Cajeputene; Kautschin

CAS NUMBER: 138-86-3

MOLECULAR FORMULA: $C_{10}H_{16}$

MOLECULAR WEIGHT: 136.23

CHARACTERISTICS: *Form:* Liquid; *Color:* Colorless; *Odor:* Pleasant, lemon-like

PHYSICAL PROPERTIES: *Specific gravity:* 0.8422 (20 C); *Refractive index:* 1.4744 (20 C); *Boiling point:* 176–176.4 C; *Solubility:* Soluble in alcohol; insoluble in water

DERIVATION: Occurs in various ethereal oils, particularly in oils of lemon, orange, caraway, dill, bergamot, peppermint, and spearmint

LINALOOL

SYNONYMS: 3,7-Dimethyl-1,6-octadien-3-ol; 2,6-Dimethyl-2,7-octadien-6-ol; Linalol

CAS NUMBER: 78-70-6

MOLECULAR FORMULA: $C_{10}H_{18}O$

MOLECULAR WEIGHT: 154.25

CHARACTERISTICS: *Form:* Liquid; *Color:* Colorless; *Odor:* Sweet, intense floral

PHYSICAL PROPERTIES: *Specific gravity:* 0.859–0.867 (25/25 C); *Refractive index:* 1.4610–1.4640 (20 C); *Optical rotation:* ±2°; *Flash point:* 175 F (TCC); *Solubility:* Soluble in alcohol, ether; insoluble in water

DERIVATION: Occurs in oils of Ceylon cinnamon, sassafras, orange flower, bergamot, ylang ylang, rosewood, petitgrain, linalol wood; synthetically made from geraniol; made synthetically from geraniol

WARNING AND CAUTION: Combustible; nontoxic

LINALYL ACETATE

SYNONYMS: 3,7-Dimethyl-1,6-octadien-3-yl acetate; Bergamol
CAS NUMBER: 115-95-7
MOLECULAR FORMULA: $C_{12}H_{20}O_2$
MOLECULAR WEIGHT: 196.28
CHARACTERISTICS: *Form:* Liquid; *Color:* Colorless; *Odor:* Bergamot
PHYSICAL PROPERTIES: *Specific gravity:* 0.908–0.920 (25/25 C); *Refractive index:* 1.450–1.458 (20 C); *Optical rotation:* –1 to +1°; *Boiling point:* 108–110 C; *Solubility:* Soluble in alcohol, ether, diethyl phthalate, benzyl benzoate, mineral oils; slightly soluble in propylene glycol; insoluble in water, glycerin
DERIVATION: Action of acetic anhydride on linalool in presence of sulfuric acid
WARNING AND CAUTION: Combustible; low toxicity

LINALYL BENZOATE

SYNONYMS: 3,7-Dimethyl-1,6-octadien-3-yl benzoate
MOLECULAR FORMULA: $C_{17}H_{22}O_2$
MOLECULAR WEIGHT: 258.37
CHARACTERISTICS: *Form:* Liquid; *Color:* Yellow-brownish; *Odor:* Heavy tuberose
PHYSICAL PROPERTIES: *Specific gravity:* 0.980–0.999 (25/25 C); *Refractive index:* 1.5050–1.200 (20 C); *Flash point:* 208 F (TCC); *Solubility:* Soluble in 1 part 90% ethyl alcohol

LINALYL BUTYRATE

SYNONYMS: 3,7-Dimethyl-1,6-octadien-3-yl butyrate; Linalyl isobutyrate
CAS NUMBER: 78-35-3
MOLECULAR FORMULA: $C_{14}H_{24}O_2$
MOLECULAR WEIGHT: 224.34
CHARACTERISTICS: *Form:* Liquid; *Color:* Yellow; *Odor:* Fruity
PHYSICAL PROPERTIES: *Specific gravity:* 0.893–0.904 (25/25 C); *Refractive index:* 1.4510–1.4560 (20 C); *Flash point:* > 212 F (TCC); *Solubility:* Soluble in 3 parts 80% ethyl alcohol
DERIVATION: Found in lavender oil; synthetically from acetone

LINALYL FORMATE

SYNONYMS: 3,7-Dimethyl-1,6-octadien-3-yl formate
MOLECULAR FORMULA: $C_{11}H_{18}O_2$
MOLECULAR WEIGHT: 182.26
CHARACTERISTICS: *Form:* Liquid; *Color:* Slightly yellow; *Odor:* Fruity, rose, bergamot
PHYSICAL PROPERTIES: *Specific gravity:* 0.915–0.924 (25/25 C); *Refractive index:* 1.4550–1.4580 (20 C); *Boiling point:* 100–103 C; *Flash point:* 190 F (TCC); *Solubility:* Soluble in 6 parts 70% ethyl alcohol, 1 part 80% ethyl alcohol; insoluble in water
DERIVATION: Synthetically from acetone
WARNING AND CAUTION: Combustible; low toxicity

LINALYL PROPIONATE

SYNONYMS: 3,7-Dimethyl-1,6-octadien-3-yl propionate
MOLECULAR FORMULA: $C_{13}H_{22}O_2$
MOLECULAR WEIGHT: 210.32
CHARACTERISTICS: *Form:* Liquid; *Color:* Colorless to slightly yellow; *Odor:* fresh bergamot, lily of the valley
PHYSICAL PROPERTIES: *Specific gravity:* 0.895–0.902 (25/25 C); *Refractive index:* 1.4500–1.4550 (20 C); *Flash point:* 196 F (TCC); *Solubility:* Soluble in 8 parts 70% ethyl alcohol, 2 parts 80% ethyl alcohol, most fixed oils, mineral oils, propylene glycol; insoluble in glycerin
DERIVATION: Found in lavender oil; synthetically from acetone
WARNING AND CAUTION: Combustible; low toxicity

MAGNESIUM CARBONATE

MOLECULAR FORMULA: $MgCO_3$
MOLECULAR WEIGHT: 485
CHARACTERISTICS: *Form:* Powder, light bulk; *Color:* White; *Odor:* Odorless
PHYSICAL PROPERTIES: *Specific gravity:* 3.0 (25/25 C); *Refractive index:* 1.52 (20 C); *Solubility:* Soluble in water and in diluted acids with effervescence; insoluble in alcohol
DERIVATION: By mixing solution of magnesium sulfate and sodium carbonate, and filtering
WARNING AND CAUTION: Low toxicity

MALIC ACID

SYNONYMS: Hydroxybutatenedioic acid; Hydroxysuccinic acid; Apple acid
CAS NUMBER: 6915-15-7
MOLECULAR FORMULA: $C_4H_6O_5$
MOLECULAR WEIGHT: 134.09
CHARACTERISTICS: *Form:* Crystals; *Color:* Colorless; *Odor:* Sour
PHYSICAL PROPERTIES: *Specific gravity:* 1.601 (*dl*), 1.595 (20.4 C) (*d* or *l*); *Boiling point:* 150 C (*dl*), 140 C (*d* or *l*); *Melting point:* 128 C (*dl*); 100 C (*d* or *l*); *Solubility:* Soluble in alcohol, water; slightly soluble in ether; insoluble in benzene
DERIVATION: From natural unripe apples and other fruits; synthetically by catalytic oxidation of benzene, by heating with steam under pressure
WARNING AND CAUTION: Combustible; low toxicity

MALONIC ACID

SYNONYMS: Methanedicarbonic acid; Propanedioic acid; Methanedicarboxylic acid
CAS NUMBER: 141-82-2
MOLECULAR FORMULA: $C_3H_4O_4$
MOLECULAR WEIGHT: 104.06
CHARACTERISTICS: *Form:* Crystals, triclinic small; *Color:* White
PHYSICAL PROPERTIES: *Specific gravity:* 1.63 (25/25 C); *Melting point:* 132–134 C; *Solubility:* Soluble in alcohol, ether, water

DERIVATION: From monochloroacetic acid with potassium cyanide and hydrolysis; from malic acid; from diethyl malonate; from lignous wastes
WARNING AND CAUTION: Highly toxic; strong irritant

MALTOL

SYNONYMS: 3-Hydroxy-2-methyl-4-pyrone; 3-Hydroxy-2-methyl-4H-pyran-4-one; 3-Hydroxy-2-methyl-γ-pyrone; Larixinic acid; Palatone; Veltol
CAS NUMBER: 118-71-8
MOLECULAR FORMULA: $C_6H_6O_3$
MOLECULAR WEIGHT: 126.11
CHARACTERISTICS: *Form:* Crystalline powder; *Color:* White; *Odor:* Caramel, butterscotch, fruity, strawberry
PHYSICAL PROPERTIES: *Solubility:* Soluble in alcohol, propylene glycol; slightly soluble in water
DERIVATION: Found and isolated from bark of young larch trees (*Larix decidua mill.*); in pine needles (*Abies alba mill., pinaceae*); in chicory, wood tars and oils, roasted malt

MENTHOL

SYNONYMS: Isopropyl-4-methylcyclohexan-2-ol; Hexahydrothymol; 3-*p*-Menthanol; Peppermint camphor; 3-Hydroxymenthane; Mentha camphor; 5-Methyl-2-(1-methylethyl) cyclohexanol; *p*-Menthanol; 1-Menthol; Methylhydroxyisopropylcyclohexane; *p*-Menthan-3-ol
CAS NUMBER: 89-78-1
MOLECULAR FORMULA: $C_{10}H_{20}O$
MOLECULAR WEIGHT: 156.27
CHARACTERISTICS: *Form:* Crystals or granules; *Color:* Colorless; *Odor:* Peppermint; *Taste:* Peppermint
PHYSICAL PROPERTIES: *Specific gravity:* 0.890 (25/25 C); *Refractive index:* 1.458 (25 C); *Optical rotation:* –50° (10% alcohol solution); *Boiling point:* 212 C; *Freezing point:* 41–43 C; *Flash point:* 200 F (TCC); *Solubility:* Soluble in 3 parts 70% alcohol, chloroform, ether, petrol ether, glacial acetic acid; slightly soluble in water
DERIVATION: From peppermint oil and other mint oils; synthetically by hydrogenation of thymol
WARNING AND CAUTION: Moderate irritant

MENTHONE

SYNONYMS: 1-*p*-Menthan-3-one; 5-Methyl-2-(1-methylethyl) cyclohexanone; 1-Methyl-4-isopropylcyclohexan-3-one; 4-Isopropyl-1-methylcyclohexan-3-one; 3-*p*-Menthanone; Terpinene; 3-Hydroxymenthene
CAS NUMBER: 1074-95-9
MOLECULAR FORMULA: $C_{10}H_{18}O$
MOLECULAR WEIGHT: 154.25
CHARACTERISTICS: *Form:* Oily liquid; *Color:* Colorless; *Odor:* Slightly peppermint; *Taste:* Bitter

PHYSICAL PROPERTIES: *Specific gravity:* 0.888–0.895 (25/25 C); *Refractive index:* 1.4480–1.4530 (20 C); *Optical rotation:* –15 to +15°; *Boiling point:* 207 C; *Flash point:* 170 F (TCC); *Solubility:* Soluble in 3 parts 70% ethyl alcohol, organic solvents; slightly soluble in water

DERIVATION: Found in oils of peppermint, Japanese mint, pennyroyal, geranium, and many other oils

WARNING AND CAUTION: Combustible; low toxicity

MENTHYL ACETATE

SYNONYMS: 5-Methyl-2-(1-methyl) cyclohexanol acetate; Menthol acetic ester; 1-Isopropyl-4-methylcyclohex-2-yl acetate

CAS NUMBER: 89-48-5

MOLECULAR FORMULA: $C_{12}H_{22}O_2$

MOLECULAR WEIGHT: 198.31

CHARACTERISTICS: *Form:* Liquid; *Color:* Colorless; *Odor:* Menthol

PHYSICAL PROPERTIES: *Specific gravity:* 0.922–0.927 (25/25 C); *Refractive index:* 1.447 (20 C); *Optical rotation:* –72.47′ to –73.18′; *Boiling point:* 227 C; *Flash point:* 198 F (TCC); *Solubility:* Soluble in alcohol, ether; slightly soluble in water

DERIVATION: From peppermint oil; by boiling menthol with acetic anhydride in presence of sodium acetate

WARNING AND CAUTION: Combustible; low toxicity

METHYL ACETATE

CAS NUMBER: 79-20-9

MOLECULAR FORMULA: C_3H_6O

MOLECULAR WEIGHT: 74.08

CHARACTERISTICS: *Form:* Liquid, volatile; *Color:* Colorless; *Odor:* Fragrant, apple

PHYSICAL PROPERTIES: *Specific gravity:* 0.92438 (25/25 C); *Refractive index:* 1.3619 (20 C); *Boiling point:* 54.05 C; *Freezing point:* –98.05 C; *Flash point:* 15 F (TCC); *Solubility:* Soluble in alcohol, ether, water

DERIVATION: By heating methyl alcohol and acetic acid in presence of sulfuric acid, and distilling

WARNING AND CAUTION: Flammable; explosive

METHYL ANTHRANILATE

SYNONYMS: 2-Aminobenzoic acid methyl ester; Methyl 2-aminobenzoate; Neroli oil, artificial; Methyl *o*-aminobenzoate

CAS NUMBER: 134-20-3

MOLECULAR FORMULA: $C_8H_9NO_2$

MOLECULAR WEIGHT: 151.16

CHARACTERISTICS: *Form:* Liquid; *Color:* Pale yellow with bluish florescence; *Odor:* Grape

PHYSICAL PROPERTIES: *Specific gravity:* 1.167–1.175 (15 C); *Refractive index:* 1.5820–1.5840 (20 C); *Boiling point:* 135 C; *Freezing point:* 23.8 C; *Solubility:* Soluble in 60% alcohol, propylene glycol; slightly soluble in water

DERIVATION: Occurs in neroli, ylang ylang, bergamot, jasmine, grape juice; by

heating anthranilic acid and methyl alcohol in presence of sulfuric acid, and distilling
WARNING AND CAUTION: Combustible

METHYL BENZOATE
SYNONYMS: Niobe oil; Benzoic acid methyl ester; Essence of niobe; Oil of niobe
CAS NUMBER: 93-58-3
MOLECULAR FORMULA: $C_8H_8O_2$
MOLECULAR WEIGHT: 136.15
CHARACTERISTICS: *Form:* Liquid; *Color:* Colorless; *Odor:* Fruity, ylang ylang
PHYSICAL PROPERTIES: *Specific gravity:* 1.085–1.088 (25/25 C); *Refractive index:* 1.5150–1.5180 (20 C); *Boiling point:* 98–200 C; *Freezing point:* –12.3 C; *Flash point:* 181 F (TCC); *Solubility:* Soluble in 4 parts 60% ethyl alcohol, ether, methanol, fixed oils; insoluble in water
DERIVATION: Found in oils of clove, ylang ylang, jonquil, tuberose; heating methyl alcohol and benzoic acid in presence of sulfuric acid; passing dry hydrogen chloride through a solution of benzoic acid in methanol
WARNING AND CAUTION: Combustible

METHYL BUTYRATE
SYNONYMS: Butanoic acid methyl ester
CAS NUMBER: 623-42-7
MOLECULAR FORMULA: $C_5H_{10}O_2$
MOLECULAR WEIGHT: 102.13
CHARACTERISTICS: *Form:* Liquid; *Color:* Colorless
PHYSICAL PROPERTIES: *Specific gravity:* 0.898 (20 C); *Refractive index:* 1.3879 (20 C); *Boiling point:* 102 C; *Freezing point:* –95 C; *Flash point:* 14 F (TCC), 57 C (CC); *Solubility:* Soluble in alcohol, ether; slightly soluble in water
WARNING AND CAUTION: Flammable; moderately toxic

METHYL CINNAMATE
SYNONYMS: Methyl 3-phenyl propionate; Methyl cinnamylate
CAS NUMBER: 103-26-4
MOLECULAR FORMULA: $C_{10}H_{10}O_2$
MOLECULAR WEIGHT: 162.19
CHARACTERISTICS: *Form:* Crystals; *Color:* White; *Odor:* Strawberry
PHYSICAL PROPERTIES: *Specific gravity:* 1.0415; *Boiling point:* 259.6 C; *Freezing point:* 34 C; *Solubility:* Soluble in 1 part 80% alcohol, ether, mineral oil; insoluble in water
DERIVATION: Found as constituent in oil of galanga; by heating methyl alcohol, cinnamic acid, and sulfuric acid, and distilling
WARNING AND CAUTION: Combustible; low toxicity

METHYL HEPTENONE
SYNONYMS: 6-Methyl-5-heptene-2-one
CAS NUMBER: 409-02-9

MOLECULAR FORMULA: $C_8H_{14}O$
MOLECULAR WEIGHT: 126.20
CHARACTERISTICS: *Form:* Liquid; *Color:* Colorless; *Odor:* Sharp citrus-lemongrass
PHYSICAL PROPERTIES: *Specific gravity:* 0.846–0.851 (25/25 C); *Refractive index:* 1.4380–1.4420 (20 C); *Boiling point:* 173–174 C; *Freezing point:* –67.1 C; *Solubility:* Soluble in alcohol, ether; insoluble in water
DERIVATION: From oil of lemongrass or by oxidation of secondary alcohol
WARNING AND CAUTION: Combustible; low toxicity

METHYL HEPTYNE CARBONATE

SYNONYMS: Methyl 2-octynoate; Heptyne carboxylic acid methyl ester; Folione
CAS NUMBER: 111-12-6
MOLECULAR FORMULA: $C_9H_{14}O_2$
MOLECULAR WEIGHT: 154.21
CHARACTERISTICS: *Form:* Liquid; *Color:* Colorless; *Odor:* Strong violet
PHYSICAL PROPERTIES: *Specific gravity:* 0.919–0.924 (25/25 C); *Refractive index:* 1.446–1.490 (20 C); *Flash point:* 192 F (TCC); *Solubility:* Soluble in 6 parts 70% ethyl alcohol, 2 parts 80% ethyl alcohol, most fixed oils, mineral oils
DERIVATION: From heptaldehyde
WARNING AND CAUTION: Combustible; low toxicity

METHYL IONONE

SYNONYMS: α-Methyl ionone; β-Methyl ionone; δ-Methyl ionone; Irone; Raldeine; Cyclocitrylidene methyl ethyl ketone
MOLECULAR FORMULA: $C_{14}H_{22}O$
MOLECULAR WEIGHT: 206.33
CHARACTERISTICS: *Form:* Liquid; *Color:* Colorless to amber yellow; *Odor:* Floral
PHYSICAL PROPERTIES: *Specific gravity:* 0.926–0.939 (25/25 C); *Refractive index:* 1.501–1.504 (20 C); *Boiling point:* 144 C; *Flash point:* 217 F (TCC); *Solubility:* Soluble in alcohol; insoluble in water
DERIVATION: Oil of orris; several isomers are available as α, β, δ, γ, and mixtures. The constants are approximately as above specified

METHYL ISOEUGENOL

SYNONYMS: Propenylveratrole; Isoeugenol methyl ether; 1,2-Dimethoxy-4-propenylbenzene; Propenyl guaiacol
CAS NUMBER: 93-16-3
MOLECULAR FORMULA: $C_{11}H_{14}O_2$
MOLECULAR WEIGHT: 178.23
CHARACTERISTICS: *Form:* Liquid; *Color:* Colorless to slightly yellow; *Odor:* Spicy, carnation, sweeter than eugenol
PHYSICAL PROPERTIES: *Specific gravity:* 1.047–1.053 (25/25 C); *Refractive index:* 1.5650–1.5690 (20 C); *Boiling point:* 262–264 C; *Flash point:* >212 F (TCC); *Solubility:* Soluble in 2 parts 70% ethyl alcohol, ; insoluble in mineral oil, glycerol
WARNING AND CAUTION: Combustible; low toxicity

METHYL ISOVALERATE

SYNONYMS: 3-Methylbutanoic acid methyl ester
MOLECULAR FORMULA: $C_6H_{12}O_2$
MOLECULAR WEIGHT: 116.16
CHARACTERISTICS: *Form:* Liquid; *Color:* Colorless; *Odor:* Valerian
PHYSICAL PROPERTIES: *Specific gravity:* 0.881 (20 C); *Boiling point:* 116–117 C; *Solubility:* Soluble in alcohol, ether; slightly soluble in water

METHYL NAPHTHYL KETONE

SYNONYMS: α and β-Naphthyl methyl ketone; α and β-Acetonaphthylene; 1′ and 2′-acetonaphthone; Oranger liquid (trademark)
MOLECULAR FORMULA: $C_{12}H_{10}O$
MOLECULAR WEIGHT: 170.21
CHARACTERISTICS: *Form:* Liquid; *Color:* Amber; *Odor:* Sweet neroli, grape
PHYSICAL PROPERTIES: *Specific gravity:* 1.110–1.116 (25/25 C); *Flash point:* > 212 F (TCC); *Solubility:* Soluble in 7 parts 70% ethyl alcohol, 2 parts 80% ethyl alcohol
DERIVATION: A mixture of α and β-naphthyl methyl ketone, in which the α-isomer predominates

METHYL PHENYL ACETATE

SYNONYMS: Methyl α-toluate
MOLECULAR FORMULA: $C_9H_{10}O_2$
MOLECULAR WEIGHT: 150.18
CHARACTERISTICS: *Form:* Liquid; *Color:* Colorless; *Odor:* Musky, honey
PHYSICAL PROPERTIES: *Specific gravity:* 1.062–1.066 (25/25 C); *Refractive index:* 1.5050–1.5080 (20 C); *Flash point:* 193 F (TCC); *Solubility:* Soluble in 7 parts 60% ethyl alcohol, 2 parts 70% ethyl alcohol, fixed oils; insoluble in water

METHYL SALICYLATE

SYNONYMS: Methyl *o*-hydroxybenzoate; Oil of wintergreen synthetic; Gaultheria oil; Wintergreen oil; Betula oil; Sweet birch oil; Teaberry oil; 2-Hydroxybenzoic acid methyl ester
CAS NUMBER: 119-36-8
MOLECULAR FORMULA: $C_8H_8O_3$
MOLECULAR WEIGHT: 152.15
CHARACTERISTICS: *Form:* Oily liquid; *Color:* Colorless, yellowish, reddish; *Odor:* Wintergreen, sharp
PHYSICAL PROPERTIES: *Specific gravity:* 1.180–1.185 (25/25 C); *Refractive index:* 1.5350–1.5380 (20 C); *Boiling point:* 222 C; *Freezing point:* –8 C; *Flash point:* 210 F (TCC); *Solubility:* Soluble in 7 parts 70% ethyl alcohol, glacial acetic acid; slightly soluble in water
DERIVATION: From wintergreen oil, leaves of Gaultheria; by heating methanol and salicylic acid in presence of sulfuric acid; by esterification of salicylic acid with methanol; by distillation of gaultheria or bark of *Betula lenta*; it is a constituent of many fruit juices, e.g., apple, grape, raspberry, cherry

WARNING AND CAUTION: Combustible; highly toxic; restricted by FDA for food use

NEROL

SYNONYMS: *cis*-3,7-Dimethyl-2,6-octadien-1-ol; 2,6-Dimethyl-2,6-octadien-8-ol
CAS NUMBER: 106-25-2
MOLECULAR FORMULA: $C_{10}H_{18}O$
MOLECULAR WEIGHT: 154.24
CHARACTERISTICS: *Form:* Liquid; *Color:* Colorless; *Odor:* Sweet rose, neroli
PHYSICAL PROPERTIES: *Specific gravity:* 0.875–0.880 (25/25 C); *Refractive index:* 1.4730–1.4780 (20 C); *Boiling point:* 224–225 C; *Flash point:* 198 F (TCC); *Solubility:* Soluble in 9 parts 50% ethyl alcohol
DERIVATION: Found in many essential oils, mostly in neroli oil; iodization of geraniol with hydriodic acid and alcoholic soda

NEROLIN

SYNONYMS: β-Naphthyl ethyl ether; β-Naphthol ethyl ether; Ethyl 2-naphthyl ether; 2-Ethoxynaphthalene; Bromelia; Nerolin 11
MOLECULAR FORMULA: $C_{12}H_{12}O$
MOLECULAR WEIGHT: 172.23
CHARACTERISTICS: *Form:* Crystals; *Color:* White; *Odor:* Neroli, orange blossom
PHYSICAL PROPERTIES: *Freezing point:* 35 C; *Solubility:* Soluble in 5 parts 95% ethyl alcohol; insoluble in water
DERIVATION: From β-naphthol and ethyl alcohol in presence of sulfuric acid
WARNING AND CAUTION: Combustible

γ-NONYL LACTONE

See Aldehyde C-18

γ-OCTALACTONE

SYNONYMS: γ-Hydroxyoctanoic acid lactone
MOLECULAR FORMULA: $C_8H_{14}O_2$
MOLECULAR WEIGHT: 142.20
CHARACTERISTICS: *Form:* Liquid; *Color:* Colorless to slightly yellow; *Odor:* Strong coconut-like
PHYSICAL PROPERTIES: *Specific gravity:* 0.970–0.980 (25/25 C); *Refractive index:* 1.4430–1.4470; *Flash point:* > 212 F (TCC); *Solubility:* Soluble in 3 parts 50% ethyl alcohol, 2 parts 60% ethyl alcohol, 1 part 70% ethyl alcohol

PHENYL ACETATE

SYNONYMS: Acetylphenol; Acetic acid phenyl ester
CAS NUMBER: 122-79-2
MOLECULAR FORMULA: $C_8H_8O_2$
MOLECULAR WEIGHT: 136.14
CHARACTERISTICS: *Form:* Liquid; *Color:* Colorless; *Odor:* Phenolic
PHYSICAL PROPERTIES: *Specific gravity:* 1.073 (25/25 C); *Refractive index:* 1.5030

(20 C); *Boiling point:* 195–196 C; *Flash point:* 176 F (TCC); *Solubility:* Soluble in alcohol, chloroform, ether, glacial acetic acid; slightly soluble in water
DERIVATION: From phenol and acetyl chloride; by heating triphenyl phosphate with potassium acetate and alcohol
WARNING AND CAUTION: Combustible; low toxicity

PHENYLACETIC ACID

SYNONYMS: α-Toluic acid; Benzeneacetic acid
CAS NUMBER: 103-82-2
MOLECULAR FORMULA: $C_8H_8O_2$
MOLECULAR WEIGHT: 136.14
CHARACTERISTICS: *Form:* Crystals; *Color:* White; *Odor:* Floral
PHYSICAL PROPERTIES: *Specific gravity:* 1.0809 (25/25 C); *Boiling point:* 262 C; *Freezing point:* 74 C; *Solubility:* Soluble in alcohol, ether; slightly soluble in water
DERIVATION: Found in oil of rose, neroli, and tobacco leaf; from benzyl cyanide refluxing with sulfuric acid; leaflets on distillation in vacuo
WARNING AND CAUTION: Combustible; toxic

PHENYL ETHYL ACETATE

SYNONYMS: Phenethyl acetate; β-Phenethyl acetate; 2-Phenylethyl acetate; Benzylcarbinyl acetate
CAS NUMBER: 103-45-7
MOLECULAR FORMULA: $C_{10}H_{12}O_2$
MOLECULAR WEIGHT: 164.21
CHARACTERISTICS: *Form:* Liquid; *Color:* Colorless; *Odor:* Rose, peach-like
PHYSICAL PROPERTIES: *Specific gravity:* 1.030–1.034 (25/25 C); *Refractive index:* 1.4970–1.5010 (20 C); *Boiling point:* 226 C; *Flash point:* > 212 F (TCC); *Solubility:* Soluble in 2 parts 70% ethyl alcohol, ether, fixed oils
DERIVATION: Interaction of ethyl acetate and aluminum phenyl ethylate; interaction of acetic anhydride and phenylethyl alcohol in the presence of sodium acetate
WARNING AND CAUTION: Combustible

PHENYL ETHYL ALCOHOL

SYNONYMS: Phenethyl alcohol; 2-Phenylethanol; Benzyl carbinol; β-Phenyl ethyl alcohol; β-Hydroxyethyl benzene
CAS NUMBER: 60-12-8
MOLECULAR FORMULA: $C_8H_{10}O$
MOLECULAR WEIGHT: 122.16
CHARACTERISTICS: *Form:* Liquid; *Color:* Colorless; *Odor:* Floral odor, rose, characteristic; *Taste:* Burning
PHYSICAL PROPERTIES: *Specific gravity:* 1.017–1.020 (25/25 C); *Refractive index:* 1.5310–1.5330 (20 C); *Boiling point:* 219 C; *Freezing point:* –27 C; *Solubility:* Soluble in 50% ethyl alcohol, fixed oils, glycerol; soluble 1 part in 50 parts of water
DERIVATION: By reduction of phenylacetic ethyl ester by sodium in absolute alcohol; by action of ethylene oxide on phenyl magnesium bromide, with hydrolysis
WARNING AND CAUTION: Highly toxic by inhalation

PHENYL ETHYL ANTHRANILATE

SYNONYMS: Phenethyl anthranilate; Benzylcarbinyl anthranilate; Phenylethyl *o*-aminobenzoate
CAS NUMBER: 133-18-6
MOLECULAR FORMULA: $C_{15}H_{15}NO_2$
MOLECULAR WEIGHT: 241.29
CHARACTERISTICS: *Form:* Liquid; *Color:* Colorless; yellowish with time; *Odor:* Grape-orange
PHYSICAL PROPERTIES: *Specific gravity:* 1.14 (25/25 C); *Solubility:* Soluble in alcohol
WARNING AND CAUTION: Combustible; nontoxic

PHENYL ETHYL BUTYRATE

SYNONYMS: Phenethyl butyrate; Benzylcarbinyl butyrate
MOLECULAR FORMULA: $C_{12}H_{16}O_2$
MOLECULAR WEIGHT: 192.26
CHARACTERISTICS: *Form:* Liquid; *Color:* Colorless; *Odor:* Rose
PHYSICAL PROPERTIES: *Specific gravity:* 0.991–0.994 (25/25 C); *Refractive index:* 1.4880–1.4920 (20 C); *Flash point:* 212 F (TCC); *Solubility:* Soluble in 1 part 90% ethyl alcohol, 2 parts 80% ethyl alcohol
WARNING AND CAUTION: Combustible; nontoxic

PHENYL ETHYL PROPIONATE

SYNONYMS: Phenethyl propionate; β-Phenethyl propionate; Benzyl carbinyl propionate
CAS NUMBER: 120-45-6
MOLECULAR FORMULA: $C_{11}H_{14}O$
MOLECULAR WEIGHT: 178.23
CHARACTERISTICS: *Form:* Liquid; *Color:* Colorless to slightly yellow; *Odor:* Fruity, lily, rose
PHYSICAL PROPERTIES: *Specific gravity:* 1.010–1.014 (25/25 C); *Refractive index:* 1.493–1.496 (20 C); *Flash point:* > 212 F (TCC); *Solubility:* Soluble in 4 parts 70% ethyl alcohol, ether
WARNING AND CAUTION: Combustible; low toxicity

PROPYL ACETATE

SYNONYMS: Acetic acid *n*-propyl ester
CAS NUMBER: 109-60-4
MOLECULAR FORMULA: $C_5H_{10}O_2$
MOLECULAR WEIGHT: 102.13
CHARACTERISTICS: *Form:* Liquid; *Color:* Colorless; *Odor:* Pear
PHYSICAL PROPERTIES: *Specific gravity:* 0.836 (20 C); *Refractive index:* 1.3844 (20 C); *Boiling point:* 101.6 C; *Flash point:* 14 C; *Solubility:* Soluble in alcohol, ether
DERIVATION: From acetic acid and *n*-propyl alcohol in the presence of sulfuric acid; from acetic acid and mixture of propene in the presence of zinc chloride catalyst
WARNING AND CAUTION: Flammable; moderately toxic

PROPYL PROPIONATE

SYNONYMS: Propanoic acid propyl ester
CAS NUMBER: 106-36-5
MOLECULAR FORMULA: $C_6H_{12}O_2$
MOLECULAR WEIGHT: 116.16
CHARACTERISTICS: *Form:* Liquid; *Color:* Colorless
PHYSICAL PROPERTIES: *Specific gravity:* 0.883 (20 C); *Refractive index:* 1.3935 (20 C); *Boiling point:* 122–124 C; *Freezing point:* –76 C; *Flash point:* 174 F (OC); *Solubility:* Soluble in alcohol, ether, most organic solvents; slightly soluble in water
WARNING AND CAUTION: Combustible

RHODINOL

SYNONYMS: 3,7-Dimethyl-7-octen-1-ol; *l*-Citronellol; Reuniol; Roseol
CAS NUMBER: 6812-78-8
MOLECULAR FORMULA: $C_{10}H_{20}O$
MOLECULAR WEIGHT: 156.26
CHARACTERISTICS: *Form:* Oily liquid; *Color:* Slightly yellow; *Odor:* Rose, warm
PHYSICAL PROPERTIES: *Specific gravity:* 0.860–0.880 (25/25 C); *Refractive index:* 1.4630–1.4730 (20 C); *Optical rotation:* –5 to –9°; *Boiling point:* 114–115 C; *Flash point:* > 212 F (TCC); *Solubility:* Soluble in 5 parts 60% ethyl alcohol, ether, mineral oils; slightly soluble in water; insoluble in glycerin
DERIVATION: A mixture of *l*-citronellol and geraniol from geranium; from Reunion geranium oil
WARNING AND CAUTION: Combustible; low toxicity

SAFROLE

SYNONYMS: 4-Allyl-1,2-methylenedioxybenzene; Methylene ether allyldioxybenzene; Methylene ether *m*-allylprocatechin; 5-(2-Propenyl)-1,3-benzodioxole; Allyl catechol methylene ether; Allyldioxybenzene methylene ether; *m*-Allylpyrocatechin methylene ether; Allyl pyrocatechol methylene ether; Shikimol; 1-Allyl-3,4-methylenedioxybenzene
CAS NUMBER: 94-59-7
MOLECULAR FORMULA: $C_{10}H_{10}O_2$
MOLECULAR WEIGHT: 162.18
CHARACTERISTICS: *Form:* Oily liquid; *Color:* Colorless to pale yellow; *Odor:* Sassafras, camphor
PHYSICAL PROPERTIES: *Specific gravity:* 1.100–1.107 (15 C); *Refractive index:* 1.5363–1.5385 (20 C); *Freezing point:* 11 C; *Flash point:* > 212 F (TCC); *Solubility:* Soluble in alcohol, chloroform, ether; slightly soluble in propylene glycol; insoluble in water, glycerin
DERIVATION: From oil of sassafras or camphor oil 75%; constituent of many essential oils
WARNING AND CAUTION: Highly toxic by ingestion; strong irritant

SUCCINIC ACID

SYNONYMS: Butanedioic acid; Amber acid; Ethylenesuccinic acid; Ethylenecarboxylic acid

CAS NUMBER: 110-15-6
MOLECULAR FORMULA: $C_4H_6O_4$
MOLECULAR WEIGHT: 118.09
CHARACTERISTICS: *Form:* Crystals; *Color:* Colorless; *Odor:* Odorless; *Taste:* Acid
PHYSICAL PROPERTIES: *Specific gravity:* 1.552 (25/25 C); *Boiling point:* 235 C; *Melting point:* 185 C; *Solubility:* Soluble in alcohol, ether, methanol, acetone, glycerol; slightly soluble in water; insoluble in benzene, carbon disulfide, carbon tetrachloride, petroleum ether
DERIVATION: Fermentation of ammonium tartrate; occurs in amber and other resins as a colorless monoclinic prism
WARNING AND CAUTION: Combustible; low toxicity

SUGAR

SYNONYMS: Sweet carbohydrate; Sucrose; Glucose (from grape); Cane (*Saccharum officinarum*)
CHARACTERISTICS: *Form:* Crystalline; *Taste:* Sweet
PHYSICAL PROPERTIES: *Solubility:* Soluble in water
DERIVATION: The sugar cane is from a bamboo in tropical and subtropical regions around the world; juice from the cane is boiled to remove the water and produce grains of sugar

TARTARIC ACID

SYNONYMS: Dihydroxysuccinic acid; 2,3-Dihydroxybutanedioic acid
CAS NUMBER: 133-37-9
MOLECULAR FORMULA: $C_4H_6O_6$
MOLECULAR WEIGHT: 150.1
CHARACTERISTICS: *Form:* Crystals or crystalline powder; *Color:* Colorless
PHYSICAL PROPERTIES: *Specific gravity:* 1.7598 (25/25 C); *Melting point:* 170 C; *Solubility:* Soluble in alcohol, ether, water, glycerol; insoluble in chloroform
DERIVATION: From maleic anhydride and hydrogen peroxide; from wine residues; occurs in many fruits, free and combined with potassium, calcium, or magnesium
WARNING AND CAUTION: Low toxicity

TERPINEOL

SYNONYMS: Lilacin; Terpinelol; α-: *p*-1-Menthene-8-ol; 1-Methyl-4-isopropyl-1-cyclohexen-8-ol; β-: *p*-8-Menthen-1-ol; 1-Methyl-4-isopropenyl-cyclohexan-1-ol
CAS NUMBER: 98-55-5 (α)
MOLECULAR FORMULA: $C_{10}H_{18}O$
MOLECULAR WEIGHT: 154.25
CHARACTERISTICS: *Form and Color:* Colorless liquid or transparent crystals of low melting point; *Odor:* Sweet, lilac
PHYSICAL PROPERTIES: *Specific gravity:* 0.931–0.936 (25/25 C); *Refractive index:* 1.4825–1.4850 (20 C); *Optical rotation:* –10 to +10°; *Boiling point:* 214–224 C; *Freezing point:* 6–12 C; *Flash point:* 195 F (TCC); *Solubility:* Soluble in 2 parts 70% ethyl alcohol, 3 parts 60% ethyl alcohol; slightly soluble in water, glycerin
DERIVATION: Found in several essential oils; by heating terpin hydrate with

phosphoric acid and distilling or with dilute sulfuric acid, using an azeotropic separation; fractional distillation of pine oil
WARNING AND CAUTION: Combustible

TERPINYL ACETATE
CAS NUMBER: 80-26-2
MOLECULAR FORMULA: $C_{12}H_{20}O_2$
MOLECULAR WEIGHT: 196.29
CHARACTERISTICS: *Form:* Liquid; *Color:* Colorless
PHYSICAL PROPERTIES: *Specific gravity:* 0.955–0.962 (25/25 C); *Refractive index:* 1.4640–1.4660 (20 C); *Flash point:* 212 F (TCC); *Solubility:* Soluble in 3–5 parts 70% ethyl alcohol
DERIVATION: From cajeput oil, melaleuca, cardamom, Siberian pine needle

THEOBROMA OIL
SYNONYMS: Cacao butter; Cocoa butter
CHARACTERISTICS: *Form:* Solid; *Color:* Yellowish-white; *Odor:* Chocolate; *Taste:* Chocolate
PHYSICAL PROPERTIES: *Specific gravity:* 0.858–0.864 (100/25 C); *Refractive index:* 1.4537–1.4585 (40 C); *Melting point:* 30–35 C; *Solubility:* Soluble in chloroform, ether; slightly soluble in ethyl alcohol; insoluble in water
DERIVATION: From roasted seeds of theobroma cacao, sterculaceae; from the cacao bean, by expression, decoction, or extraction by solvent
WARNING AND CAUTION: Combustible; low toxicity

γ-UNDECALACTONE
See Aldehyde C-14 pure

VANILLIN
SYNONYMS: 4-Hydroxy-3-methoxybenzaldehyde; Methoxyprotocatechuic aldehyde; Protocatechualdehyde-3-methyl ether; Methylprotocatechuic aldehyde; Vanillic aldehyde; 3-Methoxy-4-hydroxybenzaldehyde
CAS NUMBER: 121-33-5
MOLECULAR FORMULA: $C_8H_8O_3$
MOLECULAR WEIGHT: 152.15
CHARACTERISTICS: *Form:* Crystalline needles; *Color:* White; *Odor:* Sweetish
PHYSICAL PROPERTIES: *Specific gravity:* 1.056 (25/25 C); *Boiling point:* 285 C; *Melting point:* 81–83 C; *Solubility:* Soluble in 2 parts 95% ethyl alcohol, chloroform, ether, carbon disulfide, glacial acetic acid, pyridine, water
DERIVATION: It occurs in vanilla bean extract and in many balsams and resins; from lignin contained in sulfite waste pulp liquor; made also from eugenol or guaiacol
WARNING AND CAUTION: Combustible; low toxicity

WINE RESIDUE (GREEN PURE LEES, OIL)
CHARACTERISTICS: *Form:* A distinctive appearance, odor, and flavor is imparted by producers

PHYSICAL PROPERTIES: Naturally fermented grape juice contains 6–22% alcohol
DERIVATION: The fermented juice of grapes, and of other fruits or plants
WARNING AND CAUTION: Flammable; low toxicity

YARA YARA

SYNONYMS: 2-Methoxynaphthalene; β-Naphthol methyl ether; Methyl β-naphthyl ether; β-Naphthyl methyl ether; Methoxynaphthalene
MOLECULAR FORMULA: $C_{11}H_{10}O$
MOLECULAR WEIGHT: 158.20
CHARACTERISTICS: *Form:* Power, crystals; *Color:* Colorless to white; *Odor:* Fruity, acacia, orange
PHYSICAL PROPERTIES: *Solubility:* Soluble in alcohol, ether; insoluble in water
DERIVATION: By heating β-naphthol and methyl alcohol in presence of sulfuric acid; by methylating β-naphthol with dimethyl sulfate
WARNING AND CAUTION: Combustible

Chapter XIII: BOTANICAL REFERENCES FOR THE FORMULARY

ABSINTHE (WORMWOOD)

BOTANICAL: *Family: Compositae; Genus: Artemisia; Species: Absinthium, Vulgaris, Tridentata* (sage brush, Western U.S.), *Judaica* (reported in the bible), *Arborescenses* (reported in the bible)

HABITAT/SOURCES: Europe

NOTES: Aromatic plant with a bitter taste used in making "absinthe" and in flavoring some wines. Essential oil from leaves of *Artemisia absinthium*, with constituents tunjone and derivatives. A pale-yellowish-green liquid with high alcoholic content. Absinthe produces deterioration of the brain. It is prohibited in the U.S. and in some other countries.

ACACIA

BOTANICAL: *Family: Leguminosae; Genus: Acacia; Species: Greggii*

HABITAT/SOURCES: Tropical trees

NOTES: Some species in Africa produce gum arabic

AGARIC

BOTANICAL: *Family: Agaricaceae; Genus: Agaricus; Species: Campestris*

NOTES: A fungus of cultivated mushrooms

ALLSPICE, OIL

BOTANICAL: *Family: Myrtaceae; Genus: Pimenta; Species: Officinalis*

HABITAT/SOURCES: Tropical America

NOTES: Also called "pimento."

"Spice" is the name given to food seasonings from plants. Spices have a sharp taste and odor and may stimulate appetite and digestion. Common spices are allspice, cinnamon, clove, ginger, mace, mustard, nutmeg, and pepper.

ALMOND

BOTANICAL: *Family: Rosaceae; Genus: Prunus; Species: Amygdalus, Communis, Amara* (bitter)

HABITAT/SOURCES: Mediterranean regions

BOTANICAL REFERENCES FOR THE FORMULARY

ALOE

BOTANICAL: *Family: Liliaceae or Aloaceae; Genus: Aloe; Species: Vera*
HABITAT/SOURCES: Warm countries, especially South Africa
PART USED: The leaves of some aloes, as the "Barbados aloe" have a bitter juice
NOTES: The juice is dried and used in medicine as a purgative. It produces stimulating effect on the intestine and the liver.

AMBER

NOTES: A resin with brown to dark orange-yellow color. It is mostly found along the shores of the Baltic Sea, from trees buried under ground or water millions of years ago.

AMBERGRIS

NOTES: Grayish waxy material formed in the intestine of sperm whales. It is found floating in the sea or ashore. It is employed as fixative for perfumes because it has a sweet-earth odor after exposure to air. Initially it has a disagreeable odor.

ANGELICA

BOTANICAL: *Family: Umbelliferae; Genus: Angelica; Species: Archangelica; Officinalis*
HABITAT/SOURCES: Central Europe
PART USED: The aromatic seeds, leaves, stems, and oil from the roots
NOTES: Used in medicine and as a flavoring

ANGOSTURA

BOTANICAL: *Family: Rutaceae; Genus: Galipea, Cusparia; Species: Officinalis, Trifoliata, Febrifuga*
NOTES: Angostura is the former name of the city "Bolivar" of Bolivia

ANISE

BOTANICAL: *Family: Umbelliferae; Genus: Pimpinella; Species: Anisum*
HABITAT/SOURCES: China, U.S.S.R., Spain
PART USED: Seeds
NOTES: Annual herb. The seeds have a spicy taste. Anise star, seeds of *Illicium verum*, family *Magnoliaceae*, is a source of anise oil. "Anisette" is a French dimunitive name for anise.

APPLE

BOTANICAL: *Family: Rosaceae; Genus: Malus* (wild, Europe, Asia); *Species: Pumila* (cultivated), *Sylvestris* (wild), *Baccata*

APRICOT

BOTANICAL: *Family: Rosaceae; Genus: Prunus; Species: Armeniaca*

ASAFETIDA

BOTANICAL: *Family: Umbelliferae; Genus: Ferula; Species: Foetida, Rubicaulis*

SYNONYMS: Asafoetida; Asant; Devil's dung; Food of the Gods
CHARACTERISTICS: *Form:* Lumps or tears; *Odor:* Garlic; *Taste:* Bitter acrid
PHYSICAL PROPERTIES: *Solubility:* Soluble in 50% ethyl alcohol; trituration with water yields a milky emulsion
DERIVATION: Gum resin obtained as an exudation of the decapitated rhizome and roots: 60% ethereal oil, 40% resin consisting of ester of asaresinotanoli and ferulic acid, pinene, vanillin, with about 25% gum
HABITAT/SOURCES: Iran, Turkestan, Afghanistan

AUBEPINE (HAWTHORN)
BOTANICAL: *Family: Rosaceae; Genus: Crataegus* (English); *Species: Mollis* (down), *Monogyna* (white or pinkish flower and red fruit), *Crus-Galli* (cockspur); *Species: Oxyacantha* (English)

AVOCADO
BOTANICAL: *Family: Lauraceae; Genus: Persea; Species: Americana*

BALM
BOTANICAL: *Family: Labiatae; Genus: Melissa; Species: Officinalis*
NOTES: A spicy aromatic plant

BANANA
BOTANICAL: *Family: Musaceae; Genus: Musa; Species: Sapientum* (sweet yellow), *Paradisiaca* (plantain)

BARBECUE
NOTES: Highly seasoned vinegar sauce

BARBERRY
BOTANICAL: *Family: Berberidaceae; Genus: Berberis* (Thunbergii, Japanese); *Species: Vulgaris* (Julianae, wintergreen)

BENEDICTINE
NOTES: A liqueur originally made by the Benedictine Italian monks.

BENZOIN
BOTANICAL: *Family: Estiracaceae; Genus: Styrax; Species: Benzoin*
HABITAT/SOURCES: Islands of Sumatra and Java in Indonesia
NOTES: A soft, fragrant resin from the Benzoin tree. A synthetic benzoin is made from benzaldehyde and sodium cyanide dissolved in alcohol

BERGAMOT
BOTANICAL: *Family: Rutaceae; Genus: Citrus, Monarda* (wild); *Species: Bergamia, Aurantium*
HABITAT/SOURCES: Italy, South America, western Africa

EXTRACTION: Oil from the green peels of the fruits by cold expression

BILBERRY
BOTANICAL: *Family: Ericaceae; Genus: Vaccinium; Species: Myrtillus* (European), *Whortleberry* (European)

BITTERS
NOTES: Alcoholic liquid made generally with herbs or roots and used in cocktails or as a tonic

BLACKBERRY
BOTANICAL: *Family: Rosaceae; Genus: Rubus; Species: Occidentalis*

BLACK CURRANT
BOTANICAL: *Family: Sassifragaceae; Genus: Ribes; Species: Nigrum*
NOTES: Used mainly for soft drinks or jams

BLUEBERRY
BOTANICAL: *Family: Ericaceae; Genus: Vaccinium; Species: Corymbosum* (high), *Pennsylvanicum* (low)
HABITAT/SOURCES: North America
EXTRACTION: Juicy blue, purplish or blackish berries

BOUQUET
NOTES: Flowers fastened together in a bunch. A distinctive and characteristic compound of aromatic products.

BOUVARDIA
BOTANICAL: *Family: Rubiaceaes; Genus: Bouvardia; Species: Densiflora, Heterophylla, Leiantha, Longiflora, Scabra, Teniufolia, Ternifolia*

BRANDY
NOTES: A strong alcoholic beverage distilled from wine or from fermented fruit juice. The alcoholic content is 45–55%.
See also COGNAC.

BREAD
NOTES: A food made from flour, water, and a leavening agent and baked in loaf form. It is considered the necessary food for the sustaining of life.

BUTTER
NOTES: A solid emulsion of the fat from milk by churning.

BUTTERSCOTCH
NOTES: A candy made with butter, brown sugar, corn syrup, and water.

CACAO
BOTANICAL: *Family: Sterculiaceae; Genus: Theobroma; Species: Cacao*
HABITAT/SOURCES: Tropical evergreen trees
NOTES: The seeds of cacao beans are used for making chocolate, cocoa, and cocoa butter

CAKE
NOTES: A sweet mixture of flour, liquid, eggs, and other ingredients, in loaf or rounded form, and generally baked with a leaven.

CALAMUS
BOTANICAL: *Family: Acoraceae; Genus: Acorus; Species: Calamus*
HABITAT/SOURCES: Tropical Asia
PART USED: Palm with aromatic roots (sweet flag)

CAMPHOR
BOTANICAL: *Family: Lauraceae; Genus: Cinnamomum; Species: Camphora*

CANANGA
See YLANG YLANG

CAPER
BOTANICAL: *Family: Capparidaceae; Genus: Capparis; Species: Spinosa*
HABITAT/SOURCES: Mediterranean regions

CAPSICUM
BOTANICAL: *Family: Solanaceae; Genus: Capsicum; Species: Fastigiatum, Annuum, Frutescens*
HABITAT/SOURCES: Tropical plants

CARAMEL
NOTES: A combination of sugar, butter, cream or milk, and flavoring made as a candy and cooked to a thicker consistency.
Burnt sugar, used for coloring.

CARDAMOM
BOTANICAL: *Family: Zingiberaceae; Genus: Elettaria; Species: Cardamomom*
PART USED: Fruit
NOTES: Fruit of several plants of the ginger family

CARNATION
BOTANICAL: *Family: Caryophyllaceae; Genus: Dianthus; Species: Caryophyllus*

CARROT
BOTANICAL: *Family: Umbelliferae; Genus: Daucus; Species: Carota, Sativa*

CASCARILLA
BOTANICAL: *Family: Rhamnaceae; Genus: Croton; Species: Eleuteria*
HABITAT/SOURCES: West Indies

CASHEW
BOTANICAL: *Family: Anacardiaceae; Genus: Anacardium; Species: Occidentale*
HABITAT/SOURCES: Tropical America

CASSIA
BOTANICAL: *Family: Leguminosae; Genus: Cassia, Cinnamomum, Acacia; Species: Acutifolia* (African), *Angustifolia* (Indian), *Marilandica* (wild senna), *Fasciculata* (partridge peas), *Farnesiana*
HABITAT/SOURCES: China, southeast Asia (*Cinnamomum*); West Indies, southern France (*Farnesiana*)
USES: Oil

CASTOR
BOTANICAL: *Family: Euphorbiaceae; Genus: Ricinus; Species: Communis*
HABITAT/SOURCES: Tropical Africa, Asia (native)
EXTRACTION: Oil from seeds
NOTES: Seed is poisonous

CATSUP (KETCHUP)
NOTES: A seasoned tomato purée; a variety of ketchup.

CEDRELA (CEDAR)
BOTANICAL: *Family: Pinaceae, Coniferous; Genus: Cedrus, Thuja, Chamaecyparis, Juniperus; Species: Deodara, Atlantica* (Atlas cedar), *Libani* (Lebanon cedar)

CENTAURY
BOTANICAL: *Family: Compositae; Genus: Centaura Americana; Species: Rubra*
HABITAT/SOURCES: Eurasia
NOTES: A plant with clusters of rose-purple flowers

CHAMOMILE
BOTANICAL: *Family: Compositae; Genus: Anthemis, Matricaria* (German); *Species: Nobilis, Chamomilla* (German)
PART USED: Flowers and leaves
NOTES: Small perennial plant growing to about 12 in. with many branches. The flowers and leaves smell sweet but taste bitter. The German variety grows higher (2 ft)

CHAMPAGNE
NOTES: A sparkling wine made in the old province of Champagne in France.

CHARTREUSE
NOTES: A green or yellow liqueur made from herbs and spices by Carthusian monks in the monastery near Grenoble (southeastern France)

CHEESE
NOTES: A solid or semisolid food from pressed curd of milk

CHERIMOYA
BOTANICAL: *Family: Annonaceae; Genus: Annona; Species: Cherimola*
HABITAT/SOURCES: Tropical American tree

CHERRY
BOTANICAL: *Family: Rosaceae; Genus: Prunus; Species: Avium* (sweet), *Cerasum* (sour)

CHERVIL (CICELY)
BOTANICAL: *Family: Umbelliferae; Genus: Myrrhis, Anthriscus* (Eurasia), *Chaerophyllum* (European), *Osmorhiza* (sweet); *Species: Odorata, Cerefolium* (Eurasia), *Bulbosum* (European), *Longistylis* (American)

CHOCOLATE
NOTES: The word "chocolate" is from the Mayan words meaning "warm beverage." To make chocolate, husked cacao seeds are fermented for a short period and then roasted, ground, and combined with sweetener, milk, and/or flavoring material.

CINCHONA
BOTANICAL: *Family: Rubiaceae; Genus: Cinchona; Species: Officinalis*
HABITAT/SOURCES: Peru and Bolivia
PART USED: Bark
NOTES: Trees and shrubs. The bark is used to make drugs quinine and cinchona with which malaria is treated.

CINNAMON
BOTANICAL: *Family: Lauraceae; Genus: Cinnamomum; Species: Zeylanicum, Laureirii* (tropical Asia)
HABITAT/SOURCES: Sri Lanka, Madagascar, southern India, Seychelles, Ceylon
NOTES: A spice used in flavoring. In Ceylon the bark is peeled in April and November.

CITRONELLA
BOTANICAL: *Family: Graminaceae; Genus: Andropogon* or *Cymbopogon; Species: Citratus, Nardus, Winterianus*
HABITAT/SOURCES: China, Taiwan, Indonesia, Brazil, Colombia, Guatemala
EXTRACTION: Oil from grass

CITRUS
BOTANICAL: *Family: Rutaceae; Genus: Citrus, Fortunella, Japonica,* or *Margarita*

(kumquat); *Species: Bergamot, Citron, Grapefruit, Lemon, Lime, Kumquat, Mandarin, Orange* (bitter and sweet), *Tangerine*

CLOVE
BOTANICAL: *Family: Myrtaceae; Genus: Caryophyllus; Species: Aromaticus*
HABITAT/SOURCES: Tropical
PART USED: Dried flower buds of tree

COCA
BOTANICAL: *Family: Erythroxylacae; Genus: Erythroxylon; Species: Coca*
HABITAT/SOURCES: South American tree
NOTES: The leaves contain cocaine and alkaloids. People of the Andes chew the leaves as a stimulant.

COCOA
NOTES: Roasted and ground cacao beans. Freed from the fatty oil, the powder is combined with sugar, milk, and water to make a brown to reddish beverage. Chocolate is cocoa with the fat left in.

COCONUT
BOTANICAL: *Family: Palmaceae; Genus: Cocos; Species: Nucifera*
HABITAT/SOURCES: Tropical regions
NOTES: Oil from the white flesh is used to make soaps and cosmetics.

COFFEE
BOTANICAL: *Family: Rubiaceae; Genus: Coffea; Species: Arabica*

COGNAC
NOTES: A brandy produced in the vicinity of Cognac, a town in Western France.

COLA (KOLA NUT)
BOTANICAL: *Family: Sterculiaceae; Genus: Cola; Species: Acuminata*
HABITAT/SOURCES: African trees; cultivated in tropical regions for the seeds
PART USED: Seeds
NOTES: The seed of cola contains caffeine, theobromine. The seeds are used in carbonated drinks and in pharmaceutical products.

COLOGNE
NOTES: A perfumed liquid made with alcohol and fragrant oils. It is also called "Eau de Cologne." The name refers to the city Köln of West Germany, where it was first produced commercially.

CORIANDER
BOTANICAL: *Family: Umbelliferae; Genus: Coriandrum; Species: Sativum*
NOTES: Annual herb. About 500 lb of coriander seeds gives 5 lb of oil.

CRANBERRY
BOTANICAL: *Family: Ericaceae; Genus: Vaccinium; Species: Macrocarpon* (American), *Oxycoccus* (European)
HABITAT/SOURCES: North America
NOTES: Shrubs growing in damp ground with tart red berry

CUCUMBER
BOTANICAL: *Family: Cucurbitaceae; Genus: Cucumis; Species: Sativus*

CULINARY
NOTES: Related to kitchen or cooking, used for food flavoring

CURAÇAO
NOTES: A liqueur with flavor of sour orange peels, from Curaçao, the largest island in the south Caribbean Sea.

CURRANT
BOTANICAL: *Family: Saxifragaceae; Genus: Ribes; Species: Rubrum* (red), *Nigrum* (black), *Odoratum* (golden)
HABITAT/SOURCES: Mediterranean regions
NOTES: Small, sour, seedless grape from shrubs. Used to make jam and jelly.

CYCLAMEN
BOTANICAL: *Family: Primulaceae; Genus: Cyclamen; Species: Persicum, Europaeum, Neapolitan, Africanum*

DATE
BOTANICAL: *Family: Palmaceae; Genus: Phoenix; Species: Dactylifera*
HABITAT/SOURCES: Tropical and subtropical regions

DITTANY
BOTANICAL: *Family: Labiatae; Genus: Origanum; Species: Dictamnus*
HABITAT/SOURCES: Crete
NOTES: An aromatic plant with pink flowers

EGLANTINE (WILD ROSE)
BOTANICAL: *Family: Rosaceae; Genus: Rosa; Species: Rubiginosa, Eglanteria*
SYNONYMS: Sweet briar; Sweet brier

ELDER
BOTANICAL: *Family: Caprifoliaceae; Genus: Sambucus; Species: Canadensis*
NOTES: Small trees or shrubs

ELECAMPANE
BOTANICAL: *Family: Compositae; Genus: Inula; Species: Helenum*

PART USED: Roots
NOTES: Heavy, fleshy roots with a bitter taste, similar to camphor

FENUGREEK
BOTANICAL: *Family: Leguminosae; Genus: Trigonella; Species: Foenumgraecum*
HABITAT/SOURCES: Southeastern Europe, Middle East
EXTRACTION: Resinoid from crushed seeds

FERN
BOTANICAL: *Family:* Includes 12 families; *Polypodiaceae*, most common and widely distributed; *Genus: Pteridium* (the bracken), *Adiantum* (maidenhair), *Dryopteris* (wood-fern), *Asplenium* (spleenworts), *Polypodium* (polypody), *Camptosorus* (walking-leaf), *Onoclea* (sensitive fern). Some belong to other families: *Trichomanes* (film fern), *Lygodium* (climbing fern), *Ophioglossum* (adder's tongue), *Botrychium* (rattlesnake fern). There are about 15,000 species of ferns.
NOTES: Pteridophytic ferns are flowerless and seedless, characteristically having fronds with divided leaflets and reproducing by spores in the undersurface of the fronds. They are classified in the Filicinae family.

FERNET (BRANCA)
NOTES: A liqueur made with alcohol, sugar, and essential oils. The name "Branca" refers to a specific fernet.

FIG
BOTANICAL: *Family: Moraceae; Genus: Ficus; Species: Carica*
HABITAT/SOURCES: Cultivated in Europe and Asia; wild in the Middle East, western Asia, between Syria and Afghanistan

FOUGÈRE
NOTES: French name of fern.

FRANGIPANNI
BOTANICAL: *Family: Apocynaceae; Genus: Plumeria; Species: Acutifolia, Alba, Rubra*
HABITAT/SOURCES: Tropical
NOTES: Shrubs with a milky juice and three different color flowers: yellowish, white, reddish

FUNGI (MUSHROOM)
BOTANICAL: *Family: Agaricaceae* (commonly cultivated); *Genus: Agaricus; Species: Campestris*

GALANGAL
BOTANICAL: *Family: Zingiberaceae; Genus: Alpinia; Species: Officinarum*
HABITAT/SOURCES: Eastern Asia
PART USED: Pungent, aromatic roots of plant

GARDENIA

BOTANICAL: *Family: Rubiaceae; Genus: Gardenia; Species: Jasminoides* (China)
HABITAT/SOURCES: China (native) and cultivated in various countries as shrubs and trees

GARLIC

BOTANICAL: *Family: Amaryllidaceae; Genus: Allium; Species: Sativum*

GENTIAN

BOTANICAL: *Family: Gentianaceae; Genus: Gentiana; Species: Crinita*
HABITAT/SOURCES: It grows everywhere except Africa
PART USED: Roots, which are bitter, are used in medicine
NOTES: A beautiful plant, both wild and cultivated, with about 600 species. The flowers are mostly blue, but can also be yellow and red. Many gentian flowers do not open and are called closed or bottle gentians.

GERANIUM

BOTANICAL: *Family: Geraniaceae; Genus: Pelargonium; Species: Peltatum* (ivy), *Graveolens* (rose), *Domesticus* (Lady Washington), *Robertianum* (Robert, herb), *Erodium cicutarium* (Alfilaria)
HABITAT/SOURCES: Morocco, Egypt, U.S.S.R., France, China, Reunion, Madagascar, Algeria
EXTRACTION: Oil from leaves and stalks

GERMANDER

BOTANICAL: *Family: Labiatae; Genus: Teucrium; Species: Chamaedrys*
NOTES: Aromatic plants with purplish or reddish two-lipped flowers

GIN

NOTES: A strong alcoholic liquor, distilled from grain, as rye or barley, and flavored with juniper berries

GINGER

BOTANICAL: *Family: Zingiberaceae; Aristolochiaceae* (wild), *Genus: Zingiber, Asarum; Species: Officinale, Canadense*
HABITAT/SOURCES: Tropical regions

GIROFLÉ (CLOVE)

BOTANICAL: *Family: Myrataceae; Genus: Caryophyllus, Eugenia; Species: Aromaticus, Caryophyllata*
HABITAT/SOURCES: Indonesia, Tanzania, Madagascar, Sri Lanka
EXTRACTION: Oil from dried flower buds, leaves, and twigs
NOTE: Giroflé is the French word for clove

GLACÉ

NOTES: French name for ice cream. It refers to a coated substance with sugar or gelatine applied to food on which it solidifies to a thin coating

GOOSEBERRY
BOTANICAL: *Family: Saxifragaceae; Genus: Ribes; Species: Hirtillum* (American), *Grossularia* (European), *Uva-Crispa* (Euroasia), *Physalis* (Peruvian)

GRAPE
BOTANICAL: *Family: Vitaceae; Genus: Vitis; Species: Vinifera* (European), *Labrusca* (American), *Aestivalis* (American), *Rotundifloria* (American), *Vulpina* (American)

GRAPEFRUIT
BOTANICAL: *Family: Rutaceae; Genus: Citrus; Species: Paradisi, Maxima* (shaddock tropical tree), *Grandis, Decumana*
HABITAT/SOURCES: Tropical and semitropical trees
EXTRACTION: Oil from pressing fruit peels

GREEN GAGE
BOTANICAL: *Family: Rosaceae; Genus: Prunus; Species: Domestica* (European, Italian), *Salicina* (Japanese), *Americana* (American), *Insititia* (Damson), *Myrobalan* (ornamental), *Cerasifera* (ornamental)
NOTES: A variety of plum. The name is from Sir William Gage (1724–1820), English botanist

GRENADINE (POMEGRANATE)
BOTANICAL: *Family: Punicaceae; Genus: Punica; Species: Granatum*
HABITAT/SOURCES: Semitropical shrubs or small trees, native to Africa
NOTES: Grenadine refers to mixed drinks flavored with pomegranate juice or red currants

GUAVA
BOTANICAL: *Family: Myrtaceae; Genus: Psidium; Species: Guajava*
HABITAT/SOURCES: Asian and American shrubs
NOTES: A pear-shaped fruit with yellow and pink flesh

HAWTHORN
See AUBEPINE

HAZEL NUT
BOTANICAL: *Family: Betulaceae; Genus: Corylus; Species: Americana* (North America), *Avellana* (European), *Cornuta*

HELIOTROPE
BOTANICAL: *Family: Boraginaceae; Genus: Heliotropium; Species: Arborescens* (South America)
NOTES: Small fragrant purplish flowers

HIP (ROSE HIP)
NOTES: Fresh, berry-like fruit of rose, ripened with numerous small dry seeds

HONEY

NOTES: A sweet, golden or brownish colored, viscid fluid, produced by bees from nectar of flowers. A sweet substance used in food.

HONEYSUCKLE

BOTANICAL: *Family: Caprifoliaceae; Genus: Lonicera, Banksia* (bushes, Australia); *Species: Sempervirens* (coral), *Periclymenum* (woodbine), *Tatarica* (landscaping), *Fragantissima* (landscaping)

HABITAT/SOURCES: Australian and New Zealand trees and shrubs with white or pink flowers

HOP

BOTANICAL: *Family: Cannabinaceae; Genus: Humulus; Species: Lupulus* (European), *Americanus* (wild), *Scandens* (Japanese)

HABITAT/SOURCES: Cultivated in Germany and eastern Europe

PART USED: Ripe fresh flower tops

NOTES: Contains a bitter aromatic oil from dried ripe flower. It is used in beer production.

HUCKLEBERRY

BOTANICAL: *Family: Ericaceae; Genus: Gaylussacia; Species: Baccata*

HABITAT/SOURCES: American shrubs

NOTES: Related to blueberry and whortleberry.

HYACINTH

BOTANICAL: *Family: Liliaceae; Genus: Hyacinthus; Species: Orientalis*

HABITAT/SOURCES: Cultivated in Holland in large amounts

EXTRACTION: Oil from the blossom by solvent

HYSSOP

BOTANICAL: *Family: Menthaceae; Genus: Hyssopus; Species: Officinalis*

PART USED: The seeds, flowers, and the green parts of the plant have a strong odor and taste

NOTES: A bushy evergreen shrub of the mint type.

IRIS (OIL OR CONCRETE)

SYNONYMS: Blue flag; Flag lily; Poison flag; Water flag; Orris (*Iris florentina*)

BOTANICAL: *Family: Iridiceae; Genus: Iris; Species: Pseudacorus, Versicolor* (blue flag), *Kaempferi* (Japanese), *Sibirica* (siberian), *Spuria* (butterfly), *Pumila* (dwarf bearded)

CHARACTERISTICS: *Form:* Powder, semisolid, or volatile oil; *Color:* Yellowish; *Odor:* Intense

PHYSICAL PROPERTIES: *Solubility:* Soluble in alcohol, chloroform, ether; insoluble in water

DERIVATION: From dried rhizome of *Iris florentina* or *I. carolinian*, a camphoraceous substance with iridin, isophthalic acid, gum, tannin, sugar, oil, by distillation

WARNING AND CAUTION: Combustible

JASMINE

BOTANICAL: *Family: Oleaceae, Oleander; Genus: Jasminum* (native of Asia); *Species: Officinale, Grandiflorum* (Spanish)
HABITAT/SOURCES: Cultivated in southern France, Spain, Algeria, Morocco, India, Egypt
EXTRACTION: From flowers

JONQUIL

BOTANICAL: *Family: Amaryllidaceae; Genus: Narcissus; Species: Jonquilla*
SYNONYMS: Daffodil (trumpet narcissus)
NOTES: The sweet-scented jonquil is classified as *N. odorus.*

KERNEL

NOTES: A seed in a hard husk. The inner part of a nut or edible fruit.

KETCHUP

See CATSUP

LAVENDER

BOTANICAL: *Family: Labiatae; Genus: Lavandula; Species: Officinalis, Latifolia, Vera, Spica*
HABITAT/SOURCES: Mediterranean regions, especially Spain, Morocco, southern France, Yugoslavia, U.S.S.R., Australia
PART USED: Freshly cut, flowering tops and stalks

LEMON

BOTANICAL: *Family: Rutaceae; Genus: Citrus; Species: Limon* (Asia), *Limonia, Medica*
HABITAT/SOURCES: Mediterranean regions, Brazil, Argentina, west Africa
EXTRACTION: From squeezing the peels of ripe fruits

LICORICE (LIQUORICE)

BOTANICAL: *Family: Leguminosae; Genus: Glycyrrhiza; Species: Glabra* (Mediterranean regions), *Lipidota* (wild, North America)
NOTES: The roots are used for flavoring candy, drinks, tobaccos, medicines

LILAC

BOTANICAL: *Family: Oleaceae; Genus: Syringa; Species: Vulgaris* (European shrubs)
NOTES: There are 30 species of genus *Syringa* and many varieties of cultivated shrubs

LILY

BOTANICAL: *Family: Liliaceae; Genus: Lilium* (Martagon, central Europe, and Russian mountains); *Species:* 2000 species
NOTES: One of the largest and most important plant families. There are more than 200

genus and about 2000 species

LILY OF THE VALLEY

BOTANICAL: *Family: Liliaceae; Genus: Convallaria; Species: Majalis, Montana* (wild)

LIME

BOTANICAL: *Family: Rutaceae; Genus: Citrus; Species: Aurantifolia*
HABITAT/SOURCES: Brazil, Mexico, Italy, West Indies
EXTRACTION: Pressing the peels of ripe fruits

MAGNOLIA

BOTANICAL: *Family: Magnoliaceae; Genus: Magnolia; Species: Grandiflora* (southern), *Virginiana* (swamp), *Tripetala* (umbrella tree), *Macrophylla* (big leaf), *Acuminata* (cucumber tree)
HABITAT/SOURCES: Asia and western regions shrubs and trees
NOTES: About 80 species exist

MALT (GRAIN, USUALLY BARLEY)

NOTES: Beer makers use most of the malt, usually from barley, after sprouting and distilling. It is also used to make other foods and drugs.

Malting is a process whereby grain is kept in water for 24–96 h. It is then spread on large, ventilated floors until it sprouts and grows (5–10 days). It is dried for 2–3 days from low temperature to 180 F, and aged for 4–8 weeks before use.

The starch changes into sugar and is called "maltose." It is used for sweetening various foods.

MANDARIN

BOTANICAL: *Family: Rutaceae; Genus: Citrus; Species: Nobilis, Kumquat (Cum-Quat), Madurensis, Reticulata*
HABITAT/SOURCES: Italy, Brazil, Spain, Argentina
EXTRACTION: From cold-pressed peels.

MANGO

BOTANICAL: *Family: Anacardiaceae; Genus: Mangifera; Species: Indica*
HABITAT/SOURCES: Tropical evergreen tree with rind, juice, and sweet orange-yellow flesh

MAPLE

BOTANICAL: *Family: Aceraceae; Genus: Acer* (hard); *Species: Saccharum* (sugar), *Saccharinum* (silver), *Macrophyllum* (big leaf), *Pennsylvanicum* (striped), *Spicatum* (mountain), *Rubrum* (red), *Pseudoplatanus* (sycamore), *Platanoides* (Norway), *Palmatum* (Japanese)
HABITAT/SOURCES: North temperate regions, mostly North America; trees and shrubs

MARASCA
BOTANICAL: *Family: Rosaceae; Genus: Cerasus; Species: Marasca*
HABITAT/SOURCES: European cherry tree with bitter red fruits
NOTES: See MARASCHINO

MARASCHINO
NOTES: It is a liqueur made from the fermented juice and crushed kernels of the marasca cherry. See MARASCA

MARJORAM
BOTANICAL: *Family: Labiatae; Genus: Marjorana, Origanum; Species: Hortensis, Vulgare*
NOTES: Aromatic plant with purple or white flowers and leaves

MAYONNAISE
NOTES: A creamy dressing made with egg yolks, vegetable oils, vinegar or lemon juice, beaten and seasoned.

MELON
BOTANICAL: *Family: Cucurbitaceae; Genus and Species: Cucumis melo* (musk-melon); *Citrullus vulgaris* (watermelon)
NOTES: Several varieties are widely cultivated

MENTHA
BOTANICAL: *Family: Labiatae, Lamiaceae; Genus: Mentha; Species: Piperita* (peppermint), *Spicata* (spearmint)
HABITAT/SOURCES: China, Brazil, Japan, U.S.A.
EXTRACTION: From flowering tops
NOTES: Uses limited in perfumery. Mainly used in flavoring chewing gum.

MIGNONETTE
BOTANICAL: *Family: Resedaceae; Genus: Reseda; Species: Odorata*
HABITAT/SOURCES: Mediterranean regions, widely cultivated

MIMOSA
BOTANICAL: *Family: Leguminosae, Mimosaceae; Genus: Mimosa; Species: Acacia*
HABITAT/SOURCES: Australia, southern France, Northern Italy
EXTRACTION: From flowers and twigs
NOTES: Mostly tropical

MIRABELLE (PLUM)
BOTANICAL: *Family: Rosaceae; Genus: Prunus, Prunes* (European), *Species: Domestica, Salicina* (Japanese), *Insititia* (damson)*, *Myrobalan* (ornamental), *Cerasifera* (ornamental), *Americana* (American)

* A small blue plum from Damascus, Syria; also called "bullace"

MOSS

NOTES: Soft green plant growing close together, typically in clumps on moist ground or trees. Scientifically classified as "Bryophyta musci."

MUGUET

See LILY OF THE VALLEY

NOTES: Muguet is the French name

MULBERRY

BOTANICAL: *Family: Moraceae; Genus: Morus; Species: Alba* (white), *Rubra* (red), *Nigra* (black)

NOTES: About 15 species exist

MUSK (DEER)

ZOOLOGICAL: *Family: Cervida; Subfamily: Moshinae; Genus: Moschus; Species: Moschiferus* (central and northeastern Asia)

NOTES: Musk is an oily substance with a powerful odor. It comes from a gland in a musk, a small hornless deer of the Himalaya mountains. It is used in perfumes for a persistent odor. The best quality musk is that from China, called "tong king."

NARCISSUS (DAFFODIL)

BOTANICAL: *Family: Amaryllidaceae*; *Genus: Narcissus*; *Species: Pseudo-narcissus* (daffodil), *N. tazetta* (paper white), *N. poeticus* (poet's, hybrid)

HABITAT/SOURCES: France, Morocco, Egypt

EXTRACTION: From flowers

NOTES: Daffodil (*N. pseudo-narcissus*) comprise various bulbous herbs with long, narrow leaves and short tubular fragrant yellow flowers

NECTARINE

BOTANICAL: *Family: Rosaceae; Genus: Prunus; Species: Persica*

NOTES: A variety of peach, *Prunus persica nectarina*, with a waxy smooth skin. The word "nectar" refers to a sweet liquid, secreted by flowers of various plants, from which the bees make honey.

NEROLI

NOTES: Essential oil distilled from orange flowers, used in perfumery. It is also called "orange flowers oil."

NEW MOWN HAY

SYNONYMS: Foin coupé (French for hay cut)

NOTES: A strong odor from cutting hay crops, grass, or similar growth, with a scythe or mechanical device, such as lawn mower. Hay is grass of other plants such as alfalfa or clover.

NOISETTE

SYNONYMS: Hazel nut, from noisetier, hazel tree; noisette and noisetier are French words

NOTES: A small piece of meat, especially loin. A fillet of lamb, veal, or pork, flavored with hazel nuts.

NOUGATINE

NOTES: Nougat is a confection made with sugar or honey, almond and cherries, or other nuts and fruits, mixed as a paste. The suffix "ine" is a French diminutive of the word "nougat," which refers to a confection of nuts.

NUTMEG

BOTANICAL: *Family: Myristaceae; Genus: Myristica; Species: Fragrans*
HABITAT/SOURCES: East Indies, tropics
PART USED: Seeds, kernel of fruit
NOTES: Evergreen tree growing very high (about 70 ft). After 9 years it produces about 1500–2000 nuts yearly. The seeds used as a spice, either grated or ground. The oil, called oil of mace, is from the kernels.

ONION

BOTANICAL: *Family: Liliaceae; Genus: Allium; Species: Cepa*
HABITAT/SOURCES: Cultivated worldwide

OPOPANAX

BOTANICAL: *Family: Umbelliferae, Burseraceae; Genus: Chironium, Commiphora; Species: Persicum, Katof*
NOTES: Oleoresin, from the roots of opopanax, umbelliferae of Middle East and southern Europe. Oil from opopanax, burseraceae of Syria and Arabia.

ORANGE

BOTANICAL: *Family: Rutaceae; Genus: Citrus; Species: Sinensis* (sweet), *Aurantium* (bitter)
HABITAT/SOURCES: Tropical and subtropical regions; Mediterranean regions
EXTRACTION: Oil from leaves: petitgrain. Oil from blossoming flowers of evergreen trees: neroli.
NOTES: Several evergreen trees cultivated in tropical and subtropical regions. It has fragrant flowers and fruits.

ORCHID

BOTANICAL: *Family: Orchidaceae; Genus: Cypripedium; Species: Arethusa* (American), *Calypso* (American), *Calopogon* (American), *Habenaria* (American)
HABITAT/SOURCES: Worldwide, chiefly in tropical regions

ORRIS ROOT

BOTANICAL: *Family: Iridiceae; Genus: Iris; Species: Florentina*
HABITAT/SOURCES: It is mostly produced in Italy with a center in Florence
PART USED: Oil from peeled, dried, crushed rhizomes
NOTES: Orris root is from iris. It refers to the underground stems of various European iris. It has a faint violet-like odor.

PATCHOULI

BOTANICAL: *Family: Labiatae; Genus: Pogostemon* (Asiatic); *Species: Cablin, Heyneanus*

PEA

BOTANICAL: *Family: Leguminosae; Genus: Pisum; Species: Sativa or Sativum*
HABITAT/SOURCES: Temperate zones
NOTES: Dry peas are called "arvensis."

PEACH

BOTANICAL: *Family: Rosaceae; Genus: Prunus; Species: Persica*
HABITAT/SOURCES: Temperate zones, widely cultivated; native to China

PEACH OIL

SYNONYMS: *Prunus persica*; Kernel oil; Persic oil
CHARACTERISTICS: *Form:* Liquid; *Color:* Yellow
PHYSICAL PROPERTIES: *Specific gravity:* 0.915 (25/25 C); *Freezing point:* 15 C; *Solubility:* Insoluble in water

PEAR

BOTANICAL: *Family: Rosaceae; Genus: Pyrus; Species: Communis* (European), *Pyrifolia* (Chinese, Japanese), *Ussuriensis* (Ussurian), *Calleryana* (Callery)
HABITAT/SOURCES: Widely cultivated

PEPPERMINT

BOTANICAL: *Family: Labiatae; Genus: Mentha; Species: Piperita*
HABITAT/SOURCES: Spain, Italy, Balkans, U.S.A.
EXTRACTION: From just-flowered herb, partially dried

PERSIC OIL

SYNONYMS: Peach kernel nut oil; Apricot kernel oil
CHARACTERISTICS: *Form:* Liquid; *Color:* Pale yellow; *Odor:* Almond
PHYSICAL PROPERTIES: *Specific gravity:* 0.915 (25/25 C); *Refractive index:* 1.463 (20 C); *Solubility:* Soluble in ether
DERIVATION: By expressing the blanched seeds of the peach (*Prunus persica*) or apricot (*Prunus amernica*)
WARNING AND CAUTION: Combustible; nontoxic

PICKLE

NOTES: An edible product, usually vegetable or fruit, preserved and flavored in a solution of water, saturated or strong impregnated with common salt (brine) or vinegar, often spiced.

BOTANICAL REFERENCES FOR THE FORMULARY

PIMENTO

BOTANICAL: *Family: Myrtaceae; Genus: Pimenta; Species: Officinalis*
HABITAT/SOURCES: Tropical America
PART USED: Berries
NOTES: Allspice tree has small white flowers and aromatic berries

PINE

BOTANICAL: *Family: Pinaceae; Genus: Pinus; Species: Strobus* (eastern, white), *Lambertiana* (sugar pine), *Bankisiana* (jack pine), *Palustris* (long leaf), *Ponderosa* (Ponderosa)
HABITAT/SOURCES: U.S.A., Finland, France, Portugal, U.S.S.R.
EXTRACTION: From wood chips
NOTES: Evergreen trees

PINEAPPLE (ANANAS)

BOTANICAL: *Family: Bromeliaceae; Genus: Ananas; Species: Comosus*
HABITAT/SOURCES: Tropical America

PISTACHIO (PISTACHE)

BOTANICAL: *Family: Anacardiaceae; Genus: Pistacia; Species: Vera*
HABITAT/SOURCES: Mediterranean regions and western Asia

PLUM

See MIRABELLE

POMEGRANATE

See GRENADINE

POTATOES

BOTANICAL: *Family: Solanaceae; Genus: Solanum; Species: Tuberosum*
HABITAT/SOURCES: Native to South America; cultivated worldwide

POTATOES, SWEET

BOTANICAL: *Family: Convulaceae; Genus: Ipomea or Ipoemoea; Species: Batals or Batatus*
HABITAT/SOURCES: Tropical America

PRUNELLE (PRUNE)

BOTANICAL: *Family: Rosaceae; Genus: Prunus; Species: Domestica*
NOTES: Prunes are any of several varieties of common plums which have been dried in the sun for at least 3 weeks. Prunelle is a French liqueur with plum taste and a green color.

QUASSIA

BOTANICAL: *Family: Simarubaceae; Genus: Quassia; Species: Amara*
HABITAT/SOURCES: Tropical America

PART USED: Wood and bark
NOTES: Quassia has a bitter taste from the wood and bark

QUINCE
BOTANICAL: *Family: Rosaceae; Genus: Cydonia; Species: Oblonga*
HABITAT/SOURCES: A tree native to Asia

RAISIN
NOTES: A sun-dried grape. Grapes become raisins after drying artificially or in the sun for about 2 weeks. There are four varieties of raisins: (1) Thompson, seedless; (2) Muscat, large and seed-bearing; (3) Sultana, used mainly in baking; (4) Corinthian, also called currant, smaller. Raisins are generally used for flavoring bakery products.

RASPBERRY
BOTANICAL: *Family: Rosaceae; Genus: Rubus; Species: Idaeus* (European red), *Strigosus* (American red), *Occidentalis* (American black), *Neglectus* (purple)

RHUBARB
BOTANICAL: *Family: Polygonaceae; Genus: Rheum; Species: Rhaponticum*
NOTES: A perennial vegetable producing many seeds. The rhizomes and roots have a bitter taste. Pieplant.

ROOT BEER
NOTES: An effervescent, carbonated, sweetened soft drink made with extracts of roots of many plants,

ROSE
BOTANICAL: *Family: Rosaceae; Genus: Rosa; Species: Muscosa* (moss rose), *Setigera* (climbing), *Centifolia* (moss rose)
HABITAT/SOURCES: Southern France, Algeria, Morocco, Egypt, Turkey, Bulgaria, Italy
EXTRACTION: From petals by enfleurage or steam distillation

ROSEMARY
BOTANICAL: *Family: Labiatae; Genus: Rosmarinus; Species: Officinalis*
HABITAT/SOURCES: France, Spain, Tunisia, Yugoslavia
EXTRACTION: From flowers and leaves of evergreen shrubs

RUM
NOTES: Alcoholic drink distilled from fermented molasses or sugar cane.

SAFFRON
BOTANICAL: *Family: Iridaceae; Genus: Crocus; Species: Sativus*
PART USED: Stigma
NOTES: Brilliant yellow dye and food flavoring. The plant *Crocus sativus* has a white

or purple flower with orange stigmas. The dried stigmas are used to color foods and as a cooking spice and dyestuff.

SAGE

BOTANICAL: *Family: Labiatae; Genus: Salvia; Species: Officinalis*
NOTES: Sweet odor and flavor in its leaves and stems

SAINT JOHN'S BREAD (CAROB)

BOTANICAL: *Family: Leguminosae; Genus: Ceratonia; Species: Siliqua*
NOTES: A dark evergreen tree, growing wild in the Mediterranean area. It is believed that St. John Baptist ate it when in the wilderness.

SANDALWOOD

BOTANICAL: *Family: Santalaceae; Genus: Santalum; Species: Album* (India)
HABITAT/SOURCES: Several Asian and Australian evergreen trees

SARSAPARILLA

BOTANICAL: *Family: Lilaceae; Genus: Smilax; Species: Medica, Aristolochiaefolia* (Mexico), *Aralia hispida* (North America), *Aralia nudicaulis* (North America), *Indicus* (Jamaica)
HABITAT/SOURCES: Dried roots of several kinds of smilax plants of Central and South America.
NOTES: A sweet soft drink is flavored with sarsaparilla. It contains: glucosides smilacin, parillin, resin, saponins, essential oil.

SCOTCH

NOTES: Whiskey, an alcoholic liquor distilled in Scotland and Ireland from malted barley; and from corn or rye in the U.S. and Canada; blended with 40–50 percent pure alcohol from grain.

SPICE

NOTES: Any of various aromatic and pungent vegetables used to flavor beverages and foods. They include: cloves from buds; cinnamon from bark; pepper and nutmeg from fruits; ginger from roots; mustard from seeds. Spice plants grow in tropical regions. Spices increase appetite and stimulate digestion.

STAR ANISE

BOTANICAL: *Family: Magnoliaceae; Genus: Ilicium; Species: Verum*
HABITAT/SOURCES: Eastern Asia
NOTES: An aromatic tree with purple-red flowers and anise-scented fruits. Also called "Chinese anise."

STRAWBERRY

BOTANICAL: *Family: Rosaceae; Genus: Fragaria; Species: Virginian* (American), *Chiloensis*

SWEET PEA

BOTANICAL: *Family: Leguminosae; Genus: Lathyrus; Species: Odoratus* (southern Italy)

HABITAT/SOURCES: A climbing plant, native to Italy

SUGAR

BOTANICAL: *Family: Graminaceae; Genus: Saccharum; Species: Officinarum*

HABITAT/SOURCES: Originally East Indies

NOTES: A sweet, crystalline, water-soluble material from cane sugar. It is the chief commercial source of sugar.

SYRINGA (MOCK ORANGE)

BOTANICAL: *Family: Saxifragaceae; Genus: Philadelphus; Species: Virginalis*

NOTES: Mock orange is the state flower of Idaho.

TAMARIND

BOTANICAL: *Family: Leguminosae; Genus: Tamarindus; Species: Indica*

HABITAT/SOURCES: A tropical tree

TANGERINE

BOTANICAL: *Family: Rutaceae; Genus: Citrus; Species: Nobilis* (common), *Deliciosa* (common), *Reticulata*

SYNONYMS: Citrus peel oil

CHARACTERISTICS: *Form:* Liquid; *Color:* Yellowish; *Odor:* Tangerine

PHYSICAL PROPERTIES: *Specific gravity:* 0.84–0.89 (25/25 C); *Refractive index:* 1.473–1.478 (20 C); *Solubility:* Soluble in alcohol, vegetable oils, mineral oils

DERIVATION: Expressed from the peel of tangerine, grapefruit, lemon, lime, orange

HABITAT/SOURCES: Widely cultivated

WARNING AND CAUTION: Combustible; nontoxic

TARRAGON

BOTANICAL: *Family: Compositae; Genus: Artemisia; Species: Dracunculus* (Eurasia)

NOTES: Tarragon seeds from aromatic herb are harmless. Some, however, of the same genus are poisonous.

TEA

BOTANICAL: *Family: Theaceae; Genus: Thea, Camellia* (eastern Asia)*; Species: Sinensis* (eastern Asia), *Oolong* (Formosa)

NOTES: A shrub with evergreen leaves and fragrant white flowers

THISTLE

BOTANICAL: *Family: Compositae; Genus: Carduus, Cnicus, Onopordum, Cirsium; Species: Arvense*

NOTES: Plant with sharp spines or prickles.

THYME

BOTANICAL: *Family: Labiatae; Genus: Thymus; Species: Vulgaris*
PART USED: Leaves and stems
NOTES: A fragrant garden herb or low shrub with small purplish flowers. The oil in the leaves and stems produces a scent. It is used for seasoning.

TOBACCO

BOTANICAL: *Family: Solanaceae; Genus: Nicotiana; Species: Tabacum* (tropical America)
HABITAT/SOURCES: The plant, native to America, is now cultivated worldwide.
PART USED: The leaves
NOTES: The leaves of cultivated tobacco are dried and processed for cigar, cigarettes, pipes, snuff. They contain nicotine, nornicotine, nicotianine, nicotelline, and alkaloids. The ground tobacco waste products are used for fertilizer. Tobacco is also used as insecticide.

TREFLÉ (CLOVER, TREFOIL)

BOTANICAL: *Family: Leguminosae; Genus: Trifolium, Melilotus* (white sweet clover); *Species: Pratense* (red clover), *Repens* (white clover), *Hibridum* (alsike, Swedish clover), *Incarnatum* (crimson, scarlet, Italian), *Alba, Officinalis* (yellow, sweet clover), *Indica* (sour clover)

TUBEROSE

BOTANICAL: *Family: Amaryllidaceae; Genus: Polianthes; Species: Tuberosa*
HABITAT/SOURCES: Mexico. It is extensively cultivated because of its fragrant white flowers
EXTRACTION: From the hand-picked flowers by enfleurage.

VALERIAN

BOTANICAL: *Family: Valerianaceae; Genus: Valerianella, Valeriana, Ceranthus; Species: Officinalis* (Eurasia), *Clitoria* (corn salad), *Eriocarpa* (Italian corn salad)
HABITAT/SOURCES: Poland, Hungary, France, Belgium, Japan, China, U.S.S.R.
NOTES: More than 300 different perennial or annual herbs and some shrubs. The dried and comminuted rhizomes are steam distilled.

VANILLA

BOTANICAL: *Family: Orchidaceae; Genus: Vanilla; Species: Planifolia*
HABITAT/SOURCES: Tropical
EXTRACTION: From pods
NOTES: Tropical orchids with aromatic seeds called vanilla beans; used for flavoring

VERBENA

BOTANICAL: *Family: Verbenaceae; Genus: Verbena; Species: Hybrida*
HABITAT/SOURCES: Cultivated worldwide
NOTES: About 250 species in tropical regions

VERMOUTH

NOTES: Several white wines, sweet or dry, flavored with aromatic herbs and spices

VINEGAR

NOTES: A sour liquid for seasoning food, pickling, and processing fruits, vegetables, and meats. It is a sour diluted solution of acetic acid, obtained by fermentation and used as a condiment and preservative.

VIOLET

BOTANICAL: *Family: Violaceae; Genus: Viola* (blue); *Species: Papilionacea, Pedata* (bird's foot), *Canina* (dog), *Tricolor* (pansy, wild and cultivated), *Odorata*
HABITAT/SOURCES: Italy, southern France, Africa
EXTRACTION: From leaves of the flowers

WALLFLOWER

BOTANICAL: *Family: Cruciferae; Genus: Cheirantus; Species: Cheiri*
HABITAT/SOURCES: Cultivated worldwide
NOTES: Its name derives from the fact that it grows on walls, over ruins, and along stony cliffs.

WALNUT

BOTANICAL: *Family: Juglandaceae; Genus: Juglans; Species: Regia, Nigra* (black), *Cinerea* (butternut), *Hindsii* (California), *Californica* (California)

WINE

BOTANICAL (Grapes): *Family: Vitaceae; Genus: Vitis; Species: Vinifera*
NOTES: Fermented juice from grapes and also from other fruits

WINTERGREEN

BOTANICAL: *Family: Ericaceae; Genus: Gaultheria; Species: Procumbens*
HABITAT/SOURCES: Eastern North America
NOTES: A low-growing evergreen plant with white or pinkish flowers, aromatic leaves, and spicy edible red berries

WOODRUFF

BOTANICAL: *Family: Madder; Genus: Galium, Asperula; Species: Odorata* (Eurasia)
NOTES: Small white flowers and narrow fragrant leaves; used for flavoring

WORCESTERSHIRE SAUCE

NOTES: A piquant sauce from soy, vinegar, and spices. Originally made in Worcester, England

WORMWOOD

See ABSINTHE

WORT

BOTANICAL: *Family: Graminaceae; Genus: Saccharum; Species: Officinarum*
NOTES: Plant used in infusion of fermented malt to make beer

YLANG YLANG

BOTANICAL: *Family: Anonaceae; Genus: Cananga, Canangium; Species: Odorata, Odoratum*
HABITAT/SOURCES: Madagascar, Reunion Islands, Comoro Islands, Indonesia, Malaya, Philippines
EXTRACTION: From freshly early morning-picked flowers of the tree tagalog (alang-ilang)
NOTES: Four different qualities: extra, first, second, third

ZEDOARY

BOTANICAL: *Family: Amomaceae; Genus: Amomum; Species: Curcuma*
HABITAT/SOURCES: Tropical Asia
PART USED: Dried rhizome
NOTES: Used as a stimulant, condiment, and in cosmetics.

Appendix:

LIST OF UNSAFE MATERIALS USED IN PERFUME AND FLAVOR MANUFACTURE

Page	Material	Warnings, Cautions, Notes
414	Absinthe, oil	Highly toxic by ingestion; small amount may be fatal. Its use in medicine and as a flavor in alcoholic beverages has been limited and is not allowed in the U.S.
77, 374	Acetaldehyde	Toxic in large doses
209	Acetone	Toxic; fire risk
79, 132	Acetophenone	Narcotic in high concentration
192	Allyl isothiocyanate	Highly toxic by inhalation; flammable; component of black mustard in small amount
193	Allyl mercaptan	Highly toxic by ingestion and inhalation; component of onion oil in small amount
84, 192, 326, 376	Allyl sulfide	Toxic by ingestion; it is strongly irritating to eyes and skin; component of garlic oil in small amount
24, 184	Almond bitter, oil	Use only if it is totally free of hydrocyanic acid

APPENDIX

Page	Material	Warnings, Cautions, Notes
85, 133	Amyl cinnamic aldehyde	Flammable; fire risk
88, 134, 195, 379	Benzaldehyde	Narcotic in high concentration; may cause dermatitis
210	Benzene	Toxic; fire risk
89, 134, 379	Benzyl acetate	Irritating to the eyes, respiratory tract; ingestion causes vomiting and diarrhea
135, 380	Benzyl alcohol	Outignition at 817 F
89, 136, 380	Benzyl benzoate	Avoid contact with eyes; causes skin irritation
137	Benzylidene acetone	Irritating to the skin
29	Birch tar	Poisonous
138, 381	Borneol	Causes nausea, vomiting, dizziness, mental confusion; flammable
91	Bromo styrol	Causes irritation
92	Cadinene	Low toxicity by ingestion
31, 418	Camphor	Large doses of camphor are poisonous, causing delirium and confusion
34	Cedarleaf (thuja)	Toxic—ingestion of large amounts causes convulsion, death

Page	Material	Warnings, Cautions, Notes
421	Cola	Moderately toxic
97, 142, 197	Coumarin	Toxic; it is forbidden in food products
212	n-Hexane	Toxic; fire risk
113	Methyl alcohol	Highly toxic by ingestion; it causes blindness
53	Myrrh (resinoid)	Low toxicity
50, 55, 431	Nutmeg	Ingestion of large amounts produces narcosis, delirium, death
57	Oregano	May be toxic by ingestion
58, 426, 431	Orris	Strong allergen
118	Oxalic acid	Harmful if swallowed
118	Phenyl acetic acid	Probably toxic
122	Pinene	Toxic by ingestion
217	Pokeberry	The roots of this plant are poisonous
63	Rue	Contact produces erythema, vesication; ingestion causes epigastric pain, nausea, vomiting, convulsion, death
65	Sassafras	Toxic by ingestion; not permitted for use in food and beverages (FDA)
66	Spruce (hemlock)	Low toxicity

APPENDIX

Page	Material	Warnings, Cautions, Notes
67	Tansy	Highly toxic by ingestion
129	Tiglic acid	Highly toxic by ingestion
69, 168	Turpentine (rectified)	Highly toxic by ingestion; moderately toxic by inhalation and skin absorption
18, 71, 171, 438	Wintergreen	Highly toxic by ingestion; use is restricted by FDA
72, 414	Wormwood	Permitted in vermouth only in traces because it can cause stupor, convulsion, death

Bibliography and References

Bassiri, T. 1969. *Introduction a l'etude des parfumes.* Paris: Ed Nasson et Cie.

Cerbelaud, René. 1951. *Formularie de parfumerie.* Paris: Editions Opéra.

Crooker and Henderson. 1927. Crooker and Henderson's odor arrangement. *Amer. Perfumer.* 22:325, 326.

de Navarre, Maison. 1941. *The chemistry and manufacture of cosmetics.* New York: D. Van Nostrand, Inc.

Farkas, Alexander. 1951. *Perfume through the ages: A brief history of the civilizing influence of fragrance.* New York: Psychology Library.

Fimmenore, Horace. 1926. *The essential oils.* London: Ernest Benn, Ltd.

Gattefossé, R.M. 1952. *Formulary of perfumes and cosmetics.* Trans. A.R.I.C. London: Leonard Hill Ltd.

——— 1937 *Aromatherapy, les huiles essentielles, hormones vegetales.* Paris: Libraries des Sciences, Girardot et Cie.

Gazan, M.H. 1936. *Flavours and essences: A handbook of formulas.* London: Chapman & Hall Ltd.

Gildmeister, E., and F. Hoffmann. 1913. *The volatile oils.* New York: John Wiley and Sons, Inc.

Givaudan Index. 1961. *Specifications of synthetics and isolates for perfumery.* New York: Givaudan-Delawanna, Inc.

Guenther, Ernest. 1952. *The essential oils.* New York: D. Van Nostrand, Inc.

Hack. 1969. *Hackh's Chemical Dictionary.* New York: McGraw-Hill Book Co.

Hall, Rudiger, Dieter Klemme, and Dr. Jurgen Nienhaus. 1985. *The H&R book: Guide to fragrance ingredients.* Eng. ed. London: Johnson Publications Ltd.

Hawley, Gessner G. 1971. *The condensed chemical dictionary.* 8th ed. New York: Van Nostrand-Reinhold Co.

Herstein and Jacobs. 1948. *Chemistry and technology of wines and liquors.* New York: D. Van Nostrand Co.

Jacobs, Morris B. 1947. *Synthetic food adjunct.* New York: D. Van Nostrand Co.

——— ed. 1944. *The chemistry and technology of food and food products.* Vol. 1, 2. New York: Interscience Publisher, Inc.

Jensen, H.R. 1932. *The chemistry flavouring and manufacture of chocolate confectionery and cocoa.* Philadelphia: P. Blakinston's Son and Co., Inc.

Kantack, R. 1918. *Tables of refractive indices essential oils.* London: Adam Hilger, Ltd.

Kenneth, John H. 1922. *The science of smell.* Edinburgh: Oliver and Byd.

Legrand, Amedee, ed. 1930. *Nouveau formulaire des parfums et des cosmetiques par Durvelle.* Paris: Boulevard Saint Germain.

Marmion, Daniel M. 1984. *Handbook of U.S. colorants for foods, drugs, and cosmetics.* 2nd ed. New York: Wiley Interscience Publications.

Martin, Geoffrey. 1967. *Perfumes, essential oils and fruit essences.* London: Crooby Lockwood and Sons.

Maurer, E.S. 1958. *Perfumes and their production.* London: United Trade Press.

Meroy, Joseph. 1960. *Food flavoring: Composition, manufacture and use.* Westport: Avi Publishing Co., Inc.

Moncrieff, R.W. 1967. *The chemical senses.* London: Leonard Hill.

Müller, Arno. 1950. *Internationaler Riechstoff-Kodex, International compendium of aromatic material.* Heidelberg: A. Hulting.

Parry, Ernest J. 1918. *The chemistry of essential oils and artificial perfumes.* London: Scott, Greenwood and Sons.

——— 1925. *Cyclopaedia of perfumery.* London: J. & A. Churchill.

Pearson, David. 1962. *The chemical analysis of foods.* London: J. & A. Churchill.

Redgrove, Herbert Stanley. 1928. *Scent and all about it.* London: W. Heinemann.

Rojas, Ulises. 1936. *Botanica general.* Vols. I, II, III. Guatemala City: Tipografia Nacional.

Sagarin, Edward. 1945. *The science and art of perfumery.* New York: McGraw-Hill Books.

Small Industry Research Institute. 1956. *Perfumes, flavors, and essential oils, or aromatic chemical and perfuming industries.* Stanford, Calif.: Small Business Publications.

Sornet, René. 1923. *La technique industrielle des parfumes synthetiques.* Paris: Gaultier-Villars et Cie.

Venturi, Aldo. 1946. *Le sostanze aromatiche.* Milano: Görlich.

Walter, Erich. 1916. *Manual of the essence industry.* New York: John Wiley and Sons.

Wells, F., and M. Billot. 1981. *Perfumery technology, art-science-industry.* Chichester: Ellis Horwood, Ltd.

INDEX

INDEX

INDEX

INDEX

INDEX

INDEX

INDEX

INDEX

INDEX

www.ingramcontent.com/pod-product-compliance
Lightning Source LLC
LaVergne TN
LVHW101454200926
848483LV00001B/123
* 9 7 8 0 8 2 0 6 0 3 3 4 6 *